Cultural Considerations

Drug Alerts

SAMPLE CLIENT CARE PLANS

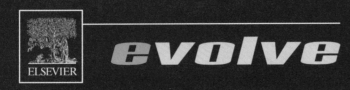

evolve

:• *To access your Online Student Resources, visit:*

http://evolve.elsevier.com/Morrison-Valfre

Evolve® Student Resources for *Morrison-Valfre: Foundations of Mental Health Care, 4th Edition,* include the following features:

- **Audio Glossary**

  Enhance your learning experience with alphabetized audio pronunciations of commonly used terms related to mental health care.

- **NCLEX-PN® Examination Style Interactive Review Questions**

  Test your knowledge with more than 300 interactive questions. Receive feedback for both correct and incorrect choices.

- **Helpful Phrases for Communicating in Spanish**

  Offer a useful tool for English-as-a-Second-Language situations.

FOUNDATIONS OF MENTAL HEALTH CARE

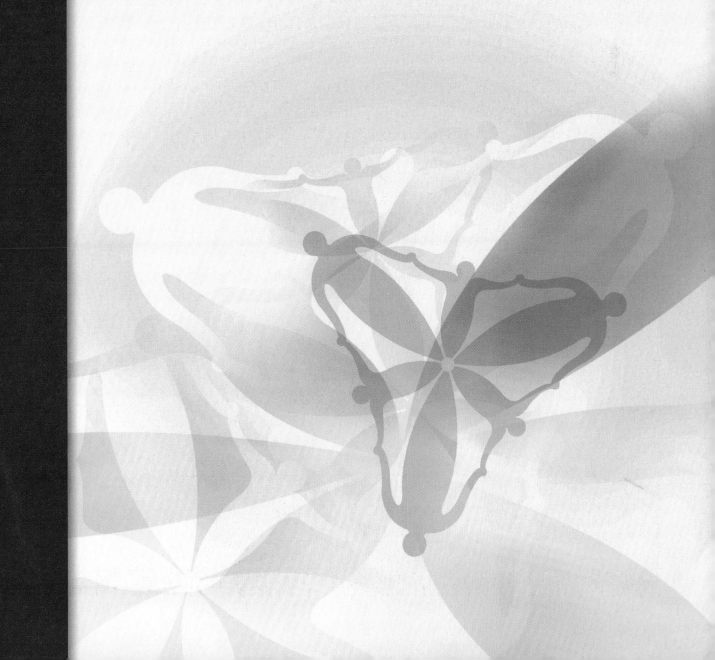

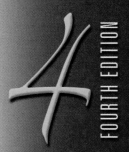

FOUNDATIONS OF MENTAL HEALTH CARE

Michelle Morrison-Valfre, RN, BSN, MSN, FNP

Health Care Educator/Consultant
Health and Education Consultants
Forest Grove, Oregon

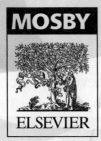

11830 Westline Industrial Drive
St. Louis, Missouri 63146

Notice

Knowledge and best practice in this field are constantly changing. As new research and experience broaden our knowledge, changes in practice, treatment and drug therapy may become necessary or appropriate. Readers are advised to check the most current information provided (i) on procedures featured or (ii) by the manufacturer of each product to be administered, to verify the recommended dose or formula, the method and duration of administration, and contraindications. It is the responsibility of the practitioner, relying on their own experience and knowledge of the patient, to make diagnoses, to determine dosages and the best treatment for each individual patient, and to take all appropriate safety precautions. To the fullest extent of the law, neither the Publisher nor the Author assumes any liability for any injury and/or damage to persons or property arising out of or related to any use of the material contained in this book.

The Publisher

Previous editions copyrighted 2005, 2001, 1997.

ISBN: 978-0-323-05644-1

Library of Congress Control Number 978-0323-05644-1

Vice President, Publishing Director: Sally Schrefer
Executive Publisher: Tom Wilhem
Managing Editor: Robin Levin Richman
Associate Developmental Editor: Jacqueline Twomey
Publishing Services Manager: Jeff Patterson
Senior Project Manager: Beth Hayes
Design Direction: Renee Duenow

Printed in the United States of America

Last digit is the print number: 9 8 7 6 5 4 3

To my beloved husband, Adolph Valfre, Jr.,
my cherished friend Marian Stoner,
and to you, dear reader,
May you leave this book richer in the knowledge
of human behavior.

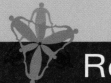

Reviewers

SALLY JASPER, MSN, RN
Instructor, Practical Nurse Program
Chemeketa Community College
Salem, Oregon

MARCIA I. JUSTICE, MNSc, RN
Instructor, Hospital Based Practical Nurse Program
St. Vincent Health System
Little Rock, Arkansas

AMY NIEPORENT, BSN, RN
Instructor
Holy Name Hospital School of Nursing
Teaneck, New Jersey

KATHY THOMAS, MSN, RN
White River Medical Center
Batesville, Arkansas

REBECCA S. UTZ, BSN, RN
Instructor, Practical Nurse Program
University of Arkansas Community College
Batesville, Arkansas

DENICE J. WISNIEWSKI, MSN, RN
Health Science Technical Education Teacher
Northeast Independent School District
Robert E. Lee High School
San Antonio, Texas

To the Instructor

Foundations of Mental Health Care, fourth edition, is intended for students and practitioners of the health care professions. Basic and advanced learners will find the information in this text useful and easy to apply in a variety of practice settings. Students in fields such as nursing, social work, respiratory therapy, physical therapy, recreational therapy, occupational therapy, rehabilitation, and medical assistance will find concise explanations of adaptive and maladaptive human behaviors as well as the most current therapeutic interventions and treatments.

Practicing health care providers—all who care for clients in a therapeutic manner—will find this book a practical and useful guide in any health care setting.

At its core, this text has three main goals:

1. To help soften the social distinction between mental "health" and mental "illness" because the difference hinges on how effectively one is coping
2. To assist nurses and other health care providers in comfortably working with clients who exhibit a wide range of maladaptive behaviors
3. To apply the concepts of holistic care when assisting clients in developing more adaptive attitudes and behaviors

Unit One, Mental Health Care: Past and Present, provides a framework for understanding mental health care. The evolution of care for persons with mental problems from primitive to current times is described. Selected ethical, legal, social, and cultural issues relating to mental health care are explored. Community mental health care is explained, followed by a chapter pertaining to theories of mental illness. To meet the ever-growing need for information on the extensive number of complementary and alternative therapies, a new chapter (Chapter 6) provides a strong base on which the health care provider can draw. Chapters on psychotherapeutic drug therapy and therapeutic modalities end the unit.

Unit Two, The Caregiver's Therapeutic Skills, focuses on the skills and conditions necessary for working with clients. Eight principles of mental health care are discussed and then applied to the therapeutic environment, the helping relationship, and effective communications. Material devoted to self-awareness encourages readers to develop introspection—a necessary component for working with people who have behavioral difficulties. Characteristics of basic human needs, personality development, stress, anxiety, crisis, and coping behaviors help readers explore behaviors common to us all. The section concludes with a description of the basic mental health assessment skills needed by every health care provider.

The clients for whom we care are the subject of **Unit Three. Mental Health Problems Throughout the Life Cycle** focuses on the growth of "normal" (adaptive) mental health behaviors during each developmental stage. The most common mental health problems associated with children, adolescents, adults, and older adults are discussed using the *Diagnostic and Statistical Manual of Mental Disorders* (DSM-IV-TR) as a framework. A chapter on dementia and Alzheimer's disease discusses the care of clients with cognitive impairments. This section is important because it explores the mental and emotional difficulties that everyone faces.

Unit Four, Clients With Psychological Problems, explores common behavioral responses and therapeutic interventions for illness, hospitalization, loss, grief, and depression. Maladaptive behaviors and mental health disorders are described in chapters on somatoform, anxiety, eating, sleeping, mood, sexual, and dissociative disorders.

The chapters in **Unit Five, Clients With Psychosocial Problems,** relate to the important social concerns of anger and its expressions, suicide, abuse and neglect, AIDS, and substance abuse. Sexual and personality disorders are also discussed. Chapters on schizophrenia and chronic mental illness focus on a multidisciplinary approach to treatment. The text concludes with a chapter titled Challenges for the Future, which prepares students for the coming changes in mental health care.

The appendices relate to standards of mental health care, a list of DSM-IV diagnoses, a tool for assessing the side effects of antipsychotic medications, and a mental status assessment tool conclude the text.

STANDARD FEATURES

- To address each mental health issue systematically, several key features are repeated throughout the text: **Objectives** stated in specific terms and a list of **Key Terms** with pronunciations and page numbers.
- The **nursing process** is applied to specific mental health problems throughout the text, with emphasis on multidisciplinary care. This helps readers understand the interactions of several health care disciplines and determine where they fit in the overall scheme of managed care.
- A **continuum of responses** describes the range of behaviors associated with each topic.
- **Development throughout the life cycle** relates to the aspect of each personality being studied.

- **Clinical disorders** include behavioral signs and symptoms based on the *Diagnostic and Statistical Manual of Mental Disorders* (DSM-IV-TR).
- **Therapeutic interventions** include multidisciplinary treatment, medical management, application of the nursing process, and pharmacological therapy.
- Each chapter concludes with **Key Points** that correlate with the learning objectives and serve as a useful review of the chapter's concepts.

LEARNING AIDS

Because the majority of mental health care takes place outside the institution, the book emphasizes the importance of using therapeutic mental health interventions during every client interaction. The following features encourage the reader's understanding and are designed to foster effective learning and comprehension:

- A new full-color design stimulates learning and calls attention to the important terms and concepts within the text.
- Selected **Key Terms** with phonetic pronunciations and a specific page reference to where the term can be found are listed at the beginning of each chapter, and each Key Term appears in color at the first mention in the text. Complete definitions are located in the Glossary. Terms with phonetic pronunciations were selected because they are either (1) difficult medical, nursing, or scientific terms or (2) other words that may be difficult for students to pronounce. The goal is to help the student reader with limited proficiency in English develop a greater command of the pronunciation of health care terminology. It is hoped that a more general competency in the understanding and use of medical and scientific language will result.
- Throughout the text, cultural aspects of various mental health principles are explored in **Cultural Considerations** boxes to encourage further thought and discussion.
- **Think About** boxes pose questions designed to stimulate critical thinking.
- **Case Studies** with thought-provoking questions encourage readers to consider the psychosocial aspects of providing therapeutic care in both community and hospital settings.
- Descriptions of each mental health disorder are drawn from **DSM-IV TR criteria.**
- Multidisciplinary **Sample Client Care Plans** demonstrate the application of the therapeutic (nursing) process to the caring for individuals with various mental health disorders.

- **Nursing diagnoses** are stated in terms approved by the North American Nursing Diagnosis Association International (NANDA-I).
- **Drug Alert** boxes prepare readers for the complexity of therapy with psychotherapeutic medications, including identifying drug interactions and potentially life-threatening side effects.
- The **holistic approach** to care offers readers a view of the "whole person" context of health care delivery.
- A **References and Further Readings** section encourage further exploration of the topics presented in the chapter. For easy access, they are grouped by chapter at the back of the book.
- The **Glossary** of Key Terms, written in an easy-to-understand format and easily loated with a color tab, follows the text.
- **Review Worksheets** encourage the use of critical thinking. Worksheets for each chapter are perforated so the sheets can be removed and submitted to the instructor, thus eliminating the need for a separate student workbook.
- Throughout the text, the liberal use of boxes, tables, and figures simplifies important concepts and stresses essential information.

ANCILLARIES
For Instructors

We recognize that educators today have limited time to prepare for classroom and clinical activities. Therefore we provide a rich collection of supplemental resources for instructors within the Evolve Resources with TEACH Instructor Resource (TIR), including:

- **TEACH Lesson Plans** with Lecture Outlines based on textbook learning objectives, provide a roadmap to link and integrate all parts of the educational package. These concise and straightforward lesson plans can be modified or combined to meet your unique scheduling and teaching needs.
- **PowerPoint Presentations** include approximately 600 slides with talking points for instructors.
- **ExamView Test Bank,** with more than 800 multiple-choice and alternate-format NCLEX-PN® Examination–Style Questions. Each question provides the correct answer, rationale, topic, client need category, step of the nursing process, objective, cognitive level, and text page reference.
- **Open-Book Quizzes** for each chapter in the textbook, with page cross references and answer guidelines.
- **iClicker Audience Response Questions** (over 160) promote learning and provide feedback for instructors in the classroom.

We provide a companion Evovle website with free student resources, including an Audio Glossary, NCLEX-PN® Examination–Style Interactive Review Questions, and Helpful Phrases for Communicating in Spanish.

FOR STUDENTS

In the Student Resources section of the Evolve website, there are over 330 **NCLEX-PN® Examination–Style Interactive Questions** with rationales for both correct and incorrect responses; Audio Glossary; and Helpful Phrases for Communicating in Spanish.

No text is written alone. The continued support of my husband, Adolph, my friend Marian Stoner, and other colleagues has provided the energy to complete this project when my own was low. The guidance, expertise, and encouragement from my editors, Robin Levin Richman, Ryan Creed, Jackie Twomey, and Beth Hayes, are much appreciated. I would also like to thank all the health care providers who so freely share their time and expertise with those who want to learn more about the dynamic and complex nature of human behavior.

MICHELLE MORRISON-VALFRE

LPN Threads

Foundations of Mental Health Care, fourth edition, shares some features and design elements with other Elsevier LPN titles. The purpose of these "LPN Threads" is to make it easier for students and instructors to incorporate multiple books into the fast-paced and demanding LPN curriculum.

The shared features in *Foundations for Mental Health Care* include the following:

- A **reading level evaluation** was performed on every manuscript chapter during the book's development.
- Cover and internal **design similarities.** The colorful, student-friendly design encourages the reading and learning of the core content.
- Numbered lists of **Objectives** that begin each chapter.
- **Key Terms** with phonetic pronunciations and page number references are provided at the beginning of each chapter. The key terms are in color as they appear in the chapter. All pronunciations were reviewed by an English as a Second Language (ESL) consultant.
- **Critical Thinking Questions** are given at the end of every Sample Nursing Care Plan.
- Bulleted **Key Points** that summarize critical concepts are listed at the end of each chapter.
- The **References and Further Readings** follow at the end of the text.
- A comprehensive **Glossary** is located at the end of the text.

And for instructors…

- **ExamView® Test Bank** with the following categories of information: Topic, Step of the Nursing Process, Objective, Cognitive Level, Client Need Category, Correct Answer, Rationale, and Text Page Reference. Located in the Evolve Resources with TEACH Instructor Resource.
- **PowerPoint Presentations with Lecture Outlines** in the Evolve Resources with TEACH Instructor Resource.

LPN Advisory Board

SHIRLEY ANDERSON, MSN
Kirkwood Community College
Cedar Rapids, Iowa

M. GIE ARCHER, MS, RN, C, WHCNP
Dean of Health Sciences
LVN Program Coordinator
North Central Texas College
Gainesville, Texas

MARY BROTHERS, MED, RN
Coordinator, Garnet Career Center School
   of Practical Nursing
Charleston, West Virginia

PATRICIA A. CASTALDI, RN, BSN, MSN
Union County College
Plainfield, New Jersey

MARY ANN COSGAREA, RN, BSN
PN Coordinator/Health Coordinator
Portage Lakes Career Center
Green, Ohio

DOLORES ANN COTTON, RN, BSN, MS
Meridian Technology Center
Stillwater, Oklahoma

LORA LEE CRAWFORD, RN, BSN
Emanuel Turlock Vocational Nursing Program
Turlock, California

RUTH ANN ECKENSTEIN, RN, BS, MEd
Oklahoma Department of Career and
   Technology Education
Stillwater, Oklahoma

GAIL ANN HAMILTON FINNEY, RN, MSN
Nursing Education Specialist
Concorde Career Colleges, Inc.
Mission, Kansas

PAM HINCKLEY, RN, MSN
Redlands Adult School
Redlands, California

DEBORAH W. KELLER, RN, BSN, MSN
Erie Huron Ottawa Vocational Education
School of Practical Nursing
Milan, Ohio

PATTY KNECHT, MSN, RN
Nursing Program Director
Center for Arts and Technology
Brandywine Campus
Coatesville, Pennsylvania

**LIEUTENANT COLONEL (RET) TERESA Y.
   MCPHERSON, RN, BSN, MSN**
LVN Program Director
Nursing Education
St. Philip's College
San Antonio, Texas

FRANCES NEU, MS, BSN, RN
Supervisor, Adult Ed Health
Butler Technology and Career Development
   Schools
Fairfield Township, Ohio

DIANNA DANCED SCHERLIN, MS, RN
National Director of Nursing
Lincoln Educational Services
West Orange, New Jersey

BEVERLEY TURNER, MA, RN
Director, Vocational Nursing Department
Maric College, San Diego Campus
San Diego, California

C. SUE WEIDMAN, RN BSN
Brown Mackie College Nurse Specialist
Forest, Ohio

SISTER ANN WIESEN, RN, MRA
Erwin Technical Center
Tampa, Florida

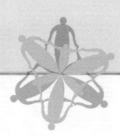

To the Student

Designed with the student in mind, *Foundations of Mental Health Care* will help you learn basic mental health nursing care with its visually appealing and easy-to-use format. The numerous special features will help you understand and apply the material.

Objectives at the start of each chapter highlight the chapter's main learning goals.

Key Terms with phonetic pronunciations and text page references are identified in color as they appear in the chapter.

New Chapter on Complementary and Alternative Therapies addresses the ever-growing use of CAM in the treatment of mental disorders.

Full-color design and illustrations enhance the visual appeal of the text.

Sample Client Care Plans with Critical Thinking Questions demonstrate the application of the therapeutic nursing process.

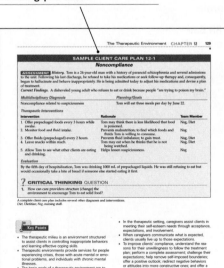

Case Studies contain critical thinking questions to help you develop problem-solving skills.

Think About Boxes contain thought-provoking scenarios and critical thinking questions.

Drug Alert boxes identify the risks and possible adverse reactions of psychotherapeutic medications.

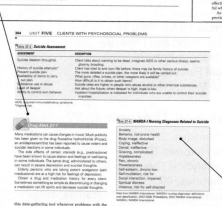

NANDA International Nursing Diagnoses relate to various disorders.

A **Glossary**, located at the back of the book and marked with an easy-to-locate color tab, provides a convenient reference to the terminology of mental health care.

Cultural Considerations address the mental health needs of culturally diverse clients.

A perforated **Review Worksheets** section (a built-in workbook) is located at the end of the book.

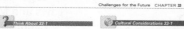

EVOLVE RESOURCES
Be sure to visit your book's Evolve website (http://evolve.elsevier.com/ Morrison-Valfre/) for an Audio Glossary, NCLEX-PN® Examination–Style Interactive Review Questions, and more!

Contents

1 The History of Mental Health Care

evolve http://evolve.elsevier.com/Morrison-Valfre/

Objectives

Upon completion of this chapter, the student will be able to:

1. Develop working definitions of mental health and mental illness.
2. List three major factors believed to influence the development of mental illness.
3. Describe the role of the church in the care of the mentally ill during the Middle Ages.
4. Compare the major contributions made by Philippe Pinel, Dorothea Dix, and Clifford Beers to the care of persons with mental disorders.
5. Discuss the impact of World Wars I and II on American attitudes toward people with mental illnesses.
6. State the major change in the care of people with mental illnesses that resulted from the discovery of psychotherapeutic drugs.
7. Describe the development of community mental health care centers during the 1960s and 1970s.
8. Discuss the shift of mentally ill clients from institutional care to community-based care.
9. Evaluate how congressional actions have affected mental health care in the United States.

Key Terms

catchment area (p. 7)

deinstitutionalization (dē-ĭn-stī-TŌŌ-shən-əl-ī-ZĀ-shən) (p. 6)

demonical exorcisms (dē-MŎN-ĭ-kəl ĔK-sōr-sīs-əms) (p. 2)

electroconvulsive therapy (ē-lĕk-trō-kŏn-VŬL-sīv THĔR-ə-pē) (ECT) (p. 6)

health-illness continuum (p. 1)

humoral (HŪ-mŏr-ăl) theory of disease (p. 2)

lobotomy (lŏ-BŎT-ə-mē) (p. 6)

lunacy (LŌŌ-nə-sē) (p. 3)

mental health (p. 1)

mental illness (disorder) (p. 1)

psychoanalysis (sī-kō-ă-NĂL-Ĭ-sīs) (p. 5)

psychotherapeutic (SI-kō-THĔR-ə-PŪ-tĭk) drugs (p. 6)

trephining (tre-PHIN-ing) (p. 2)

Mental/emotional health is interwoven with physical health. Behaviors relating to health exist over a broad spectrum, often referred to as the **health-illness continuum** (Figure 1-1). People who are exceptionally healthy are placed at the high-level wellness end of the continuum. Severely ill individuals fall at the continuum's opposite end. Most of us, however, function somewhere between these two extremes. As we meet with the stresses of life, our abilities to cope are repeatedly challenged and we strive to adjust in effective ways. When stress is physical, the body calls forth its defense systems and wards off illness. When stress is emotional or developmental, we respond by creating new (and hopefully effective) behaviors.

Mental health is the ability to "cope with and adjust to the recurrent stresses of living in an acceptable way" (Anderson and others, 2002). Mentally healthy people successfully carry out the activities of daily living, adapt to change, solve problems, set goals, and enjoy life. They are self-aware, directed, and responsible for their actions. In short, mentally healthy people cope well.

Mental health is influenced by three factors: inherited characteristics, childhood nurturing, and life circumstances. The risk for developing ineffective coping behaviors increases when problems exist in any one of these areas. If behaviors **interfere with daily activities, impair judgment,** or **alter reality,** an individual is said to be mentally ill. Simply, a **mental illness (disorder)** is a disturbance in one's ability to cope effectively. History is rich with examples of changing attitudes toward people with mental health problems.

EARLY YEARS

Illness, injury, and insanity have concerned humanity throughout history. Physical illness and injury were easy to detect with the senses. Mental illness (insanity) was something different—something that could not be seen or felt—and therefore a condition to be feared.

PRIMITIVE SOCIETIES

Although the historical record is vague, it can be assumed that some care was given to sick people. Early societies believed that everything in nature was alive

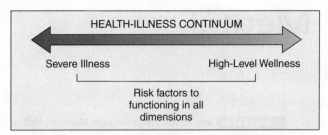

FIGURE **1-1** The health-illness continuum, ranging from high-level wellness to severe illness, provides a method of identifying a client's level of health.

with spirits. Illness was thought to be caused by the wrath of evil spirits. Therefore people with mental illnesses were possessed by demons or the forces of evil.

Treatments for mental illness focused on removing the evil spirits. Magical therapies made use of "frightening masks and noises, incantations, vile odors, charms, spells, sacrifices and fetishes" (Kelly, 1991). Physical treatments included bleeding, massage, blistering, inducing vomiting, and the practice of trephining—cutting holes in the skull to encourage the evil spirits to leave. Mentally ill individuals were allowed to remain within society as long as their behaviors were not disruptive. Severely ill or violent members of the group were often driven into the wilderness to fend for themselves.

GREECE AND ROME

Superstitions and magical beliefs dominated thinking until the Greeks introduced the idea that mental illness could be rationally explained through observation. The Greeks incorporated many ideas about illness from other cultures. By the sixth century BC, medical schools were well established. The greatest physician in Greek medicine, Hippocrates, was born in 460 BC. He was the first to base treatment on the belief that nature has a strong healing force. He felt that the role of the physician was to assist in, rather than direct, the healing process. Proper diet, exercise, and personal hygiene were his mainstays of treatment. Hippocrates viewed mental illness as a result of an imbalance of humors— the fundamental elements of air, fire, water, and earth. Each basic element had a related humor or part in the body. An overabundance or lack of one or more humors resulted in illness. This view (the humoral theory of disease) persisted for centuries.

Plato (427-347 BC), a Greek philosopher, recognized life as a dynamic balance maintained by the soul. According to Plato a "rational soul" resided in the head and an "irrational soul" was found in the heart and abdomen. He believed that if the rational soul was unable to control the undirected parts of the irrational soul, mental illness resulted. In theory, Plato anticipated Sigmund Freud by almost 2000 years.

The principles and practices of Greek medicine became established in Rome around 100 BC, but most physicians still thought that demons caused mental illness. The practice of frightening away evil spirits to cure mental illness was reintroduced, and its use continued well into the Middle Ages. The Romans showed little interest in learning about the body or mind. Most Roman physicians "wanted to make their patients comfortable by pleasant physical therapies" (Alexander and Selesnick, 1966), such as warm baths, massage, music, and peaceful surroundings.

By 300 AD, "six epidemics killed hundreds of thousands of people and desolated the land" (Alexander and Selesnick, 1966). Churches became sanctuaries for the sick, and soon hospitals were built to accommodate the sufferers. By 370 AD, Saint Basil's Hospital in England offered services for sick, orphaned, crippled, and mentally troubled people.

MIDDLE AGES
Dark Ages

From about 500 AD to 1100 AD, priests cared for the sick as the church developed into a highly organized and powerful institution. Early Christians believed that "disease was either punishment for sins, possession by the devil, or the result of witchcraft" (Ackerknecht, 1968). To cure mental illness, priests performed demonical exorcisms—religious ceremonies in which patients were physically punished to drive away the evil possessing spirit. Fortunately, these practices were tempered by the spirit of Christian charity as members of the community cared for the mentally ill with concern and sympathy.

As time passed, medieval society declined. Repeated attacks from barbaric tribes led to chaos and moral decay. Epidemics, natural disasters, and overwhelming taxes wiped out the middle class. Cities, industries and commerce disappeared. "The population declined, crime waves occurred, poverty was abysmal, and torture and imprisonment became prominent as civilization seemed to slip back into semi-barbarianism" (Donahue, 1996). Only monasteries remained as the last refuge of care and knowledge.

Throughout the Middle Ages, medicine and religion were interwoven. However, by 1130 laws were passed forbidding monks to practice medicine because it was considered too disruptive to their way of life. As a result, responsibility for the care of sick people once again fell to the community.

In the late 1100s, a strong Arabic influence was felt in Europe. Knowledge of the Greek legacy had been retained and improved upon by the Arabs. They had an extensive knowledge of drugs, mathematics, astronomy, and chemistry, as well as an awareness of the relationship between emotions and disease. The Arabic influence resulted in the establishment of learning centers, called universities. Many were devoted to the study of medicine, surgery, and care of the sick.

Problems of the mind, however, received only spiritual attention. Church doctrine still stated that if a person was insane, it must be the result of some external force—a heavenly body such as the moon. Thus the term lunacy was coined and "literally means a disorder caused by a lunar body" (Alexander and Selesnick, 1966). In time, large institutions were established, and mentally ill individuals were herded into "lunatic asylums." Magic was still used to explain the torments of the mind. A few church scholars even suggested that witches might be the source of human distresses.

Superstitions, Witches, and Hunters

The church's doctrine of imposed celibacy failed to curtail many of the clergy's sexual behaviors, and so began an antierotic movement that focused on women as the cause of men's lust. Women were thought to be carriers of the devil because they stirred men's passions. "Psychotic women with little control over voicing their sexual fantasies and sacrilegious feelings were the clearest examples of demoniacal possession" (Alexander and Selesnick, 1966). This campaign, in turn, flamed the public's mounting fear of mentally troubled people.

Witch hunting was officially launched in 1487 with the publication of the book *The Witches' Hammer*, a textbook of both pornography and psychopathology. Soon after, Pope Innocent VIII and the University of Cologne voiced support for this "textbook of the Inquisition." As a result of this one publication, women as well as children and mentally ill persons were tortured and burned at the stake by the thousands. There were few safe havens for individuals with mental illness during these troubled times.

The first English institution for mentally ill people was initially a hospice founded in 1247 by the sheriff of London. By 1330, Bethlehem Royal Hospital had developed into a lunatic asylum that eventually became infamous for its brutal treatments. Violently ill patients were chained to walls in small cells and often provided "entertainment" for the public. Hospital staff would charge fees for their "tourist attractions" and conduct tours through the institution. Less violent patients were forced to wear identifying metal armbands and beg on the streets. Insane people were harshly treated in those times, but Bethlehem Royal Hospital, commonly called Bedlam (Figure 1-2), was preferable to burning at the stake.

By the middle of the fourteenth century, the European continent had endured several devastating plagues and epidemics. One quarter of the earth's population, more than 60 million people, perished from infectious diseases during this period. The feudal system lost power and declined. Cities began to flourish and housed a growing middle class. "Luxury and misery, learning and ignorance existed side by side" (Donahue, 1996). Society was at last beginning to demand reforms. However, as the age of art, medicine, and science dawned, the hunting of "witches" became even more popular. It was a time of great contradictions.

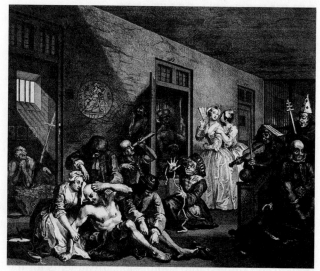

FIGURE **1-2** Bethlehem Royal Hospital in London.

THE RENAISSANCE

The Renaissance began in Italy around 1400 and spread throughout the European continent within a century. Upheavals in economics, politics, education, and commerce brought the real world into focus. The power of the church slowly declined as an intense interest in material gain and worldly affairs developed. At the same time, the medieval view of a sinful, naked body changed into a celebration of the human form by artists such as da Vinci, Raphael, and Michelangelo. Thousand-year-old anatomy books were replaced by realistic anatomical drawings. Observation, rather than ancient theories, revolutionized many of the ideas of the day.

Sixteenth-century physicians, relying on observation, began to record what they saw. Mental illness was at last being recognized without bias. By the mid-1500s, behaviors were accurately recorded for melancholia (depression), mania, and psychopathic personalities. Precise observations led to classifications for different abnormal behaviors. Mental problems were now thought to be caused by some sort of brain disorder—except in the case of sexual fantasies, which were still considered to be God's punishment or possession by the devil. However, despite great advances in knowledge, the actual treatment of mentally troubled people remained inhumane.

THE REFORMATION

Another movement that influenced the care of the sick—the Reformation—occurred in 1517. People were displeased with the conduct of the clergy and widespread abuses occurring within the Catholic Church. Martin Luther (1483-1546), a dissatisfied monk, and his followers broke away from the Catholic Church and became known as Protestants. As a result of this separation, many hospitals operated by the Catholic Church began to close. Once again the poor, sick, and insane were turned out into the streets.

SEVENTEENTH CENTURY

During the seventeenth and eighteenth centuries, developments in science, literature, philosophy, and the arts laid the foundations for the modern world. Reason was slowly beginning to replace magical thinking, but a strong belief in demons still persisted.

The 1600s produced many great thinkers. Knowledge of the secrets of nature brought a sense of self-reliance. However, many people were uncomfortable, so they once again moved toward the security of witch hunting as a means of protecting themselves from the unexplainable.

It was during the seventeenth century that conditions for mentally ill individuals were at their worst. While physicians and theorists were making observations and speculations about insanity, patients were bled, starved, beaten, and purged into submission. Treatments for the mentally troubled remained in this unhappy state until the late 1700s.

EIGHTEENTH CENTURY

During the latter part of the eighteenth century, psychiatry developed as a separate branch of medicine. Inhumane treatment and vicious practices were openly questioned. In 1792, Philippe Pinel (1745-1826), the director of two Paris hospitals, liberated patients from their chains "and advocated acceptance of the mentally ill as human beings in need of medical assistance, nursing care, and social services" (Donahue, 1996). During this period the Quakers, a religious order, established asylums of humane care in England.

In the American colonies the Philadelphia Almshouse was erected in 1731. It accepted sick, infirm, and insane patients as well as prisoners and orphans. In 1794, Bellevue Hospital in New York City was opened as a pesthouse for the victims of yellow fever. By 1816 the hospital had enlarged to contain an almshouse for poor people, wards for the sick and insane, staff quarters, and even a penitentiary.

Unfortunately, the care and treatment of people with mental illness remained as harsh and indifferent in the United States as it was in Europe. The practice of allowing poor people to care for mentally ill individuals continued well into the late 1800s and was only slowly abandoned. Actual care of mentally ill persons in the United States did not begin to improve until the arrival of Alice Fisher, a Florence Nightingale–trained nurse, in 1884.

By the close of the eighteenth century, treatments for people with mental illness still included the medieval practices of bloodletting, purging, and confinement (Figure 1-3). Newer therapies included demon-expelling tranquilizing chairs (Figure 1-4) and whirling devices (Figure 1-5). The study of psychiatry was in its infancy, and those who actually cared for insane people still relied heavily on the methods of their ancestors.

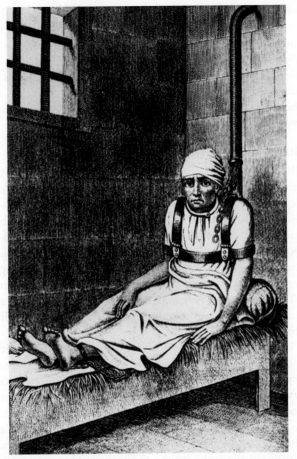

FIGURE **1-3** A patient in chains in Bedlam, London's notorious Bethlehem Royal Hospital.

NINETEENTH-CENTURY UNITED STATES

By the early 1800s the Revolutionary War had ended and the United States was a growing nation. Changes that occurred during this century had an enormous impact on the care of the mentally ill population.

One of the most important figures in nineteenth-century psychiatry was Dr. Benjamin Rush, a crusader for the insane. Dr. Rush (1745-1813) graduated from Princeton University at 15 years of age. By the time he was 31, he had been a professor of chemistry and medicine, a chief surgeon in the Continental Army, and a signer of the Declaration of Independence. His book titled *Diseases of the Mind* was the first psychiatric text written in the United States. In it, he advocated clean conditions (good air, lighting, and food) and kindness. As a result of Rush's efforts, mentally troubled people were no longer caged in the basements of general hospitals. However, only a few institutions for insane persons were actually available in the United States at this time. Mildly affected people were commonly sold at slave auctions, whereas the more violent remained in asylums that were a combination of zoo and penitentiary.

During the 1830s, attitudes toward mental illness slowly began to change. The "once insane always insane" concept was being replaced by the notion that

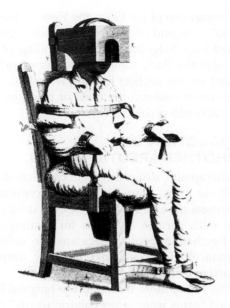

FIGURE **1-4** Tranquilizing chair.

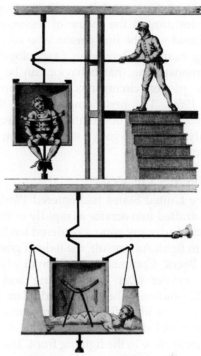

FIGURE **1-5** Circulating swing and bed.

cure may be possible. A few mental hospitals were built, but the actual living conditions for most patients remained deplorable.

It was not until 1841 that a frail 40-year-old schoolteacher exposed the sins of the system. Dorothea Dix was contracted to teach Sunday school at a jail in Massachusetts. While there, she saw both criminals and mentally ill prisoners living in squalid conditions. For the next 20 years Dix surveyed asylums, jails, and almshouses throughout the United States, Canada, and Scotland. It was not uncommon for her to find mentally ill people "confined in cages, closets, cellars, stalls, and pens … chained, naked, beaten with rods and lashed into obedience" (Dolan, 1968).

Dorothea Dix presented her findings to anyone who would listen. Her untiring crusade had results that shook the world. The public became so aroused by Dix's efforts that millions of dollars were raised, more than 30 mental hospitals throughout the United States were constructed, and care of the mentally ill greatly improved.

By the late 1800s, a two-class system of psychiatric care had emerged: private care for the wealthy and publicly provided care for the remainder of society. The newly constructed mental institutions were quickly filled, and soon chronic overcrowding began to strain the system. Cure rates fell dramatically. The public became disenchanted, and mental illness once again was viewed as incurable. Only small, private facilities that catered to the wealthy had some degree of success. State facilities had evolved into large, remote institutions that became completely self-reliant and removed from society.

By the close of the nineteenth century, many of the gains in the care for the mentally ill population had been lost. Overpopulated institutions could offer no more than minimal custodial care. Theories of the day gave no satisfactory explanations about the causes of mental problems, and current treatments remained ineffective. It was a time of despair for mentally troubled people and those who cared for them.

TWENTIETH CENTURY

The 1900s were ushered in by reform movements. Political, economic, and social changes were beginning. For the first time in history, disease prevention was emphasized. For the mentally ill population, however, conditions remained intolerable until 1908 when a single individual began his crusade.

Clifford Beers was a young student at Yale University when he attempted suicide. Consequently, he spent 3 years as a patient in mental hospitals in Connecticut. On his release in 1908, Beers wrote a book that would set the wheels of the mental hygiene movement in motion. His book, *A Mind That Found Itself*, recounted the beatings, isolation, and confinement of a mentally ill person. As a direct result of Beers' work, the **Committee for Mental Hygiene** was formed in 1909. In addition to prevention, the group focused on removing the stigma attached to mental illness. Under Beers' energetic guidance, the movement grew nationwide. The social consciousness of a nation had finally been awakened.

PSYCHOANALYSIS

In the early 1900s, a neurophysiologist named Sigmund Freud published the article that introduced the term **psychoanalysis** to the world's vocabulary. Freud believed that forces both within and outside the personality were responsible for mental illness. He developed elaborate theories around the theme of repressed sexual energies. Freud was the first person who succeeded in "explaining human behavior in psychological terms and in demonstrating that behavior can be changed under the proper circumstances" (Alexander and Selesnick, 1966). The first comprehensive theory of mental illness based on observation had emerged, and psychoanalysis began to gain a strong hold in America (see Chapter 5).

INFLUENCES OF WAR

By 1917 the United States had entered World War I. Men were drafted into service as rapidly as they could be processed, but many were considered too "mentally deficient" to fight. As a result, the federal government called on Beers' Committee for Mental Hygiene to develop a master plan for screening and treating mentally ill soldiers. The completed plan included methods for early identification of problems, removal of mentally troubled personnel from combat duty, and early treatment close to the fighting front. The committee also recommended that psychiatrists be assigned to station hospitals to treat combat veterans with acute behavioral problems and provide ongoing psychiatric care after soldiers returned to their homes.

Because of the war, a renewed interest in mental hygiene was sparked. During the 1930s, new therapies for treating insanity were developed. **Insulin therapy** for schizophrenia induced 50-hour comas through the administration of massive doses of insulin. Passing electricity through the patient's head (electroconvulsive therapy [ECT]) helped to improve severe depression, and lobotomy (a surgical procedure that severs the frontal lobes of the brain from the thalamus) almost eliminated violent behaviors. A new class of drugs that lifted spirits of depressed people, the amphetamines, was introduced. All these therapies improved behaviors and made patients more receptive to Freud's psychotherapy. Public interest was renewed, and in 1937 Congress passed the **Hill-Burton Act,** which funded the construction of psychiatric units throughout the United States.

From 1941 to 1945, the United States was immersed in World War II. Many draftees were still rejected for enlistment because of mental health problems. A large number of soldiers received early discharges based on psychiatric disorders, and many active-duty personnel received treatment for psychiatric problems.

In 1946, Congress passed the **National Mental Health Act,** which provided funding for programs in research, training of mental health professionals, and expansion of state mental health facilities. By 1949, the **National Institute of Mental Health** was organized to provide research and training related to mental illness. New approaches to the care of the mentally ill population (the therapeutic community movement, family care, halfway houses) sparked the public's enthusiasm.

The Korean War of the 1950s, the Vietnam War of the 1960s and 1970s, and other armed conflicts contributed significant knowledge to the understanding of stress-related problems. Posttraumatic stress disorders became recognized among soldiers fighting wars. Today stress disorders are considered the basis of many emotional and mental health problems.

INTRODUCTION OF PSYCHOTHERAPEUTIC DRUGS

Psychotherapeutic drugs are chemicals that affect the mind. These drugs alter emotions, perceptions, and consciousness in several ways. They are used in combination with various therapies for treating mental illness. Psychotherapeutic drugs are also called **psychopharmacologic agents, psychotropic drugs,** and **psychoactive drugs.**

"By the 1950s, more than half the hospital beds in the United States were in psychiatric wards" (Taylor, 1994). Patients were usually treated kindly, but effective therapies were still limited. Treatments consisted of psychoanalysis, insulin therapy, electroconvulsive (shock) therapy, and water/ice therapy. More violent patients were physically restrained in straitjackets or underwent lobotomy. Drug therapy consisted of sedatives (chloral hydrate and paraldehyde), barbiturates (phenobarbital), and amphetamines that quieted patients but did little to treat their illnesses.

In 1949, an Australian physician, John Cade, discovered that lithium carbonate was effective in controlling the severe mood swings seen in bipolar (manic-depressive) illness. With lithium therapy, many chronically ill clients were again able to lead normal lives and were released from mental institutions. Encouraged by the apparent success of lithium, researchers began to explore the possibility of controlling mental illness with the use of various new drugs.

Chlorpromazine (Thorazine) was introduced in 1956 and proved to control many of the bizarre behaviors observed in schizophrenia and other psychoses (Keltner and Folks, 2001). The 1950s concluded with the introduction of imipramine, the first antidepressant. Soon other drugs, such as antianxiety agents, became available for use in treatment.

As more patients were able to control their behaviors with drug therapy, the demand for hospitalization decreased. Many people with mental disorders could now live and function outside the institution. At this time, the federal government began the movement called deinstitutionalization, the release of large numbers of mentally ill persons into the community. To illustrate, 560,000 patients were cared for in state hospitals in 1955. By 1994, the number of institutionalized patients had dropped to fewer than 120,000 people (Harrington, 1999). The introduction of psychotherapeutic drugs opened the doors of institutions and set the stage for a new delivery system—community mental health care.

The 1960s were filled with social changes. With the introduction of psychotherapeutic drugs came the concept of the "least restrictive alternative." If patients could, with medication, control their behaviors and cooperate with treatment plans, then the controlled environment of the institution was no longer necessary. It was believed that people with mental disorders could live within their communities and work with their therapists on an outpatient basis.

In 1961, the Joint Commission on Mental Illness and Health published a 338-page report titled *Action for Mental Health.* The report motivated President John Kennedy to appoint a special committee to study the problem of mental illness and recommend specific actions. Recommendations from Kennedy's committee called for a bold new approach to mental health care that included the development of an entirely new entity—the community mental health center.

CONGRESSIONAL ACTIONS

As the population of people with mental illnesses shifted from the institution to the community, the demand for community mental health services expanded. To meet this demand, the federal government acted to establish a nationwide network of community mental health centers.

The **Community Mental Health Centers Act** was passed by Congress in October 1963. This act was designed to support the construction of mental health centers in communities throughout the United States. There, the needs of all people experiencing mental or emotional problems, as well as those of acute and chronic mentally ill people, would be met. Physicians (psychiatrists), nurses, and various therapists would develop therapeutic relationships with clients and monitor their progress within the community setting. Each center was to provide comprehensive mental health services for all residents within a certain geographical region, called a catchment area.

It was believed that community mental health centers would provide the link in helping mentally ill people make the transition from the institution to the community, thus meeting the goal of humane care delivered in the least restrictive way. Passage of the **Medicare/Medicaid Bill of 1965,** combined with the Community Mental Health Centers Act, led to the release of more than 75% of institutionalized mentally ill persons into the community (Morrissey and Goldman, 1984). Unfortunately, most chronically mentally ill people were "dumped" into their communities before realistic strategies, programs, and facilities were in place.

Community mental health centers expanded throughout the 1970s, but funding was inadequate and sporadic. Demands for services overwhelmed the system and non–revenue-generating services (prevention and education) were eliminated. Services for the general public dwindled, and many centers began to close their doors. Finally, in 1975, Congress passed amendments to the Community Mental Health Centers Act that provided funding for community centers based on a complex set of guidelines. The **President's Commission on Mental Health** was established in 1978 by President Jimmy Carter. Its task was to assess the mental health needs of the nation and recommend possible courses of action to strengthen and improve existing community mental health efforts. The commission's final report resulted in 117 specific recommendations grouped into four broad areas: coordination of services, high-risk populations, flexibility in planning services, and least restrictive care alternatives.

By 1980, Congress passed one of the most progressive mental health bills in history. The **Mental Health Systems Act** addressed community mental health care and clients' rights and established priorities for research and training. However, before the recommendations could be nationally implemented, the United States elected a new president and mental health reform changed dramatically.

Just as legislation that comprehensively dealt with mental health issues was about to be enacted the political climate changed. Federal funding for all mental health services was drastically reduced. The passage of the **Omnibus Budget Reconciliation Act (OBRA) of 1981** essentially repealed the Mental Health Systems Act. This resulted in **block grant funding** whereby each state received a "block" or designated amount of federal money. The state then determined where and how the money was spent. Unfortunately, many states proved less committed to mental health with the use of their block grant money. As a result, many hospitalized mentally ill people (especially the older adult population) were transferred to less appropriate nursing homes or other community facilities.

To stem the practice of inappropriate placement for the chronic mentally ill population, the Omnibus Budget Reconciliation Act of 1987 was passed. Because people with chronic mental problems could no longer be "warehoused" in nursing homes or other long-term facilities, many were discharged to the streets. As concern for a rapidly expanding federal budget deficit grew, funding for mental health care dwindled. By the late 1980s, funding was curtailed for most inpatient psychiatric care. Following the trend, most insurance companies withdrew their coverage for psychiatric care.

In 2006, the National Alliance for Mental Illness (NAMI) conducted the "first comprehensive survey and grading of state adult mental health care systems conducted in more than 15 years" (NAMI, 2006). Their results revealed a fragmented system with an overall grade of D. Recommendations focused on increased funding, availability of care, access to care, and greater involvement of consumers and their families.

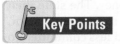

Think About 1-1

- What do you think are the most important services in a national health care plan?
- What priority would you give to care of people with mental illness?

Today, many of our population's most severely mentally ill people still wander the streets in abject poverty and homelessness as a result of federal and state funding cuts. Community mental health centers have closed their doors or drastically reduced their services. Federal funding is limited to block grants (for all health care) to each state. The original goals of comprehensive care, education, rehabilitation, prevention, training, and research were lost in the efforts to curtail costs.

Currently, lawmakers in the United States are struggling to define a new national health policy. Models for delivering cost-effective health care are being investigated, but no comprehensive plan is yet in place. Other countries, such as Canada, the United Kingdom, and Australia, are faced with similar mental health care issues. It is in all of our best interests to accept the challenge of providing for our societies' mental and physical health care needs. Think About 1-1 offers something to consider.

Key Points

- Mental health is the ability to cope with and adapt to the stresses of everyday life.
- Mentally healthy people are self-aware, directed, and responsible for their actions.
- Mental illness is an inability to cope that results in impaired functioning.
- Mental health is influenced by inherited characteristics, childhood nurturing, and life circumstances.

- The causes and treatments of mental illness were based in superstition, magical beliefs, and demonical possession from primitive societies into the 1800s.
- Priests cared for the sick and exorcised demons, but mentally troubled people were treated with care by the Christian community during the Middle Ages.
- By the late Middle Ages, large asylums housed the insane, and the belief that witches were the carriers of the devil led to the burning of thousands of women, children, and mentally ill people.
- By the 1500s, psychotic behaviors were being accurately observed and recorded, but the Reformation movement returned many insane people to the streets as church sanctuaries closed.
- During the 1800s, Americans Dr. Benjamin Rush and Dorothea Dix crusaded for the humane care of mentally ill people.
- Standards for the care of the insane population improved during the mid-1800s until huge waves of people overwhelmed the mental health care system, causing the conditions to deteriorate.
- A book written by Clifford Beers about his experience as a mental patient set the mental hygiene movement of the early 1900s into motion.
- By the 1920s, Sigmund Freud's psychoanalytical theories became a popular method for treating emotional problems.
- The First and Second World Wars pointed out the need for comprehensive mental health care.
- With the introduction of psychotherapeutic drug treatment, many psychiatric institutions closed.
- Community mental health centers were built during the 1970s, but a change in political climate left the project uncompleted and countless mentally ill people without treatment.
- Today, many legislative changes again challenge us to develop comprehensive, cost-efficient care for society's mentally ill members.

evolve   Be sure to visit the companion Evolve site at http://evolve.elsevier.com/Morrison-Valfre/ for additional online resources.

2 Current Mental Health Care Systems

Objectives

Upon completion of this chapter, the student will be able to:

1. Describe the current mental health care system in Canada, Norway, the United Kingdom, Australia, and the United States.
2. State the major difference between inpatient and outpatient psychiatric care.
3. Explain the community support systems model of care.
4. List four settings for community mental health care delivery.
5. Identify five components of the case management method of mental health care.
6. Discuss the roles and purpose of the multidisciplinary mental health care team.
7. Name four high-risk populations served by community mental health centers.
8. List five community-based mental health services for people with HIV/AIDS.

Key Terms

advocacy (ĂD-və-kə-sē) (p. 13)
case management (p. 12)
community mental health centers (p.11)
community support systems (CSS) model (p. 11)
consultation (p. 13)
crisis intervention (p. 14)
diagnosis-related groups (DRGs) (p. 17)
health maintenance organizations (HMOs) (p. 10)
homelessness (p. 17)
inpatient psychiatric care (p. 11)
multidisciplinary (MŪL-tĭ-dĭ-sĭ-plə-nă-rē) **mental health care teams** (p. 15)
outpatient mental health care (p. 11)
preferred provider organizations (PPOs) (p. 10)
psychosocial rehabilitation (p. 13)
recidivism (rē-SĬD-ĭ-vĭz-əm) (p. 11)
resource linkage (p. 13)
third-party payments (p. 10)

The delivery of a population's health care varies with the culture. Because cultures, values, and beliefs differ, international comparisons of health care systems are difficult to make. The more developed nations have complex health care systems, but almost half of all countries in the world "have no explicit mental health policy and nearly a third have no program for coping with the rising tide of brain-related disabilities" (Sherer, 2002).

MENTAL HEALTH CARE IN CANADA

By the late 1960s, Canada adopted a **government-administered health insurance plan.** Today a "single-payer arrangement" is used in the Canadian health care system, which is based on five principles: universality, portability, accessibility, comprehensiveness, and public administration. Each guiding principle is explained in Box 2-1.

Each province or territory organizes, administers, and monitors the health care delivery system of its citizens. Benefits may vary, but all Canadian citizens are eligible for diagnostic, emergency, outpatient, medical, hospital, convalescent, and mental health services. Medications for people over age 65 years are also provided. The agency responsible for the health of Canadians is the Department of National Health and Welfare. It provides technical and financial support for each provincial health care program; enforces federal food and drug laws; promotes health; and administers social welfare programs.

Canada's health care system is divided into curative and preventive operations with the major focus on cure and treatment. Preventive services, including mental health, are delivered through public health departments. "Private psychotherapy, community mental health, other day programs, and hospital psychiatric services" (Kirkpatrick, 1999) are available to every Canadian based on need.

MENTAL HEALTH CARE IN NORWAY

Like other European countries, Norway has adopted a **national insurance system.** The National Insurance Act of 1967 provides access to health care for everyone

Principles of the Canadian Health Act

1. *Universality.* Everyone in the nation is covered.
2. *Portability.* People can move and still retain their health coverage.
3. *Accessibility.* Everyone has access to the system's health care providers.
4. *Comprehensiveness.* Provincial plans cover all medically necessary treatment.
5. *Public administration.* The system is publicly run and publicly accountable.

From Edelman CL, Mandle CL: *Health promotion throughout the lifespan,* ed 5, St. Louis, 2002, Mosby.

living in Norway. Employees contribute a percentage of their wages and pay out-of-pocket fees for health care until a "payment ceiling" (about $175) is reached. Thereafter, all services are covered except adult dental care.

Financing and delivery of health care services occur on three levels. Health policy is legislated, and health service delivery is monitored by national authorities. Hospitals and specialized medical services are managed by Norway's 19 counties, whereas primary health care services are organized on the municipal level. Mental health care is available to all citizens of Norway.

MENTAL HEALTH CARE IN BRITAIN

All British citizens are provided health care through a government-managed **national health care system.** The Secretary for Social Services is responsible for setting fees for private health care providers, budgets for hospitals, and salaries for hospital physicians. Parliament allocates funds for the health care system and regulates the rates at which general practitioners are paid. Tax revenues provide most of the financing for health care.

Mental health care is available for all British citizens as part of the standard benefit package. Physician services, emergency surgeries, hospital stays, and prescription drugs, along with preventive, home, and long-term care, are all provided by the government. Eye care is not included and dental care is limited, but all other basic health care needs are provided. Private insurance is also available.

MENTAL HEALTH CARE IN AUSTRALIA

Australians are provided an interesting mix of health care plans. The government provides a **public health plan** that covers all public hospitals and physician services. Also available is a **national private plan,** which supplements the basic public plan. In addition, numerous **private insurance plans** are available for eye care, rehabilitative services, and psychiatric treatment.

National health care is financed by a tax on all citizens above a certain income. Policy and budget decisions are made at the federal level. Individual states are responsible for the administration and delivery of health care services that are available through local government agencies, semi-voluntary agencies, and profit-oriented, nongovernmental organizations. Mental health care is not provided in Australia's basic health plan, so treatment for psychiatric disorders is more common for those with large incomes or private insurance plans.

MENTAL HEALTH CARE IN THE UNITED STATES

Health care in the United States is based on the **private insurance model.** Today, more than 75% of the population is covered by private insurance or public programs (Medicare and/or Medicaid). More than 15% of U.S. citizens have no health care coverage at all.

HEALTH INSURANCE

During the 1960s, third-party payments became available. With **third-party payments,** medical costs were covered by a "third party"—usually an insurance company or the state or federal government. By the late 1970s, many employers provided insurance that included some coverage for mental health care. Mental health care was available but expensive during the 1980s. Today, health care is delivered and costs are controlled through a **managed care system** using four types of health care plans.

Fee-for-Service Plans

Clients can choose any health care provider and do not require a referral to see a specialist. Many fee-for-service plans are being replaced by other, less costly, health care plans.

Preferred Provider Organizations

During the 1980s, **preferred provider organizations (PPOs)** were established to help curtail the rapidly growing increases in health care costs. They consist of a network of physicians, hospitals, and clinics that agree to provide care for different organizations at a discount. The client may see any health care provider, without referrals, within the network, and 80% to 100% of the costs to the client are covered.

Point-of-Service Plans

Point-of-service plans are similar to PPO plans except that clients are required to obtain referrals from their primary care physicians in order to see specialists.

Health Maintenance Organizations

Health maintenance organizations (HMOs) deliver health care to enrolled clients who pay a fixed price. Health care costs are covered as long as clients receive care within the system, and referrals to specialists are required. Clients may or may not have a choice of care providers. Costs are contained by monitoring the delivery of care and limiting access to specialists and/or expensive procedures. Many HMO plans place a limit on mental health care benefits.

The distinction between public and private mental health care financing is beginning to blur. Federal funds (Medicare) and state funds (Medicaid) are being used to cover costs in both the private and public sectors. Currently, Medicare funds about 30% to 50% of all state mental health systems.

CARE SETTINGS

Mental health care is delivered primarily in community settings, and admission rates to psychiatric inpatient facilities were at an all-time low by 1983. However, by 1988, hospitalizations for mental illness were on the rise and emergency departments saw huge increases in clients with psychiatric problems. Today there are more people in need of care than there are treatment settings.

INPATIENT CARE

Individuals are admitted to inpatient psychiatric care on the basis of need. The severity of the client's illness, the level of dysfunction, the suitability of the setting for treating the problem, the level of client cooperation, and the client's ability to pay for services all enter into the decision regarding inpatient psychiatric care.

Clients who receive inpatient care remain at the institution for 24 hours per day. There, all aspects of the environment focus on providing therapeutic assistance. Inpatient psychiatric care settings provide clients with safe, stable, and therapeutic surroundings. Discharge occurs when client behavior has appropriately improved and treatment goals have been attained. Clients may be discharged into the community, to a group home or other structured setting, or to another institution for long-term psychiatric care.

The most important advantage of inpatient psychiatric care is that it provides clients with a safe and secure environment where they can focus on and work with the problems that brought them there. Clients may also be committed to psychiatric care by way of the criminal justice system. The legal aspects of involuntary commitment are discussed in Chapter 3.

OUTPATIENT CARE

As the emphasis shifts from institutional to community mental health care, the demand for outpatient psychiatric service grows. An outpatient mental health care setting is a facility that provides services to people with mental problems within their home environments. Outpatient psychiatric clients are able to remain within their communities, associating with the real world.

Community-based mental health care occurs within a dynamic society. Supervision is limited, and the responsibility for controlling behavior lies squarely with the individual. Clients are assessed in relation to their environment, and therapies are designed to assist them in functioning appropriately within their communities. Unfortunately, the number of outpatient psychiatric care facilities in the United States is being rapidly outpaced by the mental health needs of a nation undergoing many changes.

Mentally ill people make use of community services only sporadically. Many wait until major problems occur before seeking treatment. When services are used, a "Band-Aid" approach that treats only the presenting complaint is often used. As a result, many mentally ill individuals who end up in the emergency departments of general hospitals or county jails are in need of inpatient psychiatric care. Today it is estimated that "between 600,000 and one million jail admissions annually are mentally ill" (Harrington, 1999).

Unable to cope in the community setting, people with chronic psychiatric problems often return to institutions or use community services on a revolving-door basis. This behavior pattern is known as recidivism and means a relapse of a symptom, disease, or behavior. Recidivism is a major problem in mental health care. It is associated with negative treatment outcomes, staff frustration, and inappropriate use of services. Lower rates of recidivism are seen in communities where coordination and cooperation among community agencies and mental hospitals exist.

Psychiatry and mental health care policies are based on the medical treatment model: identify the symptom and then treat it. This point of view became inadequate once clients were released into the community. A broader, community-oriented, more flexible outlook was needed.

Community Support Systems Model

For mentally ill people to function well within their communities, a wide range of support services is necessary. The community support systems (CSS) model views clients holistically—as individuals with basic human needs, ambitions, and rights. The goal of the CSS model is to create a support system that fosters individual growth and movement toward independence through the use of coordinated social, medical, and psychiatric services. Effective community support systems are consumer-oriented, culturally appropriate, flexible enough to meet individual needs, accountable, and coordinated. A typical program may include services such as health care, housing, food, income support, rehabilitation, advocacy, and crisis response (Figure 2-1).

The most successful community mental health centers have forged strong links with community agencies, services, and government. Other centers have developed slowly, but the CSS model of mental health care is proving to be one of the most comprehensive and workable concepts for the future.

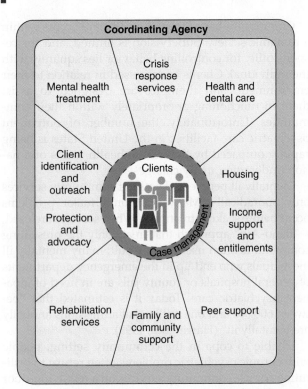

FIGURE **2-1** Community support system.

From Haber J and others: *Comprehensive psychiatric nursing*, ed 5, St. Louis, 1997, Mosby.

Box 2-2 *Examples of Community Services*

SERVING INDIVIDUALS
Rape crisis centers
Churches and synagogues
Employment, job-training agencies
Recreational clubs
Adult education programs
Literacy programs
Mediation groups
Meals on Wheels
Colleges and universities
Mental health agencies

SERVING FAMILIES
Women, Infants, and Children (WIC)
Children's groups (e.g., Camp Fire Girls)
Nutritional services
Church groups
Community "Welcome Wagon"
Recreation centers
Day care centers for young, disabled, or elderly people
Family-planning agencies
Family recreation centers and groups
Shelters for victims of domestic violence

SERVING THE COMMUNITY
Environmental groups
Education groups (e.g., American Lung Association, March of Dimes)
Utility companies
Community emergency shelters
Government agencies
Police and fire departments
Fair housing bureau or agency
Prisons
Performing arts centers
Public forests and parks

DELIVERY OF COMMUNITY MENTAL HEALTH SERVICES

Mental health services and support systems are available through a variety of community agencies, support groups, and civic organizations. Services focus on prevention, maintenance, treatment, and rehabilitation of mental health problems. Some agencies or groups limit their focus to one area (e.g., Alcoholics Anonymous focuses on treatment of alcohol addiction). Individuals, families, and communities benefit from the activities of various groups. Box 2-2 lists examples of commonly available community services.

COMMUNITY CARE SETTINGS

Community mental health services are based on the needs of specific populations. Also, mentally ill people must be treated in the least restrictive manner. Therefore several services are available in various settings throughout the community. See Table 2-1 for examples.

With short institutional stays and the release of people with chronic mental illness into the community, the need for home psychiatric care providers to fill the gap between institution and community is rapidly growing. Psychiatric clinical nurse specialists (CNSs) ease the transition from hospital to home for clients and their families and assist clients in navigating the mental health care system. They also provide psychosocial crisis interventions and collaborate with clients, families, and other professionals to deliver the most appropriate and cost-accountable psychiatric care. Case Study 2-1 illustrates the role of the mental health CNS in the home care setting.

CASE MANAGEMENT SYSTEMS

Defined as a holistic system of interventions, case management is designed to support the transition of mentally ill clients into the community. The major components of case management are psychosocial rehabilitation, consultation, resource linkage (referral), advocacy, therapy, and crisis intervention. Clients are involved with the assessment, planning, and evaluation of their care. Goals are stated as client outcomes. Success is measured in terms of client satisfaction, improved coping behaviors, and appropriate use of services. The overall goal of case management is a successfully functioning client who is able (with support) to avoid relapse and achieve productive patterns of living. A look at each component of case management may help clarify the process.

Table 2-1	*Community Mental Health Care Delivery*		
SETTING	**FOCUS/SERVICES**	**STAFF MEMBERS**	**COMMENTS**
Emergency care (community hospital emergency departments [EDs], emergency psychiatric clinics)	Stabilization, assist with the crisis, refer to appropriate community resources	Nurses, social workers, therapists, psychologists, psychiatric technicians	Many chronically mentally ill use ER settings as entries into the mental health care network
Residential programs (group homes)	Offer a protected, supervised environment within the community	Home care providers, therapists, nurses, technicians, physician	Provide food, shelter, clothing, supervision, counseling, vocational training, socialization
Partial hospitalization (day treatment centers)	Provides care and treatment for clients who are too ill to be independent—clients are gradually introduced into the community	Psychologists, therapists, nurses, counselors, social workers, technicians	Multidisciplinary care and treatment have led to client success and proven the effectiveness of these programs
Psychiatric home care	Delivers care to clients and families in their homes; helps clients and families transition from institution to home; crisis interventions; referral to resources	Psychiatric clinical nurses (CNSs), home care providers	Collaborates with client, family, other mental health professionals to provide ongoing care
Community mental health centers	Services include crisis intervention, family counseling, education, care for the chronically mentally ill, medical care, vocational and skills training	Psychologists, therapists, nurses, counselors, social workers, technicians	Lack of adequate financing has resulted in fragmented services

CNSs, Clinical nurse specialists; *ER,* emergency room.

Psychosocial Rehabilitation

Use of multidisciplinary services to help clients gain the skills needed to carry out the activities of daily living as actively and independently as possible best describes psychosocial rehabilitation. Clients are first assessed for physical, social, emotional, and intellectual levels of function. Then specific plans for teaching needed skills are developed. If clients are capable of work, vocational rehabilitation is offered.

The psychosocial rehabilitation model of care encourages decision making, thus empowering clients. This empowerment fosters a sense of self-esteem and mastery that results in improved coping abilities. As clients feel the success of making their own decisions, they are encouraged to take control over other areas of their lives. Education is also a strong component of psychosocial rehabilitation because mastering daily living skills motivates clients to more productive and independent ways of functioning.

Consultation

In mental health care, consultation is defined as a process in which the assistance of a specialist is sought to help identify ways to work effectively with client problems. The case management system relies on the expertise of psychiatrists, nurses, psychologists, social workers, counselors, and various therapists to find ways for clients to receive the services and support that help them to achieve their goals. For example, a nurse might work with a client on personal grooming skills while a social worker locates supported housing and a

vocational counselor seeks out an appropriate work setting. By covering all the bases, care providers hope to maintain clients in the least restrictive setting (the community) and assist them with their needs.

Resource Linkage

The process of matching clients' needs with the most appropriate community services best describes resource linkage. Health care providers have traditionally referred clients to other services, but resource linkage adds the component of periodic monitoring. The advantages of coordinating and linking services are several: clients can be more easily moved into different programs because background information moves with them; duplication of services is avoided; and as the clients' level of functioning improves, services can be tailored to support the new, more effective behaviors. With resource linkage, the focus for treatment of clients is on care instead of the more traditional emphasis on psychiatric symptoms and illness (see Think About 2-1).

Advocacy

A critical concept of case management, advocacy is providing the client with the information to make certain decisions. Advocacy for mentally ill people involves more than other areas of health care. Advocates work to protect clients' rights, help to clarify expectations, provide support, and act on behalf of clients' best interests. Every person involved in mental health care can act as an advocate by supporting community efforts and policies that encourage healthy living practices.

Case Study 2-1

Joanne is a 59-year-old woman with severe depression, anorexia, and suicidal ideation. The psychiatric home care referral was an effort by her husband to prevent nursing home placement. Joanne presented with a 30-year history of scleroderma (a disfiguring skin condition), numerous surgeries and hospitalizations, and a 10-year psychiatric history with numerous suicide attempts. She has severe anxiety and agoraphobia (fear of crowds and open spaces). Her anorexia was severe, with her weight at 77 pounds. Medical and psychiatric problems were interwoven, and she needed comprehensive intervention. The clinical nurse specialist (CNS) served as case manager.

Because Joanne could not leave home and needed medication management, a psychiatrist made home visits. Companion services were supplied while the husband was at work. The husband was actively involved in the decision making regarding his wife's care, but he needed supportive interventions.

Over a 4-month period, Joanne progressed from a severely withdrawn, suicidal person to someone who was dealing with her panic attacks, agoraphobia, and scleroderma. Her weight had increased to 90 pounds. Although she would continue to cope with a chronic illness, her hopelessness was gone, and her ability to function in her daily life had markedly improved. She was able to continue living in her home and community with the help of community mental health services.

• What follow-up care would you plan for Joanne?
• What activities would help Joanne meet her social needs?

Modified from Mellon SK: Mental health clinical nurse specialist in home care for the 90s, *Issues Ment Health Nurs* 15:229, 1994.

Think About 2-1

You are a health care provider who has recently moved to this area. As a staff member in a community mental health clinic, you are responsible for helping refer clients to appropriate agencies.

• How would you go about locating agencies in the community that provide services for mentally ill individuals?

Therapy

Therapy is provided for each client based on assessed needs, client cooperation, and available services. Medications may be included as part of the overall plan of treatment. Therapies may include the use of counseling, support groups, vocational rehabilitation programs, and techniques to assist clients with problem-solving and adaptive behaviors.

Crisis Intervention

The crisis intervention component of case management is crucial to the success of the client. People with chronic mental dysfunction have great difficulty in coping with stress. What may be bothersome or inconvenient to us could provoke a crisis in someone with mental illness. When problems, frustration, anxiety, or even loneliness become too intense, a crisis erupts. The client becomes unable to cope and retreats into the safety of his or her illness. Crisis intervention describes a short-term, active therapy that focuses on solving the immediate problem and restoring the client's previous level of functioning. Crisis services help stabilize the client, prevent further deterioration, and support the client's readjustment process. The use of crisis services also results in better distribution of resources. Emergency department visits decrease, rehospitalization is prevented, and law enforcement resources are better focused on those who break the law instead of apprehending mentally ill individuals. For clients with severe, treatment-resistant mental illness, a new approach, known as **continuous intensive case management,** is being used.

A new, highly flexible model of care, known as **assertive community treatment (ACT),** provides "medical, psychosocial, and rehabilitation services by a community-based team that operates seven days a week, 24 hours a day" (Salkever and others, 1999). The team usually consists of a social worker, psychiatrist, addictions counselor, and four clinicians (two social workers and two registered nurses). Clients are seen individually and in supportive therapy groups. They attend day treatment programs or pursue vocational training. Many clients live in supervised housing arrangements. Table 2-2 provides a summary of the continuous care team's treatment activities. In short, care teams direct the client's treatment during all encounters with the mental health care system.

Intensive case management programs have demonstrated that clients with chronic and severe mental illness can be effectively stabilized within the community with appropriate support systems. As the pressures of increased demand for services and cost restrictions force the system into trying new approaches, mental health care professionals must not lose sight of the most important element in the equation—the client.

MULTIDISCIPLINARY MENTAL HEALTH CARE TEAM

Professionals working within the mental health system have various educational backgrounds. In the past, each would work with clients from his or her particular point of view or specialty. This approach resulted in disjointed, fragmented care. In some cases care providers worked at cross-purposes, leaving clients unsure and confused. The need for coordinated assessment and treatment was filled by the multidisciplinary mental health care team concept.

CARE TEAM

The main purpose of the team approach to treating mental illness is to provide effective client care. The mental health care team "provides a forum where

Table 2-2 *Continuous Care Team Treatment Strategies*

SETTING	MENTAL HEALTH CARE TEAM INTERVENTIONS
Community	Meets with clients 2-4 times per week
	Accompanies client to appointments and other community activities
	Helps with daily living/social skill needs
	Monitors medications
	Nurtures relationships with persons interested in client's well-being
	Encourages client to call team instead of using ER
Emergency room	Prearranges for ER staff to notify clinician on arrival of continuous care client
	Conducts assessment of client and planning of care jointly with ER physician
	Avoids unnecessary hospitalizations
Hospital	Care team psychiatrist and primary therapist remain in charge of the client's case
	Helps with decisions regarding admission, treatment, and discharge
	Coordinates treatment with inpatient staff

Modified from Arana JD, Hastings B, Herron E: Continuous care teams in intensive outpatient treatment of chronic mentally ill patients, *Hosp Community Psychiatry* 42:503, 1991.
© American Psychiatric Association. Reprinted by permission.
ER, Emergency room.

psychiatrists, social workers, psychologists, nurses, and others can democratically share their professional expertise and develop comprehensive therapeutic plans for clients" (Haber and others, 1997). The team approach can also be cost-effective by preventing duplication of services and fragmentation of care. Clients and their significant others contribute to the plan of care and remain actively involved throughout the course of treatment.

Multidisciplinary mental health care teams exist in both inpatient and outpatient settings. The number of team members may vary, but the core of the team is usually composed of a psychiatrist, a psychologist, a nurse, and a social worker. Other team members, known as adjunct therapists, join the team as needed.

Each team member holds a degree or certificate in a specialized area of mental health. This approach allows clients to be assessed and treated from various points of view. As data are compiled, a broad, hopefully holistic picture of the client emerges and individualized therapeutic plans are developed. Table 2-3 identifies team members, their educational preparation, and their function.

CLIENT AND FAMILY

No discussion of the mental health team is complete without including the client. As the consumers of services and the focus of therapeutic interventions, clients contribute important information that may make the difference between success or failure of therapeutic plans. Including clients and their families in the treatment process reflects a fundamental change in attitude toward those with mental illness and their families.

Mental illness today is considered to be a manageable, even treatable, complex of disorders.

CLIENT POPULATIONS

Community mental health care was originally designed to provide prevention, education, and treatment services for all members living within an area. Community mental health services for the general public include crisis interventions, working with businesses to decrease costs and improve the effectiveness of mental health programs, and providing aid for individuals and families to adjust to life difficulties.

However, certain groups of people are at a high risk for developing mental health problems in every community, large or small. They include more obvious populations, such as homeless people, and more subtle high-risk groups, such as children, families, adolescents, older people, and people who are human immunodeficiency virus (HIV) positive. Clients living in rural areas present a challenge because of distances among services.

Clients with HIV infection or acquired immunodeficiency syndrome (AIDS) are using community mental health services in ever-growing numbers. People with AIDS face overwhelming physical, emotional, and social consequences. Mental health problems associated with HIV disease include organic problems, such as impairments in memory, judgment, or concentration progressing to dementia. Psychosocial problems include anxiety, depression, adjustment disorders, increased substance abuse, panic disorders, and suicidal thoughts. In addition, many researchers believe that stress directly affects the immune system. Fear of AIDS may hasten the onset of complications. AIDS-related anxiety can increase everyday apprehensions in the lives of many noninfected people.

Comprehensive community mental health services for people with HIV/AIDS are not yet available in all areas. Treatment facilities that offer comprehensive services focus on persons with AIDS, their families and friends, and the general public. Clinicians accept referrals from other agencies, provide mental status and suicide risk assessments, offer crisis intervention services, and provide individual or group therapies for clients with HIV/AIDS. Family members and significant others are encouraged to join support groups. Some mental health care centers train family members in techniques for keeping clients oriented or on task. Respite care (time off for the caregiver) services are sometimes coordinated through the center. Some mental health care centers work with interested community groups to provide prevention strategies and education about AIDS for all citizens of the community.

Clients living in rural areas present a special challenge for mental health care providers. Small villages, settlements, and farms dot the country landscape of the United States and Canada. In the United States,

Table 2-3 *Mental Health Team Members*

TEAM MEMBER	EDUCATIONAL PREPARATION	RESPONSIBILITIES AND FUNCTIONS
Psychiatrist	MD with residency in psychiatry	Physician; leader of the team; responsible for administration and planning; diagnostic and medical functions are main tasks
Clinical psychologist	PhD in clinical psychology	Specializes in study of mental processes and treatment of mental disorders; performs diagnostic testing; treats clients
Psychiatric social worker	Master's degree in social work (MSW)	Evaluates families; studies environmental and social causes of illness; conducts family therapy; admits new clients
Psychiatric nurse	Master's degree; advanced level preparation; baccalaureate degree; diploma nurse; associate degree nurse; licensed practical nurse	Responsible for client's activities of daily living/ environment management and individual, family, and group psychotherapy; coordinates care team activities; supervises technicians and psychiatric assistants; active in various community roles
Psychiatric assistant or technician	High school education; special on-job training in setting of employment	Supervised by professional nurse; assists in providing basic needs of clients; carries out nursing functions; maintains the therapeutic environment; supervises leisure-time activity; assists with individual/group therapy
Occupational therapist	Advanced degree in occupational therapy (OT)	Assesses potential for rehabilitation; provides socialization therapy and vocational retraining
Expressive therapist	Advanced degree and specialized training in art therapy	Helps make use of spontaneous creative work of the client; works with groups; encourages members to analyze artwork; adjunct to care team in diagnosis and treatment of children
Recreational therapist	Advanced degree and specialized training in recreational therapy	Provides leisure-time activities for clients; teaches hospitalized clients useful pastimes; uses pet therapy, psychodrama, poetry, and music therapy
Dietitian	Advanced degree and special training in dietetics (RD)	Provides attractive, nourishing meals; helps treat food-related illnesses
Auxiliary personnel (housekeepers, volunteers, clerks, secretaries)	Various backgrounds and on-job training	Assists clients with activities of daily living and other practical jobs; can be invaluable in helping clients
Chaplain	Seminary pastoral counselor or rabbinical education	Attends to the spiritual needs of clients and families; pastoral, marital counseling

Modified from Haber J and others: *Comprehensive psychiatric nursing,* ed 5, St. Louis, 1997, Mosby.

rural residents define and relate to health differently from people in cities. Children and adolescents living in rural areas have less access to services. Mental health care providers (e.g., nurses, therapists) who work in rural areas cope with clients of all ages and with all types of problems. They are also expected to provide and coordinate comprehensive mental health care with few available resources.

Other populations, such as **families, the elderly, children,** and **adolescents,** are vulnerable to mental health problems. Community mental health services are a vital link to the well-being of a population. Social and economic changes will continue to influence community mental health care, but as the system matures, the goal of individualized, holistic mental health care for all people should not be forgotten.

IMPACT OF MENTAL ILLNESS

Mental illness affects everyone directly or indirectly. Many people personally know someone with behavioral problems. Indirectly, mental illness costs taxpayers

millions of dollars as the costs of care and number of clients continue to escalate. As a result of several national armed conflicts, veterans are flooding the system with stress-related disorders. Today, health care reform is part of an overall strategy to distribute scarce resources and control expenses.

INCIDENCE OF MENTAL ILLNESS

Worldwide, one quarter of the world's population will experience a mental illness during their lifetime (Sherer, 2002). Although exact statistics are unavailable, it is estimated that at any given time "at least 19% of adults in the United States (and) 7.5 million children" (National Mental Health Association, 1999) suffer from mental-emotional disorders. Chronic severe mental disorders, such as schizophrenia and depression, have emerged as major challenges to treatment. Substance abuse has become a national problem. The incidence of Alzheimer's disease and other dementias is expected to increase threefold over the next 15 years. Social problems such as AIDS, homelessness, violence, and abuse occur with mental problems. Millions of divorces each year place families in crisis situations. It is easy to see why there are growing numbers of mentally troubled people in today's society.

ECONOMIC ISSUES

The nationwide movement to treat people with mental illness in the least restrictive environment is part of a plan to reduce mental health care costs while still providing ongoing care. Unfortunately, funding has not kept pace with the need for services.

To control costs, Congress in 1983 established the **Health Care Financing Administration,** which developed a cost-containment method whereby health care providers are paid at predetermined rates. A group of more than 400 diagnosis-related groups (DRGs) classifies each illness. Medicare, the funded health plan for elderly and disabled people, adopted these groups. Payment guidelines, based on clients' average lengths of inpatient stay, determine each DRG. If clients are not discharged from hospitals within the specified time, funding is stopped and the facility or client becomes responsible for payment. Today, mental health facilities provide services for more than 54 million mentally troubled people in the United States. Mental health care cost taxpayers $99 billion dollars in 1996 (U.S. Surgeon General, 2002).

Mental illness also influences economics in less direct ways. Unemployed, homeless, and troubled families cost society in many more ways than dollars. Loss of productivity and unfulfilled potential are difficult to appraise financially. Clearly, economic issues have and will continue to play a major role in the availability and delivery of mental health care.

SOCIAL ISSUES

Many social problems are related to mental illness. Changing lifestyles, work patterns, family structures, and health are a few of the many changes that influence a society. Mentally ill individuals, however, are likely to be struggling with more basic issues, such as poverty, homelessness, and substance abuse.

By 2001, nearly 12% of U.S. citizens lived below the poverty line. This means that almost 33 million people, with 6.8 million poor families, live without life's basic necessities (Procter and Dalaker, 2002). A significant number are incapable of making a living as a result of mental problems. They exist along the fringes of society, attempting to meet the most basic needs of food, shelter, and clothing. Within this environment of poverty, hopelessness grows, and it becomes easier to retreat into one's mental illness than face the grim reality of poverty.

After a time, homelessness becomes poverty's companion. The National Academy of Sciences defines homelessness as the lack of a regular and adequate nighttime dwelling. Millions of U.S. citizens are homeless on any given day. About 10% of the homeless are older than 60 years. Many are families, and as many as

85% of the homeless population suffer from addictions or mental disturbances (Walker, 1998).

Homelessness is a national problem that continues to grow. The actual number of homeless people is difficult to count because with no regular housing they tend to melt into society and disappear into the world of soup kitchens and temporary shelters. In the past, most homeless people were single men, usually with alcohol problems. However, today's statistics present a different picture. Women, children, and families now account for many of the homeless people.

Several factors contribute to homelessness. Social conditions, such as a lack of low-income housing, public assistance eligibility requirements, and the movement of chronically mentally ill people into communities that lack adequate support systems, have all had an adverse impact on homelessness. Community resources relating to available housing, steady employment, and welfare services affect homeless people. Family dysfunction, poverty, and health status all relate to the homeless problem.

Many families live from paycheck to paycheck, with just enough money to scrape by until the next check. Even a small event can trigger a crisis. An increase in the rent, for example, may force a family out of their home. Most community mental health centers offer services for homeless people. Currently, short-term strategies for working with the **homeless** population include temporary shelters, assisted-housing programs, and volunteer efforts such as Habitat for Humanity.

Society's use of mind-altering chemicals has resulted in many mentally ill individuals becoming addicted to "recreational drugs," such as crack, cocaine, LSD, and heroin. When used in combination with prescribed psychotherapeutic drugs, overdoses, permanent psychotic states, and death may occur. Street drugs also cost money. It is not uncommon for people with mental problems to spend money on drugs before they buy food. Addicted people with mental disorders suffer from two separate disorders, with each compounding the severity of the other. Illicit drugs and mental illness become a vicious circle.

The current mental health care system in the United States is undergoing major changes as budgets decline, social issues emerge, and needs for treatment grow. Organization and technology may address some of the system's problems, but provider-client contact is and will remain the core of mental health treatment.

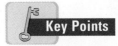

Key Points

- The health care systems of many developed countries are undergoing financial challenges.
- Canada's health care system is administrated by each province under the guidance of the Department of National Health and Welfare and includes coverage

for most medical, hospital, convalescent, and mental health services.

- Norway has a national insurance system that provides access to health care for everyone and covers all services, including mental health care.
- All British citizens are provided health care through a government-managed national health care system.
- Australians are provided a mix of health care plans that include a public health plan, a supplemental national private plan, and private insurance plans.
- Funds for health care in the United States are provided through federal (Medicare) and state (Medicaid) programs, private insurance coverage, and direct client payments.
- Mental health care is offered in inpatient and outpatient (community) care settings.
- The community support systems (CSS) model for mental health care is an organized network of people committed to assisting those with mental illness within the community setting.
- Community mental health care settings include psychiatric clinics, general hospitals, residential care programs, day treatment facilities, and psychiatric home care.
- Case management is a holistic system of interventions designed to support the integration of mentally ill clients into the community.

- Psychosocial rehabilitation is the use of multidisciplinary services to help clients learn the skills and supports needed to carry out the activities of daily living as actively and independently as possible.
- Psychosocial rehabilitation, consultation, resource linkage, advocacy, crisis intervention, and therapy are the basic components of the case management system.
- Intensive case management may use continuous care or assertive community treatment (ACT) teams who assume responsibility for the client in and out of the hospital.
- Community mental health services serve high-risk populations, such as children, people in crisis situations, homeless individuals, clients with HIV/AIDS, clients living in rural areas, and elderly people.
- Mental health services are commonly delivered by the multidisciplinary care team—a group of physicians, nurses, psychologists, therapists, and their assistants who each contribute to the client's plan of care and treatment.
- Social and economic issues must be considered when discussing mentally troubled persons.

evolve Be sure to visit the companion Evolve site at http://evolve.elsevier.com/Morrison-Valfre/ for additional online resources.

3 Ethical and Legal Issues

Objectives

Upon completion of this chapter, the student should be able to:

1. State the differences among values, rights, and ethics.
2. Explain the purpose of the Patient Care Partnership.
3. List six steps for making ethical decisions.
4. Identify the legal importance of practice acts.
5. Describe the process of involuntary psychiatric commitment.
6. Name four areas of potential legal liability for mental health care providers.
7. Know the difference between the legal terms *negligence* and *malpractice*.
8. Discuss three legal responsibilities that relate to nursing and health care providers.

Key Terms

assault (p. 25)
attitudes (p. 19)
autonomy (aw-TŎN-ə-mē) (p. 21)
battery (p. 25)
belief (p. 19)
beneficence (b-NĔ-fə-sən[t]s) (p. 22)
civil law (p. 23)
codes of ethics (p. 22)
confidentiality (KŎN-fĭ-DĔN-shē-ĂLĭ-tē) (p. 25)
contract law (p. 23)
controlled substances (p. 25)
criminal law (p. 23)
defamation (dĕf-ə-MĀ-shən) (p. 25)
duty to warn (p. 26)
elopement (ĭ-LŌP-mənt) (p. 26)
ethical dilemmas (p. 22)
ethics (p. 21)
false imprisonment (p. 25)
felonies (p. 23)
fraud (p. 25)
informed consent (p. 26)
invasion of privacy (p. 25)
involuntary admission (p. 24)
laws (p. 23)
libel (p. 25)
malpractice (p. 26)
misdemeanors (MĬS-dĭ-MĒ-nərs) (p. 23)
morals (p. 19)
negligence (p. 26)
nonmaleficence (nŏn-mə-LĔF-ə-sən[t]s) (p. 22)
parity (p. 21)

The Patient Care Partnership: Understanding Expectations, Rights and Responsibilities (p. 21)
professional (nurse) practice acts (p. 23)
reasonable and prudent care provider (p. 26)
right (p. 20)
slander (p. 25)
standards of practice (p. 24)
tort law (p. 23)
value (p. 19)
values clarification (p. 20)

Health care professions are defined by certain beliefs, rights, and principles that serve as the basis for ethical and legal concepts. The framework for delivering appropriate therapeutic interventions is rooted in these concepts.

Attitudes, beliefs, values, and morals influence who we are. To be effective with mentally ill clients, we must first appreciate these concepts within ourselves and then understand them as they apply to our clients and their support persons.

VALUES AND MORALS

Attitudes are ideas that help shape our points of view. The term can also describe one's outlook, such as "He has a cheerful attitude." A **belief** is a conviction that is intellectually accepted as true whether or not it is based in fact. A **value** is something that is held dear, a feeling about the worth of an item, idea, or behavior. Values are formed in childhood. They shape our reactions, influence our behaviors, reflect the society in which we live, and are often used as a basis for making decisions. Values are individual, and they may change.

Morals reflect one's attitudes, beliefs, and values. One's morals define right or wrong behavior. Once established, morals become deeply ingrained and are not easily changed.

ACQUIRING VALUES

As children grow, they observe and take on the reactions of others in their environment. These adopted reactions become our earliest attitudes. Preschool children learn the difference between right and wrong behaviors and adopt the family's beliefs and traditions. As attitudes and beliefs develop, values begin to form.

Children are exposed to a variety of values at school. They develop work habits, learn to solve problems, interact with others, and make decisions. Parental values are still modeled because the family remains the major source of values until adulthood.

During the teen years, adolescents begin to identify their own significant values. By early adulthood, an individual value system is established. Adults may feel secure with their values or discard them for new ones. Older adults may feel threatened by the changing social values, but they tend to hold onto their own value systems.

Culture, society, personality, and experiences all shape our values. How values are shared largely depends on the sociocultural environment. Most societies use a combination of methods to transmit values (Potter and Perry, 2001). These methods are outlined in Table 3-1.

People who choose to work in the health care professions usually arrive with strong personal values. Human values important in caregivers include a concern for the welfare of others (**altruism**), respect for the uniqueness and worth of people (**human dignity**), **equality, justice, truth, freedom,** and **acceptance.** Caring is the foundation of health care, for if we do not care, we will be unable to effectively treat, teach, or work with clients.

VALUES CLARIFICATION

Every society has a value system. Habits, customs, and traditions are important to traditional societies. Modern societies rapidly change, and people are often not aware of their values until they experience difficulties and their values are questioned.

Values clarification is a step-by-step process to help identify significant values. The process helps care providers become aware of how their own values affect interactions with clients. Values clarification involves three steps: choosing, prizing, and acting (Table 3-2).

To illustrate, let us assume that you are working at the local clinic. Today a large, scruffy man who has not bathed in weeks presents himself for care. There is a wild look in his eyes, and he is arguing with himself as he approaches you. What you really want to do is run, but you must cope with this client. How does the value of caring apply here?

First, you have freely **chosen** to care about people; otherwise you would have selected another line of work. Second, you **prize** the value of caring because your clients see you as compassionate and concerned. Third, you **act** on your values by accepting the unkempt, scruffy man as a person worthy of care. You ask him what you can do to help. He begins to cry and tells you that since the death of his wife and children in a house fire, no one has cared if he lives or dies. By acting on your value (caring), you have touched this person and paved the way for him to improve his situation.

You have chosen to care. You cherish the value of caring enough to act, even when that value is threatened. Be clear about **your values.** Be aware of your **client's values** because they are the guidelines for one's lifestyle, conduct, and relationships.

RIGHTS

A **right** is described as a power, privilege, or existence to which one has a just claim. Rights have several roles in society; they can be used as expressions of power, to justify actions, and to settle disputes. Rights help define social interactions because they contain the principle of **justice;** they equally and fairly apply to all citizens. For example, we all have the right to be respected as human beings and treated with dignity. Rights also have obligations. You have the right to drive down the road, but inherent in this right is the obligation to obey traffic laws.

Table 3-1 *How Values Are Transmitted*

MODE OF TRANSMISSION	DEFINITION
Modeling	Copying an example—One person behaves in the ideal or preferred manner, while the other copies the behavior.
Moralizing	Sets standards for right and wrong—Choice is not allowed.
Laissez-faire	Unrestricted choices—No direction is given. One is free to explore and learn from experiences. This mode of transmission may result in confusion or frustration.
Reward/punishment	Rewards valued behaviors and punishes undesirable acts; authoritarian—Children learn that strength is right. This mode of transmission may send the message that violence is acceptable.
Responsible choice	A balance of freedom and restriction—One may choose among stated options. New behaviors and consequences are explored.

Modified from Potter PA, Perry AG: *Fundamentals of nursing: concepts, process, and practice,* ed 5, St. Louis, 2001, Mosby.

Table 3-2 *Values Clarification Process*

STEP	PROCESS
Choosing	Consider all possible alternatives. Consider all possible consequences. Choose freely without pressure or coercion from others.
Prizing	Cherish or prize the choice. Share choice with others. Reaffirm importance of value.
Acting	Make value a part of behaviors (internalize value). Generalize value to all situations. Repeatedly act with consistent behavioral pattern.

CLIENT RIGHTS

The 1972 **Patient's Bill of Rights** states that all clients have the rights to respectful care, privacy, confidentiality, continuity of care, and relevant information. It also addresses clients' rights to examine their bills, refuse treatment, and participate in research. A revised document, The Patient Care Partnership: Understanding Expectations, Rights, and Responsibilities, was adopted in 2003. Statements of rights now exist for the old, young, disabled, pregnant, dying, developmentally disabled, and mentally ill—the most vulnerable people in society.

People with mental illness tend to lose their rights in two ways. First, the problems with which they are coping require energy. Sometimes reality eludes them. Many are not able to recognize their rights, much less exercise them. Second, the mental health delivery system can impose limits on clients' abilities to exercise their rights. To protect their rights, the Mental Health Systems Act Bill of Rights was passed by the U.S. Congress in 1980. This bill served as a pattern from which state bills of rights for the mentally ill population were developed. For an example of a client's right to treatment, see Box 3-1.

Currently, 23 states have enacted mental health parity laws that require insurance companies to include coverage for mental illness that is equal to the coverage for physical illness. However, only nine states include treatment for substance abuse in their parity laws.

CARE PROVIDER RIGHTS

The rights of nurses and other care providers relate to respect, safety, and competent assistance. Care providers have the right to **respect** as individuals. Nurses have the right to full and equal participation as members of the health care team. All health care providers have the right to set standards for quality and develop policies that affect client care.

Every health care provider has the right to function within a **safe** environment. This applies to both the physical environment (i.e., properly maintained equipment) and the affective or emotional environment. Care providers who strive to minimize the physical and emotional stresses of the working environment are exercising their right to function safely.

The right to **competent assistance** includes the right to receive assistance from people who are capable of performing at the stated level. For example, the certified nurse assistant (CNA) who is assigned to work with a nurse is able to function adequately and safely as a nursing assistant. Health care providers need to exercise their rights. By doing this, we remind the system of the therapeutic values inherent in the caregiver-client relationship.

Box 3-1 *Example of the Right to Treatment*

In 1957, Mr. Donaldson was involuntarily committed, on his father's initiation, to a Florida state hospital for care, treatment, and maintenance. For 14 years before his commitment, he was gainfully employed. Despite the fact that Mr. Donaldson posed no danger to himself or others, his requests for ground privileges, occupational training, and an opportunity to discuss his case with the superintendent, Dr. O'Connor, or others were denied. During his 15 years of confinement, he was not provided with any treatment.

Mr. Donaldson frequently requested his release, which the superintendent was authorized to grant even though "Mr. Donaldson was lawfully confined, because even if he continued to be mentally ill, he posed no danger to himself or others. Between 1964 and 1968, Mr. Donaldson's friend requested on four separate occasions that Mr. Donaldson be released into his custody. These requests, and requests made by a halfway house on Mr. Donaldson's behalf, were all denied by Dr. O'Connor, who believed that Mr. Donaldson should be released into his parents' custody. Dr. O'Connor further believed that Mr. Donaldson's parents were too old and infirm to care for him adequately.

In *O'Connor v. Donaldson* (1975), the court found that Mr. Donaldson's care was merely custodial because he received no treatment. He was not dangerous, community alternatives were available for him, and the physician's refusal to release him was "malicious." The Federal Court of Appeals ruled that Mr. Donaldson had a constitutional right to treatment and awarded him $38,000 in damages.

From Varcarolis EM, Carson VB, Shoemaker NC: *Foundations of psychiatric mental health nursing: a clinical approach*, ed 5, Philadelphia, 2006, Saunders.

ETHICS

Ethics is a set of rules or values that govern right behavior. Ethics reflect values, morals, and principles of right and wrong. The purpose of ethical behavior is to protect the rights of people. Health care ethics focus on the moral aspects of health care availability, delivery, and policy. They are also called **biomedical ethics, bioethics,** or **medical ethics.**

ETHICAL PRINCIPLES

Ethical principles are the concepts that form the basis for professional codes of ethics (Edelman and Mandle, 2002). They are the behaviors that define what is good or right conduct. Ethical codes serve two purposes: (1) they act as guidelines for standards of practice and (2) they let the public know what behaviors can be expected from their health care providers.

The concepts of autonomy, beneficence, nonmaleficence, and justice are the main ethical principles on which codes of ethics are established. Remember these principles. They will serve you well as you encounter the many ethical situations inherent in health care.

Autonomy refers to the right of people to act for themselves and make personal choices, including refusal of treatment. Caregivers who practice the principle of autonomy encourage clients to participate in informed decision making. The procedure known as informed consent promotes autonomy by providing relevant information and choice for the client.

Beneficence means to actively do good. Actions that promote client health are beneficent. Choosing the action that is the most therapeutic for the client is an example of beneficence.

The principle of nonmaleficence can be stated in three words: **do no harm.** Perhaps it is the most important ethical principle of the caregiving professions. Although nurses must sometimes carry out procedures that result in pain, they are considered in light of the benefits gained. Therapeutic interventions are delivered only after client safety and comfort are considered. Nonmaleficence ensures that clients will not be harmed during care.

Justice implies that all clients are treated equally, fairly, and respectfully. Because health care resources are limited, the application of justice can be difficult. However, all clients deserve respect and a share of the available resources.

The concepts of confidentiality, fidelity, and veracity are other important ethical principles. The client's rights to privacy, truth, and duty are protected by these ethical principles. **Confidentiality** is the duty to respect private information. It is a legal and ethical duty of health care providers to keep all information about clients limited to only those directly involved with care. Sharing private information not only is unethical but also may be grounds for legal action.

Fidelity is the obligation to keep your word. Telling the client that you will return in 10 minutes is a promise. Keep that appointment because your client relies on you and your credibility grows or diminishes depending on how well you keep your promises. Do what you say, or do not say it.

The final principle, **veracity,** is the duty to tell the truth. Be careful here. Answer client's questions honestly, but remember to stay within your standards and limitations of practice. It is not within your realm, for example, to discuss the disease prognosis or lead a client toward a certain decision.

CODES OF ETHICS

Codes of ethics for practical (vocational) and registered nurses have been developed by the International Council of Nurses, the American Nurses Association, the National Federation of Licensed Practical Nurses, and the Canadian Nurses Association (Box 3-2). Codes of ethics have been developed for other health care professions and may differ slightly, but all are based on the same ethical principles. Provide information to clients, be truthful, and support your clients, but consult your supervisor if there is any question of appropriateness. It is important to practice with ethical principles in mind.

Box 3-2 | *ICN Code of Ethics for Nurses*

1. NURSES AND PEOPLE

The nurse's primary responsibility is to those requiring nursing care.

The nurse promotes an environment in which human rights, values, customs, and spiritual beliefs of the individual, family, and community are respected.

The nurse ensures that the client receives sufficient information on which to base consent for care and treatment.

The nurse holds in confidence personal information and uses judgment in sharing that information.

The nurse shares with society the responsibility for initiating and supporting actions to meet health and social needs of the public, in particular those of vulnerable populations.

The nurse shares the responsibility to sustain and protect the natural environment from depletion, pollution, degradation, and destruction.

2. NURSES AND PRACTICE

The nurse carries personal responsibility and accountability for nursing practice, and for maintaining competence by continual learning.

The nurse maintains a standard of personal health such that the ability to provide care is not compromised.

The nurse uses judgment regarding individual competence when accepting and delegating responsibility.

The nurse at all times maintains standards of personal conduct which reflect well on the profession and enhance public confidence.

The nurse, in providing care, ensures that the use of technology and scientific advances are compatible with the safety, dignity, and rights of people.

3. NURSES AND THE PROFESSION

The nurse assumes a major role in determining and implementing acceptable standards of clinical nursing practice, management, research, and education.

The nurse is active in developing a core of research-based professional knowledge.

The nurse, acting through professional organizations, participates in creating and maintaining safe, equitable social and economic working conditions in nursing.

4. NURSES AND CO-WORKERS

The nurse sustains a cooperative relationship with co-workers in nursing and other fields.

The nurse takes appropriate action to safeguard individuals, families, and communities when their health is endangered by a co-worker or any other person.

Modified from the International Council of Nurses: *The ICN code of ethics for nurses,* Geneva, Switzerland, 2006, The Council.

ETHICAL CONFLICT

In today's world of advanced technologies and complex situations, no clear-cut answers exist for complicated questions that arise. Ethical dilemmas (conflicts) exist when there is uncertainty or disagreement about the moral principles that endorse different courses of action.

In health care, ethical dilemmas arise when problems cannot easily be solved by decision making, logic, or use of scientific data. Answers to ethical dilemmas usually have a broad impact. Because of this, many health care institutions have established **bioethics committees** to study, educate, and assist staff members in coping with ethical dilemmas.

Most of the time, no clear-cut solutions exist for ethical dilemmas. Although each ethical dilemma is unique, the method for making ethical decisions can be applied to all situations. Guidelines for dealing with such dilemmas are given in Box 3-3. "Making ethical decisions in an orderly systematic manner increases one's ability to deal with the dynamic and sometimes complex issues relating to ethics. The quality of care depends on the skills and ethical integrity of the practitioner" (Morrison, 1993).

LAWS AND THE LEGAL SYSTEM

Every health care provider must be familiar with the basic concepts of the legal system. Laws are the controls by which a society governs itself. They are derived from rules, regulations, and moral and ethical principles. Laws apply to every member of society.

GENERAL CONCEPTS

Laws exist at every level of government. In the United States, federal law defines the organization of the government. Federal law is based on the U.S. Constitution. Laws at the state level are derived from the state's constitution and apply to citizens living within its boundaries. Local and city laws evolve from state law.

Laws change as society changes, but they are all based on the principles of justice (fairness), change, standards, and individual rights and responsibilities. Laws have several functions in our society. They define relationships, describe appropriate and objectionable behaviors, and explain what kind of force is applied to maintain rules. Laws help provide solutions for many social and legal problems, and they serve to protect the rights of people while defining the limits of acceptable behaviors.

There are two types of law: public law and private law. **Public law** focuses on the relationship between the government and its citizens. The division of public law that is of importance to caregivers is known as criminal law. Its main function is to protect the members of society. Serious crimes, known as felonies, are punishable by death or imprisonment. Less serious crimes are called misdemeanors, with punishments ranging from fines to prison terms of less than 1 year.

Private law is commonly called civil law. Its function is to deal with relationships between individuals.

Box 3-3   *Guidelines for Making Ethical Decisions*

1. *Identify all elements* of the situation. Gather data. Identify each person involved in the decision-making process.
2. *Assume good will.* All care providers want a satisfactory resolution to the problem. When working with emotionally charged issues, remember that there is no need for competition.
3. *Gather relevant information.* Thoroughly assess lifestyle, preferences, wishes, and support systems. Try to form an "ideal picture" of the resolution for the dilemma.
4. *List and order values.* Decide which ethical principles are most important in the situation. List them in order of importance, then determine a plan or course of action.
5. *Take action.* Implement the plan. Monitor any changes.
6. *Evaluate* the effectiveness of the plan.

Modified from Potter PA, Perry AG: *Fundamentals of nursing: concepts, process, and practice,* ed 5, St. Louis, 2001, Mosby.

Two important types of civil law for caregivers are contract law and tort law. Contract law deals with agreements between individuals or institutions. These agreements or contracts may be written or implied. For example, on employment, health care providers enter into contracts with the employing institution.

"A tort is a legal wrong that is committed against the person or the property of another individual" (Morrison, 1993). Tort law relates to individuals' rights and includes the need to be compensated for a wrong. Tort law is especially important for caregivers because many potential legal problems exist in every health care setting. Figure 3-1 lists the areas of law that are most significant for care providers.

LEGAL CONCEPTS IN HEALTH CARE

Each health care profession is governed by rules and standards. Nursing, for example, is regulated by state boards of nursing that define the practice of nursing and regulate the profession through licensing procedures and disciplinary actions. Each state's board of nursing identifies the limits and scope of practice through a series of regulations known as that state's **nurse practice act.** Nurses need to be familiar with their state's nurse practice act because it is the **legal framework for practice in that state.** Other health care providers are responsible for knowing their state's governing regulations. Caregivers are legally responsible for their actions. They are expected to know what is contained within their professional (nurse) practice acts.

Institutional policies also help to define health care practices. **Policies** are statements that define a course of action. **What** is to be done is stated in policies. **How** a task or skill is to be performed is defined in the

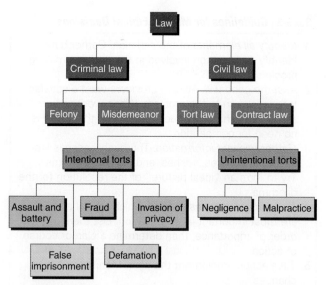

FIGURE **3-1** Laws important for health care providers.

institution's **procedure manual. Job descriptions** define the job, its functions, its qualifications, and to whom the caregiver reports. Guidelines for sound health care delivery can be found in each state's practice act; professional standards; and the employing institution's policies, procedures, and job descriptions.

A **standard** is a measurement for comparison by which one evaluates an action. Standards of practice are usually developed by each specific health care discipline. Standards of nursing practice, for example, are a set of guidelines that provide measurable criteria for nurses, clients, and others to evaluate the quality and effectiveness of nursing care. Psychiatric mental health standards for nursing practice can be found in Appendix A.

LAWS AND MENTAL HEALTH CARE

Historically, people with mental illnesses were afforded few legal rights. Only recently have mental health clients been able to exercise their claims to fair and adequate treatment in settings helpful to their care. Nurses and their colleagues need to be aware of clients' legal rights to freedom, privacy, and choice. Laws relating to mental health issues "attempt to balance the basic rights of the individual against society's interest in being protected from persons who, because of mental disorder, present a threat of harm" (Keltner, Schwecke, and Bostrom, 2007).

CLIENT-CAREGIVER RELATIONSHIP

An awareness of the obligations in the client-caregiver relationship ensures safe, legal practice. From a legal point of view, the caregiver and client enter into an **implied contract** on acceptance of service. The caregiver provides services that are accepted by the client. This idea of contractual obligations is one legal aspect of the caregiver-client relationship. Two other important aspects are liability and standards of care.

The concept of **liability** states that care providers are legally responsible for their professional obligations and behaviors. It includes the obligation to remain competent, maintain a current knowledge base, practice at a level appropriate to one's education, and practice unimpaired by drugs, disability, or illness.

Clients still retain their legal rights when they enter the mental health care system. The 1980 Mental Health Systems Act states that mentally ill individuals have rights to obtain information and treatment within a supportive, humane environment. The Patient Self-Determination Act of 1991 gives clients the right to make decisions about their care (Loewy, 1998). Individuals who are admitted to psychiatric facilities retain the right to vote, to buy and sell property, and to possess a driver's license.

People with mental illness may be unaware of their legal rights or unable to exercise them. Clients' judgments may be limited as the result of their illness and/or medications. It is important to recognize and safeguard clients' legal rights because behind every mental disorder lives a real person.

ADULT PSYCHIATRIC ADMISSIONS

The decision to seek psychiatric care, whether made by the client, family, or community, is difficult. When the client originates the request for mental health services, it is considered a **voluntary admission.** Because they are often aware of their problems, most voluntarily admitted clients are active participants in their treatments and have a low potential for violence. Voluntarily admitted clients may legally discharge themselves at any time.

When individuals engage in behavior that is harmful to themselves or others, the involuntary admission process is undertaken. The 1953 Act Governing Hospitalization defines an involuntary admission as a process for institutionalization initiated by someone other than the client. Involuntary psychiatric admissions provide a protected, therapeutic environment, which is usually necessary for the client's safety. Clients may stay for days to years.

Physicians, police, and representatives of a county administrator may commit an individual for emergency treatment without a warrant, but a court order is usually required for long-term stays. Procedures for psychiatric commitment in the United States vary from state to state. Each state establishes standards for commitment, but most laws allow involuntary commitment only if the person is dangerous to self or others or cannot function in a reasonable manner. Most states have similar procedures for involuntary admissions.

The commitment process begins when a formal petition is filed. The client is then assessed by one or two physicians, and a determination is made to either release or hospitalize the person (Stuart, 2005). If the person is hospitalized, the length of stay may be on an emergency, temporary, or indefinite basis. Clients who are indefinitely hospitalized must be gravely disabled and unable to provide for themselves. Indefinite commitments are most often an action of the courts that usually provide a guardian or conservator to protect the client's rights. They are subject to yearly review, and clients retain the right to consult a lawyer and petition the court for discharge. Figure 3-2 illustrates the process of involuntary commitment.

AREAS OF POTENTIAL LIABILITY

Mental health care providers are placed in the unique position of balancing their clients' rights with the need to protect society. Many legal issues relate to the care of mentally ill individuals, and an awareness of the potential liabilities helps safeguard caregivers' as well as clients' rights.

The most common crimes in health care settings are homicide, controlled substance violations, and theft. Legally, **homicide** is the killing of a human being, whereas **murder** is killing with intent. For example, a nurse who mistakenly gives a client the wrong drug that causes death may have committed homicide. However, a nurse who knowingly administers a lethal drug may be guilty of murder.

The Controlled Substances Act of 1970 was passed by Congress to regulate the supply and distribution of certain powerful drugs. **Controlled substances** currently include narcotics, stimulants, depressants, hallucinogens, and some tranquilizers. As agents of the physician, nurses administer controlled drugs. They are responsible for adhering to their institution's policies and procedures regarding storage, distribution, and documentation of controlled substances.

Robbery, theft, and **larceny** all describe the taking of another person's personal property. Clients who lose valuable items can hold the agency liable for theft. Ensuring that a valuables disposition list is completed for every client is an important protection against theft.

Fraud is the giving of false information with the knowledge that action will be taken based on the information. For example, a technician documents that a treatment was given when it was not. The physician then bases a decision on the client's lack of response. The technician is guilty of fraud. Practicing with the utmost honesty is the best protection against fraud.

Defamation is defined as a false communication that results in harm. It is subdivided into two categories: written defamation, or **libel**, and verbal defamation, referred to as **slander**. Psychiatric care providers should base their communications on objective data and clinical observations, not judgments or opinions.

Assault is any act that threatens a client. No physical contact need occur, just a threatening action. Telling a client that he or she will be physically forced to do something if uncooperative is an example of assault. **Battery** is when touching occurs without the client's permission. The best prevention against assault or battery is clear

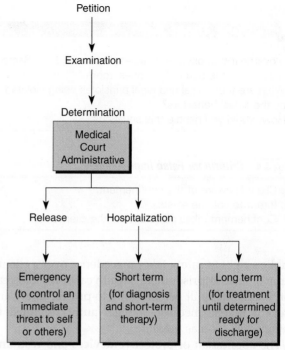

FIGURE 3-2 The involuntary commitment process.

communication. Make sure clients understand what you intend to do before you begin.

Another important area of potential liability relates to **invasion of privacy**. "The right to privacy includes privacy related to the body, confidential information and the right to be left alone" (Morrison, 1993). An invasion of privacy occurs when a client's space, body, or belongings are violated. Although caregivers must be continually vigilant to protect a client's privacy, those rights may occasionally be outweighed by the need to ensure safety. For example, a client who behaves suicidally may have personal belongings searched for potentially dangerous objects.

The client's right to privacy also includes **confidentiality**, which is the sharing of information about the client only with those persons who are directly involved in care. Discussing any client with noninvolved people constitutes a breach of confidentiality (see Think About 3-1).

All mental health care providers can protect the client's privacy by treating each person with dignity and respect. Caregivers who work in inpatient settings need to orient clients to their environment and inform them of their privacy rights and how those rights may be restricted.

Detaining a competent person against his or her will constitutes **false imprisonment**. Any time a client's freedom of movement is restrained the potential for liability exists (Box 3-4). Both physical force and verbal intimidation are included in the concept of false imprisonment. For example, threatening a client with confinement constitutes grounds for false imprisonment.

Involuntarily committed clients may make false imprisonment claims in some states, but usually the

Think About 3-1

You overhear two psychiatric aides discussing Mrs. Samson while making the bed in Mr. Jones' room.
• What are the ethical and legal principles being violated by the aides' behaviors?
• How would you handle this situation?

| Box 3-4 | *Criteria for False Imprisonment* |

1. Client is aware of the confinement.
2. Intent to confine exists.
3. Confinement takes place against the client's will.

---

public's right to safety takes precedence over a client's claim of false imprisonment. Health care providers can confine mentally ill persons only to protect safety and prevent injury; medical or legal authority must be obtained as soon as possible.

The application of **protective devices and restraints** may constitute false imprisonment. Restraints must be used **only** to protect the client, not for staff convenience. The least restrictive measures should first be attempted and documented. A written medical order for restraints must be on file in the client's chart. Once restraints have been applied, the caregivers have an increased obligation to observe, assess, and monitor the client every 15 minutes. The restraints must be removed, one limb at a time, and the limb exercised every 2 hours. All observations and actions must be documented. Restraints are removed as soon as the client's behavior is under control.

The concepts of both negligence and malpractice are rooted in the "reasonable and prudent person" theory. Negligence is defined as the omission (or commission) of an act that a reasonable and prudent person would (or would not) do. For example, a public swimming pool owner who did not repair a slide that then caused a child's injury could be guilty of negligence.

The concept of malpractice usually applies to professionals and is defined as a failure to exercise an accepted degree of professional skill that results in injury, loss, or damage. To be considered negligent, professional misconduct must meet four requirements:
1. The care provider owed a duty to the client.
2. The care provider did not carry out the duty (breach).
3. The client was injured as a result of the care provider's action or inaction (proximate cause).
4. Actual loss or damage resulted from the actions.

To illustrate, a suicidal client is to be continuously observed (duty). The staff goes to lunch, leaving the client alone (breach of duty). During this time, the client commits suicide (proximate cause) and dies (damage). The staff is guilty of malpractice because no reasonable and prudent caregiver would leave a client unattended in a similar situation.

CARE PROVIDERS' RESPONSIBILITIES

The main responsibility of mental health care providers is to help clients cope with their problems. Dignified, humane treatment includes the protection of rights as human beings, citizens, and clients. Mental health clients have specific rights to treatment, refusal of treatment, informed consent, examination by the physician of their choice, confidentiality, and freedom from restraints. Informed consent is an agreement between the client and caregivers that documents knowledge of and agreement to treatment. The client must be aware, informed, and capable of consenting. Mental health clients are presumed competent and able to consent to treatment. Obtaining consent for treatment is the physician's responsibility, but nurses often assist in the process. Other legal issues that relate to psychiatric care include elopement and the duty to warn.

A special situation, known as elopement, sometimes arises during hospitalization when clients run away or elope from the institution. Caregivers who fail to prevent client elopement may be held liable if the client is injured as a result of the elopement. Keeping clients under supervision, plus accurate documentation of client behaviors and therapeutic actions, can prevent elopement from occurring.

All caregivers have the duty to warn. In situations where serious harm or death may occur, mental health professionals have a duty to protect potential victims from possible harm. For example, if your client states that he intends to kill his barber, you have a duty to warn the barber. Contact the client's physician and your supervisor, and be sure to document the situation.

In some states nurses have a duty to report certain information. Examples of reportable data include suspected incidents of abuse, gunshot wounds, and certain communicable diseases. The rights of the client are sometimes balanced by the right of the public to be protected.

Documentation in client records is used in court to prove or disprove a claim. Each client record should be completed in ink, be dated and timed, and be legible and complete. Data must be objective with client statements in quotation marks. Documentation should reflect the nursing process, standards of care, and client responses. Accurate, objective documentation is one of the best defenses against potential legal problems.

THE REASONABLE AND PRUDENT CAREGIVER PRINCIPLE

The law judges professional actions by asking, "What would a reasonable and prudent care provider do under similar circumstances in a similar situation?" Then a comparison between behaviors is made. Engage in "reasonable and prudent" care by following standards of practice and the employing agency's policies, procedures, job descriptions, and contracts. Safe practice is based on your knowledge of the limits that define caregiving in your practice setting. Health care providers have the overall responsibility to practice in a competent, safe manner. This involves an active pursuit of new knowledge plus a willingness to conduct oneself according to ethical and legal standards. Areas of potential liability exist in many situations, and laws are not always clear when dealing with mental illness. To practice safely and effectively be aware of your actions and develop an alertness to potential problems.

Key Points

- Societies share common values, morals, and rights that serve as foundations for making decisions.
- Values clarification is a three-step process to identify one's significant values.
- Rights are defined as powers or privileges to which one has a just claim.
- Clients' rights are addressed by the federal Mental Health Systems Act Bill of Rights and by each state in its state patient's bill of rights.
- Health care providers have the rights to practice their professions in safety and with respect and competent assistance.
- Ethics is a shared set of codes, rules, or laws that govern right behavior.
- Ethical principles for health care professionals have been organized into codes of ethics based on primary and secondary ethical principles.

- The six-step ethical decision-making process helps health care providers in resolving ethical dilemmas.
- Laws are the controls by which a society governs itself. They function to define relationships, describe acceptable behaviors, maintain rules, and protect the public.
- Legal concepts that govern health care providers are found in state practice acts; standards of practice; and institutional policies, procedures, and job descriptions.
- The involuntary psychiatric commitment process consists of petitioning, examination, and a determination to either release or hospitalize.
- Areas of potential legal liability for mental health care providers include crimes, fraud, libel, slander, assault and battery, invasion of privacy, false imprisonment, negligence, and malpractice.
- Negligence is a failure to exercise an accepted degree of professional skill or learning that results in injury, loss, or damage.
- Health care practitioners have a legal responsibility to practice (1) in a safe, competent manner, (2) accurate and objective record keeping, and (3) within one's legal limitations. Nurses have the added responsibility to dispense controlled substances according to procedures.
- Care providers who work with mentally ill clients need to be aware of the potential liabilities inherent in client care situations.

evolve Be sure to visit the companion Evolve site at http://evolve.elsevier.com/Morrison-Valfre/ for additional online resources.

CHAPTER 4

Sociocultural Issues

evolve http://evolve.elsevier.com/Morrison-Valfre/

Objectives

Upon completion of this chapter, the student will be able to:

1. Compare the concepts of culture, ethnicity, and religion.
2. Explain the consequences of stereotyping mental health clients.
3. Describe seven characteristics of culture.
4. Identify three ways in which culture influences health and illness behaviors.
5. List the six components of cultural assessment.
6. Explain the importance of recognizing clients' spiritual or religious practices.
7. Identify four topics to be included in the assessment of a client who is a refugee.
8. Integrate cultural factors into a holistic plan of therapeutic care.

Key Terms

cultural competence (KŎM-pa-tens) (p. 32)
culture (p. 28)
disease (p. 30)
environmental control (p. 33)
ethnicity (ĕth-NĬS-ĭ-tē) (p. 28)
extended family (p. 34)
gender roles (p. 34)
illness (p. 30)
norms (p. 29)
nuclear (NOO-klē-er) **family** (p. 34)
prejudice (p. 29)
race (p. 28)
refugee (p. 35)
religion (p. 28)
role (p. 29)
spirituality (SPĬR-ĭ-choo-Ă-lĭ-tē) (p. 28)
stereotype (STĔR-ē-ō-tīp) (p. 29)
territoriality (TĔR-ĭ-TÔR-ē-ĂL-ĭ-tē) (p. 33)

Culture has a profound influence on mental illness and its treatment. Mental illness is defined within a cultural context. What may be appropriate behavior in one culture might be considered insanity in another. This is an important point because an awareness of each client's cultural background helps us understand the client as a whole person and improves our therapeutic effectiveness.

NATURE OF CULTURE

An accurate understanding of any person is incomplete without consideration of the cultural, ethnic, and religious concepts that define and guide one's life. Simply put, culture is a total way of life. It is the learned pattern of behavior that shapes our thinking and serves as the basis for social, religious, and family structure. Culture is a **shared** system of values that provides a framework for who we are.

Race is a biological term that describes a group of people who share distinct physical characteristics, such as skin color, facial features, and hair texture. Ethnicity is a social term associated with the customs, cultural habits, and socialization patterns of a particular (ethnic) group. Ethnic groups function as subsocieties within a larger society and play important roles in preserving cultures. The values, traditions, expectations, and customs of each ethnic group are passed from one generation to another. Ethnicity contributes to one's point of view because ethnic groups function as focal points for evaluating the value systems of other groups. A recent multicultural study in Great Britain revealed that ethnicity is "an important factor in influencing perceptions of schizophrenia" (Orrell, 2002).

Spirituality and religion play important roles in the concept of culture. The term spirituality refers to a belief in a power greater than any human being. Religion relates to a defined, organized, and practiced system of worship. Religious groups may have values that range from allowing for individual variation to requiring a commitment to place the religion before family, work, and friends. Often mental health clients have religious components to their illnesses. "Delusions of religiosity" may be ingrained in the illness. The challenge for caregivers is to "balance pathological behavior with appropriate cultural expression of religion" (Taylor, 1994).

CHARACTERISTICS OF CULTURE

Culture is an abstract concept, composed of the values, beliefs, roles, and norms of a group. Large multicultural societies have many cultural variations and subgroups. Health caregivers have varied cultural backgrounds themselves. Knowing how one's own culture relates to clients' cultural backgrounds is key to establishing effective care.

Cultural values strongly influence thinking and actions. A culture's **belief system** develops over generations, formed by the feelings and convictions that are believed to be true. Belief systems can be found in a culture's political, social, and religious practices. Conflicts in cultural value systems can lead to mental illness. People may also express one value and then act out another. Observing behaviors, rather than merely listening, allows caregivers to gain a more accurate picture of the client's values. Because people of different cultures respond in various ways to time, activity, relationships, the supernatural, and nature, learning about the client's cultural values is an important area of health care.

Beliefs about mental health have a strong impact on the outcome of treatment. When people believe in the treatment and in their care providers, successful outcomes are much more frequent. Know and respect the client's beliefs. Some things that you find strange may be of great cultural importance to the client.

Values and beliefs help define norms, which are a culture's behavioral standards. Norms are the established rules of conduct that define which behaviors are encouraged, accepted, tolerated, and forbidden within a culture. Simply put, norms are the rules for behavior. A role is an expected pattern of behaviors associated with a certain position, status, or gender. Cultures commonly describe roles based on age, gender, marital status, and occupation. Individuals within the culture are expected to fill their roles and conform their behaviors to meet the expectations defined by the role. Some cultures have clearly defined role expectations, whereas other cultures define their roles with vague and ambiguous terms.

"A stereotype is an oversimplified mental picture of a cultural group" (Haber and others, 1997). Some beliefs are passed on through generations and tend to color the perceptions and influence the behaviors of people who hold them. Stereotyping may take negative, positive, or traditional forms. The extreme form of negative stereotyping is called prejudice. Stereotyping occurs when one assumes that all members of a culture behave in the traditional manner.

Stereotypes develop unconsciously in many people, especially those who have had little exposure to culturally diverse groups. Health care providers need to know and understand their own racial, ethnic, religious, and social stereotypes. Clients, especially those with mental problems, are very sensitive to discrimination. If they sense such treatment, they will resist receiving care. By removing stereotypes, each person can be treated as an individual with the respect and dignity that is his or her right. Caregivers who assess the behaviors of culturally different clients without personal biases are better able to distinguish adaptive behaviors from dysfunctional ones (see Case Study 4-1).

Cultures vary greatly in values, beliefs, and behaviors, but they all share several characteristics. Table 4-1 presents a brief description of the main characteristics of culture.

Case Study 4-1

Hauni is a 22-year-old woman who recently arrived from Sumatra. She has been ill for 3 days and arrives at the clinic with a friend. Although Hauni speaks English, the nurse who is obtaining her history must frequently repeat her questions. With patience, Hauni responds to the questions, but she immediately freezes when Dr. Dankin enters the examination room. Although she feels very ill, she refuses to be examined. Sensing the client's uneasiness, the nurse confers with Dr. Dankin, who recommends that the case be turned over to Dr. Linda Smith. Hauni responds immediately to Dr. Smith, even to the point where she becomes talkative.
- What difference did the recognition of the client's cultural background make in her care?
- What do you think would have happened if the client's culture was not considered?

Culture is a social phenomenon. It is **learned** through life experiences and **transmitted** or passed from one generation to another through language, symbols, and practices. Culture is **shared.** Values, beliefs, and standards of behavior are known to all members and allow children to learn right from wrong and adjust their behaviors according to the cultural norms. Culture is **integrated** into an interwoven framework of political, social, religious, and health practices. Because a culture reflects its members, it is **dynamic,** changing, and adaptive. Cultural habits are **satisfying.** They fill a need within the society and result in gratification. Last, an individual's behavior may or may not represent the culture. Individual behaviors may differ from the major behavioral patterns and still be tolerated to a certain extent. When a person's actions go beyond a culturally acceptable point, they are considered eccentric, maladaptive, or deviant. Each of these characteristics helps to explain the framework of a culture. To deliver holistic, effective mental health care, all care providers must assess the impact and meaning that each cultural characteristic holds for the client.

INFLUENCES OF CULTURE

People base many health decisions on both scientific and cultural values. As a result, many individuals seek health care from folk healers as well as medical practitioners.

HEALTH AND ILLNESS BELIEFS

The practice of Western medicine is based on scientific treatment methods and tends to disregard that which cannot be explained by research. Providers of health care are specifically licensed and trained in one area of expertise. Health care is offered in institutions and is often delivered in an impersonal, assembly-line manner.

Table 4-1 *Characteristics of Culture*

CHARACTERISTICS	DESCRIPTION	EXAMPLE
Culture is learned.	A learned set of shared values, beliefs, and behaviors—not genetically inherited.	Cuban family members learn that humor is a way of making fun of people, situations, or things called *chateo*. It includes exaggeration, jokes, and satirical expressions or gestures.
Culture is transmitted.	Passed from one generation to another.	In Asian cultures the concept of family extends both backward and forward. An individual is seen as a product of all generations from the beginning of time. The concept is reinforced by rituals such as ancestor worship and family record books. Personal actions reflect on all generations.
Culture is shared.	A shared set of assumptions, values, beliefs, attitudes, and behaviors of a group. Members predict one another's actions and react accordingly.	In the Arab culture a woman will not make eye contact with a man other than her husband. All decisions are made by her husband. Because a woman may not be touched by another man, health care may be provided only by another woman.
Culture is integrated.	Includes religion, politics, economics, art, kinship, diet, health, and patterns of communication. All are interrelated.	In Ireland and the United States, the primary cultural force and national unifier of Irish culture has been the Catholic Church. The parish, rather than the neighborhood, has traditionally defined the family's social context.
Culture contains ideal and real components.	Behavior may diverge from ideal behavior and still be acceptable.	The American mainstream culture condemns the drinking of alcohol on a daily basis. However, those who do so but "hold their liquor well" are regarded with only minimal disapproval.
Culture is dynamic and continuously evolving.	Cultural change is an ongoing process. All aspects do not change at the same time. Habits and newer behaviors are easier to alter than deep-rooted values and beliefs.	Italian-American values regarding the family roles of men and women are often more traditional than those of other men and women in the workplace.
Individual behavior is not necessarily representative of the culture.	Although culture defines the dominant values, beliefs, and behaviors, it does not determine all the behaviors in any group. Variation from the major pattern of behavior is called eccentric behavior. The meaning of this behavior to the culture will determine if it is regarded as normal, eccentric, or deviant.	Male and female roles are strictly defined in traditional Greek culture. Women are secondary; the man is the head of the family. Men work and provide for their families; it is a dishonor if the wife works outside the home. Within this cultural context, a Greek woman who is a proponent of the feminist movement might be viewed as eccentric or deviant.

Modified from Haber J: *Comprehensive psychiatric nursing*, ed 5, St. Louis, 1997, Mosby.

Folk medicine, "on the other hand, embodies the beliefs, values and treatment approaches of a particular cultural group" (Edelman and Mandle, 2002). Its foundation is based on empirical knowledge—observation and experience without an understanding of cause or effect. Folk practitioners explain disease culturally as an imbalance of energies. Caregivers may receive training through an experienced practitioner, religious groups, or self-study. Care is provided in the home or community in a personal, individualized manner. Providers of health care within the Western system of medicine need to know about clients' folk medical practices, because many people seek out professional care only after seeking folk healing (Table 4-2).

Traditional health beliefs involve explanations of the causes of health and disease. For example, Navajo and traditional African American cultures view health as a state of harmony with nature. The mind and body are one and function in harmony with the earth and the supernatural. Disease is caused by a state of disharmony.

Chinese cultures consider health to be a balance of positive and negative energy forces (yin and yang). An imbalance of yin or yang results in disease. Hispanics feel that good health is a gift from God, sprinkled with good luck. Illness is an imbalance of the hot and cold body properties and is considered God's punishment (D'Avanso and Geissler, 2003). Low-income families define health as the ability to work. Illness is seen as unpreventable. Throughout the years, millions of people have sought health care from alternative (folk) sources. Understanding and respecting the client's cultural health beliefs and practices promote effective treatment for those who seek science-based health care.

Illness Behaviors

Disease is a condition in which a physical dysfunction exists, whereas **illness** includes social, emotional, and intellectual dysfunctions. Culture has no impact on disease, but illness and its attendant behaviors are strongly influenced by culture.

Table 4-2 Comparison Between Folk and Western Health Care Systems

CRITERIA	WESTERN	FOLK
Philosophy of care	Curative	Curative
Approach to care	Fragmented specialization Often impersonal	Personalized
Setting for services	Institutions	Homes, community, other social places
Treatments	Technology Approved pharmacological agents	Herbs, charms, amulets, massage, meditation
Providers	Licensed professionals	Healers, shamans, spiritualists, priests, other lay unlicensed therapists
Support for care	Other ancillary personnel and agencies	Family, relatives, friends
Payment for services	Third-party insurers Personal funds	Negotiable
Philosophy of health	Influenced by the professional's definition and dealt with in terms of illness and treatment	Reflected as a quest for harmony with nature
Definition of disease	Result of cause-effect phenomena; cure is achieved by scientifically proven methods	Imbalance between person and physical, social, and spiritual worlds

From Edelman CL, Mandle CL: *Health promotion throughout the lifespan*, ed 5, St. Louis, 2002, Mosby.

When the signs and symptoms of illness appear, an individual may choose one of four courses of action: (1) do something to relieve the symptoms, (2) do nothing, (3) vacillate without taking any real action, or (4) deny the existence of the problem. Several studies have compared the illness behaviors of men from various cultural backgrounds. Results revealed that Italian Americans sought medical help when relationships were affected by the illness. Irish Americans sought help for their symptoms only after receiving approval of others. Americans of Anglo-Saxon origin required medical assistance only when their symptoms interfered with specific activities.

Illness behaviors are also affected by beliefs (e.g., Christian Scientists do not seek medical help for illness) and culture. For example, if headaches are considered a sign of weakness, to seek treatment would be to act counter to the cultural heritage. To be effective, health care providers must assess each client's attitudes and behaviors relating to illness.

On Mental Illness

Clients and their care providers may have very different belief systems about mental disorders. Members of a culture may define normal and abnormal behaviors differently from those outside the culture. To illustrate, in several cultures the practice of altered states of consciousness or trances is considered acceptable. Health care providers need to understand their clients' cultural definitions of mental health and illness.

Cultural descriptions of mental dysfunction are classified as **naturalistic** illness or **personalistic** illness. According to Haber and others (1997), "naturalistic illnesses are caused by impersonal factors without regard for the individual." Forces that exist outside the individual cause mental illness. Personalistic illnesses are seen as aggression or punishment directed toward a specific person. Examples include voodoo, witchcraft, and the evil eye.

Beliefs in witchcraft are widespread in Haitian, Puerto Rican, and African American cultures. Spells, hexes, and incantations are used to cause a person injury, illness, or even death. The practice of voodoo calls the spirits of the dead back to the world of the living to bless or curse specific people. The chosen individual "takes on" or internalizes the behaviors associated with the hex. Mental illness in these cultures is considered to be the result of witchcraft, magic, or evil spells.

Stress and Coping

All cultures classify their members by gender and age. Age and gender roles contain certain norms, status, and expectations. Some cultures, for example, value elderly people and respect their acquired wisdom, whereas others consider their elders as nonproductive burdens. Clearly, the role of elders in the latter example is associated with more stress. Adolescence in many cultures can be a stressful time. Societies that clearly define adolescence and its roles tend to be less stress inducing than cultures that lack a clear definition.

Women are often placed in stressful roles as a result of their culture. Traditional Greek culture, for example, sees the man as the breadwinner for the family. A Greek wife who works brings embarrassment to the entire family group. A great deal of stress would result for a working woman in this culture.

Stress is associated with various culturally defined roles. Ways of coping with stress are also culturally determined. Crying, screaming, and other displays of emotion are viewed as healthy outlets in one culture, whereas others expect quiet, unemotional responses to stress. Caregivers who are aware of clients' cultural stresses and their associated behaviors are better able to assist them in developing more effective coping skills.

CULTURAL ASSESSMENT

Cultural competence is the process of continually learning about the cultures with which we work and developing cross-cultural therapeutic health care skills. "A culturally-competent mental health practitioner is one whose behaviors and attitudes promote effective resolution of a mental health issue for someone who is different, culturally, from him/herself" (Jackson, 2002). Transcultural nursing is the use of culturally sensitive therapeutic interventions. The professional care provider does not impose personal cultural values on others. He or she is an active listener and analyst who develops effective care plans based on the insights, knowledge, and beliefs of the client's culture. All care providers must guard against the tendency to transfer their own cultural expectations onto clients or make generalizations based on their own cultural attitudes. Each client is uniquely molded by his or her culture.

Cultural assessments are tools that allow us to learn how clients perceive and cope within their worlds. Several tools have been developed, but all include six areas of assessment: communication, environmental control, space and territory, time, social orientation, and biological factors (Figure 4-1) (Giger and Davidhizar, 2004). Box 4-1 summarizes the cultural assessment found in the *Diagnostic and Statistical Manual of Mental Disorders,* Fourth Edition, Text revision (DSM-IV-TR).

COMMUNICATION

People of all cultures communicate. The process of communication, however, involves more than just the use of language. Communication is a complex, interwoven tapestry of voice, gesture, and touch. Both verbal and nonverbal components of communication have cultural meaning. To assess a client's cultural communications refer to Box 4-2.

Clients communicate their emotional states based on their cultural backgrounds. In some cultures, verbal expressions of emotion are approved, whereas other cultures value communicating indirectly and may resent the frankness of mental health care providers. Clients require sensitivity if we are to effectively understand each other. We all communicate; some of us are just louder than others.

Cultural traditions, practices, and kinship systems also communicate. A society's religious practices communicate its basic beliefs. Attitudes toward children, family, health care, and dying are all communicated through cultural behaviors. It is wise to learn the important customs of a culture if one is caring for its members (see Cultural Considerations 4-1).

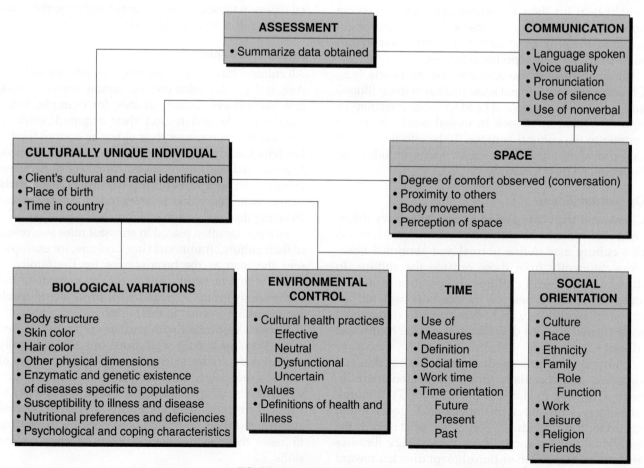

FIGURE **4-1** Cultural assessment.

ENVIRONMENTAL CONTROL

Environmental control focuses on the individual's ability to perceive and control the environment. Does the client feel that the power to effect change lies within, or is everything the result of fate, chance, or luck? What are the client's values relating to the nature of humanity, the supernatural, health, and illness? How are the causes and treatments for mental illnesses viewed?

Environmental control includes an assessment of clients' **cultural health practices.** What is their definition of "good health," and what is done to maintain health? When alternative (folk) practices are assessed, both clients and their care providers increase the potential for success.

SPACE, TERRITORY, AND TIME

The concepts of space and territory are included in a cultural assessment. **Space** is the area that surrounds the client—an invisible "bubble" that travels with a person. The physical distance that a person maintains between oneself and others is influenced by one's culture. People consciously maintain a "comfortable" distance from each other. Mental health clients often have additional perceptions about space. For example, some clients feel the need to be physically **closer** to people for feelings of safety and security. Space comfort areas are divided into four distances: public, social, personal, and intimate (Figure 4-2). Observe and respect your client's degree of comfort at each distance and his or her use of surrounding space.

Some clients have a need to establish a territory. **Territoriality** is the need to gain **control** over an area of space and claim it for oneself. For many, a territory helps to provide a sense of identity, security, autonomy, and control over the environment. People will protect their territory (even if it is the size of a hospital bed), and health care providers can be casually careless about invading these precious spaces. Caregivers, especially nurses, need to know and respect the client's territorial space if culturally appropriate care is to be given.

The concept of **time** is rooted in a culture's basic orientation. Cultures oriented to the past (e.g., Chinese, Amish) strive to maintain the customs and traditions of previous generations. Present-oriented cultures focus on current daily events but may not follow a schedule. Many American Indians are present oriented but not to time. Cultures with future time orientations use today as a tool for meeting future goals. Schedules are established, and people are oriented to the time of day. An example of a future-oriented culture is the middle class of the United States and Canada. Western society's concept of time is linear. For some cultures the linear concept of time is difficult to understand.

Box 4-1 *DSM-IV-TR Cultural Assessment*

Use a narrative summary for the following categories:
- Cultural **identity** of the client
- Cultural **explanations** of the problem or illness
- Cultural factors relating to **psychosocial environment**
- Cultural factors relating to **level of functioning**
- Cultural elements of the **relationship** between client and care provider
- **Overall cultural assessment** for diagnosis, planning, and care

Modified from American Psychiatric Association: *Diagnostic and statistical manual of mental disorders,* ed 4, text revision, Washington, DC, 2000, The Association.

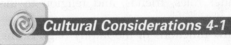
Cultural Considerations 4-1

Your client is a Xhosa from Southeastern Africa. His people believe that displeasing the ancestors results in illness.

Explain how this information will affect the client's therapeutic care plan.

Box 4-2 *Cultural Communication Assessment*

VERBAL COMMUNICATIONS	NONVERBAL COMMUNICATIONS

Language
  Dialect
  Pronunciation
  Voice quality
  Rate of speech
  Style of speech
  Volume of speech
  Use of small talk, laughter
 	
Music
Written language
  Formal usage
  Regional usage
 	
Communicates emotions verbally
  More verbally oriented
	Touch
	  Use of touch
	  How touch is perceived and received
	
	Space
	  Interpersonal distance
	  Use of silence, eye contact, facial gestures (e.g., smiles, frowns)
	  Communicates emotions nonverbally
	  More behaviorally oriented

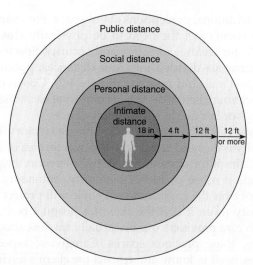

FIGURE **4-2** Space and distance zones.

Clients with mental dysfunctions frequently have misperceptions about time. An inability to tell the difference between day and night can exist, and difficulty following schedules is common. Problems with time may be based in the client's cultural orientation or psychiatric illness. Until the caregiver can discover the difference, the delivery of effective care is difficult.

SOCIAL ORGANIZATION

To assess a client's social orientation, one must consider how the family unit and its importance in the society are culturally defined. The family unit imparts the culture's important traditions, beliefs, values and customs. Social orientation also includes the meaning of work, gender roles, friends, and religion to the client.

Although the functions of the family (e.g., caring for the young, providing identity, security) remain similar among most cultures, the size and composition differ. Middle-class Americans live within a nuclear family unit consisting of parents and one or more children. In many cultures, aunts, uncles, grandparents, cousins, and/or godparents are also included in the family. This family unit is called an extended family, and its importance to the client is usually significant. To illustrate, the Inuit people of Alaska view any separation from the family as traumatic. Many groups—such as traditional Chinese, Mexicans, and Puerto Ricans—believe the family to be the supreme social organization. Family causes take priority in these cultures. When care providers fail to consider the whole family, culturally sensitive care goals cannot be achieved.

Gender roles are expected behavioral patterns based on gender. The traditional roles for men and women in one society may collide with the expectations of another. Women who have learned to fill a serving, passive gender role may have great difficulty assuming the assertive and outspoken role of the modern Western woman. Be sensitive to this area of assess-

ment. Few women will identify themselves as having a culturally based gender role conflict. Mental health problems more frequently seen in women include eating disorders, phobias, and depression. Men, on the other hand, tend to demonstrate more violent and abusive behaviors. Cultural norms that identify gender roles often encourage the expression of conflict in different ways.

Assessment of social orientation also includes the client's **religious beliefs** and practices. Religious beliefs and practices serve many functions in a culture. They bind people together in a common belief system. Religion helps to explain the unexplainable, such as unexpected deaths or natural catastrophes, and it helps to provide meaning and guidance for living.

Religious beliefs and practices vary widely. Attitudes toward health, illness, death, burials, procreation, food, and stress all have religious components. Although it is impossible to discover the inner workings of every religion, it is necessary to be aware of the religious practices of those clients with whom you frequently interact. Table 4-3 lists the world's major religions by size.

BIOLOGICAL FACTORS

The final area of cultural assessment focuses on the biological or physical differences that exist among different cultural groups. When assessing the client's cultural group for biological factors, consider the following: physical, enzymatic, and genetic variations; susceptibility to disease; and psychological characteristics.

Physical variations include differences in body structure, eyes, ears, noses, teeth, muscle mass, and skin color. People of some races are taller than others. For example, African Americans are usually taller than Asian Americans. The shape of the eyelids and nose varies from one racial group to another. Teeth may also vary in size and shape: "Australian aborigines have the largest teeth in the world, as well as four extra molars" (Giger and Davidhizar, 2004). In contrast, white Americans tend to have small teeth. Certain muscles of the wrist and foot are absent in some racial groups. Differences in skin color range from pale white to black. Mongolian spots, for example, are bluish discolorations of the skin that may be found in black, Asian, Mexican, and American Indian newborns. In this case, knowing the client's cultural background may prevent possible misdiagnosis because Mongolian spots can be mistaken for bruises resulting from child abuse.

A person's **genetic makeup** is largely determined by racial group. Physical appearance, metabolic activities (see Drug Alert 4-1), enzyme functions, and susceptibility to disease are all influenced by racial factors. To illustrate, sickle cell anemia is commonly found in African Americans but rarely in white Americans. Lactose (milk) intolerance is very common

Table 4-3	*World's Largest Religions*
RELIGIOUS BODY	**NUMBER OF ADHERENTS**
Christianity	2.1 billion
Islam	1.5 billion
Agnostic/Athiest	1.1 billion
Hinduism	900 million
Buddhism	376 million
Jehovah's Witnesses	15,374,986
Church of Jesus Christ of Latter-day Saints	11,394,522
Seventh-day Adventists	11,300,000
New Apostolic Church	10,260,000
Ahmadiyya	10,000,000

From Hunter P: *Largest religious bodies,* www.adherents.com/ Religions_By_Adherents.html.

in black, American Indian, and Asian groups, yet is rare in northern European whites. Tuberculosis is common in American Indians, and diabetes is rare in Eskimos.

Certain **psychological characteristics** may be related to different cultural groups. A low socioeconomic status can affect mental health when housing, education, and health care are substandard. Feelings of insecurity can result when a client's views of health care are threatened. The Hmong people of Laos, for example, believe that "losing blood saps strength and may result in the soul leaving the body, causing death" (Rairdan and Higgs, 1992). Therefore great anxiety is produced in a Hmong client when blood is drawn. Cultural factors do affect mental health. Nurses and their colleagues must become aware of group differences if they are to consistently deliver culturally appropriate mental health care.

CULTURE AND MENTAL HEALTH CARE

No society is immune to mental disorders, but research is needed to study mental illness from a worldwide perspective. The definition and treatments of mental illness vary among cultures. To understand and treat clients from diverse backgrounds, the concept of cultural competence has evolved. As the name implies, cultural competence seeks to deliver appropriate client care based on knowledge of the client's culture.

It is important here to understand the unique status of refugees. By definition, a refugee is a person who, **because of war or persecution,** flees from his or her home or country and seeks refuge elsewhere. Many refugees have seen or experienced imprisonment, torture, and harrowing escapes. Some have lost family members, and all must learn to cope within a new and strange reality.

When assessing a person who is a refugee, be alert to the possibility of **stress-related problems.** In addition to the routine cultural assessment, tactfully obtain the

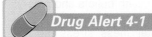
Drug Alert 4-1

Culture and ethnicity play a role in the actions of medications. "There are dramatic ethnic differences in the metabolism of psychotropic medications and the effects of drugs on target organs" (Flaskerud, 2000). Monitor clients closely for side effects and adverse reactions to their medications.

Think About 4-1

You are on vacation in Bali when you suddenly become ill with a high fever, vomiting, and diarrhea. After a long search, you finally locate a hospital. You enter the building and find that everything is strange and uncomfortable. You cannot even speak the language, but you know you must be treated.
- How do you feel about this situation?
- What would you do to cope?

following information: **immigration history, a history of the flight and arrival in the new country, time in the new country, and who or what was lost** (Lipson, 1993). Because of a usually traumatic history, higher incidences of depression, anxiety, and stress disorders occur in refugee groups. Be sensitive to the special circumstances of refugees.

Clients from other cultures may evaluate their health care differently. Haitian Americans, for example, may feel that improvement in health was not the result of good care but the mystical healing power of tree leaves kept close to the body. There exist many such customs and beliefs (see Think About 4-1). If sensitive health care providers are able to view clients as unique, dynamically functioning individuals, then culturally effective health care is one step closer to becoming a reality.

Key Points

- Culture is a learned pattern of behaviors, values, beliefs, and customs shared by a group of people.
- Ethnicity is a social term associated with the customs, cultural habits, and socialization patterns of a particular (ethnic) group.
- Religion relates to a defined, organized, and practiced system of worship.
- Stereotyping is basing one's behavior on an oversimplified mental picture of a cultural group. Clients who sense such biases during treatment will resist receiving care.
- Culture is learned, transmitted, shared, integrated, dynamic, and satisfying.

- Culture influences people's health beliefs and practices, including clients' definitions of health and illness, attitudes about mental illness, stress and coping behaviors, and illness behaviors. Each area needs to be assessed.
- Cultural assessments focus on six areas: communication, environmental control, space and territory, time, social orientation, and biological factors.
- Religious beliefs and practices function to bind people together in a common belief system, help explain the unexplainable, and provide meaning and guidance for living.
- Religious beliefs and practices vary widely. Attitudes toward health, illness, death, burials, procreation, food, and stress all have religious components and implications for health care providers.
- Working with refugees requires extra sensitivity because of their frequently traumatic experiences and losses. In addition to the routine cultural assessment,

obtain information about immigration history, a history of the flight and arrival in the new country, time in the new country, and who or what was lost.
- Because no universal descriptions of mental health and illness exist, the definition and treatment of mental illness vary among cultures.
- Culturally competent health care seeks to deliver the diverse therapeutic actions necessary for appropriate, effective client care.
- When caregivers are able to consistently view each client as a unique, dynamic individual functioning within a sociocultural context, then culturally appropriate health care will become a reality.

---

evolve Be sure to visit the companion Evolve site at http://evolve.elsevier.com/Morrison-Valfre/ for additional online resources.

evolve http://evolve.elsevier.com/Morrison-Valfre/

Objectives

Upon completion of this chapter, the student will be able to:

1. Explain how theories can be applied to mental health care.
2. Discuss three psychoanalytical therapies that resulted from Freud's work.
3. Identify how developmental, humanistic, and behavioral theories differ in their viewpoints.
4. Discuss how Maslow's human needs theory can be used in the care of clients with emotional problems.
5. Compare and contrast the main concepts of systems, cognitive, and sociocultural theories.
6. Describe the concept of homeostasis.
7. Explain how Selye's theories of stress and adaptation influence the delivery of health care.
8. Analyze how psychobiology is adding to our knowledge about mental health care.
9. Examine how nursing theories apply to mental health care.
10. Describe three kinds of psychotherapy used in the treatment of mental disorders.
11. Explain the difference between psychotherapies and somatic therapies for treating mental illness.

Key Terms

affective (p. 41)
closed system (p. 44)
cognition (kŏg-NĬ-shŭn) (p. 45)
cognitive (p. 41)
defense mechanisms (p. 38)
ego (p. 38)
equilibrium (Ē-kwĭ-LĬB-rē-ŭm) (p. 44)
homeostasis (HŌ-mē-ō-STĀ-sĭs) (p. 46)
id (p. 38)
inferiority (p. 40)
libidinal (lĭ-BĬD-ĭ-nəl) **energy** (p. 38)
life space (p. 44)
model (p. 37)
neuropeptides (NOOR-ō-PĔP-tīds) (p. 48)
neurotransmitters (NOOR-ō-TRĂNS-mĭ-tĕrs) (p. 48)
open system (p. 44)
personifications (pĕr-SŎN-ĭ-fə-KĀ-shən) (p. 40)
phototherapy (p. 50)
psyche (SĪ-kē) (p. 40)
psychoanalysis (SĪ-kō-ə-NĂ-lĭ-sĭs) (p. 38)
psychobiology (p. 47)

psychoneuroimmunology (PNI) (SĪ-kō-NOO-rō-ĬM-ū-NŎL-ŏ-jē) (p. 48)
psychotherapy (p. 38)
soma (SŌ-mə) (p. 40)
somatic (sō-MAT-ĭk) **therapies** (p. 50)
stressor (p. 46)
superego (p. 38)
theory (p. 37)

A theory is defined as a statement that explains or describes a relationship among events, concepts, or ideas. Early theories evolved through observations and deductions. Modern theories are developed through observations and research. Many theorists use models to help explain their ideas more simply. A **model** is an example or pattern that helps explain a theory. For instance, a model of an airplane can be used to explain the theory of flight.

Models and theories about human behavior help explain various aspects of people. They also describe the psychodynamics of basic needs, drives, conflicts, perceptions, values, attitudes, belief systems, and cultural influences that shape every individual. Helping professionals use theories as frameworks for describing relationships among people and various aspects of their environments.

HISTORICAL THEORIES

Symbolic and magical thinking was used to explain the workings of the world for many centuries. The belief that mentally ill people were possessed or controlled by evil spirits persisted until the late 1800s when radical new ideas were introduced.

DARWIN'S THEORY

Charles Darwin (1809-1882) was a naturalist whose theory of evolution had a lasting impact on the emerging field of psychiatry. Basically, Darwin's theory stated that only the fittest organisms would adapt and survive and that, through the process of **natural selection**, increasingly superior creatures evolved. In this way, nature culls the weak and preserves the strong.

Darwin's theory led to the persistent belief that people who were impaired or unsuccessful were, by nature, lower on the evolutionary scale. Poverty, disease, alcoholism, and mental illness were all claimed to be the product of inferior genetic makeup. High incidences of tuberculosis, rickets, infant mortality, and low adult life expectancies all indicated that nature was at work. This popular theory might have continued for many years had not the work of new theorists challenged the commonly held beliefs of the time.

PSYCHOANALYTICAL THEORIES

By the middle 1800s, physicians everywhere were exploring new treatments for mental illness. Dr. Joseph Breuer (1842-1905) used hypnosis along with a new method of "talking out" symptoms. A brilliant young neurosurgeon, Sigmund Freud, heard of this and sought to work with the distinguished physician.

By 1902, Freud had become convinced of the talking cure's value because he felt that unconscious thoughts and emotions had a strong impact on behavior. He called his approach to therapy psychoanalysis, which means to explore the unconscious. Weekly discussions about psychoanalysis, attended by a number of Freud's colleagues (e.g., Alfred Adler, Otto Rank, Carl Jung), later provided the framework for several radical new theories.

Freud's theories focused on behaviors of which the patient was unaware. His study of the mind's unconscious processes evolved into theories about the development, structure, and dynamics of the personality. These ideas made psychoanalysis the most influential set of theories in the early twentieth century.

For the next 30 years Freud developed and tested his theories. By the 1920s, the definition of psychoanalysis had broadened into three areas: Freud's theories of personality, a therapy for certain emotional disorders, and a method for investigating the workings of the mind. Today the term psychotherapy is used to describe a therapy relating to mental illness. Freud's theories that are important to health care providers relate to personality development, dynamics, and defenses.

Freud believed that the mind was made up of three interacting structures, which he labeled id, ego, and superego. The id is a storage site for early childhood experiences and the instinctual drives for self-preservation, reproduction, and association with others. Freud stated that the id is governed by the "pleasure principle." It seeks out immediate pleasure or avoidance of pain without regard to outcome. Because infants demand immediate attention, they are often described as "bundles of id."

The ego is the part of the mind in active awareness, the conscious mind. The ego develops when the child becomes aware of "self," usually around 2 years. The reality-based ego gradually gains control over the impulsive id and develops into the personality that copes with the external world.

The superego is the last to develop. Attitudes, values, role expectations, taboos, rules, ideals, and standards help form the superego. There are two parts to the superego: the conscience, which punishes through guilt and anxiety when behaviors move away from its standards, and the ego **ideal,** which rewards with feelings of satisfaction and well-being for "good" behaviors. The superego is not based in reality. It uses internal standards that were learned early in life. These standards, according to Freud, are primarily stored in the **unconscious,** where they remain unavailable to awareness but still influence the ego. The superego controls the id because of its strict and rigid moralistic rules. Freud stated that the ego must maintain the delicate balance of meeting id and superego needs within the limitations of the real world. The mentally healthy adult is said to be one who has achieved a dynamic balance among all the elements of the personality.

Freud's **theory of personality development** has the central theme of sexual instinct growth through four stages from newborn to adult. He believed that the most powerful motivation was the drive to reproduce and described this drive, which he called libidinal energy, as the need to seek sexual pleasure. Freud's stages became known as the **psychosexual theory** of personality development. Emotional disturbances, according to Freud, arise from five sources: (1) instinctual-biological drives, (2) early childhood experiences, (3) deeply buried unconscious experiences and attitudes, (4) fixations (anxieties) arising from earlier psychosexual stages of development, and (5) defensive maneuvers that help prevent the person from changing.

Freud believed that all individuals have conflict embedded within themselves and thus use psychological tools to help to lessen negative feelings. He called these defense mechanisms and defined them as "psychological strategies by which persons reduce or avoid negative states such as conflict, frustration, anxiety, and stress" (Corsini, 1994) (Table 5-1). Defense mechanisms are used to avoid negative emotional states. Individuals are not consciously aware of their use. No matter which mechanism is used, the goal is to reduce uncomfortable negative emotions. Commonly used defense mechanisms include denial, fantasy, projection, and repression. See Chapter 18 for a more complete discussion of defense mechanisms.

Psychoanalytical Therapies

Early therapies based on Freud's work were designed to assist patients in working through anxieties that resulted from unconscious, repressed conflicts. Freud used **dream analysis** to delve into patients' symptoms. He believed that, during sleep, the individual's censor (superego) is less active; therefore the unconscious (id) could express itself in dreams. Therapy centered around interpreting the dream's symbols to discover the unconscious wishes that were causing the conflicts.

Table 5-1 *Common Defense Mechanisms*

MECHANISM	DEFINITION	EXAMPLE
Compensation	Attempt to overcome feelings of inferiority or make up for deficiency	A girl who thinks she cannot sing studies to become an expert pianist.
Conversion	Channeling of unbearable anxieties into body signs and symptoms	A boy who injured an animal by kicking it develops a painful limp.
Denial	Refusal to acknowledge conflict and thus escapes reality of situation	A child covered with chocolate refuses to admit eating candy.
Displacement	Redirecting of energies to another person or object	A husband shouts at his wife, the wife then berates her child, who then scolds the dog.
Dissociation	Separation of emotions from situation; isolation of painful anxieties	A soldier casually describes the battle in which he lost his legs.
Fantasy	Distortion of unacceptable wishes, behaviors	A teenager doing poorly in school daydreams about owning a private jet airplane.
Identification	Taking on of personal characteristics of admired person to conceal own feelings of inadequacy	Teenage adolescents dress and behave like the members of a popular singing group.
Intellectualization	Focusing of attention on technical or logical aspects of threatening situation	A wife describes the details of nurses' unsuccessful attempts to prevent the death of her husband.
Isolation	Separation of feelings from content to cope unemotionally with topics that would normally be overwhelming	A soldier humorously describes how he was seriously wounded in combat.
Projection	Putting of one's own unacceptable thoughts, wishes, emotions onto others	A woman is afraid to leave her house because she knows people will ridicule her.
Rationalization	Use of a "good" (but not real) reason to explain behavior to make unacceptable motivation more acceptable	A student justifies failing an examination by saying that there was too much material to cover.
Reaction formation	Prevention of expression of threatening material by engaging in behaviors that are directly opposite to repressed material	A young man with homosexual feelings, which he finds to be threatening, engages in excessive heterosexual activities.
Regression	Coping with present conflict, stress by returning to earlier, more secure stage of life	A 4-year-old boy whose parents are going through a divorce starts to suck his thumb and wet his pants.
Restitution	Giving back to resolve guilt feelings	A man argues with his wife and then buys her roses.
Sublimation	Unconscious channeling of unacceptable behaviors into constructive, more socially approved areas	A hostile young man who enjoys fighting becomes a football player.
Substitution	Disguising of motivations by replacing inappropriate behavior with one that is more acceptable	A man who is attracted to pornography campaigns to ban adult bookstores in his community.
Suppression	Removal of conflict by removing anxiety from consciousness	A woman with a family history of breast cancer "forgets" her appointment for a mammogram.
Symbolization	Use of an unrelated object to represent hidden idea	A girl who feels insignificant draws a picture of her family in which she is the smallest character.
Undoing	Inappropriate behavior that is followed by acts to take away or reverse action and decrease guilt and anxiety	A man physically abuses his wife and then cleans her wounds and nurses her back to health.

The technique of **free association** soon followed. The patient was presented with a series of words or phrases and then asked to state the first words that came to mind. The therapist would then "interpret" each response and give the patient the "real" meaning behind each association.

Psychoanalysis was the main form of therapy for Freud and many of his followers. The process lasted for many sessions, sometimes for years. Therapist and patient would develop and work through an intense **transference relationship** in which the patient actually transferred emotions associated with significant people in the past to the therapist. To achieve a cure in psychoanalysis, the patient must first recall past events and then develop insight into the meaning of each event.

Many of Freud's theories are challenged today. However, his contributions have influenced the fields of psychiatry, psychology, the humanities, education,

history, and the social sciences. Freud's revolutionary theories "brought about a new level of awareness and, for better or worse, a permanently altered image of humankind" (Corsini, 1994).

Analytical Psychotherapy

Carl Jung, the founder of analytical psychotherapy, differed from Freud in two basic respects: (1) Jung believed that the energy that Freud labeled sexually based was actually a more general life energy, and (2) Jung believed that personality could change during adulthood and is actually influenced by future plans, goals, and dreams (Jung, 1968). Jung divided the mind into three levels: the conscious ego, the personal unconscious, and the deeper collective unconscious, which stores all the experiences of humans' ancestral past. The parts of the collective unconscious he called **archetypes.** He also coined the terms **extroversion** and

introversion to describe outward-going and inward-focused personalities.

Jung's concept of the self focused on the importance of balance and wholeness. His ideas became known as the **analytical theory.** Jung used traditional psychoanalytical techniques but believed that the primary effort in life was to gain more awareness. He helped patients understand their problems and conflicts by uncovering the symbolic meanings of their disorders. The analytical view of psychotherapy did not survive as a separate discipline, but many of its concepts remain.

OTHER THEORIES

By the early 1900s, it was generally agreed that people were more than just physical bodies. The term psyche was borrowed from Plato and used to define the mental or spiritual part of an individual (as compared with the term soma, which relates to the body). It was a time for several new, but related, theories about the nature of humans.

Individual Psychotherapy

Alfred Adler graduated from the Vienna School of Medicine in 1895 and attended Freud's weekly discussions on psychoanalysis. By 1918 he had developed a new way of thinking that became known as individual psychology (also called Adlerian psychology). Adler's personality theory states that the human infant, because of dependency and helplessness, starts out in this world in a position of inferiority (of being inadequate or less than others). The child must learn to master his or her world by assessing the environment and reaching certain conclusions. Each person wants to belong, to be considered as significant, and to be treated as an individual. Thus, as children grow, they find where they fit within the family. Adler believed that the perception of children's positions within the family helped to create the evaluations of self and other people that become incorporated into adult lifestyle and that exert influence throughout life.

Adler theorized that the general goal of life is to gain mastery over the environment by coping with the tasks of work, belonging, social interactions, and interacting with members of the other gender. Later Adler added two additional life tasks, those of self and spirit. The task of **self** states that people must define themselves and find meaning in their lives. Tasks of the **spirit** include considerations of religious, philosophical, and spiritual questions.

Adlerian or individual therapy views individuals as total organisms, functioning within the environment. Therefore behavior becomes meaningful only when viewed within the social setting. Because all behavior is goal directed, people are capable of perceiving and assessing events to arrive at conclusions. However, each individual perceives the world from a unique point of view. To understand a person, the therapist "must be able to see with his eyes and listen with his ears" (Adler, 1964).

Adlerian proponents also believe that people have the ability to make choices and are responsible for their behavior. They dislike the use of labels and do not consider people with mental dysfunctions as mentally ill. Clients are referred to as "discouraged." Therapy is designed to encourage them to assume responsibility for directing their lives in more positive ways.

The concept of a **value system** was introduced by Adler. The concepts of choice, individual responsibility, and finding the meaning in life evolved and later became the foundation for the humanistic school of psychology.

Other therapists during the early twentieth century also broke with the Freudian tradition. Karen Horney (1855-1952), an early follower of Freud, stressed the importance of social and environmental conditions on personality development. Her concept of **basic anxiety** stated that a child's isolation is not inherited but results from culture and social upbringing.

Erich Fromm (1900-1980) stressed human loneliness as the motivation for social interaction. His general theme of productive love is seen in many of his writings. Fromm also developed several personality or character types.

Interpersonal Psychology

Harry Stack Sullivan's (1892-1949) theory emphasizes the social nature of people and the critical role of anxiety in personality formation. He viewed the personality as a pattern of interpersonal relationships. Mental health problems were considered to be the result of distorted images of certain relationships. Sullivan called these distorted images personifications and believed that the images and behavioral patterns from one relationship spilled over or transferred into other relationships. Therapy is a matter of assisting the client in discovering which personifications are unhealthy and substituting more effective behavioral patterns.

A central theme of Sullivan's theory is the concept of **anxiety,** which he defined as a vague feeling of uneasiness felt in response to stress. Sullivan also described six stages of psychological interpersonal development, beginning with infancy and ending with late adolescence. Many forms of therapy have benefited from his theories.

DEVELOPMENTAL THEORIES AND THERAPIES

Using Freud as a foundation, many theorists offered their views of psychological development. Jean Piaget and Erik Erikson attempted to understand the relationships among the body, mind, and society throughout the life cycle. One of the most commonly used theories in health care is Erikson's eight stages of psychosocial development, which represents the first attempt to explain human behavior throughout the entire life cycle.

COGNITIVE DEVELOPMENT

Jean Piaget (1896-1980) devised a theory of intellectual (cognitive) development. He stated that personality is the result of interrelated cognitive and emotional (affective) functions. Growth is an increasing intellectual ability to organize and combine experiences. Piaget observed that certain behaviors occurred in steps at certain age-groups, so he divided these patterns into four main stages of intellectual growth (Table 5-2). Piaget believed that children struggle to find a balance between themselves and their environments. Although no specific therapies are based on Piaget's work, his theories have become essential in the understanding of intellectual growth and development.

PSYCHOSOCIAL DEVELOPMENT

Erik Erikson (1902-1994) described the human life cycle in eight stages (Table 5-3), with each stage marked by a developmental or core task—a normal crisis that must be confronted and resolved. As each crisis is resolved, it leaves an impression that contributes to one's total personality. The uniting of the personality occurs as each **developmental psychosocial task** is mastered. Erikson believed that success in one developmental stage prepares individuals to move into the next stage. Poorly resolved core tasks continue to haunt their owners until they are mastered. Case Study 5-1 presents a person with an inadequately resolved developmental task. Erikson's theory is commonly used by caregivers as a framework for assessing and planning individualized client care.

Theories of personality development are important for health care providers. By understanding where clients are in their development, we are better able to provide effective health care and individually tailored emotional support.

BEHAVIORAL THEORIES AND THERAPIES

The foundation for behaviorism lies in the assumption that **all behavior is learned.** The behavioral school of thought states that behavior is the result of past learning, current motivation, and biological differences. Learning is a behavioral change that results when individual actions repeatedly prove successful and are reinforced. Dysfunctional behaviors are the result of learned maladaptive behaviors. A mechanical approach to human behavior is taken by focusing only on objective, observable, and measurable behaviors. The influence of the environment is stressed, but all behaviors are seen as responses to stimuli. Four important figures were instrumental in establishing the behavioral movement: Pavlov, Watson, Skinner, and Wolpe.

Ivan Pavlov (1849-1936) was the director of the physiology department at the Institute of Experimental Medicine in Saint Petersburg, Russia. There he pioneered research methods to evaluate the responses of dogs to various stimuli and discovered that a given behavior was the response to a given stimulus. His famous experiment of conditioning dogs to salivate when they heard a bell demonstrated the mechanical aspects of behavior. Pavlov then went on to discover that behaviors were more likely to be repeated when they were rewarded and they faded when ignored. His work on **conditioning** laid the foundation for the American behavioral movement.

The behavioral school of thought was established in the United States during the 1920s by John B. Watson (1878-1958). He developed the basic viewpoint for behaviorism: psychology is an objective science—the science of behavior. Watson published two books on behaviorism, and, when he died in 1958, his views were a strong force in American psychology.

Table 5-2 *Piaget's Stages of Intellectual (Cognitive) Development*

DEVELOPMENTAL STAGE	AGE	DEVELOPMENTAL TASK	DESCRIPTION
Sensorimotor	Birth–2 yr	To recognize permanence of objects	Unable to do things or distinguish self from environment; reflexes evolve into repeated actions that become coordinated movements; learns that objects in environment are still present even when they are not seen, touched, tasted; begins goal-directed and imitative behavior
Preoperational	2-7 yr	To develop symbolic mental abilities	Thinking limited; centered on self; learns to use language as tool; establishes routines; thought is focused on only one part of situation; cannot understand more than one dimension of object; justifies own behavior at all costs
Concrete operations	8-11 yr	To develop logical, objective thinking	Understands numbers, length, mass, area, weight, time, and volume; can see interrelations; able to reflect and discover relationships in environment
Formal operations	12-15 yr	To learn to think abstractly	Able to consider all possibilities of situation; can think in terms of probability and proportions; uses problem-solving approach to conflicts

Table 5-3 *Erikson's Stages of Psychosocial Development*

CORE TASK AND DEVELOPMENTAL STAGE	AGE	ASSOCIATED QUALITY	DESCRIPTION
Oral-sensory (infancy)	Birth–1 yr	Trust/mistrust Associated quality: hope	Dominated by biological drives and needs; learns to trust that needs will or will not be met; learns to trust or mistrust others and world in general
Anal-muscular (early childhood)	1-3 yr	Autonomy/shame and doubt Associated quality: will (to do the expected)	Demands for self-control influence feelings of self-confidence vs. shame and doubt in own abilities; ego is developing; parallel play
Genital-locomotor (preschool years)	3-6 yr	Initiative/guilt Associated quality: purpose	Actively explores environment; activities are directed with purpose; conscience develops; cooperative play; uses fantasy; imitates adults; beginning to evaluate own behavior
Latency (school age)	6-12 yr	Industry/inferiority Associated quality: competence (learning skills of adult)	Site of learning moves from home to school; masters skills and tasks valued by teachers and society; learns to behave according to rules; develops confidence and perseverance; practices self-restriction
Puberty (adolescence)	12-18 yr	Identity/diffusion Associated quality: fidelity (commitment to value system)	Combines experiences to form sense of personal identity; forms sexual relationships; plans for future; feels confused and indecisive; if successful with prior crises, will develop strong sense of identity; peer groups important
Young adulthood	18-25 yr	Intimacy/isolation Associated quality: love	If has strong sense of identity, is willing and able to unite own identity with another; develops devotion; commits to relationships, career If weak sense of identity, has impersonal, short-term relationships; shows prejudice; becomes socially isolated
Middle adulthood	25-65 yr	Generativity/stagnation Associated quality: caring	Strives to actualize identity that was formed in earlier stages; generates or produces children, ideas, products, services; is creative, productive, concerned for others; demonstrates caring through parenting, teaching, guiding others; adults who do not care become stagnant, self-indulgent, absorbed in themselves
Maturity	65 yr–death	Integrity/despair Associated quality: wisdom (to accept one's life and value contribution that one has made)	Adjusts to changes; senses flow of time, past, present, and future; accepts worth and uniqueness of own life as it was and is; finds order and meaning in own life; despairs when life is viewed as waste; adults who focus on what "might have been" blame others, feel a sense of loss and contempt for others

Case Study 5-1

Susan is an attractive 42-year-old housewife and mother of four teenage children. She has been married to Jeff, a long-haul truck driver and her high school sweetheart, for 22 years. The family is well respected in the community, and Susan frequently volunteers for charitable projects. The children are considered well behaved and polite. In all respects, Susan is a model wife, mother, and community member. Last week, however, Susan announced her unhappiness, left everything behind, and ran away with a 25-year-old traveling salesman.

• How would Erikson's theory of psychosocial development explain Susan's behavior?

B. F. SKINNER

Burhus Fredrick Skinner (1904-1990) was one of the most influential minds of the twentieth century. As a crusader for objective psychology, he stated that only observed behaviors in current situations were open to analysis and pursued this idea by developing the theories of operant conditioning, positive and negative reinforcement, and shaping (Skinner, 1963).

Skinner's first research efforts were focused on developing a set of learning principles. He believed that all organisms moved toward pleasure and away from pain, and his theory proposed that continual rewards strongly enforce desired behaviors, whereas negative reinforcements weaken and fade out undesirable behaviors. The process of guiding patients to replace unacceptable responses with more desirable behaviors was called **shaping,** whereas the overall approach to changing observable behavior became known as **operant** conditioning.

By 1953, Skinner published his book titled *Science and Human Behavior*. Throughout the 1960s, Skinner crusaded for improvements in the U.S. educational system. He developed the concept of **programmed learning,** a process where new knowledge is broken down to small bits of information and presented at the learner's pace. Today, programmed learning techniques are commonly used in business and industrial training courses.

OTHER BEHAVIORAL THERAPIES

During the 1960s, Joseph Wolpe explained neuroses and anxiety as conditioned responses. Researchers Dollard and Miller developed their **stimulus-response theory,** which emphasized reward as the most important element in forming new behavioral responses. Today's behavioral therapists believe that emotional problems stem from poor learning, conditioning, dysfunctional self-thinking, lack of skills, avoiding anxious situations, and misconceptions about reality. Therapeutic techniques focus on understanding the client's current behavior. The "past" is important only as it affects present actions.

Behavioral therapists teach clients to change dysfunctional thought and behavioral patterns by using **behavior modification therapies** to replace undesirable behaviors with more appropriate actions. They also provide social skills and **assertiveness training,** which teaches clients to express themselves in constructive, nonaggressive ways. The behavioral school also promotes continual research as a tool for refining and improving treatment strategies.

HUMANISTIC THEORIES AND THERAPIES

By the mid-1950s, the two main schools of thought in the study of human behavior were the psychoanalytical and the behavioral. Critics, however, believed that something was missing, and several began to look at human nature from a different point of view. This new outlook evolved into the field of humanistic psychology.

Humanistic theories are an important part of many of today's therapies because they emphasize the **total** individual. All realms of the human condition are considered important. Humanists also believe in the innate goodness of human nature and focus on the positive aspects of humanity. In short, people are holistic and multidimensional (many-sided) individuals—adapting to stress within a changing environment. These ideas serve as the foundation for the concept of holism and the model of comprehensive health care delivery.

PERLS AND GESTALT THERAPY

The first contribution to the humanistic movement was made by Fredrick Perls (1893-1970), a German-born physician who worked with brain-injured soldiers after World War I. He studied psychoanalysis, but it was his years of work with his clients that sparked the idea of the gestalt, which means "whole." From this concept, Perls developed his psychotherapy, which he termed **gestalt** therapy. Perls accepted the notion of unresolved past conflicts, but he also stressed the present, freedom, responsibility, and attempts to become whole (or "actualized"). Perls' gestalt therapy paved the way for further exploration into human nature.

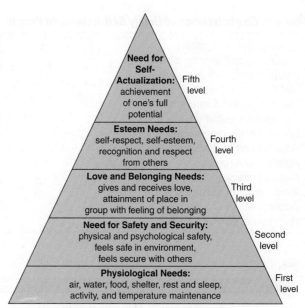

FIGURE **5-1** Maslow's hierarchy of needs.

MASLOW'S INFLUENCE

Abraham Maslow (1908-1970) had a strong impact on the practice of nursing and health care. His ideas about holistic psychology were published extensively in theories of personality, motivation, self-actualization, and human nature. The core concept of Maslow's theories is that human nature is essentially good and contains the inherent potential for self-fulfillment (Maslow, 1971). He explored how people cope with and adapt to their situations. His investigations of people who function at highly successful levels led to a theory of motivation that has become widely adopted throughout the health care professions.

Maslow grouped human needs into a hierarchy or ranking (Figure 5-1). Lower-order needs include physical and social requirements. Physical needs for air, water, food, elimination, and reproduction take first priority. The individual will perish if these needs are not filled. Second-priority needs relate to safety, security, and protection. Love and belonging needs come next. Everyone needs to feel accepted as part of a family or group. People who are lonely or isolated have unfulfilled belonging needs. Last are the needs for esteem, which include the needs for self-respect and the respect of others.

Higher-order needs for optimal functioning include aesthetic and self-actualization needs. Aesthetic needs relate to the values of beauty, goodness, order, justice, and simplicity, whereas self-actualization needs encourage individuals to develop to their highest potential.

To understand the nature of self-actualized people, Maslow studied individuals who were highly successful. He found they had several similar characteristics (Box 5-1). Maslow also believed that when needs go unmet illnesses can develop.

Today, Maslow's hierarchy of needs serves as a basis for planning and prioritizing client care. To illustrate,

| Box 5-1 | *Characteristics of Highly Self-Actualized People* |

Comfortable with reality
Expresses self spontaneously
Independent, self-directing
Has emotional depth
Has a high social interest
Expresses creativity
Shows democratic values
Accepts self and others
Able to solve problems
Needs privacy and detachment
Identifies with humanity
Appreciates life
Has gentle sense of humor

Think About 5-1

The client, a 22-year-old woman, has been admitted with anxiety, an inability to retain food or fluids, and shortness of breath. She has no health insurance and has lived alone since her recent divorce.
- Using Maslow's hierarchy, list the client's problems (unmet needs) in order of priority.

maintaining a client's airway (a physical need) takes priority over a need for socialization. Many clients in today's health care environments are experiencing unmet basic needs. Every nurse should be able to accurately assess and plan therapeutic interventions according to the client's **most critical unmet needs** (see Think About 5-1). Maslow was instrumental in the development of humanism, but he also gave us the tools for designing effective health care.

ROGERS' CLIENT-CENTERED THERAPY

Carl Rogers (1902-1987) developed a new approach to psychotherapy. During his work as a child guidance therapist, he became influenced by the theories of Otto Rank, a psychoanalyst who thought that people have a self-directing ability that emerges during therapy. Rank broke from the traditional techniques of therapy by stating that the client should direct the therapeutic relationship using the therapist as a guide to self-understanding. Inspired by Rank's ideas, Rogers began work on a new system of psychotherapy.

Rogers also built on Maslow's work by stressing the goal of self-actualization. He believed that the goal of therapy is to assist clients in becoming increasingly more aware of their experiences and emotions. Rogers thought that the therapeutic relationship should foster an open and trusting climate in which clients can safely and freely express themselves. The therapist's task is to reflect clients' feelings and support work toward healthy functioning and self-actualization.

The efforts of Rogers have benefited the disciplines of nursing, pastoral counseling, and education. He

also worked with many leaders, policymakers, and groups experiencing conflict. However, his greatest legacy was his focus on the positive, achieving side of human nature, which gave people permission to accept themselves.

CURRENT HUMANISTIC THERAPIES

Many humanistic theories are with us today. The concept of **holism** has led to the development of a holistic health care model in which each client is viewed as a unique person functioning within a changing environment. The concept of **basic needs** is used to plan and prioritize health care, to allocate scarce resources, and to assist clients in achieving their best.

Several therapies have evolved from the humanistic movement. Everett Shostrom developed a system of therapy based on the goal of self-actualization rather than cure. His **actualizing therapy** assists clients in learning to trust their inner or "core" selves despite life's negative influences.

Viktor Frankl's psychotherapy is based on a person's need to search for meaning and values in life. He called his system **logotherapy,** based on the Greek word for "meaning." His ideas of human worth and dignity grew out of his 3-year experience in a concentration camp (after having lost his entire family) during World War II.

Newer therapies continue to evolve, but each will be grounded in the basic premise of humanism: people are dynamic, multidimensional beings who strive for personal fulfillment.

SYSTEMS THEORIES

Systems theorists view humans as functioning within a set of related units (called **systems**). Royce and Powell (1983) developed the "open and closed systems" concept. They defined an open system as having boundaries that are permeable, passable, and accessible. Energy and information pass easily among open systems, and the organism grows and flourishes. A closed system has rigid, impermeable boundaries that shut out information and energy. If the system remains closed, the organism eventually will die.

Kurt Lewin (1890-1947) developed a **field theory** that proposed that behavior must be considered within the total situation. He rejected notions of past, future, or cause and effect and focused only on the immediate situation. People were systems who interact with other systems across boundaries. His concept of equilibrium states that each system attempts to maintain a balance, or steady state, within itself and among other systems.

Lewin also developed the concept of life space—the psychological field or space in which one moves. Life space includes oneself, other people, and objects. Behavior is viewed as a function of life space. Lewin also proposed the concept of **psychological tension,** which results from the interaction of opposing systems. Although his work is complex, Lewin's theories influenced the development of several therapies.

In 1960, Maxwell Maltz published a popular book titled *Psycho-cybernetics*, which explained how "positive thinking" works by programming one's behavior to achieve a desired self-image. Systems theories differ from other approaches. Systems theorists believe that behavior originates **within** the organism. All creatures are open systems with input, output, and regulating feedback mechanisms. People are open systems in a state of continual exchange, interacting within themselves, with other people, and with their environments.

COGNITIVE THEORIES AND THERAPIES

The word cognition is a general term that means "to know." It includes the mental activities of attention, language, imagery, memory, perception, and problem solving. The development of modern cognitive psychology began in the 1890s with the work of Paul DuBois, a Swiss psychologist who believed that mental illness resulted from incorrect ideas. His **rational psychotherapy** changed the incorrect ideas through the use of reason and logic. Alfred Adler's **individual therapy** and Jean Piaget's work contributed to cognitive psychology by demonstrating the importance of intellectual factors in human development.

Albert Bandura's **social learning theory** established a relationship between cognition and behavior. His work focused on the importance of learning through the use of symbols, imitation, and one's capacity for self-regulation through reflection and control. People learn by observing the outcomes of various situations (Bandura, 1986). These observations then develop into expectations and emotions. As a result, people compare themselves with others and make judgments based on their expectations and emotions. Thus our decisions act to determine our behaviors.

The main goal of all cognitive therapies is to replace dysfunctional beliefs and thoughts in order to cause a change in personal viewpoints. Clients develop successful self-control strategies by attacking dysfunctional behaviors and then learning specific coping skills. Current cognitive therapeutic techniques are grouped into three categories: cognitive restructuring, coping skills, and problem-solving skills.

COGNITIVE RESTRUCTURING THERAPIES

During the 1950s, Alfred Ellis developed a theory, called **rational-emotive-behavioral therapy (REBT),** and treatment based on the irrational beliefs and unrealistic expectations people hold of themselves. He felt that it was not the event itself but the value placed on the event that determined behavior. The goals of REBT are to help clients (1) gain insight into the irrational beliefs that cause their disturbed behaviors, (2) cease actively reinforcing the disturbed behaviors, (3) monitor the effects of their thoughts, and (4) adopt more appropriate outlooks by practicing more effective thoughts. By 1979, Aaron Beck introduced **cognitive therapy** to help clients recognize their self-defeating tendencies and replace them with more adaptive thinking. Donald Meichenbaum's **self-instructional training** takes a different approach to cognitive therapy. He believes that undesirable behaviors are the result of faulty instructions given in childhood. Therapy consists of using imagery, modeling, and anxiety control techniques to adopt new self-talk patterns. Today, **cognitive remediation** is used to help brain-injured children develop concentration, organization, and confidence (Graves, 2007).

COPING SKILLS THERAPIES

Several models have been introduced to teach clients how to develop more successful daily living skills. During the 1970s, Joseph Cautela described the process of **covert modeling**—the act of mentally rehearsing a difficult performance or event before actually doing the activity. This mental practice has been used by sport psychologists to improve the performance of their players. **Coping skills training** is similar to covert modeling except that anxiety is first induced and then the client is trained to "relax the images away." Coping skills taught by cognitive therapists include training in anxiety management, assertiveness, progressive relaxation, and techniques to reduce physical responses to stress.

PROBLEM-SOLVING THERAPIES

Some cognitive therapists see the cause of dysfunctional emotions as an inability to successfully solve problems. **Problem-solving therapy** teaches clients to solve their problems in more constructive and satisfying ways. Box 5-2 lists the steps in the problem-solving process. Note the similarities between this and the nursing (therapeutic) process.

REALITY THERAPY

William Glasser, MD, (1925-) founded the Institute for Reality Therapy to educate people about his therapeutic techniques. Glasser's theory, like Maslow's, states that people are born with certain basic needs. He thought that the most important needs are to be loved and belong, followed by needs to gain self-worth, respect, and recognition. Glasser believed that the problems of mental illness are rooted in failures within the social areas of functioning. He described people with mental illness as irresponsible and believed that values, ethics, and morals provide the basis for right behaviors. His "three Rs" of therapy encourage clients to do what is "realistic, responsible, and right" (Glasser, 1965).

Reality therapists help clients to examine and evaluate the effectiveness of their behaviors and then develop

---

Box 5-2 *Problem-Solving Process*

1. State the problem.
2. Collect information about the problem.
3. Identify the causes or patterns of the problem.
4. Examine all possible options.
5. Choose the best option, and apply it to the problem.
6. Examine the outcomes of the option's application.
7. Evaluate and revise actions based on outcomes.

---

more effective ways to satisfy their needs. Therapists and clients plan behavioral changes, and then contracts are made and both agree to abide by them. The use of contracts builds rapport, trust, and commitment. Reality therapy has become a valuable tool in treating chemical dependency problems. Glasser's methods have also been taught to thousands of educators who follow the principles of his book *Schools Without Failure.*

SOCIOCULTURAL THEORIES

Theories that focus on the social nature of people were introduced in the early twentieth century with the inquiries of George Mead. He believed that the social setting was extremely important in the development of one's self-concept. Mead stated that as children learn the rules and norms of their society, they take on approved behaviors. Breaking the rules results in social rejection and labeling if behaviors do not fall within acceptable social limits. Mead's concepts encouraged theorists to consider the social aspects of behavior.

MENTAL ILLNESS AS MYTH

In the 1950s, Thomas Szasz published a series of books and articles attacking the concepts of mental illness by arguing that deviant (different) behaviors were culturally defined. Szasz stated that all societies have individuals whose behaviors are considered abnormal and ways of controlling their more undesirable members. Many societies do this by labeling people as "mentally ill" and removing them to institutions where they are taught to conform to more socially approved behaviors (Szasz, 1974). According to Szasz, **people are responsible for their behavior.** Even those labeled mentally ill have the choice to take part in the labeling process by allowing it to occur. He also strongly stated that mental illness is not an illness but a socially defined condition.

Szasz believed that clients should be able to choose their therapist and treatment, define the problems they wanted to solve, and work with the therapist to change. Therapy was completed when the client felt satisfied with the changes. His perspective has sparked a reexamination of the moral, legal, and political aspects of modern psychiatry.

The field of **community psychology** has evolved to focus on promoting changes in society at the community level. Community therapists work with local groups and organizations to improve social conditions, such as hunger, homelessness, teen pregnancies, and social conflict.

BIOBEHAVIORAL THEORIES

Biobehavioral theories follow the medical model, which states that illness is the result of abnormalities in the structure, function, or chemistry of the body. A history, physical examination, laboratory tests, imaging techniques, and electroencephalograms (EEGs; brain wave recordings) are used to assist in diagnosis. The problem-solving approach is then applied to the data, and treatment plans are developed. Therapy is considered effective when the cause of the problem has been eliminated. Today, the fields of **behavioral medicine** and **psychobiology** are dedicated to uncovering new knowledge about the inner chemical and biological workings of the body.

HOMEOSTASIS

Walter Cannon, in the 1920s, was the first to consider the physical aspects of mental illness. His research on changes in the body's physiology during emotion led to the observation that the body always attempts to stabilize itself. Cannon believed that an emotion is a reaction that causes the body to use its resources. He described an **emergency syndrome,** which consists of a total body response that results in fright, fight, or flight behaviors when the individual is challenged or threatened. Cannon introduced the concept of homeostasis, which he defined as the tendency of the body to achieve and maintain a steady internal state. Disease, in his view, was the fight to maintain the body's homeostasis (balance) within an open system. The concept of homeostasis has also been applied to family systems, holistic health, and world ecology.

STRESS ADAPTATION THEORY

Hans Selye (1907-1982) was educated in France, Italy, Germany, and Canada. During his many years of study, he repeatedly observed students who were "just feeling sick." This led him to study Cannon's emergency syndrome and launched him toward years of research into the physical and biochemical changes associated with stress. The results of his studies led Selye to believe that many physical problems (e.g., hypertension, arthritis, coronary artery disease) are related to an inability to control stress (Selye, 1976).

Selye defined a stressor as a nonspecific response of the body to any demand placed on it. One's daily dose of stressors created what Selye called the "wear and tear" on the body. His studies revealed that people respond to stress in the same physical manner regardless

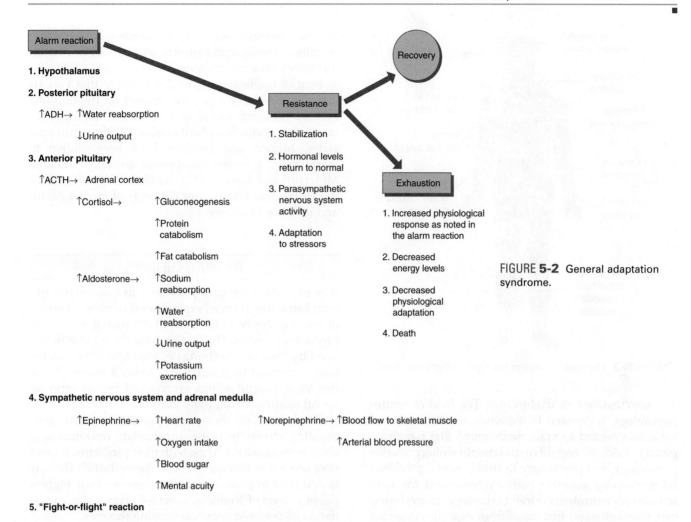

FIGURE **5-2** General adaptation syndrome.

of the stressor. Selye's stress adaptation theory (also called the **general adaptation syndrome**) describes the body's physical responses to stress and the process by which people adapt. The general adaptation syndrome consists of three stages: alarm, resistance, and exhaustion (Figure 5-2).

When stress is first perceived, the brain triggers an **alarm** reaction that releases hormones that prepare the body to stand and defend itself or run away from the threat, the **fight-or-flight response** (Figure 5-3). If the individual successfully adapts by coping with the stress, the body's heightened level of functioning returns to its usual state. However, if the stress cannot be resolved, the body continues to function at a high metabolic rate and progresses toward the next stage of adaptation.

The stage of **resistance** is the body's optimal attempt to cope with the stress. All coping skills and defense mechanisms are mobilized. Problem solving becomes difficult. The individual becomes more susceptible to other, unrelated stresses. He or she either adapts to the stress or progresses to the body's final attempt at homeostasis, the stage of **exhaustion.**

When stressors are overwhelming or last too long, the individual's resources become depleted and the organism begins to exhaust itself. Body processes break down as glands fail to produce the elevated levels of hormones required to meet the threat. Thinking becomes illogical and distorted. Problem solving and communications are ineffective. Unless the stress is removed or adapted to, the individual continues to use all physical and emotional resources until death from exhaustion results. Chilling examples of Selye's general adaptation syndrome are seen in the accounts of prisoners of war and concentration camp survivors of World War II. Selye's work reminds us that effective health care can neither be given nor received if stress levels are ignored.

PSYCHOBIOLOGY

"Psychobiology is the study of the biochemical foundations of thought, mood, emotion, and behavior" (Wilson, 1994). By applying the latest imaging technology and biochemistry, researchers are exploring human mental experiences and emotional states to learn about mood disorders, schizophrenia, language problems, and other conditions. Research is spawning new fields of study, theories, and therapies. Psychobiological theories about the causes of mental illness relate to genetics, neurotransmitter activity, viruses, fetal development,

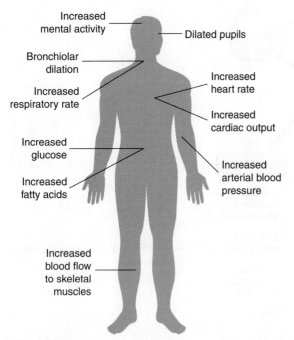

FIGURE **5-3** Physical findings of the fight-or-flight response.

and immune system dysfunction. The field of **neuropsychology** is devoted to the study and treatment of behaviors related to brain functioning. The interdisciplinary field of **cognitive psychophysiology** blends psychology and physiology to study mental processes by monitoring selective body systems, and the new science of **neurobehavioral toxicology** is exploring behavioral changes that result from exposure to toxins in the environment.

PSYCHONEUROIMMUNOLOGY

In the early 1960s, Jonas Salk developed a model of disease that encompassed the genetic, neurological, immune, and behavioral systems. Robert Ader (1981) later built on this model. His studies of the effects of stress on the immune system led him to coin the term **psychoneuroimmunology (PNI)**, the study of interactions among the body's central nervous system, its immune system, and aspects of the personality.

Ader's studies demonstrated that anxiety and depression can decrease immune system functions. Other researchers found that pain-relieving mechanisms in the brain could be activated by the body. Pain control by activating the opiate pathways in the brain has been seen in athletes, yogis, and women during labor. Some nurses are using this knowledge to help clients cope with severe pain by teaching them to turn on the body's pain-relieving mechanisms.

Research into **neurotransmitters** (the body's chemical messenger system) uncovered the existence of **neuropeptides**, neurotransmitters composed of amino acid strings. Further research found that these amino acid strings actually connect the endocrine, immune, and nervous systems. It is believed this neurobiochemical system provides the pathway for emotional reactions.

As research continues, there is mounting evidence that emotions, stress, and attitudes all have an impact on the body's immune response.

Studies are beginning to demonstrate that various interventions have a positive impact on the immune system. Research found that relaxation exercises increase the production of antibodies. Positive emotional states, humor, and laughter have been shown to increase an immune component in saliva (Dillon, Minchoff, and Baker, 1985). As the results of new research become known, our concepts of mental health and illness will change.

NURSING THEORIES

It is important for care providers to understand human behaviors from a helping point of view. Theories of nursing apply to the care of emotional as well as physical problems. The first nursing theory was developed by Florence Nightingale, who saw illness as the body's attempt to repair itself. Today's nursing theories view people as biopsychosocial beings who respond to stress in uniquely individual ways.

The focus of the therapeutic process in nursing is on assisting clients in using appropriate resources and abilities to effectively cope with their problems. Nurses may use many therapeutic techniques, but all therapy is designed to assist clients in achieving their highest possible level of wellness. Table 5-4 gives a brief explanation of the most common nursing theories.

As research increases our knowledge, our understanding of mental illness will broaden and new therapies will be introduced. Current mental health therapies are grouped into two basic categories: psychotherapy and somatic therapy.

PSYCHOTHERAPIES

Psychotherapy is the treating of mental and emotional disorders by psychological, rather than physical, means. Psychotherapies began with Freud's psychoanalysis and now include behavior therapies, cognitive therapies, crisis intervention, and hypnosis. Psychotherapeutic sessions take place on an individual basis or in a group setting.

INDIVIDUAL THERAPIES

Clients who work on a one-to-one basis with a therapist are involved in individual therapy. During **psychoanalysis**, clients analyze the meaning of certain behaviors and symbols and learn to cope by understanding the meaning or significance of their behaviors.

Client-centered psychotherapy is based on the premise that "every person has within themselves the resources for constructive change" (Smoyak, 1993).

Table 5-4 *Summary of Nursing Theories*

THEORIST	GOAL OF NURSING	FRAMEWORK FOR PRACTICE
Hildegard Peplau—1952	To develop interpersonal interaction between client and nurse	Interpersonal model emphasizes relationship between client and nurse
Ida Orlando—1954	To respond to client's behavior in terms of immediate needs	A nursing situation composed of client behavior, nurse reaction, and nurse action
Virginia Henderson—1955	To help client gain independence as rapidly as possible	Henderson's 14 basic needs
Dorothy Johnson—1968	To reduce stress so that client can recover as quickly as possible	Adaptation model based on seven behavioral subsystems
Martha Rogers—1970	To help client achieve maximal level of wellness	"Unitary man" evolves along life process—humanistic nursing
Imogene King—1997	To use communication to reestablish positive adaptation to environment	Nursing process as dynamic interpersonal state between nurse and client
Dorothea Orem—1971	To care for and help client to attain self-care	Self-care deficit theory
Betty Neuman—1995	To assist individuals, families, and groups to attain and maintain maximal level of wellness by purposeful interventions	Systems model of nursing practice having stress reduction as its goal; nursing actions in one of three levels: primary, secondary, or tertiary
Myra Levine—1970	To use conservation activities aimed at optimal use of client's resources	Adaptation model of human as integrated whole based on "four conservation principles of nursing"
Sister Callista Roy—1979	To identify types of demands placed on client and client's adaptation to them	Adaptation model based on four adaptive modes: physiological, psychological, sociological, and independence
Madeleine Leininger—1978	To care for individuals and groups in a culturally specific method meeting their health conditions	Cultural sensitivity with attention to the social structure through ethnonursing care
Jean Watson—1979	To promote health, restore clients to health, and prevent illness	Philosophy and science of caring: caring is an interpersonal process with interventions that result in meeting human needs

From Potter PA, Perry AG: *Fundamentals of nursing*, ed 6, St. Louis, 2005, Mosby.

Here the therapist expresses empathy to encourage growth and healthy change. Mobilizing the client's inner resources through the therapeutic relationship is the goal of client-centered therapy.

Cognitive therapy helps clients identify and correct their distorted thinking and dysfunctional beliefs. The therapist's role is focused on solving the problem within a limited time. Recently, **brief-term therapy** has been introduced in the United States. Studies have demonstrated that 6 to 12 sessions of therapy can be effective. The focus of therapy is on the problem that faces the client at the moment. Brief-term therapy has been effective for managing depression, stress, and marriage and family problems.

Behavioral therapy is tailored to each person's needs, behavior, and environment. Behavior modification techniques are used by therapists and clients to define positive behaviors and reinforce behavior changes. Behavior modification has proven effective with developmentally disabled persons and those with severe forms of mental illness.

GROUP THERAPIES

Group psychotherapy was developed after World War II because of a shortage of psychiatrists. The central tasks of any therapeutic group are to (1) relieve emotional discomfort and human misery and (2) cause psychological and behavioral changes.

Group therapy gatherings follow the medical model. Membership in the group is limited by the therapist. Group members are called "patients" who consider themselves "ill" and consequently exhibit "sick" behaviors. The goal of the therapist is to help "cure" patients of their problems.

Self-help groups are limited to those who share a common problem, symptom, or life situation. Examples include Alcoholics Anonymous (alcohol use problems), Synanon (drug use problems), Reach for Recovery (for postmastectomy women), and support groups for families of persons with mental illness.

T-groups evolved from systems theories. During the 1950s, basic skills training (BST) groups were formed by the National Education Association and the Research Center for Group Dynamics at M.I.T. to study the dynamics of group behavior. Professionals from different disciplines began to adapt T-group concepts to their fields. Therapists with a client-centered clinical focus developed the **encounter group,** which uses a professional trainer to encourage intense group interaction. Other practitioners focused on small work groups and productivity.

Last, **consciousness-raising groups** use the interactions among their members as a vehicle for achieving behavioral changes. The group is supportive of change, allowing individuals to analyze their interactions and then "try out" new behaviors with people from varied backgrounds.

Group therapy causes changes in behavior through one or more change mechanisms (Table 5-5). The evidence compiled over 35 years demonstrates that

Table 5-5 *Group Change Mechanisms*

THERAPEUTIC MECHANISM	DESCRIPTION
Expressiveness	Group members share emotional expression of positive and negative emotions.
Experience of intense emotion	Generating intense group emotion activates individual issues.
Altruism	The experience of helping others improves low self-esteem and poor self-concept.
Self-disclosure	The sharing of deeply personal material involves risk and develops trust.
Cognitive factors	Intellectual knowledge leads to a deeper understanding of self.
Communion	Groups foster a sense of oneness and belonging.
Discovering similarities	Relief is experienced when individuals discover that their problems are not unique.
Experimentation	Working with new behaviors within the low-risk group setting encourages change.
Feedback	Receiving information about how one is perceived by others is unique to groups.
Feelings of hope	Groups help individuals feel and believe that they can change with the group's help.

many groups do provide benefits for their members. Emotional support for one another appears to be an effective therapeutic tool.

ONLINE THERAPY

A number of therapists have established online therapy practices. Various therapies and services, ranging from answering a single question to ongoing counseling, are offered. Critics feel online therapy may be unethical and ineffective. Proponents see it as a way to reach individuals who are otherwise unable to seek counseling. Web therapy has sparked fierce debates about its usefulness. Currently, the American Psychological Association is studying the issue.

SOMATIC THERAPIES

The word **somatic** refers to the body. Historically, therapies for people with psychological distresses have been divided into those that work primarily with the mind (psychotherapies) and those that affect the body (**somatic therapies**). This division will soon fade as our knowledge of emotion and human physiology evolves.

Today, the somatic treatment of mental illness is growing with the introduction of new therapies based on biochemical and physiological research. Drug treatment therapy and electroconvulsive therapy were

established years ago and are still in use today. Biofeedback and phototherapy are relatively recent developments. Acupuncture as a therapy for addictions is the application of an ancient treatment method to modern problems.

PHARMACOTHERAPY

The use of drugs to change behavior dates back centuries, but it was not until the 1950s that medications for the control of mental illness were widely available. Currently, there are several groups of medicines that affect the mind. See Chapter 7 for a more detailed discussion.

FUTURE DEVELOPMENTS

New therapies are currently being introduced. Feminist and **women's therapy** grew from the feminist movement of the 1970s; **creative aggression therapy** teaches clients to redirect their aggression and "fight fairly"; and **movement therapy** attempts to bring the body in tune with itself to restore balance. Therapies that complement traditional medicine, such as acupuncture, are being successfully used to treat mental health discomforts. Theories about the nature of human beings and their environments will continue to develop faster than our ability to make sense of it all. Evolving theories and their research activities now flow across many fields of study. Our understanding of human nature will continue to expand and encourage us to explore the most complex of all worlds, the one inside the self.

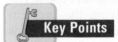 **Key Points**

- Theories and models help to explain human development and behavior.
- Charles Darwin's theories led to the belief that mental illness was the result of inferior genetic makeup and a lower place on the evolutionary scale.
- Sigmund Freud's study of the unconscious processes of the mind evolved into theories about the structure, development, defenses, and dynamics of the personality.
- Analytical psychology was founded by Carl Jung, who recognized the spiritual and creative powers of people as well as their potential for growth.
- Alfred Adler's individual therapy focuses on the ideas of choice, individual responsibility, and finding the meaning in life.
- Harry Stack Sullivan's interpersonal psychology described six stages of social development and believed that the therapist's role was to sensitively assist clients in understanding how distorted images contribute to the anxiety and isolation in their lives.
- Jean Piaget's theory of cognitive development describes four stages of intellectual and emotional growth.

- Erik Erikson's stages of psychosocial development state that, as each developmental (core) task is mastered, individuals build and unite their personalities.
- The foundation for behavioral theories and their therapies is that all behavior is learned and is seen as responses to stimuli.
- Ivan Pavlov developed the concept of conditioning.
- John B. Watson stated that psychology was the objective science of behavior and began the movement known as behaviorism.
- B.F. Skinner's experiments found that positive reinforcement enforced behaviors, whereas negative reinforcement weakened behaviors.
- Behavioral therapies today assist clients in learning how to change their dysfunctional thoughts and behavioral patterns. Examples include behavior modification techniques, assertiveness training, and training in the social skills.
- Humanistic theories view the individual as a multidimensional person who adapts to stress within a dynamic environment while striving for self-fulfillment.
- The concept of gestalt led Fredrick Perls to develop a system of therapy that stressed the present, personal freedom, and attempts to become a whole person.
- Maslow's hierarchy of needs categorizes physical and psychological requirements for functioning and describes the characteristics of successful, highly self-actualized people.
- Carl Rogers built on Maslow's work by stressing the goals of self-actualization and awareness.
- Current humanistic theories have led to holistic health care, planning based on priorities of human needs, and therapies designed to assist clients in taking charge of their lives.
- Systems theories view humans as functioning within a set of interacting and related units called systems.
- Cognitive theories focus on the importance of intellectual factors in human development and function.

- Cognitive restructuring, coping skills techniques, and problem-solving skills help clients develop successful self-control strategies by attacking dysfunctional behaviors and then learning specific coping skills.
- Glasser's reality therapy teaches people how to fill their needs in effective, satisfying, and appropriate ways.
- Sociocultural theories focus on the impact of a society on its people's behaviors and view mental illness as the result of social conditions.
- Thomas Szasz states that mental illness is a culturally defined myth with which people cooperate.
- Biobehavioral theories follow the medical model, which states that illness is the result of abnormalities in the structure, function, or chemistry of the body.
- The concept of homeostasis was developed during the 1920s by Cannon, who found that the body has a tendency to achieve and maintain a steady internal state.
- The general adaptation syndrome, described by Hans Selye, consists of the stages of alarm, resistance, and exhaustion.
- Psychobiology is the study of the biochemical bases of thought, mood, emotion, and behavior.
- Psychoneuroimmunology is the study of the interactions among an individual's central nervous system, immune system, and personality.
- Nursing theories view people as biopsychosocial beings who respond to stress in uniquely individual ways.
- Research has demonstrated that emotions affect immune functions.
- Current treatments for mental health problems include various individual and group psychotherapies and somatic therapies, such as medications, biofeedback, phototherapy, and acupuncture.

---

evolve Be sure to visit the companion Evolve site at http://evolve.elsevier.com/Morrison-Valfre/ for additional online resources.

Upon completion of this chapter, the student will be able to:

1. Explain the major difference between alternative and complementary therapies.
2. Analyze how the concept of holistic care relates to integrative medicine.
3. State the purpose of the National Center for Complementary and Alternative Medicine (NCCAM).
4. Examine what is meant by the term *whole medical systems.*
5. List three biologically based practices.
6. Discuss the basic premise of mind-body medicine.
7. Identify the theory underlying energy medicine therapies.
8. Describe four mental health problems that may be helped by complementary and alternative medicine (CAM) therapies.
9. Examine seven alternative approaches to mental health care.
10. Specify two precautions relating to CAM therapies.

Key Terms

acupuncture (ăK-ū-PŬNK-chŭr) (p. 57)
allopathic (ăl-ō-PĂTH-ĭk) (p. 52)
alternative medicine (p. 52)
aromatherapy (ă-RŌ-mă THĔR-ă-pē) (p. 54)
Ayurveda (Ā-yŭr-vā-dă) (p. 53)
biofeedback (p. 57)
chelation (kē-LĀ-shŭn) (p. 55)
chiropractic (kī-rō-PRĂK-tĭk) (p. 55)
complementary (KŎM-plĕ-MĔN-tĕ-rē) medicine (p. 52)
dietary supplements (p. 54)
electromagnetic fields (EMF) (p. 58)
expressive therapy (p. 56)
Eye Movement Desensitization and Reprocessing (EMDR) (p. 55)
homeopathy (hō-mē-ŎP-ă-thē) (p. 54)
hypnosis (p. 56)
integrative medicine (p. 52)
massage (p. 55)
meditation (p. 56)
naturopathy (nā-chŭr-ŎP-ă-thē) (p. 54)
prayer (p. 57)
Qi Gong (kē Gŏng) (p. 58)
Reiki (RĪ-kē) (p. 58)
spirituality (SPĬR-ĭ-tū-ĂL-ĭ-tē) (p. 57)
therapeutic (thĕr-ă-PŪ-tĭk) touch (p. 58)
traditional Chinese medicine (TCM) (p. 54)
whole medical systems (p. 53)

There are many systems of treatment for physical and mental problems in our world today. Some are very old and rooted in the cultures of their practitioners and people. Other systems and practices are more recent developments. Some practices are rooted in objective (empirical) data, whereas others use energy fields as a basis for treatment. All, however, share the common goal of relieving pain and improving the quality of life.

DEFINITION OF TERMS
Allopathic Medicine

The mainstream of health care practices in the modern world is based on **allopathic** methods of treatment. Allopathic practitioners use medical and surgical methods to treat disease and injury by finding what is "wrong" and "fixing" it. Allopathic medicine is based upon observation, scientific research, and objective explanations. Physicians (MDs), nurses, psychologists, and therapists receive years of special training before they are allowed to practice.

Complementary Medicine

Complementary medicine includes practices and treatments that agree or "work with" allopathic therapies. They are used **along with** common medical treatments. Massage, for example, may ease pain and relax an injured body part. Complementary medicine practitioners usually undergo some type of formal training. Many medical practices are culturally based. Practitioners may or may not be formally educated.

Alternative Medicine

Alternative medicine refers to practices and treatments that are used **instead of** conventional (allopathic) medicine. People with cancer who use special herbs or follow a certain diet to treat the problem are examples.

Integrative Medicine

Integrative medicine attempts to blend the most effective practices and treatments from both conventional and alternative treatment systems. Emphasis is on the interrelationship among body, mind, and spirit.

Holistic Care

Most current mental health care delivery systems are diagnosis and treatment oriented. Traditionally, most people received mental health care only after the onset of behavioral signs and symptoms. This resulted in acute conditions that were more difficult and expensive to treat. Emphasis was rarely on prevention or early diagnosis.

Since the 1980s, researchers have found that emotions cause chemical changes within the body that in turn affect the physical state. As health care models were developed to recognize the interrelatedness of mind, body, and environment, a movement (known as holism) began to emerge.

The word *holism* is derived from the Greek word *holos,* meaning "whole." Holism today views a person as more than just the sum of his or her parts. The concept of holism helps to blend many aspects of mental health care. The primary goal of holistic mental health care providers is to "help clients develop strategies to achieve harmony within themselves and with others, nature, and the world" (Rawlins, Williams, and Beck, 1993). This statement reflects the holistic concept of care. We are no longer content to treat the illness. We are learning to treat the whole person (Figure 6-1).

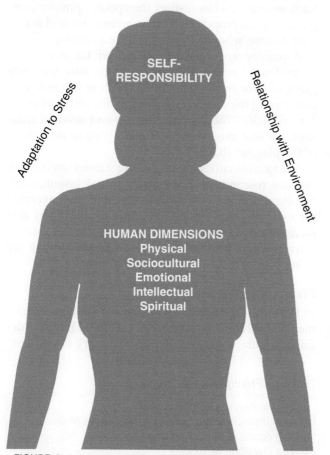

FIGURE **6-1** Holistic health care concepts: relationship with human dimensions, self-responsibility, adaptation to stress, and environment.

NATIONAL CENTER FOR COMPLEMENTARY AND ALTERNATIVE MEDICINE

The National Center for Complementary and Alternative Medicine (NCCAM) is a part of the U.S. National Institute of Health. The organization is "dedicated to exploring complementary and alternative healing practices in the context of rigorous science" (NCCAM, 2007c). Simply put, NCCAM seeks scientific validation for CAM therapies. It also acts as an information resource center for an interested public. For the sake of discussion, CAM therapies can be divided into two basic groups, body-based CAM and energy-based CAM.

Recent studies "suggest that from 50% to 80% of people suffering from mental disorders use CAM" (Pellegrini and Ruggeri, 2007). As you can see, it is important for health care providers to be familiar with CAM therapies and their most appropriate uses.

BODY-BASED CAM THERAPIES

These therapies focus on working with the body's natural abilities to heal itself. They include a variety of therapies. Some, such as Chinese medicine, are very old, whereas others are of more recent origin. Here we will briefly discuss the most commonly used CAM therapies.

WHOLE MEDICAL SYSTEMS

Whole medical systems are built on complete systems of theory and practice. They include modern, Western medicine as well as osteopathy, homeopathy, naturopathy, and culturally based systems such as ayurveda and Oriental medicine. Several systems have developed outside of Western medicine, and some are much older. Table 6-1 presents examples of three main culturally based healing systems. All systems, however, teach that wellness is a state of balance (physical, mental, spiritual) and illness is an imbalance. Herbal and natural remedies, along with good diet, exercise, and meditation/prayer, will correct the imbalance.

Ayurveda

Ayurveda is a healing system that was developed in India and literally means "the science of life." Ayurvedic medicine is described as "knowledge of how to live." Focus is on the innate harmony of the body, mind, and

Table 6-1 *Examples of Culturally Based Healing Systems*

ORIENTAL SYSTEMS	INDIAN SYSTEMS	AMERICAN INDIAN SYSTEMS
Acupuncture	Ayurveda	Sweat lodges
Shiatsu	Yoga	Talking circles
Reiki	Meditation	Cleansing rituals

spirit. Therapies such as diet, meditation, herbs, yoga, exposure to sunlight, and controlled breathing are designed to restore balance, thus healing the individual.

Homeopathy

Homeopathy is "a therapeutic method that uses natural substances in micro-doses to relieve symptoms" (Boiron, 2007). It is based on the "principle of similars." Its founder, German physician Samuel Hahnemann (1755-1843), developed treatments for his patients by choosing a very small portion of a substance that matched the patient's symptoms. Only one substance at a time is used, and the effects are closely monitored. Although the NCCAM has found homeopathy to be unproven by scientific studies, there is anecdotal evidence as illustrated in Case Study 6-1.

Naturopathy

Originating in Europe, naturopathy views disease as an alteration in the process by which the body heals itself. The term *naturopathy* means "nature disease." Its focus is on the six principles described in Box 6-1. Practitioners use several therapies, including diet, herbs, nutritional supplements, hydrotherapy, massage, joint manipulation, and lifestyle counseling.

Traditional Chinese Medicine

Traditional Chinese medicine (TCM) can trace its beginnings to 200 BC. It is based on the view that the body is a delicate balance of opposing forces: **yin** and

Case Study 6-1

Judy was a 33-year-old businesswoman with obsessive-compulsive disorder and complicated grief stemming from the unexpected loss of her 3-year-old daughter. She had been taking high doses of antidepressant medications but still felt that life was not worth living. She still blamed herself for the accident that took her beloved daughter and now was overprotective of her older child. Judy's overwhelming burden of guilt focused her thoughts of suicide.

Her obsessive-compulsive behaviors, with her since being sexually abused at age 7, increased dramatically. She began washing her hands 40 times a day and developed a constant fear of germs. The thought of contracting acquired immunodeficiency syndrome (AIDS) terrified her. She dreamed of being attacked and would not fall asleep until early morning. She started losing her hair and was compulsively eating candy.

Upon consulting a naturopath, Judy was started on one homeopathic supplement. Within 3 weeks Judy's psychiatrist recommended she stop taking her antidepressant drugs. With continued therapy from both practitioners, Judy was able to control her compulsive behaviors and obsessions with guilt and suicide.

Modified from Ullman J, Ullman R: Healing with homeopathy, *Townsend Letter* 2:7, 2007.

yang. Yin is cold, slow, and passive, whereas yang is hot, fast, and active. Health is a balance between these two energies. Mental or physical problems arise when an imbalance of these vital energies **(qi)** results. This leads to blockage of energy and blood along the energy pathways **(meridians).**

Treatments are chosen based on individual diagnosis. They include acupuncture, the use of herbs, food therapy, massage, and body manipulation. The Chinese *Materia Medica* is an extremely old reference book of herbs and other medicinal substances.

BIOLOGICALLY BASED PRACTICES

Biologically based practices attempt to improve the human condition through the use of substances extracted from nature. Treatments with these substances include aromatherapy, dietary supplements, and herbal therapies. Some are based on sound scientific evidence. Other therapies await the outcome of research before their usefulness can be examined.

Aromatherapy

Certain scents evoke certain responses in people. Aromatherapy, which means treatment using scents, is the use of essential oils to promote health and well-being. Most essential oils are obtained from extracts or essences of flowers, herbs, trees, fruits, bark, grasses, and seed. Each essential oil has distinct therapeutic, physical, and psychological properties. Certain aromas are said to prevent disease, whereas others produce a calming effect.

Aromatherapy has been practiced for over 6,000 years. Early Greeks, Romans, and Egyptians used fragrant oils for massage, bathing, healing the sick, and embalming the dead. "Hippocrates, the father of modern medicine, used aromatherapy and scented massage. He also used aromatic fumigations to rid Athens of the plague" (ICBS, 2007).

Today, aromatherapy is gaining greater acceptance because research is demonstrating that essential oils can exert specific effects on the individual. Lavender, for example, was found to promote relaxation and increase alpha brain waves, whereas jasmine increased alertness and beta brain waves. Further studies are being conducted.

Dietary Supplements

In 1994, the U.S. Congress passed the Dietary Supplement Health and Education Act (DSHEA), which defined a dietary supplement as a "dietary ingredient"

Box 6-1 *Principles of Naturopathy*

1. The healing power of nature
2. Identification and treatment of the cause of disease
3. The concept of "do no harm"
4. The physician as teacher
5. Treatment of the whole person
6. Prevention

supplement to the diet. Ingredients in dietary supplements can include "vitamins, minerals, herbs or other botanicals, amino acids, and substances such as enzymes, organ tissues, glandulars, and metabolites" (NCCAM, 2007a). In addition, the Food and Drug Administration does not impose the same standards on dietary supplements as they do on prescription drugs. Care must be exercised when considering dietary supplements. Good nutrition, though, can help combat both mental and physical problems.

Herbal Products

The use of certain plants (herbs) to treat disease and alleviate suffering is an ancient, multicultural practice. Almost every culture uses some kind of plant substance to treat the sick. There are thousands of herbal treatments worldwide, but few are scientifically proven using clinical studies. Therefore it becomes difficult to predict adverse effects or interactions with pharmaceutical medications or to judge the safety of using the herb. Research is currently studying the health claims of many commonly used herbal products.

BODY-BASED PRACTICES

CAM practices that involve moving some part of the body are termed body based. These practices focus on moving the body into an improved state of function through treatment.

Chiropractic Treatment

The relationship between body structure (the spine) and function is the subject of study for chiropractic care. Practitioners use a therapy called manipulations to help improve the relationship and help the body heal.

Chelation

The chemical EDTA was synthesized in the 1930s by German scientists. Because of its ability to bind with heavy metals, "proponents claim that EDTA chelation therapy is effective against atherosclerosis and many other serious health problems. However, there is no scientific evidence that this is so" (Green, 2007). Current international studies are being conducted to see if chelation therapy is effective.

Eye Movement Desensitization

In 1987, Francine Shapiro, PhD, a practicing psychologist in Palo Alto, California, introduced a new therapy to treat posttraumatic stress disorder (PTSD). Eye Movement Desensitization and Reprocessing (EMDR) uses controlled eye movements to help reprocess traumatic memories. At first the therapy was dismissed by the scientific community, but published studies in more than 25 scientific journals are proving the value of EMDR. The therapy is gaining popularity. "It has been endorsed by government mental health agencies in the United Kingdom and Israel, and is in wide use throughout the United States and Europe" (Glaser, 2006). EMDR has been used to help victims of 9/11, Hurricane Katrina, and the 2004 South Asia tsunami.

Basically, the clients identify a problem, such as flashbacks or nightmares of the event. They also state what they would like to have happen instead. Then the therapist moves his or her hand or a baton in a certain pattern and clients follow the movement with their eyes while recalling the disturbing event. Each "set" lasts 15 to 20 seconds and ends with clients describing how their self-perceptions have changed. Some clients are helped with one treatment, others require several. Most experience fewer negative emotions associated with the event after treatment.

"Many therapists think EMDR helps the rational left side of the brain to 'knit' a disturbing memory from the emotional right side. Often, therapists describe this as processing" (Glaser, 2006). EMDR is proving to be a useful tool for treating those who suffer from the effects of overwhelming trauma.

Massage

Massage is the manipulation of muscles and connective tissue to relax the body and enhance well-being. It is one of the oldest healing arts, with written records in China that date back 3000 years. Massage reduces stress, promotes relaxation, and improves circulation. It improves sleep, concentration, and energy. Many people with depression and anxiety are helped by the relaxing powers of massage.

Phototherapy

A relatively new development in somatic therapy is the use of bright lights for the treatment of depression. Phototherapy, also known as light therapy, has been used with success in the treatment of seasonal affective disorder (SAD). During the winter months when the available daylight hours are fewer, many people become irritable, unable to concentrate, and even depressed. Researchers found that exposure to full-spectrum light for at least 20 minutes per day resulted in an improvement of depressive symptoms (Rosenthal, 1993). Phototherapy appears to be a promising form of treatment for some disorders, but further studies and research are needed to determine its long-term effectiveness.

ENERGY-BASED CAM THERAPIES

Energy-based therapies base their practices upon two types of energy fields: the veritable and the putative (Table 6-2). Practitioners of energy medicine believe that illness results when the body's energies are out of balance. Therapies are intended to restore the amount and flow of body energy.

MIND-BODY MEDICINE

Followers of mind-body medicine believe that the mind and spirit have the ability to affect the body and its functions. The concept of the mind influencing illness and bodily functions is an old one. Traditional Chinese and Ayurvedic medicine practiced the concept 2000 years ago. Hippocrates, the father of allopathic medicine, believed that the mental, moral, and spiritual aspects of the patient must be considered if treatment was to be successful. This mind-body approach was followed well into the sixteenth century, when Renaissance science directed itself into separating the emotional and spiritual dimensions of humans from the body. As discoveries were made and technologies developed, the purpose became control over nature. Curing the illness became more important than healing the soul. The disease-based model and its search for pathologic conditions became the dominant view.

However, in the 1920s, the work of Howard Cannon revealed the "fight or flight" response and demonstrated a direct relationship between stress and neuroendocrine responses in the body. During World War II, physician Henry Beecher found the **placebo** effect when he injected wounded soldiers with saline instead of morphine and found that much of their pain was controlled. Later research found that as much as 35% of a therapeutic response to any medical procedure could be the result of the client's belief (Beecher, 1959).

Since the 1960s, research into the mind-body connection has been extensive. Much of the evidence demonstrates positive effects related to psychological functioning and improved quality of life. Plus, the risks of mind-body therapies are minimal.

Expressive therapies, such as music or dance, are thought to help people express thoughts and emotions that they are unable to state verbally. Hypnotherapy, meditation, prayer, and spiritual healing are believed to promote relaxation, decrease stress, and relieve emotional or physical pain.

Expressive Therapy

The use of creative activities to decrease stress is not new. Drawing, painting, and sculpting may help release inner conflicts and repressed emotions. Some mental health providers use expressive therapy to help diagnose and treat people with depression, schizophrenia, and trauma related to abuse. Dance and music therapy are helpful for those who are recovering from abuse to gain a sense of ease with their own bodies. Listening to music stimulates the body's neurotransmitter production (opiates and endorphins), which results in "feeling good." Music and sound therapy have successfully been used to treat stress, depression, grief, schizophrenia, and autism.

Hypnotherapy

The traditional definition of hypnosis is the induction of a relaxed, trancelike state in which the individual is receptive to appropriate suggestions. Brain scans of hypnotized persons document different patterns than those who are merely dozing. A typical hypnotherapy session lasts an hour or so. The therapist speaks softly and helps the client become deeply relaxed and tuned out to outside distractions. Once the client reaches "a state of hyperconcentration, the therapist makes suggestions" (Glower, 2005) that can alter the way one thinks and behaves. Smokers, for example, who use hypnosis are more likely to quit successfully. Hypnotherapy is being used to treat gastrointestinal problems, irritable bowel syndrome, pain, headaches, addictions, phobias, and anxiety. Self-induced hypnotic therapies are **relaxation** and **visualization.**

Hypnosis has everyday practical uses also. Bierman (a full-time emergency department physician) focuses on the concepts of human patterns and consciousness. He believes that hypnosis is just **ideas** and **responses.** His work with acutely traumatized clients demonstrates the power of the health care providers' words and actions (Bierman, 1995). Case Study 6-2 illustrates the use of Bierman's response-evoking hypnosis.

Meditation

Meditation has been used in Eastern religions for more than 2500 years. It has gained popularity in the West as a tool for combating stress. Many therapists who recommend meditation for their clients meditate daily themselves. There are many techniques for meditation, but all share four common elements: concentration, retraining the attention to one item while excluding all other thoughts, mindfulness, and an

Case Study 6-2

Larry, an alert 6 year old, arrives at the clinic knowing that he will be on the receiving end of a "shot." He dreads the sight of the approaching nurse and begins to whimper. The nurse smiles and says, "I would like you, Larry, to hold still and look very closely at the circle over there. Tell me whether it's getting bigger or smaller, and really look! Just look hard, and tell me ..." By this time, the injection has been given. "But I don't see it," says Larry. "That's right," says the nurse, "and you didn't feel it either!"

- What do you think made the outcome of this situation so positive?

Table 6-2 *Comparison of Energy Fields*

VERITABLE ENERGY	PUTATIVE (BIOFIELD) ENERGY
• Uses mechanical vibration (sound) electromagnetic forces.	• Based on concept that humans are infused with a form of energy.
• Can be measured.	• Cannot be measured.
• Uses wavelengths and frequencies to treat clients.	• Readjusts the energy flow to treat clients.

altered state of consciousness (Figure 6-2). The physical effects of twice-daily meditation include "slower heart rate, decreased blood pressure, lower oxygen consumption, and increased alpha brain wave production" (Moore, 1994). Meditation techniques have been used successfully in the fields of education, business, medicine, and mental health care.

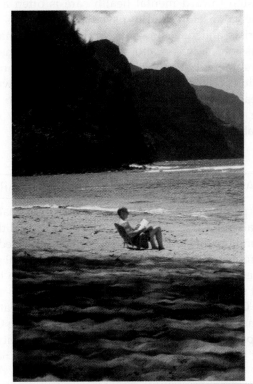

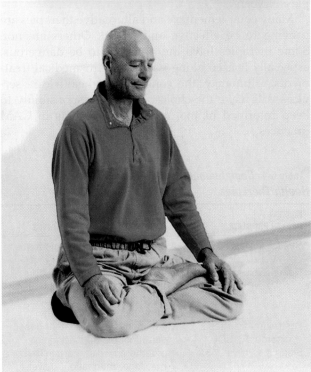

FIGURE **6-2** Meditation can assume many forms.

Prayer and Spiritual Healing

Prayer is the most commonly used CAM therapy in the United States. NCCAM (2007b) defines **prayer** as "an active process of appealing to a higher spiritual power, specifically for health reasons." **Spirituality** has a broader meaning that includes an individual's sense of meaning and purpose in life. Several studies are now being conducted to look at how prayer affects immune system functions and emotional well-being.

ENERGY MEDICINE

Practitioners of energy medicine believe in a vital, life-force energy that flows through the human body. This life force is known by many names (Table 6-3). Although these energies have not been proven scientifically, therapists "claim they can work with this subtle energy, see it with their own eyes, and use it to effect changes in the physical body and influence health" (NCCAM, 2007b). For the purposes of discussion, energy medicine is divided into two parts: biofield therapies and bioelectromagnetic field therapies.

Biofield Therapies

These are among some of the most used but unmeasured CAM therapies. Examples include acupuncture, biofeedback, Qi Gong, Reiki, therapeutic touch, and color therapy.

Acupuncture. For more than 2000 years, a treatment in Oriental medicine has cured disease and alleviated suffering. **Acupuncture** is defined as the inserting of fine needles into the skin along specific sites on the body. These sites travel along energy channels called **meridians.** Stimulating these points is thought to restore the energy or qi balance within the body. More Western explanations of acupuncture relate to the release and movement of neurotransmitters, neuropeptides, and hormones. Acupuncture has been successfully used for the treatment of drug addictions and is proving to be a cost-effective and safe form of therapy.

Biofeedback. **Biofeedback** teaches clients to control their physical responses by providing visual or auditory information about autonomic body functions. Body functions, such as respiration, pulse, or skin responses, are monitored by machines while clients practice relaxation techniques and change the monitored data. For example, changes in respiratory or pulse rates that can be seen on a graph provide clients

Table 6-3	*Life Force Energy*

NAME	CULTURE
Qi	Traditional Chinese medicine
Ki	Japanese kampoo system
Doshas	Ayurvedic medicine
Also called: biofields, etheric energy, *fohat*, homeopathic resonance, *mana*, orgone force, and *prana*	

with objective feedback and encouragement. Biofeedback has proven very useful in treating anxiety, hypertension, insomnia, headaches, and attention deficit disorders.

Qi Gong. Qi is the Chinese name for vital energy, therefore Qi Gong is a system of movement, regulation of breathing, and meditation designed to enhance the flow of qi throughout the body.

Reiki. The word **Reiki** comes from the Japanese words **rei,** meaning "God's Wisdom" or "Higher Power," and the word **ki,** which is "life force energy." Reiki is a life force energy that flows through one's body. When it is low, we are stressed or sick. When it is in abundance, we feel healthy and happy. Practitioners of Reiki use a "laying on of the hands" to promote relaxation and promote healing.

Therapeutic Touch. Therapeutic touch is based upon the practice of laying on of the hands. The healing energies of the therapist encourage the body's energies to return to a balanced state. Healers pass their hands over the body to identify the blockages or energy imbalances. The therapist then strengthens and reorients the body energies, thus restoring the biofield. Therapeutic touch is effective in stress-related conditions such as migraine headaches and anxiety. Caution should be exercised, however, as mental health problems such as paranoia, hallucinations, or delusions are associated with an impaired sense of touch.

Color Therapy. High-intensity light has been used to successfully treat SAD. Color therapy is still being studied, but practitioners believe that the energy fields that surround each of us (auras) are filled with constantly changing energies of color. When one is sick the aura is discolored. Color therapists scan the energy centers (chakras) for imbalances and expose the body to the appropriate healing color to help heal the physical problem and rebalance energies.

Electromagnetic Field Therapies

Standard medicine has used electromagnetic field energy for years in magnetic resonance imaging (MRI), radiation therapy, cardiac pacemakers and more. However, the use of that energy to treat illness with electromagnetic field (EMF) is still under study.

Magnetic therapy uses magnets placed over painful areas to relieve pain. **Repetitive transcranial magnetic stimulation (TMS)** has been successfully used to treat severe depression. **Pulsating electromagnetic therapy** enhances bone healing and is claimed to be effective with sleep disorders and headaches. **Millimeter wave therapy** has been used in Russia and other Eastern European countries to treat both physical and psychiatric illnesses. Exposure to low-power millimeter waves is thought to increase immunity and improve well-being. The main courses of action for these therapies are well not understood. Further investigations are being conducted.

TECHNOLOGY-BASED CAM APPLICATIONS

With the increasing use of electronic devices, mental health advice is just a click away. **Telemedicine** uses video and computer technology to deliver health care to remote areas and consult with experts. Practitioners can speak to and observe clients directly with webcams. **Telephone counseling** uses active listening skills to provide information and referrals. The first step toward mental health care is often a telephone counselor. **Radio psychiatry** provides psychiatrists and psychologists who offer information, discussion, advice, and referrals in response to callers' mental health questions. **Electronic communications** offer a wide range of information as well as a means of communicating with others who may share the same problems. Treatment is now even available online.

CAM APPROACHES TO MENTAL HEALTH CARE

More people are seeking help for their emotional and mental problems through the use of nonmedical therapies and treatments. In fact, surveys have indicated that the number of "office visits to alternative medical practitioners already exceeds the number of visits to traditional medical physicians" (Sarnat, 2001). Table 6-4 lists some CAM therapies currently being used to treat several mental health problems. Partnerships among CAM therapists and the traditional medical community are being formed in several areas of the United States. Many European nations have used some CAM therapies for years.

Many complementary and alternative therapies are proving to be effective and useful. Others are not. Some therapies have the potential to be dangerous, especially if used along with standard medical treatments. Ultimately, the consumer of health care services will make the choice. It is our responsibility to keep informed of the latest developments in CAM practices.

Table 6-4 *Complementary and Alternative Mental Health Therapies*

MENTAL HEALTH PROBLEM	COMPLEMENTARY AND ALTERNATIVE MEDICINE THERAPIES
Stress, anxiety	Aromatherapy, diet, certain herbs, massage,
Depression	Meditation, prayer, acupuncture, biofeedback, Reiki, therapeutic touch, music, dance, yoga, phototherapy, naturopathy
Posttraumatic stress disorder (PTSD)	Meditation, eye movement desensitization, biofeedback, yoga
Sleep disorders	Aromatherapy, diet, certain herbs, massage, meditation, prayer, progressive relaxation

CAM MENTAL HEALTH THERAPIES

Alternative approaches to mental illness emphasize the interactions of the body, mind, and spirit. Some therapies have long histories. Many remain unproven and controversial. The National Mental Health Information Center discussed several approaches to achieving mental wellness.

Animal-Assisted Therapy

Animals are consistent and nonjudgmental. They are always accepting and help ease loneliness. Assistance dogs have helped people with physical disabilities for years. "More recently, assistance dogs have been trained to aid those with certain conditions, such as severe social anxiety, young people with autism, and individuals prone to seizures" (Vaughn, 2007). Working with animals has been found to promote socialization, increase empathy, encourage responsibility and commitment, and foster communication.

Culturally Based Healing

Acupuncture has successfully treated individuals with stress, anxiety, and depression. It has been used in children with hyperactivity and attention-deficit disorders. Some therapists use it to assist the client with detoxification from alcohol or drugs. Yoga and meditation relieve stress and anxiety. Remember that one's culture has a profound effect on the outcome of treatment.

Diet and Nutrition

Eliminating some foods may have an impact on mental health problems. For example, eliminating wheat and milk products may reduce the severity of symptoms for those with schizophrenia. Certain herbal and vitamin treatments may ease the discomforts of depression and hyperactivity.

Expressive Therapies

Art, music, and dance all help to release emotions and foster self-awareness. Individuals recovering from abuse find that movement therapy helps them to "reconnect," to gain a sense of ease and comfort with their own bodies. Music stimulates the body to release neurotransmitters that increase well-being. Music therapy has been used to treat depression, grief, autism, and schizophrenia.

Pastoral Counseling

Ministers, pastors, priests, and rabbis offer prayer and therapeutic listening. Many are not trained therapists, but most are wise in offering support and comfort. Pastoral counselors work within a religious community where members work to help and support each other.

Self-Help Groups

People with related problems find great support and understanding with others with similar experiences. Those who "have been there" are invaluable resources for empowering others toward recovery. Box 6-2 describes the characteristics of self-help groups.

Stress Reduction and Relaxation

Learning to control the body's **fight-or-flight response** helps us to avoid the negative effects of stress. Techniques such as **guided imagery** and **creative visualization** teach the user to achieve a deep state of relaxation and then create a mental scenario of healing and wellness. Depression, alcohol and drug addictions, panic disorders, phobias, and stress have been treated with these techniques. Biofeedback offers objective evidence of relaxation. It has proven to be a useful tool in helping people with severe anxiety, phobias, and panic attacks.

WORDS OF CAUTION

Many CAM approaches to mental health care are based on years of observation, testing, and successful treatment. Many CAM therapies are relatively new and unproven by data. Because we practice within an allopathic (traditional medical) framework, we use data derived from studies to draw conclusions. The National Center for Complementary and Alternative Medicine at the National Institutes of Health was created to evaluate alternative treatment methods. Consult them frequently at www.nccam.nih.nil.gov/health for new information about CAM practices. Think About 6-1 offers food for thought.

ADVERSE EFFECTS

Some CAM therapies may have adverse or unwanted effects, especially if combined with traditional treatments. Prescription drugs can interact with certain herbs. Chelation therapy can deplete the body of potassium. Allergic reactions may result from inappropriate use of diet supplements or foods. Sometimes the individual is masking a serious need for medical help with an ineffective CAM therapy. It is important to fully explore a CAM therapy before engaging in any of its practices.

Box 6-2 *Characteristics of Self-Help Groups*

Members have similar needs.
Purpose is to assist help people cope with a life-changing event such as addiction, abuse, death, diagnosis of a mental illness.
Membership in group is voluntary, confidential, and anonymous.
Groups are informal, nonprofit, and free.
Meetings are facilitated by a survivor or one familiar with the shared experience(s).
Groups provide support, education, and ongoing encouragement.

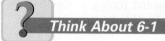

Think About 6-1

You are monitoring the response of a client who is taking an antipsychotic drug. He informs you that he has been taking an herbal preparation for his hallucinations and is now ready to stop taking his prescribed medications.
• How would you respond to him?

IMPLICATIONS FOR CARE PROVIDERS

The use of CAM therapies to treat mental health problems must be approached with caution. Always consult your supervisor and the client's primary care provider before suggesting anything to the client. Many times the whole picture is not apparent, and doing no harm is the caregiver's first priority.

If a CAM therapy is used in your environment, learn as much as possible about it, including both the negative and positive aspects. Many changes and new discoveries are on the horizon as we attempt to learn more about each other and our complexities.

Key Points

• Allopathic practitioners use medical and surgical methods to treat disease and injury by finding what is "wrong" and "fixing" it.
• Complementary medicine includes practices and treatments that agree or "work with" allopathic therapies. They are used along with common medical treatments.
• Alternative medicine refers to practices and treatments that are used instead of conventional (allopathic) medicine.
• Integrative medicine attempts to blend the most effective practices and treatments from both conventional and alternative treatment systems. Emphasis is on the interrelationship among body, mind, and spirit.
• The primary goal of holistic mental health care providers is to help clients develop strategies to achieve harmony within themselves and with others, nature, and the world.
• The National Center for Complementary and Alternative Medicine (NCCAM), a part of the U.S. National Institutes of Health, is dedicated to exploring complementary and alternative healing practices.

• Whole medical systems are built on complete systems of theory and practice and include Western medicine, osteopathy, homeopathy, naturopathy, and culturally based systems such as Ayurveda and Oriental medicine.
• Biologically based practices use substances extracted from nature. Treatments include aromatherapy, dietary supplements, and herbal therapies.
• Body-based practices focus on moving the body into an improved state of function through treatment. They include chiropractic treatment, chelation, eye movement desensitization, massage, and phototherapy.
• Energy-based therapies base their practices upon two types of energy fields: the veritable and the putative.
• Followers of mind-body medicine believe that the mind and spirit have the ability to affect the body and its functions.
• Mind-body therapies include expressive therapies, such as music or dance, hypnotherapy, meditation, prayer, and spiritual healing.
• Practitioners of energy medicine believe in a vital, life force energy that flows through the human body.
• Energy medicine is divided into two areas: biofield therapies and bioelectromagnetic field therapies.
• Biofield therapies are among some of the most used but unmeasured CAM therapies.
• Examples of biofield therapies are acupuncture, biofeedback, Qi Gong, Reiki, therapeutic touch, and color therapy.
• Current bioelectromagnetic field theories operate on the theory that energy can treat illness.
• Magnetic therapy, repetitive transcranial magnetic stimulation (TMS), pulsating electromagnetic therapy, and millimeter wave therapy are bioelectromagnetic applications of the theory.
• Technology-based approaches to mental health care include telemedicine, telephone counseling, and radio psychiatry.
• The use of CAM therapies to treat mental health problems must be approached with caution because some CAM therapies may have adverse or unwanted effects.

evolve Be sure to visit the companion Evolve site at http://evolve.elsevier.com/Morrison-Valfre/ for additional online resources.

Objectives

Upon completion of this text, the student will be able to:

1. Briefly explain how psychotherapeutic medications affect human beings.
2. Identify four classifications of psychotherapeutic medications.
3. Discuss three classes of antianxiety agents and the side effects associated with each.
4. Prepare a list of three teaching points for clients who are beginning antidepressant therapy.
5. Explain the three major guidelines for care of clients taking lithium.
6. Identify one central nervous system and three peripheral nervous system side effects of antipsychotic (neuroleptic) drug therapy.
7. Describe five care guidelines for clients receiving psychotherapeutic drugs.
8. Discuss three topics for teaching clients about their medications.
9. Explain how informed consent and noncompliance relate to psychotherapeutic medications.

Key Terms

affective disorders (p. 64)
akathisia (ĂK-ə-THĒ-zhə) (p. 68)
akinesia (Ă-kĭ-NĒ-zhə) (p. 68)
antipsychotics (ĂN-tĭ-sĭ-KŎT-ĭks) (p. 67)
autonomic nervous system (ANS) (p. 62)
central nervous system (CNS) (p. 62)
drug-induced parkinsonism (DRŬG-ĭn-doost PĂHR-kĭn-sən-ĭz-əm) (p. 68)
dyskinesia (DĬS-kĭ-NĒ-zhə) (p. 68)
dystonia (dĭs-TŌN-nē-ə) (p. 68)
extrapyramidal (ĔKS-trä-pĭ-RĂM-ĭ-däl) **side effects (EPSEs)** (p. 67)
hypertensive crisis (p. 65)
informed consent (p. 71)
lithium (LĬTH-ē-əm) (p. 66)
mania (p. 65)
monoamine oxidase inhibitors (MAOIs) (MŎN-ō-ə-MĒN ŎK-sĭ-dās ĭn-HĬB-ĭ-tors) (p. 64)
mood disorders (p. 64)
neuroleptic malignant syndrome (NMS) (NOOR-ō-LĔP-tĭk mə-LĬG-nənt SĬN-drōm) (p. 68)
neuron (p. 62)
neurotransmitter (NOOR-ō-TRĂNS-mĭ-tĕr) (p. 62)
noncompliance (p. 70)

parasympathetic (PAIR-ə-SĬM-pə-THĔT-ĭk) **nervous system** (p. 62)
peripheral (pĕ-RĬF-ĕr-ăl) **nervous system (PNS)** (p. 62)
psychotherapeutic (SĬ-kō-thĕr-ə-PYŪ-tĭk) **drugs** (p. 61)
sympathetic nervous system (p. 62)
tardive dyskinesia (TĂR-dĭv DĬS-kĭ-NĒ-zhə) (p. 68)

Psychotherapeutic drugs are powerful chemicals that produce profound effects on the mind, emotions, and body (Keltner and Folks, 2005). They were first discovered as side effects of other drugs, such as antihistamines for allergies. In 1949, lithium was found to be effective in treating the mania of bipolar illness. The 1950s brought the use of chlorpromazine (Thorazine) into the therapeutic regimen. The tranquilizer meprobamate (Miltown) became so popular in 1955 that drugstores were "required to place signs in the window when they sell out" (Keltner, Schwecke, and Bostrom, 2007). By the early 1960s, tricyclic antidepressants, monoamine oxidase inhibitors (MAOIs), and haloperidol (Haldol) had been placed on the market. The antianxiety drug diazepam (Valium) became extremely popular, and soon it was the most often prescribed medication in the world. Newer psychotherapeutic drugs have been introduced, and even more will be available in the future. Health care professionals who work with these drugs must remember that psychotherapeutic medications are powerful chemicals with many, sometimes severe, side effects.

HOW PSYCHOTHERAPEUTIC DRUG THERAPY WORKS

Psychiatric medications act mainly on the body's nervous system by altering the delicate chemical balances within that system. Most psychotherapeutic medications interrupt the chemical messenger (neurotransmitter) pathways within the brain by suppressing major nerve pathways that connect the deeper brain to the frontal lobes and limbic system.

The frontal lobes of the brain are the source of the higher human functions, such as love, creativity, insight, planning, judgment, and abstract reasoning. The limbic system is responsible for emotions, motivation, memory, and the fight-or-flight response. When these areas of the brain are affected by medications, profound changes in behavior result. People usually experience more stable moods, but **many higher brain functions are impaired.** As with all medications, there is a trade-off between therapeutic effects and unwanted reactions. One of the primary responsibilities of health care providers (especially nurses) is to recognize therapeutic versus unwanted effects.

The human nervous system consists of an intricate network of structures that activates, coordinates, and controls all the functions of the body. All parts of the nervous system work together. It is important to remember that if a drug affects one part of the nervous system it will, without a doubt, have an impact on the other activities of the system. Figure 7-1 illustrates the divisions of the nervous system.

The central nervous system (CNS) is composed of the brain and spinal cord. Together they control all the motor and sensory functions of the body. Information about movement travels from the brain down through the spinal cord, reaches the appropriate muscle group, and results in movement. Sensory information (e.g., touch, temperature, position) is relayed in the opposite direction: from the muscles and other body areas, up through the spinal cord, and into the brain. Throughout this process, the CNS combines all incoming (sensory) and outgoing (motor) data.

The peripheral nervous system (PNS) is composed of the 31 spinal cord nerves plus the 12 pairs of cranial nerves. The peripheral nervous system is further divided into a "motor" system and an "autonomic" (automatic) system. Each spinal nerve contains motor and sensory neurons (nerve cells). The motor portion of the spinal nerve activates heart, muscles, and glandular secretions, whereas sensations of touch, temperature, pain, and spatial perception are transmitted by the sensory portion. The cranial nerves carry a mixture of information; some nerves are mainly motor, others carry mainly sensory information, and a few perform both motor and sensory functions.

The autonomic nervous system (ANS) is responsible for regulating the vital functions of the body. The activities of the heart muscle, smooth muscles, and glandular secretions are all controlled "automatically" by this remarkable system. Two divisions of the autonomic nervous system, the sympathetic and parasympathetic systems, work together to monitor and govern "automatic" body responses.

The sympathetic nervous system prepares the body for immediate adaptation through the fight-or-flight mechanism. The heart rate and output increase, which moves blood into the muscles. Vessels to the stomach and other nonvital organs constrict and detour blood to the skeletal muscles. The pupils of the eyes dilate to improve visual acuity, and the bronchioles of the lungs expand to allow for greater exchange of airflow. Increases in blood sugar and fatty acid levels provide glucose for fuel, and all digestive and excretory processes are slowed. The result is greater cellular energy production and increased mental activity. Physically,

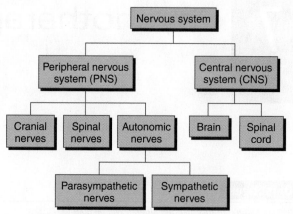

FIGURE **7-1** Divisions of the nervous system.

the body is preparing to protect itself. People who are highly stressed demonstrate many sympathetic nervous system responses.

The parasympathetic nervous system is designed to conserve energy and provide the balance for the sympathetic system's excitability. The main functions of this system are to monitor and maintain control over the "regulatory" processes of the body, which it accomplishes by governing smooth muscle tone and glandular secretions. Parasympathetic stimulation slows the heart rate, decreases circulating blood volume, relaxes sphincters, and increases intestinal and glandular activity. Respiratory, circulatory, digestive, excretory, and reproductive functions respond to parasympathetic messages. The parasympathetic nervous system uses the neurotransmitter acetylcholine to do its work, and it is often referred to as the cholinergic nervous system.

As you can see, the sympathetic and parasympathetic divisions of the autonomic nervous system act in opposite ways. Fortunately, this excite-calm interaction provides a balance. Organs are rich in both adrenergic (sympathetic) and cholinergic (parasympathetic) receptor sites, and this allows the organism to maintain itself in a state of balance, or **homeostasis.** Table 7-1 lists the physical responses to parasympathetic and sympathetic nervous system stimulation. It is wise to be familiar with these responses because many people who take psychotherapeutic medications demonstrate side effects related to autonomic nervous system functions.

The basic unit of the nervous system is the neuron, or nerve cell. Its function is to transmit electrical information to other neurons. Electrical information traveling through a neuron generates a chemical messenger called a neurotransmitter. Although nerve cells are found in great abundance throughout the body, they are not physically connected to each other. Each neuron is separated by a small space or gap called a **synapse.** Neurotransmitters travel across this gap, open a channel for the electrical information to pass, and then quickly become inactivated. Neurotransmitters are divided into four groups: monoamines, cholinergic group, amino acids, and neuropeptides. Many psychotherapeutic drugs

Table 7-1 *Autonomic Nervous System Actions*

TISSUE	PARASYMPATHETIC (CHOLINERGIC OR MUSCARINIC) RESPONSE	SYMPATHETIC (ADRENERGIC) RESPONSE
Eye	Constriction (miosis)	Dilation (mydriasis)
	Accommodation (focus on near objects)	
Glands	Increased salivation (copious, watery)	Increased sweating*
	Increased tears and secretions of respiratory and gastrointestinal tract	Increased salivation (thick, contains proteins)
Heart	Decreased rate	Increased rate
	Decreased strength of contraction	Increased strength of contraction
	Decreased conduction velocity through the atrioventricular node	Increased conduction velocity through the atrioventricular node
Bronchioles	Smooth muscle constriction (restricts airways)	Smooth muscle relaxation (opens airways)
Blood vessels	Constriction of vessels in heart (not a prominent effect in humans)	Dilation of vessels in heart and skeletal muscle
	Dilation of vessels in salivary gland and erectile tissues	Constriction of vessels in skin, viscera, salivary gland, erectile tissues, kidney
Gastrointestinal tract		
Smooth muscle	Contraction	Relaxation
Sphincters	Relaxation	Contraction
Urinary bladder		
Fundus	Contraction	Relaxation
Trigone and sphincter	Relaxation	Contraction
Uterus		Contraction
Liver		Glycogenolysis

Modified from Clark JF, Queener SF, Karb VB: *The pharmacologic basis of nursing practice*, ed 6, St. Louis, 2000, Mosby.
*Acetylcholine is the neurotransmitter for this response.

alter the flow of message exchanges in or around the synapse. The study of the neurochemistry of behavior has already altered the way in which mental-emotional problems are considered.

CLASSIFICATIONS OF PSYCHOTHERAPEUTIC DRUGS

The four classes of psychotherapeutic medications are (1) antianxiety agents; (2) antidepressants and (3) antimanics, which are used to treat mood or emotional disorders; and (4) antipsychotics, which help curb the hallucinations and loss of reality experienced by individuals with psychotic disorders.

Millions of people are currently being treated with psychotherapeutic drugs. People receiving psychotherapeutic (also called psychotropic) medications must be routinely monitored for effectiveness, side effects, and life-threatening adverse reactions. Because of this need for close monitoring, nurses and all other care providers must be knowledgeable about the roles that these powerful chemicals play in treating mental illness.

ANTIANXIETY MEDICATIONS

Anxiety is common to us all, but when it interferes with one's ability to function it becomes an anxiety disorder. In today's world, anxiety disorders are a common mental health problem. A thorough discussion of anxiety and its treatments can be found in Chapter 18. Here we consider the antianxiety medications that are a usual part of the therapeutic treatment plan.

Antianxiety agents are drugs that reduce the psychic tension of stress. They are also referred to as anxiolytics

or "minor tranquilizers." Medications in the antianxiety group are divided by their chemical formulas into categories. Table 7-2 lists the major drugs used for anxiety and depression.

The benzodiazepines have "dominated clinical practice for more than three decades" (Keltner and Folks, 2005) in the treatment of anxiety disorders. They are effective, are generally well tolerated, and do not affect sleeping patterns (a common problem with many psychotherapeutic drugs). Benzodiazepines are prescribed to provide sedation, induce sleep (called a hypnotic), prevent seizures, and prepare clients for general anesthesia, but they are mainly used to decrease anxiety.

People with high levels of anxiety have low levels of a neurotransmitter called gamma-aminobutyric acid (GABA). Benzodiazepines act by increasing GABA activity, which results in decreased anxiety. They are fast acting, with the onset of action occurring within 1 hour. The drug exerts its action (duration) for about 4 to 6 hours. Thus clients experience relief from symptoms within hours.

Benzodiazepines are metabolized by the liver and excreted by the kidneys. People with impaired liver or kidney function must be carefully monitored if this drug class is prescribed. Pregnant and nursing women are usually not treated with benzodiazepines because these medications enter the breast milk. Caution must also be used when administering antianxiety agents to older or debilitated adults because of their slower metabolism.

The side effects of benzodiazepines are usually minimal, but they include fatigue, sedation, dizziness, and orthostatic hypotension (a drop in blood pressure on standing). Because long-term use of antianxiety

Table 7-2 | *Antianxiety and Antidepressant Medications*

DRUG CLASS	EXAMPLES	COMMENTS
Azaspirones (for anxiety)	Buspirone (BuSpar)	Takes 2-4 wk to relieve symptoms of anxiety; not habit forming; does not impair memory, balance, or cause sedation; minimal side effects
Benzodiazepines (for anxiety)	Triazolam (Halcion), lorazepam (Ativan), chlordiazepoxide (Librium), diazepam (Valium), flurazepam (Dalmane)	Oldest anxiolytic; fast acting; main side effect is drowsiness; potential for dependency; withdrawal symptoms if stopped abruptly
Beta-blockers (for anxiety)	Propranolol (Inderal), atenolol (Tenormin)	Used to treat social phobias; reduces palpitations, sweating, tremors, blood pressure, and heart rate
Tricyclics (TCAs) (for depression, anxiety)	Amitriptyline (Elavil), desipramine (Norpramin), doxepin (Sinequan Triadapin), imipramine (Tofranil), nortriptyline (Aventyl)	Takes 2-3 wk to take effect; side effects: drowsiness, dry mouth, dizziness, weight gain, impaired sexual function; treats anxiety, depression, posttraumatic stress disorder (PTSD), obsessive-compulsive disorder
Monoamine oxidase inhibitors (MAOIs) (for depression)	Phenelzine (Nardil), tranylcypromine (Parnate), selegiline (Carbex)	Not often prescribed because of serious adverse reactions and interactions with food and drugs; strong dietary restrictions
Selective serotonin reuptake inhibitors (SSRIs) (for depression)	Fluvoxamine (Luvox), fluoxetine (Prozac), paroxetine (Paxil), sertraline (Zoloft)	First choice for treating anxiety, depression, other problems; side effects: gastrointestinal (GI) distress, headache, dizziness, sexual dysfunction
Atypical antidepressants (for depression)	Mirtazapine (Remeron), bupropion (Wellbutrin), maprotiline (Ludiomil), trazodone (Desyrel)	Agitation can occur with bupropion; common side effects: sleepiness, increased appetite, weight gain, dizziness
Selective serotonin/ norepinephrine reuptake inhibitors (SSNRIs) (for depression)	Nefazodone (Serzone), venlafaxine (Effexor)	Side effects: nausea, dry mouth, dizziness, sedation, sweating, anorexia; monitor blood pressures

drugs can result in dependence, therapy for clients is usually limited to a few months.

The antianxiety agent called buspirone (BuSpar) differs from benzodiazepines in several ways. First, it belongs to a different chemical class, the azaspirones, and does not cause the sleepiness or muscle relaxation associated with benzodiazepines. Second, therapeutic effects are not seen for 3 to 6 weeks after beginning treatment. Buspirone has less potential for abuse; however, clients are still cautioned to avoid alcohol. Third, the potential for overdose is lessened because the drug has a wide dosage range. Side effects are few: lightheadedness, dizziness, headache, and nausea (Keltner and Folks, 2005).

A new drug, called pregabalin (Lyrica) is currently being introduced to treat several kinds of anxiety disorders as well as seizures and neuropathic pain. Side effects are fewer than those of other antianxiety drugs, so clients are more likely to comply with treatment.

Antianxiety drugs have several drug interactions, including CNS depression when they are combined with other CNS depressants, such as alcohol and street drugs (Skidmore-Roth, 2007). The combination can produce serious, even fatal, reactions. Concentrations of the cardiac drug digoxin may be increased during treatment with antianxiety medications, so clients taking this medication must be routinely assessed for signs or symptoms of digoxin toxicity.

Antacids should not be taken because they interfere with absorption of the antianxiety agent into the bloodstream.

Nursing care for clients receiving antianxiety agents includes frequent assessments for therapeutic actions and side effects. Many of these drugs are prescribed on an "as needed" (prn) basis. Medications used on this basis require accurate client assessments, good judgment, repeated evaluations of the medication's effects, and objective documentation.

ANTIDEPRESSANT MEDICATIONS

Feelings of great joy and deep sadness are common human experiences. We are all familiar with these emotional extremes and think of them as the natural highs and lows of everyday life, but when one's mood begins to interfere with the ability to perform the routine activities of daily living, intervention is needed. Mood disorders are ineffective emotional states, ranging from deep depression to excited elation. They are also called affective disorders because the word *affect* means emotions. The major mood disorders are discussed in Chapter 21.

Basically, antidepressant medications exert their action in the body by increasing certain neurotransmitter activities. Based on their chemical formula, antidepressants are divided into categories: tricyclic antidepressants, monoamine oxidase inhibitors (MAOIs), selective serotonin reuptake inhibitors (SSRIs), atypical antidepressants, and selective serotonin/norepinephrine reuptake inhibitors (SSNRIs) (see Table 7-2).

The physician's first choice for the treatment of depression is often an antidepressant. Antidepressants are also indicated for bipolar disorders, panic

Table 7-3 *Drug Interactions With Monoamine Oxidase Inhibitors*

TYPE OF INTERACTION	SIGNS/SYMPTOMS
Anticholinergic reactions	Dry mouth, decreased tearing, blurred vision, constipation, urinary hesitancy or retention, excessive sweating
Hypertensive crisis	Throbbing, radiating headache, stiff neck, palpitations, tightness in chest, sweating, dilated pupils, very high blood pressure and pulse rate
CNS depression	Changes in level of consciousness; sedation, increasing lethargy, disorientation, confusion, agitation, hallucinations, lower seizure threshold

CNS, Central nervous system.

Box 7-1 *Dietary and Drug Interactions With Monoamine Oxidase Inhibitors*

MEDICATIONS TO AVOID

Prescription and over-the-counter drugs: Nasal and sinus decongestants; cold, allergy, and hay fever remedies; inhalants for asthma; weight-loss pills, pep pills, stimulants; narcotics, local anesthetics

Any medication should be approved by the physician

Illicit drugs: Cocaine, any amphetamine (uppers)

FOODS TO AVOID

Alcoholic drinks: Beer, ale, red wines (Chianti), sherry wines, liqueurs, cognac

Dairy products: Aged cheese, sour cream

Fruits and vegetables: Avocados, bananas, fava and broad beans, canned figs, any overripe fruit

Meats: Pickled or smoked, bologna, chicken or beef liver, dried fish, meat tenderizer, salami, sausage

Other foods: Large amounts of caffeinated coffee, tea, or cola; chocolate; licorice; soy sauce; yeast

Modified from American Psychiatric Association: *Diagnostic and statistical manual of mental disorders*, ed 4, text revision, Washington, DC, 2000, American Psychiatric Association.

Box 7-2 *Side Effects of SSRI Antidepressants*

Dry mouth, nausea, vomiting constipation, diarrhea, anorexia, differences in taste; headache, changes in alertness, tremor, dizziness, weakness, fatigue, increased sweating; sexual dysfunction; visual disturbances; urinary disturbances

SSRI, Selective serotonin reuptake inhibitor.

disorders, obsessive-compulsive disorders, enuresis (bed-wetting), bulimia, and neuropathic pain. Antidepressants have been used with success in post-traumatic stress disorder, organic mood disorders, attention-deficit/hyperactivity disorder, and conduct disorders in children.

Antidepressants interact with a variety of other substances. Because they block the destruction of specific major neurotransmitters, higher levels of these chemicals circulate throughout the body. Ingesting foods or drugs that contain certain chemicals produces more neurotransmitters, which can result in overstimulation of the nervous system. Antidepressant drug interactions can produce serious cardiovascular and blood pressure reactions as well as CNS depression. Table 7-3 describes the more serious drug interactions encountered with the MAOI antidepressants.

Antidepressant medications require 1 to 4 weeks before symptom relief is noticed. However, side effects may be experienced soon after beginning therapy. Some side effects are a nuisance, such as a dry mouth. Others, such as a **hypertensive crisis** (a sudden, severe elevation in blood pressure) can be life threatening. **Anticholinergic side effects** include dryness of the mouth, nose, and eyes; urinary retention; and sedation. These discomforts can be so bothersome that some people refuse to take their medications regularly. Clients should be routinely monitored for physical and behavioral changes. Those experiencing postural hypotension should be protected from falls. Kidney and liver function should be assessed and monitored monthly. Any signs of toxicity (e.g., headache, stiff neck, palpitations) should be reported to the physician immediately.

Clients should also be assessed for changes in attitudes and suicidal gestures. Frequently, depressed people attempt suicide when taking antidepressants because of increased energy levels that can lead to a renewed interest in suicide. Take precautions to protect clients if you believe that they may be suicidal. Changes in a client's behavior may indicate a thera-

peutic improvement, a drug side effect, a drug-food interaction, or an emerging psychosis. Good communication with clients helps to assess subtle changes that may indicate problems.

Clients, no matter which medications they are taking, must be taught about their drug therapy. Instructions should include information about dosages, actions, and wanted and unwanted effects. Those who are taking MAOIs must understand their dietary and drug restrictions. Box 7-1 lists the foods and medications that must be avoided while taking MAOIs.

SSRIs are the first choice in treatment for many physicians because their side effects are more manageable (Box 7-2). Because of this, SSRIs are indicated for both short- and long-term therapy.

ANTIMANIC MEDICATIONS

Mania is a state characterized by excitement, great elation, overtalkativeness, increased motor activity, fleeting grandiose ideas, and agitated behaviors. Some therapists refer to mania as agitated depression because it frequently occurs with severe depression. Antidepressant drug therapy helps clients cope with their depression, but it has little effect during the manic stage of behavior.

Lithium is a naturally occurring salt. In 1949, lithium was found to be effective in the treatment of mania, but as a result of reports of fatal side effects, the drug was not available in the United States until 1970. Lithium is the mainstay treatment of the manic phase of bipolar depression. Newer products are currently available for clients who do not respond or cannot tolerate lithium therapy. Box 7-3 lists the major antimanic medications.

Lithium is currently used in the United States for the treatment of manic episodes. Because lithium stabilizes mood, it is indicated for the treatment of acute mania and as a prophylaxis (preventative) for clients with bipolar disorders. Lithium has also been investigated for the treatment of drug abuse, alcoholism, phobias, and eating disorders. Therapy is contraindicated (not prescribed) for pregnant women and people with kidney failure. Clients with physical health problems must be carefully monitored.

Lithium is well absorbed into the bloodstream and excreted faster than sodium by the kidneys. For this reason, clients who are taking lithium must be cautioned about balancing their salt intake, fluid intake, and activity. Lithium interacts with a variety of other drugs. For a list of significant drug interactions associated with antimanic drugs, consult a drug reference.

The difference between therapeutic and toxic levels of lithium is minimal. The drug is usually well tolerated by most clients, but how well the drug is excreted varies from client to client. The "narrow therapeutic index" of lithium requires close observation of client responses. If the blood levels are too low, manic behavior returns; however, if levels are too high, an uncomfortable and possibly life-threatening toxicity may result. Lithium levels higher than 1.5 mEq/L are considered toxic.

Clinical improvement commonly takes as long as 3 weeks. Clients in the acute manic stage usually require the addition of antipsychotic or sedative medications until the effects of lithium take hold. Clients are monitored monthly for thyroid and kidney functions because long-term use of lithium can cause altered thyroid function (hypothyroidism) and loss of the kidney's ability to concentrate urine. Great care must be taken to frequently assess and monitor each client's responses to each medication because undesirable effects are present with every medication the client receives.

The major guidelines for care of clients taking lithium relate to three areas: helping with the prelithium workup, educating the client to maintain stable blood levels of the drug, and monitoring the client for side effects and possible toxic reactions.

The prelithium workup consists of a complete physical, history, electrocardiogram (ECG), and numerous blood studies. Nurses are responsible for obtaining a complete functional assessment that describes the client's habits and activities of daily living. They should also review the results of all diagnostic tests. Data from these assessments are used to plan appropriate care and forecast potential problems.

Stabilizing lithium levels involves teaching the client and family about the following: expected side effects, the difference between common side effects and those requiring immediate notification of the physician, and coping with the lifestyle changes required by this medication. Box 7-4 lists the most important guidelines for clients who are receiving lithium.

Make sure the client and family understand each bit of information. Ask them to repeat what they have learned, apply it to several "what if" situations, and describe the appropriate actions for each side effect.

Box 7-4 *Guidelines for Clients Taking Lithium*

To achieve a therapeutic effect and prevent lithium toxicity, clients taking lithium should be advised of the following:
1. Lithium must be taken on a regular basis at the same time daily. If you miss a dose wait until the next scheduled time to take the lithium.
2. When lithium treatment is started, mild side effects may develop, such as fine hand tremor, increased thirst and urination, nausea, anorexia, and diarrhea or constipation. Some foods, such as celery and butter fat, may have an unappealing taste. Most side effects will pass with time.
3. Serious side effects of lithium include vomiting, extreme hand tremor, sedation, muscle weakness, and dizziness. The physician should be notified immediately if any of these effects occur.
4. Lithium and sodium compete for elimination from the body through the kidneys. An increase in salt intake increases lithium elimination, and a decrease in salt intake decreases lithium elimination. Thus it is important that the client maintain a balanced diet, liquid, and salt intake. The client should consult the physician before making any dietary changes.
5. Various situations can require an adjustment in lithium doses; for example, the addition of a new medication to the client's drug regimen, a new diet, or an illness with fever or excessive sweating.
6. Blood for determination of lithium levels should be drawn in the morning approximately, 8 to 14 hours after the last dose was taken.

Box 7-3 *Commonly Prescribed Antimanics*

GENERIC NAME	TRADE NAME
carbamazepine	Tegretol
clonazepam	Klonopin
lithium	Carbolith, Duralith, Eskalith-CR, Lithane, Lithotabs
valproic acid	Depakene*
lamotrigine	Lamictal
gabapentin	Neurontin

*Depakene has not yet been approved by the Food and Drug Administration for treatment of mania.

Modified from Keltner NL, Folks DG: *Psychotropic drugs*, ed 3, St. Louis, 2001, Mosby.

Reinforce the information with written instructions. The informed client is a more willing participant in treatment.

ANTIPSYCHOTIC (NEUROLEPTIC) MEDICATIONS

Antipsychotics are also called major tranquilizers or neuroleptics. Most antipsychotic medications are available in tablet, liquid, and injectable forms. Each class of antipsychotics has profound effects on the most complex of all body systems—the brain and nervous system.

Most antipsychotic drugs are used to treat the symptoms of major mental disorders, such as schizophrenia, acute mania, and organic mental illnesses. They are also used to treat some resistant bipolar (manic-depressive), paranoid, and movement disorders. A few antipsychotics are used to treat nausea, vomiting, and intractable hiccups. Box 7-5 lists the most common antipsychotic drugs.

The psychosis called schizophrenia is associated with two groups of symptoms: Type 1, positive schizophrenic symptoms, and Type 2, negative schizophrenic symptoms (Table 7-4). Antipsychotic medications appear to be much more effective in controlling the positive symptoms of acute schizophrenia. Their use for clients with chronic brain disorders remains controversial because these drugs block already depleted dopamine (a neurotransmitter) pathways.

Antipsychotic medications interact with many other chemicals. For example, antacids hinder the absorption of antipsychotic drugs, so they must be administered 2 hours after the oral antipsychotic. Alcohol, antianxiety medications, antihistamines, antidepressants, barbiturates, meperidine (Demerol), and morphine produce severe CNS depression when mixed with antipsychotics. As a health care provider, you are responsible for the safety of your clients. Research every medication and over-the-counter drug for possible interactions with the prescribed antipsychotic, and monitor your clients' responses to each drug. If drug references do not contain enough information, consult the pharmacist or physician.

The side effects and adverse reactions of antipsychotic medications are numerous and troublesome for the client. Both the central and peripheral nervous systems are affected by antipsychotics. Extrapyramidal side effects (EPSEs) are defined as abnormal movements produced by an imbalance of neurotransmitters in the brain. The most common EPSEs are listed in Box 7-6.

Peripheral nervous system side effects include dry mouth, blurred vision, photophobia (sensitivity to bright light), tachycardia, and hypotension. Caregivers must protect clients from falls during the first few weeks of therapy because the chance for low blood pressure (hypotension) is greatest when clients stand or change positions suddenly. These hypotensive episodes cause tachycardia (rapid heartbeat) as the body attempts to adapt to a lower blood pressure. Antipsychotic drugs affect each person uniquely. They are powerful medications that must be administered with great care.

Box 7-5 | *Commonly Prescribed Antipsychotics*

GENERIC NAME	TRADE NAME
PHENOTHIAZINES	
chlorpromazine	Thorazine
fluphenazine	Prolixin
mesoridazine	Serentil
perphenazine	Trilafon
prochlorperazine	Compazine
promazine	Sparine
thioridazine	Mellaril
trifluoperazine	Stelazine
triflupromazine	Vesprin
BUTYROPHENONE	
haloperidol	Haldol
MISCELLANEOUS	
clozapine	Clozaril
loxapine	Loxitane
molindone	Moban
olanzapine	Zyprexa
quetiapine	Seroquel
risperidone	Risperdal
thiothixene	Navane

CLIENT CARE GUIDELINES

Nurses and those who administer psychotherapeutic drugs have five basic responsibilities relating to these medications: (1) to assess clients, (2) to coordinate care,

---

Table 7-4 | *Positive and Negative Symptoms of Schizophrenia*

	TYPE 1: POSITIVE SYMPTOMS	TYPE 2: NEGATIVE SYMPTOMS
Signs and symptoms	Delusions, illusions, hallucinations	Anergia (lack of energy); anhedonia (inability to feel happiness or pleasure); apathy (does not care about anything); avolition (unable to choose or exert own will); flat affect (no emotional responses); will not speak unless spoken to
Anatomy and physiology	Hyperdopaminergic reactions (too much dopamine)	Nondopaminergic reactions (too little dopamine)
	Brain size and structure normal	Brain has structural changes: decreased blood flow, increased size of ventricles, decrease in size of brain
Response to antipsychotic medications	Usually good	Usually poor

Box 7-6 *Extrapyramidal Side Effects of Antipsychotics*

SIGN/SYMPTOM	DEFINITION
Akathisia	The inability to sit still
Akinesia	Absence of physical and mental movement
Drug-induced parkinsonism	Term used to describe a group of symptoms that mimic Parkinson's disease
Dyskinesia	The inability to execute voluntary movements
Dystonia	Impaired muscle tone (rigidity in the muscles that control gait, posture, and eye movements)
Neuroleptic malignant syndrome (NMS)	A serious and potentially fatal side effect with unstable vital signs, fever, confusion, muscle rigidity, tremor, incontinence
Tardive dyskinesia	Irreversible side effect of long-term treatment that produces involuntary, repeated movements of muscles in the face, trunk, arms, and legs

(3) to administer medications, (4) to monitor and evaluate client responses, and (5) to teach clients about their medications. Each area of responsibility involves careful observation and an understanding of each drug's therapeutic and adverse actions. All caregivers should be aware of their clients' medication regimens and report any unusual signs or symptoms to the nurse or physician.

ASSESSMENT

The first step of the nursing (therapeutic) process is the most important because an accurate and complete database enhances the quality and effectiveness of client care. Many nurses are very skilled with the psychosocial and mental status assessments necessary for the care of clients with mental-emotional problems. However, it is important to also remember that physical difficulties are common companions of psychic problems. See Case Study 7-1 for a vivid example of this principle.

A history should be completed for every client whether the presenting problems are of physical or mental origin. A complete health history includes a profile of the client's current living situation, family structure, and daily activities. Attention should also be paid to his or her past medical, family, and social histories. An investigation of the client's chief complaint (problem) rounds out the basic database. Laboratory and other diagnostic studies may be ordered by the physician or nurse practitioner, and special medication assessments must be conducted for clients receiving psychotherapeutic medications (Stuart, 2005). Table 7-5 offers an example of a medication history assessment tool. Assessing clients is a continual process. Good physical and psychosocial assessments add an important dimension to the client's overall plan of holistic care.

Case Study 7-1

Gary T., a 36-year-old man, is admitted to the mental health unit of the community hospital with a diagnosis of paranoid schizophrenia. He is considered a danger to others because of his aggressive and uncooperative behavior. After receiving a major tranquilizer, he spent a relatively quiet night but cried out frequently. Today, Mary S. is assigned to care for him.

After reviewing the change-of-shift report and Gary's record, Mary decides that he needs a thorough assessment, so she goes in search of her client. She is surprised to find a rather burly, bearded man lying curled on his side and whimpering quietly to himself. While knocking on the door, she introduces herself and requests a few minutes of his time. "Hardly matters," he grumbles softly.

Mary approaches his bed carefully, remembering his tendency for physical aggression. As she seats herself near his bedside, she thinks that she caught an expression of pain. Acting on this nonverbal message, Mary gently questions, "Where are you hurting?"

Gary looks straight into her eyes and says through clenched teeth, "I think it's my back or legs or something. Ever since this pain started, I've been unable to control myself. All I want to do now is make everybody who is messin' with me hurt as much as I do."

This is the clue that sends Mary on the path of assessing Gary's pain. She discovers in his past medical history that Gary had fallen off a roof about 3 months ago. The injuries had not resolved, and attempts at treatment were resulting in ever-increasing discomfort. Pain medications, even when combined with alcohol, had little effect on the pain. Mary's physical assessment reveals difficulties with walking, sitting, and changing positions. He is not able to lift his legs off the bed.

Mary knows that something is physically wrong. Her first priority of care is to help Gary find some relief from his pain. After sharing her findings with her supervisor, Mary consults the physician in charge of Gary's case, who orders several diagnostic tests. The results of the tests reveal a large herniated disk in his back. Gary is immediately transferred and prepared for surgery.

Weeks later, a large, burly man approaches Mary in the hallway. He reminds her of someone familiar, but she cannot quite place him. As he draws closer, she recognizes Gary, who has come to thank her for listening to him. "I told the others that I was hurtin', but they didn't listen, so I got upset. I guess I can be pretty rowdy when I'm hurtin'. But you listened to me and I had surgery and the pain is gone. I can be a nice guy again. If you hadn't listened to me, I'd really be crazy by now. Thanks."

Mary feels great but reminds herself to carefully and thoroughly (physically, emotionally, socioculturally, and spiritually) assess each client as a unique individual. The answer to a complex problem may lie in a simple solution, but one must be alert enough to recognize the clues.

• What do you think may have happened if Mary had not assessed a physical problem with this mental health client?

Table 7-5 | *Medication History Assessment Tool*

PSYCHOTHERAPEUTIC MEDICATIONS	OTHER PRESCRIPTIONS	OVER-THE-COUNTER DRUGS	SUBSTANCE USE
Each drug ever taken	**Each drug in past 6 mo**	**Each drug in past 6 mo**	**Alcohol, caffeine, street drugs**
Drug name?	Drug name?	Drug name?	Substance(s)?
Reason for prescription?	Reason for prescription?	Reason for taking?	When used?
When started?	When started?	When started?	
Length of time taking drug?	Length of time taking drug?	Frequency of use?	Frequency of use?
Highest daily dose?	Highest daily dose?	Highest dose?	
Effectiveness?	Effectiveness?	Effectiveness?	Effects?
Side effects, adverse reactions?	Side effects, adverse reactions?	Side effects, adverse reactions?	Side effects, adverse reactions?
Any physical changes since starting medication?	Any physical changes since starting medication?		Any problems associated with use?
Was drug taken as prescribed (compliance)?	Was drug taken as prescribed (compliance)?		

Modified from Stuart GW, Laraia MT: *Pocket guide to psychiatric nursing*, ed 5, St. Louis, 2001, Mosby.

COORDINATION

Physicians prescribe treatments; psychologists recommend therapies; and social workers, psychologists, and other health care team members propose plans of care based on their area of expertise. Nurses coordinate and ensure that each component of the treatment plan is carried out. They juggle scheduling for tests, treatments, and therapies; monitor responses to medications; teach clients and their significant others about treatments, medications, and other aspects of therapy; and encourage clients to become actively engaged in their treatment. Nurses also act as advocates, consult with other members of the treatment team throughout the client's stay, and provide care that encourages clients toward wellness.

Each health care team member coordinates client care with others. Multidisciplinary care planning meetings are held frequently to discuss client progress and problems from each specialist's viewpoint. Treatment goals are discussed, and care plans are updated as client behavior changes.

DRUG ADMINISTRATION

One traditional role of nurses is the administration of medications to clients. Today, in some facilities, this task has fallen to the certified medication aide (CMA). The term certified medical technician (CMT) is also used. CMAs or CMTs are usually nursing assistants with specialized training in the administration of certain oral medications. However, it remains the responsibility of the nurse to monitor clients for drug effectiveness and adverse reactions. Other care providers should also be aware of the actions and side effects of their clients' medications.

It is not uncommon for a client to be taking two or more psychotherapeutic drugs at the same time. In these instances, caregivers must be especially vigilant for side effects and signs of drug interactions.

MONITORING AND EVALUATING

Physicians evaluate client responses and adjust medical therapies, but care providers are in the best position to observe the physical and behavioral changes that accompany the administration of psychotherapeutic medications. All caregivers should be familiar with the major side effects and adverse reactions for each class of psychotherapeutic drugs used in their practice settings.

Interactions with other medications and substances can become life threatening. For example, when alcohol is combined with antidepressant drugs, severe CNS depression occurs. This in turn results in lethargy, progressing to respiratory depression, coma, and even death. Certain groups of people are at an increased risk for developing drug interactions, including older adults, debilitated people, people with immunosuppressed or compromised organ systems (especially liver and kidneys), and clients who have physical illnesses (Think About 7-1).

Monitoring clients' responses to their drugs is an important, potentially lifesaving intervention. Do not take this responsibility lightly, because your clients depend on your knowledge.

CLIENT TEACHING

Every individual has a right to be informed about his or her diagnosis and treatment plan. Each client must be prepared to safely take each medication, must monitor for side effects daily, and must know what course of action to take when side effects occur. See Table 7-6 for client teaching guidelines.

Nurses must be able to reach clients on their own level of understanding. To prevent miscommunication, the nurse must speak in terms that the client can grasp and proceed at a pace that allows for understanding and the formulation of questions. Most psychotherapeutic medications slow the client's ability to follow and understand a line of thought. Therefore it

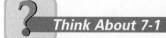

You are monitoring the responses of three clients who are taking Haldol. The first client is a 23-year-old woman, the second is a 50-year-old man, and the third is a 76-year-old man.
- Which client is at greatest risk for developing side effects?
- What are your reasons for making this choice?

Table 7-6 *Teaching Guidelines: Psychotropic Medications*

NURSING PROCESS	EXAMPLES OF ACTIONS
Assessment	Assess client for the following: Level of understanding Ability to self-administer medications Willingness to take medications on a daily basis Level of cooperation Ability to obtain and purchase medications Support of family Past medication history, including side effects of any drug taken
Planning	Nursing diagnoses: Deficient knowledge: psychotherapeutic medications Risk for noncompliance
Interventions	For each drug, teach client to recognize the following: Generic and brand names Purpose and action Therapeutic effects Dosage, route, schedule of drug Administration, what to do if a dose is missed Specific precautions (driving, operation of power equipment) Side effects and actions to take if they occur Possible drug/food interactions Signs of overdosage or underdosage Drug storage, expiration dates Provide information in written form Develop written medication schedule Reinforce other data given by care team
Evaluation	Observe client to evaluate effectiveness of teaching Reassess if any areas of instruction were not understood by client or family

is important to repeat essential points. Be sure the client comprehends by having him or her repeat the most important information.

Provide information in writing. Having a written explanation gives the client something tangible and real that can be reviewed and referred to when memory fails. Clients taking psychotherapeutic medications are likely to forget what has been taught. Preprinted drug information is helpful, but there is no substitute

for individualized client teaching. If possible, include the family or significant others. They can be very helpful in assisting the client with following the medication routine.

Helping clients and their significant others to adapt to change is a health care provider's responsibility. Psychotherapeutic medications are designed to produce behavioral changes, and these changes affect the client and people within the client's environment. A well-informed client and family are able to cope more effectively with the life changes that result from psychiatric drug therapy.

SPECIAL CONSIDERATIONS

Because psychotropic medications affect the body's nervous system, they are potentially harmful chemicals. Professionals with prescriptive authority must weigh the benefits of therapy with the possible harm that may result from the side effects or adverse reactions of a medication.

ADVERSE REACTIONS

Health care providers, especially nurses, must constantly remain vigilant for the effects of psychotherapeutic medications. Clients who are taking psychotropic drugs (especially antipsychotics) are at risk for developing the serious problems of neuroleptic malignant syndrome and tardive dyskinesia. Accurate identification of the signs and symptoms of each may prevent many complications. Detailed descriptions of these and other drug reactions are found in Chapters 31 and 32.

NONCOMPLIANCE

An informed decision made by a client not to follow a prescribed treatment program defines noncompliance. Many psychiatric clients choose to discontinue or reduce their medications because of the distressing side effects. Others have difficulty following treatment programs because of the nature of their problems. For example, paranoid or delusional people seldom cooperate with medication regimens or schedules. One study found that "about 40% of patients stopped taking their prescribed medications within one year" (Jarboe, 2002). Many outpatient clients do not take their medications as prescribed. Even clients within inpatient settings do not take their medications consistently. It is not uncommon for people to hide drugs in the cheek or pretend to swallow and then discard or hoard them. The physician should be notified in these cases, and a liquid form of the medication should be requested.

The keys to improving client compliance are education and an effective client-caregiver relationship (Balon, 2002). Work with your clients to find and eliminate the factors that lead to noncompliance. Simplify the medication routine, if possible. Teach about and monitor for side effects and adverse reactions.

INFORMED CONSENT

Another consideration relating to psychotherapeutic medications is the issue of informed consent. **Informed consent** is the process of presenting clients with information about the benefits, risks, and side effects of specific treatments, thus enabling them to make voluntary and knowledgeable decisions about their care. With the treatment of physical disorders, the process is straightforward: treatments are described, and the client makes the decision to accept or reject the plan. However, with mental disorders, the picture is not so clear. In the past, psychiatric clients who were considered a danger to themselves or others were routinely medicated without their permission.

Today, the Patient Self-Determination Act states that clients have the right to accept or refuse care and cannot be pushed, coerced, or talked into following a certain course. In 1986, the New York Court of Appeals held that "in nonemergency situations, involuntary patients cannot be forced to take psychotic medications" (Keltner, Schuecke, and Bostrom, 2001). This ruling has led to an uncomfortable compromise between client rights and people's needs to feel safe.

When clients stop taking their medications, care guidelines focus on ensuring safety and assessing for the return of symptoms. When caring for the client within an inpatient setting, caregivers should observe for any changes in behavior, be prepared for the client to become aggressive or act out, and protect the client and others from harm. If the setting is the clinic, the caregiver should instruct the client's significant others about the return of psychiatric symptoms, the signs and symptoms of side effects and adverse reactions, and the available community resources. Although care providers cannot manipulate or force clients into taking medications, they can use their rapport and communication skills to assist clients in making decisions based on complete information and sound judgment. "Agency policies about informed consent must be followed to protect the patient, staff, and agency" (Finkelman, 2000).

New drugs are being developed, ones that act more specifically, have a shorter onset, and produce fewer side effects. More treatments and therapies will be introduced. Complementary and alternative medicine will play a growing role in mental health care. It is our responsibility to safely practice within this sea of change.

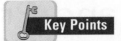
Key Points

- Psychotherapeutic medications are powerful chemical substances that produce their effects on the nervous system by interrupting the chemical messenger (neurotransmitter) pathways within the brain.
- Four classes of psychotherapeutic medications are antianxiety agents, antidepressants, antimanics, and antipsychotics.
- Drugs for the treatment of anxiety include the benzodiazepines, the azaspirones, and beta-blockers for social phobias. Their main side effects are sedation and gastrointestinal (GI) disturbances.
- Antidepressant medications treat depression and other mood disorders by increasing certain neurotransmitter activity within the brain and CNS.
- Mania and bipolar depressive illnesses are treated with lithium, a naturally occurring mood stabilizer.
- The major guidelines for care of clients taking lithium are helping with the prelithium workup, educating the client to maintain stable blood levels of the drug, and monitoring the client for side effects and possible toxic reactions.
- Antipsychotic drugs are indicated for clients with schizophrenia, acute mania, organic mental illnesses, some resistant bipolar disorders, paranoid disorders, some disorders of movement, nausea and vomiting, and intractable hiccups.
- Extrapyramidal side effects include CNS alterations that produce abnormal involuntary movement disorders. Peripheral nervous system side effects include dry mouth, blurred vision, photophobia (sensitivity to bright light), tachycardia, and hypotension.
- Clients who are receiving antipsychotics are at risk for developing the serious problems of neuroleptic malignant syndrome and tardive dyskinesia.
- Nurses who work with clients who are receiving psychotherapeutic drugs have five basic responsibilities: to assess, to coordinate, to administer, to monitor and evaluate, and to teach.
- A special medication assessment (drug history) must be conducted for clients receiving psychotherapeutic medications.
- A primary responsibility of nurses is to monitor clients for drug effectiveness and adverse reactions.
- Client education is a major role of nurses.
- Noncompliance is defined as an informed decision made by a client not to follow a prescribed treatment program.
- Informed consent is presenting clients with information about the benefits, risks, and side effects of specific treatments, thus enabling them to make decisions about their care.

evolve   Be sure to visit the companion Evolve site at http://evolve.elsevier.com/Morrison-Valfre/ for additional online resources.

8 Skills and Principles of Mental Health Care

evolve http://evolve.elsevier.com/Morrison-Valfre/

Objectives

Upon completion of this chapter, the student will be able to:

1. Describe three characteristics of a mentally healthy adult.
2. Explain how the phrase "do no harm" applies to mental health care.
3. Apply the seven principles of mental health care to client care.
4. Identify the four components of any behavior.
5. Summarize the primary purpose and six guidelines for providing safe and effective crisis intervention.
6. Illustrate how setting limits helps to provide consistency for mental health clients.
7. Describe how failure contributes to the development of insight.
8. Identify ways to prevent overinvolvement and codependency.
9. Discuss the importance of personal and professional commitments.
10. Describe four techniques for developing a positive mental attitude.
11. List ten principles for nurturing yourself and other caregivers.

Key Terms

acceptance (p. 80)
advocacy (AD-və-kə-se) (p. 79)
behavior (p. 74)
caring (p. 79)
commitment (p. 81)
consistency (p. 78)
coping mechanisms (p. 77)
crisis (p. 77)
crisis intervention (p. 77)
empathy (ĔM-pə-thē) (p. 74)
failure (p. 80)
holistic (ho-LIS-tik) health care (p. 73)
insight (p. 79)
introspection (IN-tro-SPEK-shən) (p. 80)
mentally healthy adult (p. 72)
nurture (p. 83)
principle (p. 72)
responsibility (p. 75)
self-awareness (p. 79)
stigma (STIG-mə) (p. 73)

PRINCIPLES OF MENTAL HEALTH CARE

A **principle** is a code or standard that helps govern our conduct. Principles guide decisions and actions. Professional principles provide guidelines for people who practice within the helping professions. Most health care professions are guided by standards of care, state practice acts, and principles. This chapter examines the basic principles and skills for those who work with mentally or emotionally troubled clients.

THE MENTALLY HEALTHY ADULT

The concepts of mental health and mental illness are not easily defined. Health, by its very nature, is a changing state that is influenced by genetics, behavior, and the environment. Mental health is just as dynamic—changing as the stresses of life are encountered.

Most people manage to adapt to the changes in their lives and remain contributing members of their society. Although problems may exist, mentally healthy adults are content with whom and where they are in life. They are able to love and express love freely without the fear of losing their independence. Flexibility and a willingness to try something different lead to an eagerness for learning. Life is considered important, and its special moments are cherished. Adversity is seen as a challenge or opportunity for growth. To simplify, a **mentally healthy adult** is a person who can cope with and adjust to the recurrent stresses of daily living in an acceptable way. Although mentally healthy adults experience unhappiness, anxiety, or other psychic distresses, they manage to pool their resources, rise above the negativity, and continue on with their lives.

Citizens of the industrialized cultures label a person as mentally ill only after the ability to function independently in society is impaired for a period (Giger and Davidhizar, 2004). In our culture, mental illness results when an individual's problems become so overwhelming that one is unable to carry out the activities of daily living or function independently and develops maladaptive behaviors. Other cultures have different definitions of mental illness (see Cultural Considerations 8-1 for an example of another viewpoint).

Laos is a country in southeast Asia. Its inhabitants, the Lao, believe that 32 spirits live within the body and govern its functions. Illnesses, including mental disturbances, are thought to be the result of an imbalance of the spirits, unhealthy air currents, or bad winds. Pinching or scratching parts of the body to produce red marks helps to let the bad winds out of the body and restore health. Strings are worn around the wrists, neck, ankles, or waist to prevent soul loss.

Box 8-1	*Principles of Mental Health Care*

1. Do no harm.
2. Accept each client as a whole person.
3. Develop mutual trust.
4. Explore behaviors and emotions.
5. Encourage responsibility.
6. Encourage effective adaptation.
7. Provide consistency.

MENTAL HEALTH CARE PRACTICE

A foundation of the helping professions is based on the care of the whole person. Practicing the principles of mental health care is the responsibility of all health care providers. No matter which specialty or where the setting, every caregiver helps clients cope with their problems.

The world of health care is familiar and comfortable for those who practice within its realm. The sights, sounds, and smells of the health care environment become known and familiar. Daily routines are established, and the employees all understand what behaviors are expected of them. However, to a person who is ill (disabled, stressed), visiting a medical facility can be an uncomfortable experience. Anxiety results when illness or disability affects an individual. No matter how casual a client may appear, a heightened stress level is present every time interactions with health care providers take place. Some people are so intimidated by the health care system that they wait until their problems become severe and difficult to treat. Sensitive care providers remember that clients are "out of their element" when seeking health care and need emotional support and effective care.

The skills developed when working with the mental and emotional needs of people will be used throughout your career, for yours is the profession of caring. The seven principles of mental health care listed in Box 8-1 will help guide you.

DO NO HARM

The "do no harm" principle serves as a guide for all therapeutic actions. Care providers in every setting have the responsibility to protect clients, but for caregivers working with mental health clients, this principle is especially important.

The main therapeutic tool of mental health care providers is the "self." Therapeutic use of the self can result in great improvements in clients' behaviors when the "do no harm" principle is applied. When it is overlooked or forgotten, the one who loses is the client, the very person we are obligated to protect. No matter what the circumstances, avoid any action that may result in harm to your client. The "do no harm" principle also relates to the "reasonable and prudent

nurse (caregiver)" concept found in U.S. law. It is derived from the ancient writings of Hippocrates, whose principle of "do no harm" proves to be as true and valid today as it was so long ago.

ACCEPT EACH CLIENT AS A WHOLE PERSON

People with mental problems suffer from a socially imposed stigma. The word stigma is defined as a sign or mark of shame, disapproval, or disgrace, of being shunned or rejected. Because people feel uneasy about discussing behaviors that are different, they shy away from mentally troubled individuals. One of the barriers in recovering from a mental illness is the social stigma that clients experience. Caregivers should set examples by acting as advocates for clients and educating themselves about psychiatric illnesses.

The principle of acceptance (allowing others to be who they are without passing judgment) is important in health care because you will care for many different people. Those differences do not have to be understood, but they must be accepted. You may even disapprove of clients' attitudes and behaviors, but you must accept the person because it is the **person** who is the focus of your health care activities. This section discusses a point of view that encourages the principle of acceptance.

Holistic Framework

Holistic health care is based on the concept of "whole." Understanding clients in relation to their work, family, and social environments encourages caregivers to consider their many needs and tailor individualized interventions.

In a health-oriented model, clients are assessed for their strengths and abilities. Goals of care are mutually developed. Interventions are designed for the individual, and clients receive the services most important and relevant to them. Responsibility for success is shared among clients and care providers.

Health care providers who practice holistically realize that each person must be accepted for who and what he or she is, no more and no less. Accept the person, uncomfortable behaviors and all. Search for meaning in their actions because behaviors are attempts to fill needs. Your acceptance is communicated to the clients, and your actions will eventually result in success. However, if you pass judgment, clients will sense your disapproval and therapeutic actions will fall on fallow ground.

Viewing clients holistically also involves an acceptance of their lifestyles, attitudes, social interactions, and living conditions. This can be difficult, especially when the environment or lifestyle is harmful. People with mental-emotional difficulties may display odd behaviors or verbalize unusual beliefs. They need to be accepted just as clients with physical maladies are. Our reactions to their behaviors can sometimes cloud their messages. Identify your reactions to clients. Work to develop an acceptance of each by considering the whole individual.

Caregivers may find that progress comes slowly when working with clients who are experiencing mental health problems. A holistic point of view and a focus on the positive encourage both care providers and clients to strive for success. They allow psychiatric clients respect and help us accept all people regardless of how different from ourselves they may be.

DEVELOP MUTUAL TRUST

The word *trust* means assured hope and reliance on another. Erikson's theory (see Chapter 5) lists the development of trust as the first core task of the infant. Trust is an important concept for human beings, who are social and group oriented. Trust implies cooperation, support, and a willingness to work together. Trust occurs on many levels. For example, when you drive your vehicle, you are engaging in an act of trust—you trust that oncoming drivers will stay on their side of the small, painted yellow line that divides the road. Numerous other small acts of trust occur throughout the day, but we are usually too busy to notice. Yet to care providers, the concept of trust holds much importance.

Individuals who are unable to trust cannot rely on others for help. Many people with mental-emotional problems struggle with problems of trust. Care providers must routinely demonstrate that they can be trusted. To communicate the messages of trust, remember to do what you say you will do. If you tell a client that you will return in 10 minutes, be back in 10 minutes (better yet, be there in 9 minutes). Clients soon learn which caregivers follow their words with actions. Trust begins to grow when clients know they can depend on their caregivers.

Trust is the foundation of therapeutic relationships. It forms the basis for the success or failure of all actions. People who become your clients, no matter what their diagnoses, need to trust that they will be cared for in a safe and supportive manner. The development of trust between clients and caregivers involves three concepts: caring, empathy, and advocacy (Keltner, Schwecke, and Bostrom, 2007).

For people with mental illness, caring plays an especially important role. They know, subconsciously, whether you actually care or regard them as just another client. Before trust can be developed, clients must truly believe that their nurses and other providers care. Empathy is the ability to recognize and share the emotions of another person without actually experiencing them. Empathy is a powerful therapeutic tool. If clients believe that you are willing to share their discomforts, they become more interested in learning to help themselves.

People with mental-emotional difficulties are not always capable of making informed decisions. Here caregivers intervene to ensure that the client's basic needs are being met. For example, if a client decides not to eat, the care provider may act in the client's best interest by making the food easily available. The client cannot be forced to eat, but he or she can be encouraged to make more healthful choices. Client advocacy also involves the concept of empowerment. Many mentally ill people are quite capable of taking part in their care and treatment. Some are not, but all deserve the opportunity to make the decisions they are capable of making. Nurses and other caregivers act as advocates by assisting clients through the decision-making process. Providing information and education assists clients in making appropriate decisions about their care. When clients feel that their care providers understand and act in their best interests, trust is established. The therapeutic relationship is more fully discussed in Chapter 11.

EXPLORE BEHAVIORS AND EMOTIONS

Every behavior serves a purpose and has meaning. Behaviors are attempts to fill personal needs and goals. Each of us lives within our own private world. Most people's private worlds (internal frames of reference) are agreeable with others. However, people with mental-emotional difficulties have private worlds that may be difficult for the average person to understand.

"Behavior consists of perceptions, thoughts, feelings, and actions" (Stuart and Laraia, 2005) (Figure 8-1). A disruption in any one of these areas can result in behavioral problems. Distorted perceptions, impaired thought processes, and alterations of emotional expression lead to maladaptive actions. Behaviors also must be

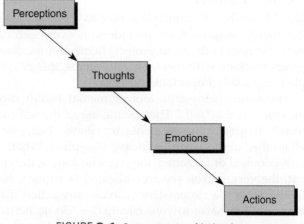

FIGURE **8-1** Components of behavior.

understood in terms of the context or setting in which they occur. A particular environment may be threatening because of uncomfortable past experiences in similar settings.

It is sometimes difficult to accurately interpret the message that a client's behavior is sending. Actions may be clouded with symbols or influenced by chemical substances. Alcohol and other drugs affect perceptions, emotional expression, and judgment, as well as behavior.

An often overlooked method of understanding the meaning of a client's behavior is to simply **ask** the individual. Many clients are willing to share themselves when (1) they have trust in you and (2) you are willing to take the time to listen. When people with mental health problems can discuss their behaviors or share their emotions, they are not looking for approval or reproach. Acceptance and a gentle exploration of what the behaviors mean to them will help clients develop and practice insight. Recognizing ineffective behaviors and replacing them with more appropriate actions constitute the first step toward gaining some control over one's situation.

Explaining how you view the client's behaviors allows for perception checks. Is the client sending the same message that you are receiving? Does each of you see the same messages in the client's symbols? If the client says he feels like a duck, do you know what he is really trying to portray? Sharing your perceptions helps clients see how their behavioral messages are being received by other people. It also allows caregivers the opportunity to gain insight into their worlds.

Some clients are unable to verbally share the meanings of their behaviors. They communicate with actions only. Caregivers must develop acute observational skills with these individuals. Repeated behaviors are often attempts to undo or fix something. Other actions can be cries for help or forms of self-punishment for wrongful deeds. The meaning of a client's behaviors may be shrouded in mystery, but time, trust, and persistent observations assist in discovering the real meanings that lie behind the messages.

ENCOURAGE RESPONSIBILITY

Responsible people are capable of making and fulfilling obligations. They are accountable for their decisions or actions. Responsibility infers that a person is able to exercise capability and accountability. Individuals who are unable to make or keep obligations are not considered to be responsible. Health care providers work with clients who exhibit a wide variety of coping styles and behaviors. Encouraging responsibility is a primary mental health intervention because it helps build self-worth, dignity, and confidence. It also assists clients in learning more successful coping behaviors. Responsibility is a cornerstone of modern societies and a goal of mental health care.

As children grow and develop the necessary skills for living within a society, so do their responsibilities. The assumption of responsibilities starts when the child begins to explore and manipulate the environment. Responsibility is learned early. The primary instructor is the family, but the social group and culture exert strong influences. As children learn about "right behaviors," they develop the responsibility to engage in them. There is a saying that states: "If the family does not teach responsibility, the school will. If the school does not teach responsibility, then the group will. If the group does not teach responsibility, then society will, and society sends irresponsible people to jail."

Many people with mental-emotional problems have difficulty behaving in responsible ways. Some have never been taught because of their dysfunctional family or childhood experiences. Others cannot remember or hold onto a logical picture long enough to be responsible. However, every person has the capacity for growth and therefore some degree of responsibility. Nurses and other professionals who work with the mentally ill population plan and implement specific interventions designed to help clients achieve their highest possible level of responsibility.

The first step in developing self-responsibility relates to care of the self. The basic physical needs of life (Maslow's lower-order needs) must be met no matter what the circumstances. Every adult and sadly many children must procure food, clothing, and shelter for themselves. People with mental-emotional problems commonly have difficulty in meeting basic needs, so lessons of self-responsibility usually begin with something as basic as caring for one's daily personal hygiene needs.

Caregivers should assess their clients' abilities to perform the skills associated with the activities of daily living. For example, sometimes the reason for poor hygiene is a lack of knowledge. A person may never have been taught to bathe frequently or brush his or her teeth after every meal. In such cases the caregiver must teach and the client must learn the basic skills of personal cleanliness. When the client assumes responsibility for basic needs, it leads to improved feelings of self-worth. When one looks good, one feels better. Small successes become positive steps that help equip clients with the skills necessary for effective functioning.

The next step in assuming self-responsibility is to be accountable for one's emotions. "I'm sorry. I lost my temper," does not excuse the action. Mental health clients frequently have poor control over their emotions (called poor impulse control). They immediately react without considering the consequences of their behaviors. Becoming responsible for one's emotions involves the willingness to identify and then "own" the problems and emotions. It also requires a willingness and determination to try new and more effective ways of coping with emotional reactions.

When clients learn to replace an unacceptable behavior with a more effective action, they achieve a degree of control over their lives. As individuals become responsible they begin to succeed. Those small successes help remove them from the role of victim and realize the value of becoming responsible.

People who seek treatment for mental or emotional problems must assume the responsibility for cooperating with and following their therapeutic plan of care. This involves a commitment to becoming actively involved by sharing personal information, being open to new ideas, and being willing to try new ways of doing things.

Clients are also responsible for the effects of their actions on others. The enjoyment of social interactions is accompanied by the responsibility of behaving appropriately. People who have problems with emotional (impulse) control can become a threat to the safety of others when their behaviors are inappropriate. It is important for caregivers to assist clients in controlling their behaviors because people who act in irresponsible ways are soon removed from social settings.

Responsibility is a fundamental concept in mental health care. It is a key to developing more effective behaviors and building self-worth. Some psychiatric therapies are designed around the concept of responsibility. For example, William Glasser's reality therapy (1998) uses responsibility as a therapeutic tool (Box 8-2).

ENCOURAGE EFFECTIVE ADAPTATION

Mental health clients may be labeled with one or more psychiatric diagnoses, but all have one thing in common—unsuccessful coping behaviors. The very nature of mental illness is characterized by actions that are not in keeping with society's definitions of appropriate behaviors. Mental health caregivers provide clients with education about and opportunities to engage in more effective behaviors.

With some mental-emotional difficulties we can speak of cures. Situational depression, for example, is frequently cured. Many cases of confusion or delirium are cured when a physical problem is discovered. However, some mental problems are chronic and force clients and their significant others to make permanent changes in how they live their lives. Despite this reality, many people with chronic illnesses (physical and mental) adapt and lead full, satisfying, and meaningful lives. Adaptation in this context is not the same as the "cure" of a medical illness. Here it means sufficient improvement to carry on everyday activities. In other words, if we can teach clients to replace maladaptive behaviors with more effective actions, they will improve in their abilities to live more successfully.

One Step at a Time

There is an old saying, "The longest journey begins with a single step." This was never as true as it is in mental health care. To people with mental-emotional problems, everything seems overwhelming. Even the simplest decisions can be monumental. People diagnosed with schizophrenia may not be able to differentiate one world from another long enough to follow a train of thought to a logical conclusion. Therefore it is important for caregivers to give instructions simply and repeat them often.

When planning therapeutic interventions, remember the importance of mastering the first item before proceeding to more complex steps. This process involves breaking down a task or concept into small and simple units. For example, the goal is for the client to arrive on time for appointments. This may involve wearing a watch, being able to tell time, remembering the appointment, and transporting oneself to the appointment. The first step in meeting the goal may be the purchase of a watch or learning to tell time.

There are two points to be made here. First, **do not assume, assess.** Using the example above, one assumes that every adult can tell time, but the results of this assessment revealed that the client could not tell time because of blurred vision. Unless the caregiver helps the client deal with the visual problems, he or she will not be successful in meeting the goal of routinely keeping all appointments. Second, remember that success is built on many small steps. Breaking each learning experience down into small units increases the chances of mastery. Make sure that the client will succeed within the first few steps. The taste of success is especially sweet in the early stages, and it encourages people to continue trying. One small, successful step soon becomes two, and those small triumphs can become symbolic of the client's potential for growth and change.

Box 8-2 **Reality Therapy**

Reality therapists do not accept the concept of mental illness. Calling people "irresponsible" rather than "mentally ill" and describing how they are irresponsible help clients develop the responsibility to satisfy their needs.

Reality therapy differs from psychoanalysis in six ways:
1. Because reality therapy does not accept the notion of mental illness, clients are not accepted into therapy as mentally ill people who have no responsibility.
2. Reality therapy works in the present with an eye on the future. It does not accept the limitations of the past.
3. Reality therapists personally relate to clients, not as aloof professionals or transference objects.
4. Reality therapists do not look for unconscious conflicts. Clients cannot excuse their behaviors based on unconscious motivations.
5. The morality of behavior is emphasized. Issues of right and wrong are defined and enforced.
6. The goal of reality therapy is to help clients help themselves fulfill their needs right now.

Crisis Intervention

When experiencing stress, people use their resources to decrease the discomfort. These efforts, called coping mechanisms, are defined as any thought or action aimed at reducing stress. We all use coping mechanisms as the tools that help us work through the ups and downs of daily living. Coping mechanisms are divided into three main types: psychomotor (physical), cognitive (intellectual), and affective (emotional). When coping mechanisms are successfully used, an individual is able to solve problems and reduce stress. These are adaptive or constructive coping mechanisms. However, when efforts to decrease stress are used without resolving the conflict, then the coping mechanism is labeled as maladaptive or destructive. Table 8-1 describes each type of coping mechanism.

A crisis is an upset in the homeostasis (steady state) of an individual. A crisis has several characteristics that separate it from other stressful situations. First, the definition of crisis is an individual matter that depends on the perception of the event, the severity of the threat, and the available coping strategies and resources. Second, a crisis occurs when an individual's usual coping mechanisms are ineffective. The crisis demands new solutions with new coping strategies. Third, crisis is self-limiting. Because human organisms cannot endure high levels of continued stress, crises are usually resolved within a short time. Fourth, a crisis usually affects more than one person. Everyone within the person's support system is affected by the crisis.

As people experience a crisis, they travel through similar stages: perception, denial, crisis, disorganization, recovery, and reorganization (Figure 8-2). Once an event is **perceived** as a crisis, an overwhelming feeling of **denial** is experienced. This emotion serves to protect the individual from sudden, intense stress. An increase in tension is felt as attempts are made to eliminate the problem. As efforts to cope are ineffective, the individual or family enters the stage of **crisis** in which everything seems to "fall apart."

During the **disorganization** phase, individuals become preoccupied with the crisis situation. Activities of daily living no longer continue. The individual becomes flooded with anxiety as attempts are made to reorganize or escape. One may blame others or pretend the situation does not exist, but nothing helps. Once all attempts to deny, solve, escape, or ignore the problem have failed, the individual slowly moves toward the recovery. This is the stage at which most people seek help.

Recovery begins when attempts to cope with the problem result in success. One success provides encouragement and builds on another, and soon the stage of reorganization is entered. Normal activities are resumed. When a crisis is successfully resolved, the individual functions at a higher level than before. Growth has taken place, and one becomes stronger and more capable.

Crises can also result in unsuccessful resolutions or pseudoresolutions. **Unresolved crises** result when maladaptive behaviors are used to hide the problem. An example is the husband who sends his wife to counseling for depression while he continues to abuse her when he drinks. **Pseudoresolution** occurs when nothing is learned from the crisis and the opportunity for growth was missed. However, new stressors may trigger buried conflicts of the unresolved crisis. The inability to solve future crises may be compounded by these old conflicts (see Think About 8-1).

The main goal of crisis intervention is to help individuals and families manage their crisis situations by offering immediate emotional support. People are then assisted in developing effective coping mechanisms, which allows time to reorganize resources and support systems.

Victims of crisis are treated in settings such as emergency departments, clinics, jails, places of worship, homes, and even over the telephone. Crisis hotlines are 24-hour telephone lines that are staffed by volunteers trained in crisis intervention techniques. Emotional

---

Table 8-1 | *Types of Coping Behaviors*

MECHANISM	DESCRIPTION	EXAMPLE
Psychomotor (physical)	Efforts to cope directly with problem	Confrontation, fighting, running away, negotiating
Cognitive (intellectual)	Efforts to neutralize threat by changing meaning of problem	Making comparisons, substituting rewards, ignoring, changing values, using problem-solving methods
Affective (emotional)	Actions taken to reduce emotional distress; no efforts are made to solve problem	Ego defense mechanisms such as denial and suppression; see Chapter 5 for other ego defense mechanisms

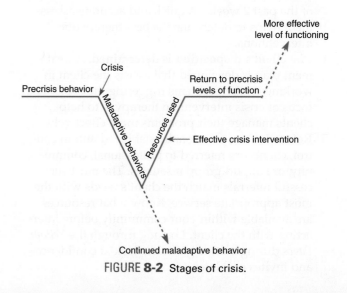

FIGURE **8-2** Stages of crisis.

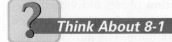

Think About 8-1

List two crises you have personally experienced.
• What coping mechanisms did you use?
• How were they successful in helping you cope?
• What did you do to resolve each crisis?
• What was learned from each experience?

support and referral to various community resources are offered to any caller.

Guidelines relating to crisis intervention have been developed by the National Institute for Training in Crisis Intervention and other organizations. Because crisis situations are high-stress encounters for all parties, the following guidelines can assist in providing safe, effective crisis interventions:

1. **Care is needed immediately.** Actions must be taken to reduce anxiety levels. Sometimes this may require only reassurance. In other situations, interventions must be taken to ensure safety and prevent harm.

2. **Control.** People experiencing a crisis are often unable to exercise control. Safety for both client and care provider must be considered. The care provider must quickly assume control but only until the client is able to recover self-control. Again, the level of control is determined by each situation. Some people are relieved that someone else is in control, whereas others resort to physical aggression during a crisis. Control is important in a crisis because without it, the client cannot be helped to work with the problems that triggered the crisis.

3. **Assessment.** Although assessment usually is the first step in the care process, the issues of immediacy, safety, and control must be considered first in crisis. Thoroughly assess the situation. Ask direct questions, such as "What happened?" Have the client explain the situation and review the events of the past 2 weeks. A quick and accurate assessment helps to determine the best therapeutic interventions.

4. **The client's disposition is determined.** A treatment plan is developed that assists the client in working on the problems triggering the crisis. The focus of crisis intervention therapy is to help clients manage their problems more effectively.

5. **Referral.** Once emotionally stabilized and in control, clients are referred to professional, community, or support group resources. The most successful referrals match the client's needs with the most appropriate service. Know what resources are available within your community before interacting with the client. Looking through the *Yellow Pages* during a crisis generates lack of confidence and invites problems.

6. **Follow-up.** Care providers must see if the referrals were actually contacted. A follow-up telephone call will often reveal new problems that prevent the client from receiving needed care.

All people experience crises. When new coping mechanisms are needed but are unavailable because of immaturity, an individual experiences a developmental or maturational crisis. Severe stresses within one's environment may cause a situational crisis. Assisting people in crisis to mobilize their resources is an important step in encouraging effective adaptation.

PROVIDE CONSISTENCY

The last principle for mental health care providers relates to the concept of consistency, which is behaviors that imply being steady and regular, dependable. People with mental illness often lack the security of someone who is there when needed. In some cases, the consistency and reliability of mental health care providers are their only stability. The link that serves as a bridge between the client's world and the world of reality is frequently the reliability of the therapeutic relationship.

The concept of consistency is usually addressed in the client's plan of care, but each therapeutic intervention must be routinely used by every member of the care team. Clients often test staff members by "playing one against the other" or attempting to manipulate the situation and gain control. However, when each care provider responds by giving the same message, clients learn that members of the care team can be relied on to do what they say they will do. Two general guidelines for providing consistency are to set limits and focus on the positive changes that clients are making.

Setting limits involves clients, staff members, and institutional policies (Chenevert, 1994). As the plan of care is developed, each rule or limitation is established. Facility policies define some limitations. The remainder relate to therapeutic activities, social interactions, and personal behaviors. Whatever the limitations, the client must be informed and willing to cooperate with the plan of care.

Each member of the care team is responsible for understanding the purpose of each limitation and the methods for enforcing them. To illustrate, the facility's policy is for all clients to remain out of bed during the day. To accomplish this, the staff informs each client every morning that the doors to the rooms will be locked by 9 AM. Then the aide makes 9 AM rounds and locks the door to each room. The clients were first informed and then reminded of the rule. Then the enforcement or actual action demonstrated that the limitation would be enforced. Something as simple as providing a routine can teach clients about the values of reliability, consistency, and stability.

This brings us to a valuable point: Do not commit yourself unless you are able to fulfill the commitment.

If your actions are not reliable, if you do not behaviorally demonstrate stability and consistency, then the therapeutic relationship will be established with great difficulty. Clients are people, and they need to know whether someone truly cares and is willing to make the connection that helps them to heal.

SKILLS FOR MENTAL HEALTH CARE

Caregivers serve as therapeutic instruments, with each interaction designed to move clients toward the goals of care. They also act as role models for good mental and physical health. They are expected to help solve problems while graciously coping with the varied personalities of many individuals. Caregivers work to instill confidence in their clients and encourage them to change and to try new behaviors within the security of the therapeutic relationship.

To practice effectively, a caregiver's approach to clients must continually be monitored and adjusted. Thought and consideration must be given to each therapeutic action. Making a positive, therapeutic use of your personality requires "a consistent, thoughtful effort directed toward developing an awareness of self and others" (Taylor, 1994).

SELF-AWARENESS

Simply defined, **self-awareness** is a consciousness of one's personality. It is the act of looking at oneself: of considering one's abilities, characteristics, aspirations, and concepts of self in relation to others. It is an awareness of one's personal and social behaviors and their impact on others (Morrison, 1993). In short, self-awareness is the ability to objectively look within.

The development of self-awareness requires time, patience, and a willingness to routinely consider one's behaviors, attitudes, and values. The rewards, however, are worth the efforts because both clients and caregivers benefit when therapeutic goals are achieved. Personally, self-awareness allows individuals to direct and mold the pattern of their lives, to be in charge of their own growth and development. Caregivers who encourage the development of self-awareness in their clients must be ready to practice it themselves. To improve self-awareness requires caring, insight, acceptance, commitment, a positive outlook, and the willingness to nurture oneself. If you are willing to put effort into these areas, you will evolve into a person who is able to use your personality to achieve therapeutic change and personal fulfillment.

CARING

Everyone has the universal human need for love. Maslow's hierarchy of needs lists the need for love and belonging as the first nonphysical requirement after safety. Without love infants fail to grow or thrive and adults become isolated, lonely, and depressed. Human beings are gregarious creatures. We are meant to live with others. Although physical appearances, behavioral patterns, and communication styles may differ, each person carries within the need to belong and be loved.

Caring is the energy on which the health care professions are built. It is defined as a concern for the well-being of another person, and it includes behaviors such as accepting, comforting, honesty, attentive listening, and sensitivity. Caring is the glue that binds individuals to each other. It is energy of the soul, freely given in hopes of helping another human being. Caring cannot be taught as a procedure or skill. It must be developed, encouraged, and molded into the therapeutic personality of the caregiver.

Caring serves as a thread that connects people and moves them toward recovery. For people with mental illness, caring plays an especially important role. They know, subconsciously, whether you actually care or regard them as just other clients. Before trust can be developed, clients must truly believe that their nurses and other providers really care. The caring qualities of empathy and advocacy are especially important when caring for mentally troubled individuals.

Empathy is the ability to recognize and share the emotions of another person without actually experiencing them. It includes an understanding of the meaning and significance of that person's behavior. It is a willingness to see the world as the client does. Clients with mental illnesses frequently live in a lonely world of personal suffering, detached from society. Empathy, in these cases, becomes a powerful therapeutic tool that can help reestablish one's self-worth and dignity.

Advocacy is the process of providing a client with the information, support, and feedback needed to make a decision (Keltner and others, 2007). Client advocacy adds the obligation to act in the client's best interest. People with mental-emotional difficulties are not always capable of making informed decisions. In cases like these, caregivers intervene to ensure that the client's basic needs are being met. For example, if a client decides not to eat, the care provider may act in the client's best interest by making the food easily available. The client cannot be forced to eat, but he or she can be encouraged to make more healthful choices. Box 8-3 lists several therapeutic actions that demonstrate caring.

INSIGHT

We all are responsible for our own growth and development, both professionally and personally. We gain insight and wisdom through experience. **Insight** is the ability to clearly see and understand the nature of things. Insight relies on common sense, good judgment, and prudence. Although not always comfortable, our insights provide us with new opportunities to take risks, explore our own potentials, and fail as

Box 8-3 *Therapeutic Actions: Caring*

Address client by Mr. or Ms. (last name) until otherwise instructed.
Respect the client's unique personality.
Do not judge the client's behaviors or attitudes.
Share often with the client that every person has the potential for change.
Show interest in the whole person, not just the diagnosis.
Customize information to the client's level of understanding.
Watch for nonverbal messages.
Promote self-esteem by recognizing and communicating that the client is a worthwhile and valuable individual.
Assess your own interactions, nonverbal actions, and communications.

Box 8-4 *Using Failure Positively*

To use failure positively:
1. Realize that failure is a necessary part of growth.
2. Give yourself permission to fail.
3. Consider failure as a learning experience.
4. Discover new options and opportunities created by the failure.
5. Expect to succeed with the next attempt.

well as succeed. For care providers, insight includes sensitivity to people, the ability to make keen observations, and a willingness to seek new knowledge.

Self-awareness is developed through the practice of introspection, which is the process of looking into one's own mind. Introspection is an analysis of self—one's feelings, reactions, attitudes, opinions, values, and behaviors. It is also a process for observing and analyzing one's behavior in various situations. Introspection allows us to "step out" of the interaction and watch our own behaviors. This process is assisted when caregivers can view themselves interacting with various clients on videotape or television. Introspection allows caregivers to identify both personal and professional learning needs. Practice **professional introspection** by keeping a small notebook. Throughout the day, jot down any questions or subjects that relate to the care of your clients—anything about which you feel you need to know more. After work, make it a point to research at least one question or topic every day. This practice will serve as a valuable aid for gaining new knowledge. Knowledge breeds competence, and from competence grows the confidence to provide the best possible care.

Personal introspection is the process of learning who you are. This type of introspection may be accompanied by emotional discomfort, but, for those individuals who can overcome their own emotional defenses, introspection serves as a valuable tool for developing self-awareness.

RISK TAKING AND FAILURE

The process of developing self-awareness includes the elements of risk and failure. If one is to grow, then one must take risks. Risk taking implies the possibility of failure. For most of us, the word *failure* has a negative meaning that implies defeat and a lack of success. However, failure can be filled with positive, growth-promoting experiences. **Failure provides the opportunity for change.** It encourages creativity, stimulates

learning, and sharpens one's judgments. Failure is a price that must be paid for improvement. When used as a learning tool, the experience of failure can provide insight and the foundation for the next step toward success. The person who never fails cannot savor the rewards of success.

How do we grow from our failures? The first and most important step is to understand that **failure is a necessary part of change.** The second step is to **give yourself permission to fail.** The odds of a person living a lifetime without a failure are about zero. Failure, learning, and growth are all partners in the development of self-awareness. The third step is to **consider your failure as a learning experience.** Examine the elements of the failure, and discover what improvements could be made. More effective actions in the future can avoid the failures of the past. The fourth and last step is to discover the opportunities that are created by failure. Often a failure opens new doors or presents a problem in an entirely different light. Examining and learning from failure can create new options and opportunities. Box 8-4 lists several suggestions for using failure as a positive experience. Remember, one fails only when one refuses to grow from the experience.

ACCEPTANCE

Although people may engage in behaviors that are considered inappropriate, every individual has worth and some degree of dignity. Each client must be given respect and the opportunity to participate in care if treatment is to be successful. Acceptance in this context means the receiving of the entire person and the world in which he or she functions.

Accepting clients does not necessarily include approving of their behaviors. This is an important distinction; you must accept the person, but you do not have to accept the behavior. Many caregivers who work with mentally and emotionally troubled clients do not hesitate to tell a client when his or her behavior is inappropriate, but no mental health caregiver should ever directly attack or correct the person. Table 8-2 presents examples of communications that focus on the difference between correcting the behavior and correcting the person. The very reason clients with mental-emotional problems seek help is to correct their ineffective behaviors. We, as their care providers, must accept the entire person as a complete package

Table 8-2 *Focus on Correcting Behavior Versus Person*

FOCUS ON BEHAVIOR	FOCUS ON PERSON
"Sam, undressing in the dayroom is inappropriate."	"Sam, I've told you not to undress in the dayroom."
"Mary, stop! No slapping is allowed here."	"Mary, stop that! Why are you slapping him?"
"I find it difficult to be here when you …"	"You're disgusting when you do that."

regardless of our own reactions. This acceptance then becomes the foundation on which other therapeutic actions are based.

BOUNDRIES AND OVERINVOLVEMENT

Caregivers are expected to give of themselves in the care of others. Today we realize that to effectively care for others, we must care for ourselves and recharge our batteries, if we are to maintain the necessary energy to therapeutically work with clients. One of the ways in which caregivers maintain their energy levels is to define their helping boundaries.

We all have limits or boundaries over which we will not cross. Personal boundaries provide order and security because they help to establish the limits of one's behavior. To illustrate, you would not think of stealing from your friends because a personal boundary limits you from doing so.

Professional boundaries define the needs of the caregiver "as distinctly different from the needs of the patient: what is too helpful and what is not; and what fosters independence vs. unhealthy dependence" (Pillette, Berck, and Achber, 1995). Once clients are stabilized, they are expected to begin functioning independently with guidance and encouragement from the members of the health care team. Professional (helping) boundaries have been crossed when caregivers become too helpful or controlling. The caregiver may feel good, but the client does not function any better as a result of the interventions.

The need for professional boundaries must be continually balanced with one's needs to be caring. To do this, care providers establish their own set of professional boundaries by defining the limits of both their personal and professional lives. The focus of the professional aspect is the client, but the focus of the caregiver's personal life is himself or herself. The boundaries of each remain distinct because one cannot focus on the client and the self at the same time.

To maintain their professional boundaries, caregivers assess relationships with their clients often. If they find themselves having difficulty in setting limits or feel that they are the only one who "really understands" a certain client (the beginnings of codependency), then cause for concern exists and help should be sought. Discussing the situation with appropriate persons helps provide perspective and increases one's therapeutic effectiveness. The therapeutic relationship is anchored in the effective management of professional (helping) boundaries. When the focus of interaction is the client and progress is being made toward the therapeutic goals, the relationship is effective and satisfying for both client and caregiver.

Detecting boundary violations is often difficult because "a person's own needs stimulate and maintain the violation" (Pillette and others, 1995). However, early detection helps prevent larger problems in the future. Frequent self-assessments assist in monitoring for problems. A delicate balance exists between knowing when to help and when not to help clients. Caregivers who are aware of this balance keep the client as the major focus of concern and maintain the professional boundaries that help individuals progress toward their therapeutic goals.

We have all had (or will have) special clients, those who have touched us deeply. Becoming overinvolved is not difficult to do. However, to thrive and grow ourselves, we must learn to walk the fine line between compassion and overinvolvement.

Caregivers are people too, complete with their own attributes and problems. It is easier to form a rapport with some clients than others. Sometimes that rapport leads to an overinvolvement because the client touches the caregiver in some special way. This initial attraction can soon result in conflict because the caregiver begins to have difficulty separating the professional relationship from the growing friendship with the client. When the client-care provider relationship begins to fulfill the caregiver's needs, codependency results. The relationship loses its therapeutic effectiveness, and the caregiver or client withdraws, left with a mix of unresolved feelings and unmet goals.

To protect yourself from becoming codependent, remember this one rule of thumb: If you show a significantly greater level of concern for one client than for others, then you are running the risk of becoming overinvolved. Recognize this risk early, and discuss it with your supervisor. Exploring your feelings in relation to the client helps to regain the balance between professionalism and compassion. Often just the personal awareness of the potential of becoming overinvolved is enough to prevent it from occurring. Compassion, empathy, and acceptance are vital elements of health care, but they must be balanced by professionalism, judgment, and therapeutic actions that meet the client's needs.

COMMITMENT

A **commitment** is a personal bond to some course of action or cause. The health care professions are undergoing radical changes. If provision of high-quality care for every person is to remain a primary goal of our society, then a strong commitment from each health care provider will be needed to maintain the focus on our clients. Caregivers must be committed to providing competent health care, no matter what the setting or circumstances.

The first and most important commitment is to yourself, the commitment to consciously take charge of your personal and professional growth. Self-commitment involves a promise to do the best you can in every situation and to be the best that you can be. Each person has a unique set of talents, an individual personality, and areas of life that need improvement. People who are committed to improving themselves are able to consider both the positive and negative aspects of their personalities without guilt or remorse. They realize their mistakes and attempt to profit from them by extracting the lessons hidden in each error. They then commit themselves to applying hard-earned lessons to new situations, which in turn enhances self-awareness and expands one's ability to cope with new experiences.

Health care providers have stronger commitments than most people. They are committed to caring about the welfare of humankind. They demonstrate this dedication by continually seeking out new knowledge, keeping up-to-date with the latest professional developments, and striving to improve their therapeutic effectiveness.

You are committed; otherwise, you would not be reading these words. Take the time to discover what you feel is most important in life. Then look behind the topic, and you will find yourself committed to a certain course of action. The exercise of describing one's commitments helps to expand self-awareness and reminds us of the interconnectedness of all human beings.

POSITIVE OUTLOOK

Distress of the human spirit can be far more damaging than a medical diagnosis. A positive, health-oriented attitude alone can make a difference in functioning. Learn to approach problems with an attitude that employs the client's strengths, assets, and resources. A focus on the positive aspects of a situation stands a greater chance of success. When it is assumed that the mental health client will succeed, clients usually live up to expectations and do just that—succeed. One small success fosters and breeds other triumphs. Keep your focus on the "can do." It can have surprising results.

One of the most effective and important tools for developing self-awareness is a positive or optimistic attitude. One's outlook affects every perception, thought, and emotion. People are attracted to individuals with positive attitudes. A person with a positive outlook radiates energy and well-being that cheers up everyone in the vicinity. On the other hand, individuals with negative attitudes tend to discourage other people from interacting with them. Their attitude of doom and gloom can even foster the development of many physical and mental problems.

Positive attitudes and thoughts can act as buffers against stress and conflict. They can prevent caregiver burnout, the syndrome that results when care providers give too much without renewing their energies. A positive outlook does not require one to be continually upbeat. The reality of each situation must be considered objectively, but there is no reason to harbor a negative attitude when a positive one is much more fulfilling. In addition, caregivers who practice positive thinking act as role models for those clients who do not cope effectively within their worlds.

Achieving and maintaining a positive outlook is especially important for caregivers who work with mentally and emotionally troubled individuals. A positive attitude is the secret weapon for coping with the adversity of life. It is the key to maintaining physical and emotional health, especially for those who share their energies therapeutically. Developing a positive attitude (Box 8-5) is a process that requires persistent and patient efforts because our current attitudes and habits are deeply ingrained. However, the process can be assisted by following these five tips:

1. **Listen to your self-talk.** Pay attention to the words you use. Each word has an emotional attachment to it. The human brain is programmed by thoughts, which become feelings, which evolve into words and actions. Many people complain of being under too much stress or pressure. No one denies that modern life contains its share of stresses. However, it is how each stressor is defined that determines your point of view. If you do not define the event as stressful, then it is not. Practice listening to yourself. You may be surprised at what you discover.

2. **Change recurrent negative themes.** Any thought, emotion, word, or action that is self-defeating needs to be replaced with a positive, empowering one. Releasing and replacing one's negative attitudes lead to greater self-esteem, awareness, confidence, and happiness, not to mention the added benefits of a highly effective immune system. Practice changing your negative themes because your outlook determines the success or failure of an action.

3. **Be your own cheerleader.** Give yourself a pep talk every morning and whenever you are coping with stresses. Present yourself with positive, inspiring thoughts. Your brain does not question your thoughts. Those stored thoughts then become the basis for actions. Positive statements uplift the spirits and help to convince you of your value.

Box 8-5 *To Develop a Positive Attitude*

1. Recognize the negative thoughts, emotions, and attitudes. Reject them and throw them out of your personality.
2. Replace each negative attitude by frequently repeating positive statements.
3. Repeat upbeat and enthusiastic words that help to build a feeling of success.
4. Visualize future successes.
5. Act the part.

4. **Visualize future successes.** Take a few moments during each day to picture yourself achieving a goal. Fantasize about the feelings associated with achievement, and think about the steps that lead to the goal. Picture yourself as a dynamic person and capable caregiver; it will help to provide the blueprint for future growth. Besides, it is fun to do.

5. **Act the part.** Visualize yourself as a person with confidence and ability. You will find that your actual level of confidence grows each time you project an image of self-assurance. Developing a positive outlook will serve you well.

NURTURING YOURSELF

A critical first step in the development of self-awareness is to recognize and tend to your own needs. To nurture someone is to encourage their development. Caregivers are expected to work hard for the welfare of their clients, but they must also care for and nurture themselves. Energy cannot be continually spent without being renewed. Care providers function at a high level of wellness to provide the energy required by their clients. You have chosen to care for others. Part of the responsibility you accepted when making this decision was to care for yourself. To effectively care for your clients you must first nurture yourself.

PRINCIPLES AND PRACTICES FOR CAREGIVERS

Health care providers seek to "instill hope, empower others, encourage independence, and help improve the other's condition. When we are unable to achieve that, unable to alleviate suffering, we often experience a sense of frustration and failure" (Sherwood, 1992). When this frustration occurs repeatedly, we become emotionally worn or burned out, as many caregivers call it. Somehow each of us must find the balance between the moral duty to care amid the stress of

> **Box 8-6** | *To Nurture Yourself*
>
> 1. Be knowledgeable.
> 2. Value each individual as a human presence.
> 3. Be responsible and accountable for your actions.
> 4. Be open to new ideas.
> 5. Connect with others. Support your colleagues.
> 6. Take pride in yourself.
> 7. Like what you do.
> 8. Recognize the moments of joy in the struggles of living. Take time to smell the roses.
> 9. Recognize and accept your own limitations, but strive to improve. At the end of the day, focus on your accomplishments rather than the things left undone.
> 10. Rest each day, and begin anew.

Modified from Sherwood G: The responses of caregivers to the experience of suffering. In Starck PL, McGovern JP, editors: *The hidden dimension of illness: human suffering*, New York, 1992, National League for Nursing Press.

constant suffering and the concern for one's well-being. Box 8-6 offers basic principles for maintaining oneself when caring for others. Using these guidelines will assist you in finding the balance between giving and renewing. Remember them, because they are keys for replenishing the energies that you so freely share with others.

To nurture yourself requires more than food, water, sleep, and activity. To nourish the part of the self from which one's therapeutic energies are drawn requires special renewal. Caregivers nurture themselves in different ways. Some turn to a special source of comfort, whereas others find renewal in the adventure of trying new things. Spending time alone recharges some nurses. Others need the challenge of physical activities, travel, or new relationships.

Recently, research has pointed out the many benefits of daily meditation for stress reduction, relaxation, and renewal (Kabot-Zinn, 1994). Basically, meditation, termed the relaxation response by Western medicine, is the practice of becoming still and quiet. Health care professionals who practice meditation for as little as 15 minutes per day find it a valuable source of renewal and stress reduction.

In this busy world, it is easy to lose sight of one simple fact: your ability to care for your clients depends on how well you care for yourself. How you choose to nurture and renew yourself is a matter of personal preference. The important thing is that you do it regularly and without guilt. A good diet, adequate exercise, and restful sleep must not be ignored, but the essence of caring must also be applied to the self. Caregivers need to be willing to accept, love, and nourish themselves as much as they do their clients.

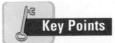 **Key Points**

- A mentally healthy adult is a person who can cope with and adjust to the stresses of daily living in a socially acceptable way. Mentally healthy adults are content with themselves, able to love and express love, flexible, eager to learn, and unafraid of adversity.
- The main therapeutic tool of mental health care providers is the "self." Therapeutic use of the self is used with the "do no harm" principle as a basis for practice.
- Understanding clients in relation to their work, family, and social environments encourages caregivers to practice holistic health care.
- The seven principles of mental health care are as follows: do no harm, accept each client as a whole person, develop mutual trust, explore behaviors and emotions, encourage responsibility, encourage effective adaptation, and provide consistency.
- Behavior consists of perceptions, thoughts, feelings, and actions.
- In mental health terms, adaptation means sufficient improvement to carry out everyday activities.

- The goal of crisis intervention is to offer immediate emotional support. Procedures for crisis intervention focus on the concepts of immediacy, control, assessment, disposition, referral, and follow-up.
- Setting and enforcing limits can teach clients about the values of reliability, consistency, and stability.
- When used as a learning tool, the experience of failure can provide insight, encourage creativity, stimulate learning, and sharpen judgment.
- To prevent overinvolvement and codependency, recognize the risk of a significantly greater level of concern for one client than for others, explore your feelings in relation to the client, and discuss it with your supervisor.
- Caregivers have the power to shape their clients' successes or failures, based on their own personal values and beliefs.
- A commitment is a bond that moves an individual to action. Self-commitment involves a promise to do one's best in every situation. Professional commitment is demonstrated by seeking out new knowledge, keeping up to date with the latest professional developments, and striving to improve one's therapeutic effectiveness.
- A positive mental attitude is developed by listening to your self-talk, changing recurrent negative themes, being your own cheerleader, visualizing future successes, and acting the part.
- Principles for nurturing yourself include the following: be knowledgeable, value each individual, be responsible and accountable, be open to new ideas, connect with others, support your colleagues, take pride in yourself, enjoy what you do, recognize the moments of joy in the struggles of living, recognize and accept your own limitations but strive to improve, and focus on your accomplishments rather than the things left undone.

---

evolve Be sure to visit the companion Evolve site at http://evolve.elsevier.com/Morrison-Valfre/ for additional online resources.

Mental Health Assessment Skills

evolve http://evolve.elsevier.com/Morrison-Valfre/

Objectives

Upon completion of this chapter, the student will be able to:

1. Identify two purposes of the mental health treatment plan.
2. List and define each step of the nursing process.
3. Describe three methods of data collection.
4. List six parts of a holistic nursing assessment.
5. Identify four guidelines for conducting effective psychiatric interviews.
6. Explain the importance of performing physical assessments of clients with psychiatric diagnoses.
7. Explain the purpose of the mental status examination.
8. List the five general categories of the mental status examination.
9. Describe the process for conducting a mental status examination.

Key Terms

affect (ĂF-ĕkt) (p. 92)
assessment (ə-SĔS-mĕnt) (p. 87)
calculation (KĂL-kyū-LĀ-shŭn) (p. 94)
data collection (p. 87)
insight (p. 94)
interview (p. 87)
judgment (p. 94)
memory (p. 93)
mood (p. 92)
nursing (therapeutic) process (p. 86)
perceptions (p. 92)
risk factor assessment (p. 88)
sensorium (sĕn-SŌ-rē-ŭm) (p. 93)
thought content (p. 93)
thought processes (p. 93)

The ability to effectively obtain and use information about clients is a vital part of the multidisciplinary treatment plan and the foundation of the nursing (therapeutic) process. Learning about clients' problems requires special abilities. Therapeutic communications, interactions, and assessment skills help care providers learn about all aspects of their clients. This chapter provides the starting point for making thorough mental health assessments. Good assessment skills are critical to quality health care. Caregivers must first learn about the person before they can provide personalized care or judge the effectiveness of any therapeutic action.

MENTAL HEALTH TREATMENT PLAN

People enter the health care system because they are distressed, disabled, or suffering. The diagnosis and treatment of people with mental health problems is challenging. Problems are not as easily identified and defined as physical disorders. According to the *Diagnostic and Statistical Manual of Mental Disorders* (DSM-IV-TR), "no definition adequately specifies precise boundaries for the concept of mental disorder" (American Psychiatric Association, 2000). The relationship between the physical and psychological self is difficult to separate. It is important to remember, however, that every psychological problem has physical effects and each physical illness has psychological effects. The wise care provider is aware of both.

When individuals first enter the mental health care system, they undergo a comprehensive assessment. Clients are interviewed by several members of the multidisciplinary health care team. Physical and psychological diagnostic testing is performed, and data are gathered from as many sources as possible. The physician provides information regarding clients' physical state and need for medications. The social worker assesses the client's family, work, and social interactions. The dietitian learns about the client's nutritional status. The psychiatrist and psychologist explore the client's emotional and cognitive (intellectual) functioning. The nurse assesses how the illness or disability affects the client's activities of daily living. Other care providers contribute information through their observations and interactions with the client.

Team members then meet to compare data, identify problems, and develop treatment approaches. When the team and the client agree on the treatment goals, a course of action is planned. Usually medical treatments (medications) are combined with psychotherapies, behavioral therapies, and other therapeutic actions. The overall treatment plan is then developed especially for the individual client. Therapeutic actions are implemented, and the client's progress toward each goal is routinely evaluated.

The mental health treatment plan serves several purposes. First, it is a guide for planning and implementing client care. Nurses are guided by the treatment plan when they develop specific nursing care plans. Psychologists, social workers, and other therapists use the treatment plan as a framework for implementing their specialized therapeutic actions.

Second, the plan serves as a vehicle for monitoring the client's progress and the effectiveness of therapeutic interventions. Clients meet often with treatment team members to discuss problems and attempts to meet their goals. Therapeutic interventions are evaluated, and the treatment plan is revised to include new information.

Third, the mental health treatment plan serves as a means for communicating and coordinating client care. It prevents costly duplication of services and provides a focus for all therapeutic activities, regardless of specialty. This increases the effectiveness of each member of the treatment team. Developing the mental health treatment plan is not a complex process, but it is always changing. Using the treatment plan allows clients and care providers the opportunity to work together to meet client goals.

DSM-IV-TR DIAGNOSIS

Most therapists who work with mentally or emotionally troubled individuals use the DSM-IV-TR (see Appendix B) to aid in diagnosis and help guide clinical practice. Clients are assessed and classified according to five categories or axes (Table 9-1). Using a multiaxial (many-category) system helps care providers gain a more complete understanding of each person. It also promotes therapeutic interventions based on individual clients. The diagnosis of mental health problems remains the responsibility of the physician, but nurses and other care providers should be familiar with the multiaxial system of psychiatric assessment. Several tools are available for assessing mental status. An example is Table 9-2, which explains the global assessment of functioning (GAF) scale.

NURSING (THERAPEUTIC) PROCESS

Each step of the nursing (therapeutic) process is designed to support goal-directed care for clients (Stuart and Laraia, 2005). The process serves as an organizational framework for effective care. It consists of five steps: assessment, diagnosis, planning, intervention, and evaluation. Using this process encourages us to focus on the client and develop appropriate and effective care measures.

The first step, **assessment,** is the data-collection step. Data relating to the client are collected from every possible source. Medical records are reviewed, a history is obtained, and observations are made. Discussions with family members or friends add to the database. Soon a picture of the client begins to emerge. Using the mass of collected information as a database, care providers plan care based on needs, abilities, preferences, and concerns of the client.

Next, data are sorted into related areas, and **problems are identified.** Each problem is then examined in detail. Problem statements and nursing diagnoses are developed. Medical diagnoses and interventions relate to the client's physical or mental dysfunctions. Nursing diagnoses and interventions focus on how the client's problems affect his or her ability to carry out the activities of daily living. Client needs are also considered when problem statements are being developed.

Table 9-1 *DSM-IV-TR Axes*

AXIS	CATEGORY	EXAMPLE
I	Clinical disorders	Mood, substance abuse, schizophrenic disorders
II	Personality disorders and mental retardation	Dependent, antisocial personality disorders Mild, moderate, severe retardation
III	General medical conditions	Heart, digestive diseases
IV	Psychosocial and environmental problems	Educational, housing, legal, economic, social environment problems
V	Global assessment of functioning (GAF)	Overall level of psychological, social, and occupational functioning

Table 9-2 *Global Assessment of Functioning Scale*

SCORE	LEVEL OF FUNCTION
100-91	**Superior functioning** in a wide range of activities; no symptoms; handles life's problems; sought out by others for many positive qualities
90-81	**Absent or minimal symptoms;** everyday problems and concerns; socially effective; generally satisfied with life
80-71	**Transient, expectable symptoms;** normal reactions to psychosocial stressors; example: difficulty focusing following an argument
70-61	**Some mild symptoms** or some difficulty in social, occupational, or school functioning; has some meaningful interpersonal relationships
60-51	**Moderate symptoms** or moderate difficulty in social, occupational, or school functioning; has few friends, conflicts with peers or co-workers
50-41	**Serious symptoms;** serious impairment in social, occupational, or school functioning; no friends; unable to keep a job
40-31	**Impaired reality testing, communication;** major impairment in several areas (work, school, family relations, mood, thinking); example: depressed man avoids friends, can't work, neglects family
30-21	**Seriously impaired judgment, communication;** inability to function in almost all areas; behavior influenced by hallucinations, delusions
20-11	**Some danger to self or others** or gross impairment in communication or occasionally fails to maintain personal hygiene; suicidal; violent; manic excitement
10-1	**Persistent danger of hurting self or others** or persistently does not maintain minimal personal hygiene; serious suicidal acts with expectation of death; recurrent violent acts

Modified from American Psychiatric Association: *Diagnostic and statistical manual of mental disorders,* ed 4, text revision, Washington, DC, 2000, The Association.

During the **planning** phase, the outcome of each problem is projected by identifying behaviors that indicate that the problem is solved. These "expected outcomes" are then used to monitor the client's progress. Specific short- and long-term goals are developed, and therapeutic actions (interventions) are planned. Then a written care plan is developed.

The **intervention** phase includes the actual delivery of the planned actions. Therapeutic interventions, carried out by all mental health care team members, guide clients toward their goals. Client responses to each intervention are monitored. Work to keep an open mind when observing the client's responses to care, and remember that many reactions are culturally determined (see Cultural Considerations 9-1).

The final phase of the process, **evaluation,** determines the effectiveness of care. By comparing expected outcomes with actual results, care providers are able to note which actions met the goals and which did not. Those actions that did not result in improvement are reassessed, and the process is begun again.

Clients are involved as partners in care. Although some individuals are unable or too discouraged to make decisions, most clients are capable of participating in some part of their care. Caregivers help clients problem solve by involving them in the care-planning process. Evaluations of both clients' and caregivers' actions allow for adjustments in the dynamic process known as "treatment." Use of the nursing (therapeutic) process requires knowledge, experience, and the practice of good judgment. Experience grows with each application of the process, and sound judgment is gained by looking at every possible side of a problem before arriving at a decision. The nursing (therapeutic) process serves as a tool for defining and solving client problems, but the tool is only as effective as the practitioner. The art of choosing the best course of action must be carefully practiced. Let the "do no harm" principle guide you as you grow.

ABOUT ASSESSMENT

Assessment includes the "gathering, verifying and communicating of information relative to the client" (Anderson, Anderson, and Glanze, 2006). Clients are

Cultural Considerations 9-1

It is considered taboo in East Indian Hindu culture for a male to extend his hand when greeting a female. Initiating direct eye contact with a woman is seen as a seductive gesture. The proper way to introduce oneself to a female Hindu client is to first greet the husband or oldest female companion. Many Hindu individuals are unwilling to give up speaking their native language, so a Hindu-English–speaking family member commonly accompanies the client.

dynamic (changing) individuals affected by more than an illness or disorder. For this reason, the holistic assessment includes gathering information about the physical, intellectual, social, cultural, and spiritual aspects of each client. The more complete the picture, the more effective the treatment approaches will be.

DATA COLLECTION

Data (information) relating to clients are grouped into objective and subjective categories. **Objective data** refer to information that can be **measured and shared.** They are gathered through the senses of sight, smell, touch, and hearing. Blood pressure readings, pulse rates, and laboratory reports that are compared with "normal" illustrate the use of objective data. When working with mental health clients, care providers obtain objective data through physical examinations, daily assessments, diagnostic testing results, and repeated observations of behaviors (Potter and Perry, 2005).

Subjective data relate to clients' perceptions. They include information that is abstract and difficult to measure or share. The experiences of pain, nausea, and anxiety, for example, cannot be measured by anyone but the individual experiencing them. Emotions and mental states are all subjective and difficult to measure. As a result, it is extremely important to document subjective information as descriptively and accurately as possible. Do not include interpretive statements (judgments). To document that the client is angry (unless he states that he is angry) is an interpretive statement or judgment. It is better to state that the client was pacing about the room while slamming his fist into the wall and swearing. When documenting subjective data, quote the client as much as possible. Subjective information is collected during the initial health history interview and during every interaction with clients. The simple question "How do you feel?" usually elicits much subjective information.

The term **data collection** refers to a variety of activities designed to gather information about a certain subject. Data-collecting methods for care providers include interviews, observational techniques, and rating scales and inventories. An **interview** is a meeting of people with the purpose of obtaining or exchanging information (Keltner, Schwecke, and Bostrom, 2007). Interviews can be formal and highly structured or informal and casual. Information gathered from formal interviews is usually documented on a standardized form. The interview is an excellent method for obtaining assessments. It also serves as the starting point for building the therapeutic relationship. Informal interviews usually occur casually and provide great opportunities to learn more about clients and their families. Caregivers use informal interview techniques when they investigate client problems or explore certain topics.

Data gathering through observational techniques is commonly used. **Observation** is the process of purposeful looking. When using observation as a data-gathering technique, caregivers must be careful to be objective. Personal bias or attitudes can alter one's perceptions and affect the objectivity of the observations. The use of observation is an excellent method for gathering information when the caregiver can remain impartial and does not pass judgment.

Physical assessment skills are important to the data-gathering process. They are used to gather data, investigate changes in physical conditions, and evaluate the effectiveness of therapeutic interventions. Physical examination skills are special methods for obtaining information about the body's functioning. The technique of observation is called inspection, which means a purposeful examination of the body. The skills of auscultation and percussion use the examiner's sense of hearing to detect sounds within the body. Finally, the technique of palpation requires the sense of touch to draw out information about temperature, texture, and pulsations of the body.

Social workers, psychologists, and other therapists frequently use rating scales and inventories. These are data-gathering tools specifically designed to bring out certain kinds of information. The results are then compared with standardized measurements. Rating scales and inventories can be very useful for focusing on specific aspects of client problems.

ASSESSMENT PROCESS

The process of assessing clients is ongoing. It begins with the client's admission to the facility or service and ends only after the client's relationship with the health care system has ended. To gain an understanding of clients, become observant and alert for information that may have an impact on care.

Holistic Assessment

The physical, social, cultural, intellectual, emotional, and spiritual areas have an impact on health. Without knowledge of these six aspects, health care providers become narrowed and limited in their effectiveness. The holistic assessment for those who work with mentally or emotionally troubled clients is the same as that used by caregivers in any setting. In psychiatric treatment situations, however, the emphasis is on mental-emotional functioning. The **psychiatric assessment** tool focuses on obtaining data about the problems, coping behaviors, and resources of clients (Table 9-3). Information collected from assessment activities serves as part of the database from which medical, nursing, and other treatment decisions are made. A risk factor assessment is required for clients who may pose a risk for violence toward themselves or others.

Risk Factor Assessment

A risk factor assessment helps "formulate a nursing diagnosis based on the identification of risk factors that potentially present an immediate threat to the

Table 9-3 *Summary Psychiatric Assessment Tool*

AREA OF ASSESSMENT	EXAMPLE
Appraisal of health/illness	Events leading to problem, definition of problem, client's goal, regular health care received
Previous psychiatric treatment	Diagnosis, type of treatment, medications, compliance, psychiatric history in family
Coping responses, physical status	Review of function in each body system, physical assessment, diet history, sleep patterns, exposure to toxic substances, activities of daily living
Coping responses, mental status	Appearance, speech, motor activity, mood, affect, interactions, perceptions, thought content and process, memory, concentration, calculations, intelligence, insight, judgment
Coping responses, discharge planning, needs	Client's ability to provide for food, clothing, housing, safety, transportation, supportive relationships, work needs, financial needs
Coping mechanisms	Adaptive mechanisms, maladaptive mechanisms
Psychosocial and environmental problems	Educational, occupational, economic, housing problems; difficulties with support group, culture, access to health care services
Knowledge deficits	Understanding of psychiatric problem, coping skills, medications, stressors

Modified from Stuart GW, Laraia MT: *Principles and practice of psychiatric nursing*, ed 8, St. Louis, 2005, Mosby.

patient" (Stuart and Laraia, 2005) or others in the vicinity. With this assessment tool, eight areas of potential risk are identified (Figure 9-1). Positive findings lead to more specific assessments and appropriate safety precautions. The risk factor assessment is completed by a registered nurse, but other health care providers assist by gathering important information and making objective observations.

THE HEALTH HISTORY

Each client is interviewed on admission to the health care service. The purpose of the history interview is to obtain data about the unique individual who is the client. It offers care providers an opportunity to introduce themselves and serves as a starting point for establishing the therapeutic relationship. During the interview, insight into client concerns, worries, and expectations is gained. The interview also offers the opportunity to obtain clues that may require further investigation. When used appropriately, the interview is a powerful method for gathering important information and establishing the therapeutic relationship.

RISK FACTOR ASSESSMENT

DIRECTIONS

The purpose of this assessment is to identify risk factors that potentially present an immediate threat to the patient. An RN must complete this assessment within the **FIRST HOUR** of the patient's encounter with the health care system.

The space labeled "Informants" should identify by name any source of information used to assess the patient. The "Reason for This Encounter" should quote the patient when possible.

The tool comprises eight (8) areas of potential risk. Positive findings in any area direct the nurse to initiate a more specific assessment or to initiate appropriate precautions. At the end of the risk factor assessment, the nurse must list the nursing diagnoses and total number of risk factors identified. A nursing care plan must be initiated immediately to address any nursing diagnosis that reflects an identified risk factor.

RISK FACTOR ASSESSMENT TOOL

Date: _____

INFORMANTS: _____
REASON FOR THIS ENCOUNTER: _____
_____
_____

RISK FACTORS:
1. Potential for Suicide/Self-Harm:

☐ yes ☐ no   Active or recent suicidal or self-harm ideation or attempt?
☐ yes ☐ no   History of suicidal or self-harm ideation or attempt?
• If yes to either question, initiate a Suicide/Self-Harm Assessment.

2. Potential for Assault/Violence:

☐ yes ☐ no   History of assaultive, destructive, or violent behavior?
☐ yes ☐ no   Does the patient express feelings of anger or aggression?
• If yes to either question, initiate an Assault/Violence Assessment.

3. Potential for Substance Abuse Withdrawal (alcohol, illicit drugs, prescription drugs, or inhalants):

☐ yes ☐ no   Have you ever felt the need to cut down on your drinking or drug use?
☐ yes ☐ no   Have people annoyed you by criticizing your drinking or drug use?
☐ yes ☐ no   Have you ever felt bad or guilty about your drinking or drug use?
☐ yes ☐ no   Have you ever had a drink first thing in the morning (eye opener)?
• If yes to any question, initiate a Substance Abuse/Withdrawal Assessment.

4. Potential for Allergic Reaction/Adverse Drug Reaction:

☐ yes ☐ no   Food
☐ yes ☐ no   Medication
☐ yes ☐ no   Other
• If yes to any question, initiate an Substance Abuse/Withdrawal Assessment.

5. Potential for Seizure:

☐ yes ☐ no   Is there a history of seizures?
• If yes to this question, initiate a Seizure Assessment.

6. Potential for Falls/Accidents:

☐ yes ☐ no   Ages 70 or older/5 or under
☐ yes ☐ no   History of confusion
☐ yes ☐ no   History of falls/accidents
☐ yes ☐ no   Sensory deficits
☐ yes ☐ no   Impaired mobility/balance
☐ yes ☐ no   Medications (check as many as apply)
     ☐ yes ☐ no   Sedatives/tranquilizers/narcotics
     ☐ yes ☐ no   Anesthetics
     ☐ yes ☐ no   Diuretics/antihypertensives
     ☐ yes ☐ no   Laxatives
     ☐ yes ☐ no   Substance abuse
     ☐ yes ☐ no   Psychotherapeutics
• If yes to two or more items, initiate Fall Precautions.

7. Potential for Elopement:

☐ yes ☐ no   Does the patient wish or intend to leave?
☐ yes ☐ no   Does the patient have a history of elopement?
• If yes to either question, initiate Elopement Precautions.

8. Potential for Physiological Instability:

☐ yes ☐ no   Existing unstable physical problem?

Vital signs: T _____ P _____ R _____

BP Stand _____ BP Sit _____ Weight _____ Height _____

• If yes to unstable problem or data out of normal range, initiate Physical Assessment.

Total number of risk factors identified (1-8) _____

IDENTIFIED NURSING DIAGNOSES:

☐ yes ☐ no   Risk for self-directed violence
☐ yes ☐ no   Risk for other-directed violence
☐ yes ☐ no   Risk for self-mutilation
☐ yes ☐ no   Risk for injury, related to _____

RN Signature_____ Date: _____ Time:_____

FIGURE **9-1** Risk factor assessment.

EFFECTIVE INTERVIEWS

The success of any client interview rests on the caregiver's ability to listen objectively and respond appropriately. To enhance your interviewing skills, follow these guidelines:

- Remember that **personal values must not cloud professional judgments.** Reacting to a client's personal appearance or behaviors can stereotype him or her and result in a negative impact on the effectiveness of the therapeutic relationship.
- **Do not make assumptions** about how you think the client feels. Discover what each event means to the client and how he or she views the situation. The experience of losing a loved one, for example, depends on how an individual interprets or perceives an event.
- Always **take into account the client's cultural and religious values and beliefs.** With mental health clients, this point cannot be emphasized enough. Caregivers must learn about their clients' cultures if they are to understand their points of view. With clients from unfamiliar cultures, it is wise to research information about the culture and its religious practices before conducting the interview.
- **Pay particular attention to nonverbal communications.** Much can be learned if one is observant. Note which subjects are avoided or quickly passed over during the interview. These behaviors can be clues that indicate a need for further investigation. Observing methods of self-expression helps the caregiver to focus on the client's unspoken signals and the messages they communicate.
- **Have clearly set goals.** Know the purpose of the interview. Is this an initial assessment interview or the investigation of a specific condition? The assessment interview is not a random discussion; it is a purposefully planned interaction with the client.
- **Monitor your own reactions** during the interview. Use self-awareness to signal when you are becoming too emotionally involved. A caregiver may identify with certain clients with similar interests or situations, but self-awareness allows one to understand the emotional responses generated by certain clients. Interviewing skills are used throughout the nursing (therapeutic) process. Work to develop and refine your interviewing skills because they are an important tool.

Sociocultural Assessment

The health history includes information about both the physical and psychological functions of an individual. The sociocultural assessment focuses on the cultural, social, and spiritual aspects of an individual. During the history interview, the care provider obtains information about a client's background and observes the client's appearance, behaviors, and attitudes (these are also included in the mental status examination).

The sociocultural assessment focuses on six areas. Clients are asked questions about their age, ethnicity (culture), gender, education, income, and belief system. Risk factors and stressors are also defined during the sociocultural assessment (National Depressive and Manic-Depressive Association, 1995). This information helps care providers develop accurate and appropriate plans of care.

Review of Systems

The holistic assessment also includes a review of each body system and its functioning. Clients are first questioned about their **general health** care, past illnesses and hospitalizations, and **family health** history. Questions then focus on the function of **each body system.** Last, the lifestyle and **activities of daily living** are assessed. Box 9-1 lists the topics covered by the health history for clients with mental health problems. Data obtained from the health history, physical assessments, and various diagnostic examinations all help complete the picture of each individual client.

PHYSICAL ASSESSMENT

Clients receive a physical examination on admission to a psychiatric service. The purpose of the examination is to discover physical problems that can be treated medically. Many alterations in behavior are often traced to a physical cause. For example, low blood sugar levels can result in confused and uncooperative behavior. Hormone imbalances, exposure to toxic substances, and severe pain can also affect behavior.

A complete physical examination is performed by a physician or nurse practitioner. The client's current health status is explored, and then each system is examined. Nurses have an obligation to assess each client's health status on a routine basis. A complete physical assessment is not needed every day, but nurses must be alert to changes in their clients' conditions. Most nurses use a systems approach or head-to-toe assessment. Both take less than 5 minutes and can be performed any time information about physical functions is needed.

Diagnostic studies for clients with mental-emotional problems include standard blood and urine tests, evaluation of electrolytes, and hormone function examinations. Many clients are screened for tuberculosis, human immunodeficiency virus (HIV), and sexually transmitted diseases. Studies such as x-ray examinations, electrocardiograms (ECGs), electroencephalograms (EEGs), and brain imaging studies (computed tomography [CT], magnetic resonance imaging [MRI], positron emission tomography [PET] scans) may be ordered. To complete the picture, the client's current mental and emotional state is assessed via a mental status examination.

Box 9-1 | *Health History for Mental Health Clients*

HEALTH CARE HISTORY
General Health Care
Regular health care provider
Frequency of health care visits
Last medical examination and test results
Any unusual circumstances of pregnancy or births
Hospitalizations and surgeries: when, why indicated,
   treatments, outcome
Family history
Diagnosed brain problem
Head trauma: Details of accidents or periods of uncon-
   sciousness for any reason—blows to the head, elec-
   trical shocks, high fevers, seizures, fainting, dizziness,
   headaches, falls
Endocrine disturbances: Thyroid and adrenal function
   particularly, diabetes, stability of glucose levels

LIFESTYLE
Eating: Details of unusual or unsupervised diets,
   appetite, weight changes, cravings, caffeine intake
Medications: Full history of current and past psychiatric
   medications in self and first-degree relatives
Substance use: Alcohol and drug use
Toxins: Overcome by automobile exhaust or natural gas;
   exposure to lead, mercury, insecticides, herbicides,
   solvents, cleaning agents, lawn chemicals
Occupation (current and past): Chemicals in workplace
   (farming, painting)
Cancer: Full history, particularly consider metastases
   (lung, breast, melanoma, gastrointestinal tract, and
   kidney are most likely to be affected); results of
   treatment (chemotherapy and surgeries)
Lung problems: Details of anything that restricts flow
   of air to lungs for more than 2 minutes or adversely
   affects oxygen absorption (brain uses 20% of oxygen
   in body), such as with chronic obstructive pulmonary
   disease, near drowning, near strangulation, high-
   altitude oxygen deprivation, resuscitation
Cardiac problems: Childhood illnesses such as scarlet
   or rheumatic fever; history of heart attacks, strokes,
   or hypertension
Blood diseases: Anemia, arteriosclerotic conditions,
   HIV, work-related accidents, military experiences
Injury: Safe sex practices, contact sports and sports-
   related injuries, exposure to violence or abuse
Presenting symptoms and coping responses:
   Description—nature, frequency, and intensity; threats
   to safety of self or others; functional status; quality
   of life

From Stuart GW: *Handbook of psychiatric nursing,* ed 6, St. Louis, 2005,
Mosby.
HIV, Human immunodeficiency virus.

Table 9-4 | *The Mental Status Examination*

General description	Appearance; speech; motor activity; interaction during interview
Emotional state	Mood; affect
Experiences	Perceptions
Thinking	Thought content; thought processes
Sensorium and cognition	Level of consciousness; memory; level of concentration and calculation; information and intelligence; judgment

From Stuart GW: *Handbook of psychiatric nursing,* ed 6, St. Louis,
2005, Mosby.

enables care providers to plan and deliver the most
appropriate care for each of their clients.

The mental status examination explores the following areas: general description, emotional state,
experiences, thinking, and sensorium and cognition
(Table 9-4).

GENERAL DESCRIPTION

Under the category of general description, the client's
general appearance, speech, motor activity, and behavior during the interaction are assessed. This category
includes everything that can be readily observed about
a client, such as physical characteristics, dress, facial
expressions, motor activity, speech, and reactions. To
assess a client's physical characteristics, observe each
part of the client's body, noting anything unusual. Describe the person's body build, skin coloring, cleanliness, and manner of dress. Does the person appear
neat and tidy or careless and unkempt? Note any body
odors. If cosmetics are used, are they appropriately
applied? Does the client's appearance match his or her
gender, age, and situation? People with depression, for
example, may look unkempt and neglected. It is not
uncommon for manic clients to dress in colorful but
bizarre clothing and wear many cosmetics and jewelry.
Document all findings. Facial expressions, eye contact,
and pupil size are noted. Do the client's facial expressions match his or her emotions and actions? Is eye
contact avoided or held for long periods? Note the size
of the client's pupils. Large, dilated pupils are seen in
people with drug intoxication, whereas small pupils
are associated with narcotic use.

Describe the rate, volume, and characteristics of the
client's speech. Note any abnormal speech patterns
(see Chapter 10).

Next, turn your attention to the client's motor activity, gestures, and posture. Observe the client's physical
movements for the level and type of activity. Note any
unusual movements or mannerisms. Is the client agitated, tense, restless, lethargic, or relaxed? Are there
any tics, grimaces, repeated facial expressions, or tremors present? Excessive body movements are seen in
individuals with anxiety or mania. They can also result from the use of stimulants or other drugs. Repeated movements or behaviors are seen in clients
with obsessive-compulsive disorders, and picking at

MENTAL STATUS ASSESSMENT

The mental status examination allows care providers to
observe and describe a client's behavior in an objective,
nonjudgmental way. It is a tool for assessing mental
health dysfunctions and identifying the causes of clients'
problems. Understanding each part of the examination

one's clothing is often seen in clients with delirium or toxic reactions.

To complete the general description, assess the client's behavior during the interaction (see Think About 9-1). How did the client relate to you? Was he or she cooperative, hostile, or overly friendly? Did the client appear to trust you? Note if the verbal messages matched the behaviors. Clients who use unconnected gestures, for example, may be hallucinating.

EMOTIONAL STATE

To assess the client's emotional state, the care provider considers the client's mood and affect. **Mood** is defined as an individual's overall feelings. Mood is a subjective factor that can be explained only by the person experiencing it. Usually people will have a basic mood, although it may change sometime during the day. To illustrate, a basically relaxed and happy person may feel disappointed by an incident during the day but soon forgets and returns to his or her commonly happy mood.

Affect is the client's emotional display of the mood being experienced. Table 9-5 explains several kinds of affect. A person's mood can range from overwhelming sadness to great elation and joy. These variations are referred to as one's range of emotion. Affect can be categorized as appropriate, inappropriate,

pleasurable, or unpleasurable. To assess a client's affect, ask what he or she is feeling and then observe the reactions. Do the responses to your questions match the subjects being discussed? Is the client overreacting, not reacting at all, or responding inappropriately? Document objective descriptions of the client's behaviors. Descriptions communicate much more information than a single medical term does.

EXPERIENCES

The category of experiences explores the client's **perceptions**, the ways in which he or she experiences the world. An individual's perceptions are often called one's frame of reference. In short, a person's perceptions help determine his or her sense of reality.

People who are having mental health problems may have difficulty in perceiving the same reality as the rest of society. Hallucinations are perceptions that have no external stimulus. The client may hear voices or see things that are not perceived by other people. Hallucinations involving taste, touch, or smell may indicate a physical problem. Visual and auditory hallucinations are associated with schizophrenia, the acute stage of alcohol or drug withdrawal, and organic brain disorders. Alterations in perceptions that have a basis in reality are called illusions. External stimuli are present, but they are perceived differently by the client. For example, a client perceives the person walking down the hall as a wolf. If a client is having illusions or hallucinations, ask him or her to describe the experience. Box 9-2 lists several questions that can help explain the client's experience.

Remember that hallucinations or illusions are very real to the person experiencing them. Caregivers cannot "talk them out of it" or tell them to ignore what they are perceiving. However, because they are so real, clients usually are willing to describe them when asked.

Think About 9-1

Cybil is being admitted to the clinic's day treatment program. She insists that she feels fine, but she will not speak, except to answer "yes" or "no" and refuses to give her caregiver eye contact.
- What messages is Cybil's behavior sending?
- How do her verbal and nonverbal messages agree or disagree?

Table 9-5 *Common Emotional Responses (Affects)*

NAME OF AFFECT	DESCRIPTION
INAPPROPRIATE RESPONSE	
Labile	Rapid, dramatic changes in emotions
Inconsistent	Affect and mood do not agree
Flat	Unresponsive emotions
PLEASURABLE RESPONSE	
Euphoria	Excessive feelings of well-being (feeling too good)
Exaltation	Intense happiness, often with feelings of grandeur
UNPLEASURABLE (DYSPHORIC) RESPONSE	
Aggression	Anger, hostility, or rage that is out of keeping with situation
Agitation	Motor restlessness, often seen with anxiety
Ambivalence	Having both positive and negative feelings
Anxiety	Vague, uneasy feeling, often from unknown cause
Depression	Sadness, hopelessness, loss that is present over time
Fear	Reaction to recognized danger

THINKING

The "thinking" section of the mental status examination focuses on the client's thought content and processes. Thought content relates to what an individual is thinking. Clients may be experiencing delusions, obsessions, phobias, preoccupations, amnesia, or confabulations.

Disturbances in thought processes relate to how a person thinks—how he or she analyzes the world and connects and organizes information. Disorders of thought processes include blocking, flight of ideas, loose associations, and perseveration. Several disorders of thought processes are listed in Table 9-6.

Another problem of thinking is **depersonalization,** a feeling of unreality or detachment from oneself or one's environment. The unreal feelings produce a dreamlike atmosphere that overtakes the individual's consciousness. One's body does not feel like one's own. Events that are dramatic or important are viewed with a detached calmness, as if the person were watching instead of participating in reality. Feelings of depersonalization can normally occur when one is anxious, stressed, or very tired. Depersonalization disorders are often seen in clients with severe depression and in some forms of schizophrenia.

Box 9-2 *Assessing Illusions or Hallucinations*

Ask the client if he or she hears voices or see things when other people are not present. If the answer is yes, ask the client to describe the experience. Questions can include the following:
- How many different voices (images) do you hear (see)?
- What do the voices say (images do)?
- Do you recognize any of the voices (images)?
- When did the voices (images) first begin? What was happening in your life at the time?
- How do you feel about the voices (images)?

Assessment of the client's thought content and process occurs throughout the entire mental status examination. Are the client's thoughts based in reality? Are ideas communicated clearly? Do the client's thoughts follow a logical order? Are there any unusual thoughts, preoccupations, or beliefs present? Does the client have any suicidal, violent, or destructive thoughts? (Forster, 1994). Are there any persistent dreams? Does the client believe that someone is intent on harming him or her (feelings of persecution)? Observe the client closely, and listen intently. Much information will be revealed during the course of the interaction.

SENSORIUM AND COGNITION

The sensorium is that part of the consciousness that perceives, sorts, and combines information. People with a clear sensorium are oriented to time, place, and person. They are able to use their memories to recall recent and remote information. Levels of consciousness and memory recall help to assess a person's sensorium.

Level of consciousness can be determined by observing the amount of stimuli it takes to arouse the client (Table 9-7). If the client cannot be awakened by verbal stimuli, notify your supervisor immediately. If the client is awake, note his or her responses to your questions, the degree of interaction, and the amount of eye contact that is being made.

Memory is the ability to recall past events, experience, and perceptions. For the purpose of testing, memory is divided into three categories: immediate, recent, and remote memory. Immediate memory is also referred to as **recall.** To assess immediate memory (recall), ask the client to remember three things (e.g., a color, an address, an object). Later in the conversation (at least 15 minutes), ask the client to repeat the three items. Recall can also be tested by having the client repeat a series of numbers within a 10-second period.

Table 9-6 *Disorders of Thinking*

DISORDER	DESCRIPTION
THOUGHT PROCESSES (HOW ONE THINKS)	
Blocking	Thoughts stop suddenly for no reason
Flight of ideas	Rapid changes from one thought to another related thought
Loose associations	Poorly organized or connected thoughts
Perseveration	Repeating same word in response to different questions
THOUGHT CONTENT (WHAT ONE THINKS)	
Delusions	False beliefs that cannot be corrected by reasoning or explanation
Obsession	Thought, action, or emotion that is unwelcome and difficult to resist
Phobias	Strong fears of certain things, places, or situations
Preoccupations	All experiences and actions are connected to central thought that is usually emotional in nature
OTHERS	
Amnesia	Inability to remember past events
Confabulation	Using untrue statements to fill in gaps of memory loss

Table 9-7 *Levels of Consciousness*

Comatose/unconscious	Unresponsive to any verbal or painful stimuli
Stuporous	Responds only to strong physical stimuli; falls asleep if not stimulated
Drowsy/somnolent	Wakens with strong verbal stimuli; falls asleep if left undisturbed
Lethargic	Can be verbally aroused; shows decreased wakefulness; may have periods of excitability alternating with periods of drowsiness
Alert	Awake and responsive; oriented to time, place, and person
Hyperalertness	Increased state of alertness or watchfulness (hypervigilance)
Mania	State of extreme excitement, elation, and activity

Recent memory includes events within the past 2 weeks. Caregivers test recent memory by asking the client to recall the events of the past 24 hours. Loss of recent memory is seen in people with Alzheimer's disease, anxiety, and depression.

Assessing **remote memory** involves asking the client questions about his or her place of birth, schools attended, ages of family members, and the person's background. This part of the mental status examination can easily be done during the nursing health history interview. It is sometimes difficult to tell if the client has accurate memories. Long-term memory loss is seen in clients with organic (physical) problems, conversion disorders, and dissociative disorders.

The level of concentration focuses on the client's ability to pay attention during the conversation. **Calculation** tests the ability to do simple math problems. Have the person count rapidly from 1 to 20; perform simple addition, multiplication, and division problems; and subtract 7 from 100, then 7 from 93, and so on. Then ask practical questions such as the number of dimes in $1.90. Note how easily the client becomes distracted during the tasks. People with mental-emotional problems commonly have difficulty with concentration and calculations. These difficulties also occur in people with physical disorders, such as brain tumors, so it is important to assess the client's ability to concentrate and do simple calculations.

During this phase of the mental status examination, the client's education level, general knowledge, ability to read, use of vocabulary, and ability to think abstractly are assessed. General knowledge can be tested by asking the person to name the past five presidents, five large cities, or the occupations of well-known people in the community. Ask the client about the last grade completed in school.

To determine **reading ability,** print a command, such as "Close your eyes," on a piece of paper. Ask the client to read it and follow the directions. During the conversation, also note the client's choice of words and their use.

Assess the client's ability to **think abstractly** by having him or her explain the meaning of several well-known proverbs, such as "a stitch in time saves nine"; "a rolling stone gathers no moss"; "when it rains, it pours"; or "people in glass houses shouldn't throw stones." Many people with mental health problems give concrete answers such as "Moss only grows on the north sides of stones" or "People who live in glass houses shouldn't throw stones because it breaks the glass."

Judgment refers to the ability to evaluate choices and make appropriate decisions. During the health history interview, observe how the client explains personal relationships, his or her job, and economic responsibilities. Assess the client's judgment by asking questions such as "What would you do if you …

• found an addressed envelope on the ground?"
• ran out of medication before the next appointment?"
• won $25,000?"

Judgment is often impaired in people with chemical dependence, intoxication, schizophrenia, mental retardation, and organic mental disorders. Document the client's responses using the client's own words whenever possible.

Insight refers to the client's understanding of the situation. What is the client's understanding of the disorder? Questions that help the caregiver assess insight include "Have you noticed a change in yourself recently?" and "What do you think is the cause of your anxiety (discomfort)?" Expect clients to have different degrees of insight. For example, a person with an alcohol problem may realize that he or she drinks too much but does not think that it is interfering with family life. Again, be sure to document the client's statements rather than your opinions.

Although the mental status examination may appear to be a lengthy process, much of it can be performed during the history interview. Checklists that address each area of the examination are available (see Box 9-3 and Appendix C for a copy of the Mental Status Assessment at a Glance).

Care providers often use parts of the mental status examination to assess clients whose mental state changes frequently. For example, the caregiver assesses the hallucinating client for thought content and process at intervals throughout the day.

Work to develop your powers of observation. Do not pass judgment or let your opinions interfere with data gathering. Remember, the results of the mental status examination can be affected by attitudes and beliefs. Learn to use assessment skills because they will serve you well in all practice settings.

Box 9-3 *Mental Status Assessment at a Glance*

1. Appearance
_____ Manner of dress
_____ Personal grooming
_____ Facial expressions
_____ Posture and gait
2. Speech
_____ Manner of response (frank, evading)
_____ Choice of words (to assess general intelligence, education, levels of function, thought)
_____ Speech disorder
3. Level of consciousness
_____ Level of alertness
_____ Orientation (time, place, person)
4. Attention span
_____ Ability to keep thoughts focused on one topic
_____ Repeat a series of numbers
_____ Serial 7s (ask client to subtract 7 from 100, 7 from 93, etc.)
5. Memory
_____ Immediate memory (ask client to repeat words after 15 minutes)
_____ Recent memory (ask client about yesterday's activities)

_____ Remote memory (ask client about dates of birth, marriage, schooling)
6. Understanding abstract relationships
_____ Understanding of proverbs (concrete or abstract)
_____ Ability to understand similarities (e.g., "How are a bicycle and an automobile alike?")
7. Arithmetic and reading ability
_____ Simple addition, subtraction, multiplication, and division (ask client to make change)
_____ Ability to read newspaper, magazine
8. General information knowledge
_____ Discuss newspaper or magazine article
_____ General information questions (e.g., "How many days in a year?" "Where does the sun set?")
9. Judgment
_____ Responses to family, work, financial problems
_____ Responses to "What would you do if ..." questions
10. Emotional status
_____ Ask "How do you feel today?" or "How do you feel about ..." questions
_____ Affect
_____ Current situation and coping behaviors

Modified from Jess LW: Investigating impaired mental status: an assessment guide you can use, *Nursing* 18:42, 1988.

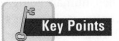 **Key Points**

- The ability to effectively obtain and use information about clients is a vital part of the multidisciplinary treatment plan.
- The mental health treatment plan is used as a guide for client care, to monitor progress and assess the effectiveness of therapeutic interventions, to communicate and coordinate clients' care, to provide a focus for all therapeutic activities, and to prevent duplication.
- Every psychological illness has physical effects, and psychological effects accompany every physical illness.
- Therapists who work with mentally and emotionally troubled individuals use the DSM-IV-TR to aid in diagnosis and help guide clinical practice.
- The nursing (therapeutic) process is a purposeful and organized approach to solving client problems that requires knowledge, experience, and the use of good judgment.
- Data-collecting methods for care providers include interviews, observational techniques, and rating scales and inventories.
- The process of assessing a client is ongoing and begins with the client's admission.
- Individuals' physical, social, cultural, intellectual, emotional, and spiritual areas of functioning are included in a holistic assessment.
- The psychiatric assessment tool includes an appraisal of the client's health, previous psychiatric treatment,

physical and mental coping responses, discharge planning needs, psychosocial and environmental problems, and needs for knowledge.
- The purpose of a risk factor assessment is to identify risk factors that may present an immediate threat to the client or others.
- The history interview is an organized conversation with a client that has the purpose of bringing out certain information about the client's health status.
- Guidelines for conducting effective interviews relate to being nonjudgmental, considering cultural factors, having clear goals, and assessing communications.
- The sociocultural assessment focuses on cultural, social, and spiritual aspects.
- The mental status examination is a tool for assessing mental health dysfunctions and identifying the causes of clients' problems.
- The mental status examination explores appearance, consciousness, behavior, speech, mood, affect, thought content, intellectual performance, insight, judgment, and perception.
- Much of the mental status examination can be performed during the history interview using checklists. Caregivers often use various parts of the mental status examination to assess clients whose mental state changes frequently.

evolve   Be sure to visit the companion Evolve site at http://evolve.elsevier.com/Morrison-Valfre/ for additional online resources.

10 | Therapeutic Communication

Objectives

Upon completion of this chapter, the student will be able to:

1. Examine two theories of communication.
2. Identify two types of communication.
3. List the five components or parts of any communication.
4. Compare the characteristics of verbal and nonverbal communications.
5. Identify three interventions for communicating with people who do not speak your language.
6. Explain eight principles of therapeutic communication.
7. Describe eight therapeutic communication skills.
8. Name three techniques for communicating with clients who have mental-emotional problems.

Key Terms

aphasia (ə-FĀ-zhə) (p. 106)
communication (p. 96)
communication style (p. 100)
disturbed communications (p. 97)
dyslexia (dĭs-LĔK-sē-ə) (p. 106)
feedback (p. 98)
incongruent (ĬN-kən-GRoo-ent) communications (p. 103)
interpersonal communications (p. 98)
intrapersonal communications (p. 98)
nontherapeutic communications (p. 103)
nonverbal communication (p. 100)
perception (pĕr-SĔP-shŭn) (p. 98)
responding strategies (p. 103)
speech cluttering (p. 106)
therapeutic (THĔR-ə-PYŪ-tĭk) communications (p. 101)
verbal communication (p. 99)

Communication is an essential component of survival for all creatures. Research has demonstrated that when insects attack a tree, it sends a chemical message to other trees in the area. Animals communicate in subtle and complex ways using both sound and movement, but the master communicator, the user of language, is the human being. Infants are born communicating with their first squall, and the elderly die listening to a world they are about to leave.

The fulfillment of human needs requires interactions with others. To meet even the most basic needs for food and water requires the cooperative efforts of people, achieved through communication and understanding. "Communication is the reciprocal exchange of information, ideas, beliefs, feelings, and attitudes between two persons or among a group of persons" (Taylor, 1994). All people communicate, but members of the health care professions modify ordinary interactions and practice therapeutic communications based on certain principles. Those who work with mentally or emotionally troubled individuals refine their therapeutic communication abilities to become highly skilled listeners "who can plan and carry out interactions specifically designed to achieve client outcomes" (Rawlins, Williams, and Beck, 1993). This chapter explores the elements and skills of therapeutically designed communication techniques.

The study of interactions between human beings has been a source of interest for centuries. Paintings on walls of caves attest to early humans' desire for communication. The introduction of the printing press during the fifteenth century made mass production of the written word possible. As people learned to read and write, learning evolved from an oral form to a visual one. Communications became more complex and a step removed from face-to-face interpersonal contact.

The inventions of the telegraph, telephone, radio, television, and computer made information available to everyone. Today, satellite communications, interactive computers, and the Internet are transporting communications and information exchanges into new and unknown realms. Tomorrow's technological developments will move us further, but the need for effective verbal and nonverbal communication skills will never be replaced by technology.

THEORIES OF COMMUNICATION

Probably one of the earliest theorists on therapeutic communications was Florence Nightingale, whose book *Notes on Nursing* emphasized the need to effectively understand and communicate with patients. However, the rest of the medical world placed little focus on the value of interacting therapeutically until the 1950s, when the publication of several theories sparked an interest in client-caregiver communications.

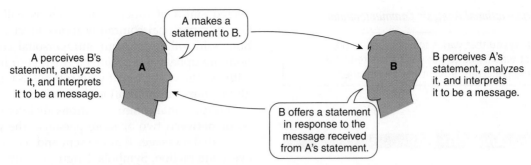

FIGURE **10-1** Ruesch's feedback loop of communication.

RUESCH'S THEORY

A theory that considers communications as the social framework for health care was developed by J. Ruesch (1961) in the late 1950s. He saw communication as a circular process in which messages traveled from within one person to another person and back again (Figure 10-1).

Events within the sender prompt the sending of a message. The message is then transmitted to another who receives it, processes it internally, and responds. Successful communications occur when agreement about the meaning of the message has been reached. Communications are unsuccessful when there is a lack of agreement or understanding about the message. Ruesch coined the term disturbed communications to describe unsuccessful interactions that result from an interference in the sending or receiving of messages, inadequate mastery of the language being used, insufficient information, or no opportunity for feedback.

Therapeutic communications are distinguished from ordinary communications by the **intent** of one of the participants **to bring about a positive change.** According to Ruesch's point of view, a therapist is one who directs communications to bring about more satisfying social relations. Therapists seek to find the nature of clients' distresses and problems. Then, with the use of therapeutic communication techniques, both client and therapist agree on the nature of the problem and what should be done about it. Many of Ruesch's ideas are useful for interacting with clients.

TRANSACTIONAL ANALYSIS

In 1964, Dr. Eric Berne, a physician with training in psychoanalysis, published *Games People Play*, which became a best-seller even though it was not intended for the general public (Berne, 1964a). In the book, Berne used the term **transactional analysis** to refer to the process of investigating what people say and do to each other. Berne also believed that three ego states exist within all of us: the parent (P) who focuses on rules and values, the child (C) who focuses on emotions and desires, and the adult (A) who bases his or her approach to the world on previous observations. These ego states make up one's individual personality, and Berne coined the term **structural analysis** to refer

to the study of the personality. Box 10-1 gives an example of each communication type.

Many of the interactions in which people engage, Berne noted, have ulterior or hidden motives used to manipulate others. He labeled these manipulations psychological games and rackets and offered his game analysis to refer to the hidden interactions that lead to a payoff.

The main goal of transactional analysis, according to Berne, is to "establish the most open and authentic communication possible between the affective (feeling) and intellectual components of the personality" (Berne, 1964b). Analyzing one's structure, transactions, and games encourages people to gain insight and determine what changes are most desirable. Because Berne (like Maslow) believed that every person needs positive feedback or "strokes" to thrive, he encouraged communications that are positive in nature. This approach is particularly valuable for nurses and other health care professionals. The focus on one's abilities fosters more effective and satisfying communications for everyone involved with the client.

NEUROLINGUISTIC PROGRAMMING

Much of the basis for neurolinguistic programming stems from the work of Milton H. Erickson, who, until his death in 1980, was considered a great medical hypnotist. To discover the keys to his success, Richard Bandler and John Grinder spent several years doing careful analyses of Erickson's extensive writings. Using their observations as a framework, they developed a method for analyzing an individual's system of communication based on the theory that any effective communication is a state of hypnosis. Effective communications alter a person's state of consciousness. Think About 10-1 presents an exercise that demonstrates this point.

By learning an individual's communication patterns, one is able to achieve more effective and fulfilling interactions. Patterns include **eye-accessing** clues (ways in which people move their eyes while thinking), **language patterns,** and the **pace** and **rhythm** of speech. Health care providers are finding neurolinguistic programming to be a powerful tool for communicating.

Box 10-1 *Transactional Analysis Communications*

Parent: "I told you that was a foolish thing to do."
Child: "I just was trying to get what I wanted."
Adult: "In the past, this is what worked for me."

Think About 10-1

Picture yourself in the forest, surrounded by tall, stately trees. You look up to see the sun filtering through the dense canopy of tree branches. Below you, the forest floor is dappled with sunlight and shade patterns dance slowly across your shoes. The air is cool and musty, damp from the mist left from the night. The world is silent except for the chirping of a lone songbird.

- What did you experience when you were reading the above paragraph?
- Did you actually experience a moment in the forest?
- Do you wish that you could go there yourself?

If your answer is "yes" to any of these questions, then the communication was successful. The pattern of communication in the paragraph altered your state of consciousness, which allowed you to share an experience. This is the "hypnosis" of neurolinguistic programming.

Other theories of communication focus on the use of body language **(kinesics)**, how people use their space **(proxemics)**, and channels of communication. Becoming familiar with several theories allows caregivers to expand and improve their communication skills and abilities.

CHARACTERISTICS OF COMMUNICATION

Communication is the act of sending and receiving information. When this definition is applied to a computer or some other mechanical mover of data, the interaction is simple. One machine contacts the other, data are exchanged, and the interaction is over. With people, however, the information exchange is much more complex. Human behaviors have strong influences on communications.

TYPES OF COMMUNICATION

People engage in two types of communications: intrapersonal and interpersonal. Each may occur singly or in combination, and each may be used in effective or maladaptive ways.

Intrapersonal communications take place **within** oneself and are commonly referred to as our "self-talk" or "self-dialogue." They are conversations that we have with ourselves when solving problems, making plans, and reacting emotionally. Intrapersonal communications are adaptive when they help us cope or focus our energies. When dysfunctional, they can result in altered states of functioning, such as hallucinations. Our intrapersonal communications affect our interactions with others. If your intrapersonal communications are upbeat and optimistic, then your interactions with clients will be too. If your self-talk is negative and glum, your communications will reflect this.

Interpersonal communications are interactions that occur **between** two or more persons—the verbal and nonverbal messages that are sent and received during every interaction. Symbols, language, culture, and behaviors have an impact on communications among people. As a result, interpersonal communications are complex and sophisticated. No matter what the communication, the importance of each message lies in its clarity. Clear communications offer a greater chance of success in every interaction.

PROCESS OF COMMUNICATION

For a successful communication to occur, five elements must be in place (Figure 10-2). There must be a **sender** who forms the message and transmits it. A **receiver** is necessary to accept the **message** and respond in return. **Feedback** refers to the responses of each person when messages are being sent and received. Last, although not an actual part of the message, the **context** or setting in which the communication takes place must also be considered.

When a message is sent, a chain of events is triggered. First, perception is needed to recognize the presence of a message. **Perception** is the use of the senses to gain information. Vision, hearing, and touch are used to sense the meaning of the communication. A person's perceptions can be affected by many factors, including past experiences, emotional states, and physical problems.

The second step of the communication process is **evaluation,** the internal assessment of the message. All overt and hidden messages are considered and then compared with past experiences. The result is an emotional **reaction** to the message and preparation to return a message to the sender.

Transmission (a response) is the last step. It includes conscious and unconscious responses to the message received. As the receiver of the message responds with a message of his or her own, the cycle begins again and is repeated with every interaction. If a person has difficulty with any step of the communication process—perceiving, evaluating, or transmitting messages—a communication problem may exist. Alert caregivers are aware of each client's process of communication and are prepared to intervene when clients are having communication difficulties.

FACTORS THAT INFLUENCE COMMUNICATION

Interaction with others is influenced by many factors, but among the most important are culture (see Chapter 4), social class, relationships, perceptions, values, and parts of the message.

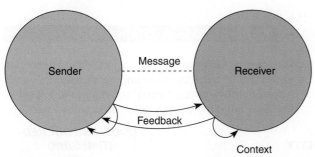

FIGURE **10-2** Components of the communication process.

Box 10-2 | *Communicating With Clients of Different Social Classes*

Show acceptance and respect for the person.
Consider the environment in which clients must cope, especially those from social classes of poverty.
Assess the client's patterns of communication, verbal and nonverbal.
Use terms the client can understand. Avoid using medical terminology.
Do not talk "up" or "down" to clients.
Ask clients to clarify any terms that are not understood.
Invite the client to take an active part in the treatment plan and its activities.

The **social class** to which one belongs has a profound influence on communications. People of various social classes interact using their own terminology, slang, clichés, speech patterns, gestures, and appearances. Variation in communication patterns can create problems for health care providers who interact with clients from social classes different from their own. Be careful not to label clients based on their communications. Communicating with clients from different social classes requires effort and patience. Both the care provider and client will feel misunderstood unless steps are taken to establish effective communication exchanges. Box 10-2 lists several therapeutic interventions for interacting with people from different social classes.

Relationships affect communications because of the level of relatedness of each person involved in the interaction. Levels of relatedness refer to the degree of intimacy, authority, and role status of the communicators. For example, people communicate differently with strangers than they do with family members.

Perceptions and **values** color communications. One's internal experiences, when combined with personal values, result in a unique frame of reference for communicating. It is important for caregivers to remember that it may be their perceptions that are impeding effective communication.

The content and context of a message have a strong impact on communications. The **content** of a message is the information being sent. The receiver is affected

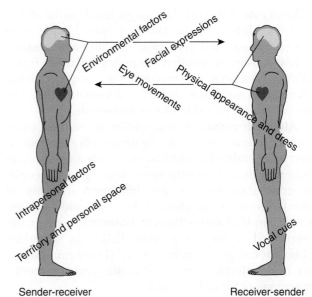

FIGURE **10-3** Factors influencing communication.

by the content and must choose an appropriate response—recognize the information, ignore the message, or change the subject. An awareness of the emotional impact related to the content of messages helps caregivers communicate more effectively.

Communications are also affected by the **context,** or environment, in which they take place. If clients are expected to share personal information, an environment that fosters privacy is necessary. The dayroom or lounge is not a place for self-disclosure. Becoming aware of the context helps to send and receive messages with greater success. Many other factors, such as one's appearance, expressions, and body movements, also have an impact on communications (Figure 10-3).

LEVELS OF COMMUNICATION

Communicating is an energy exchange that takes place on several levels. Each person involved is a unique personality who interacts on verbal and nonverbal levels at one time. Communications at both levels occur with every person-to-person interaction.

VERBAL COMMUNICATION

Verbal communication relates to anything associated with the spoken word. Verbal communications include speaking, writing, the use of language and symbols, and the arrangement of words or phrases.

For many clients with mental-emotional problems, communicating with others can be difficult. Certain clients have difficulties in perceiving. The person who is experiencing hallucinations, for example, may be unable to understand a message is being sent because the communications within the inner world are drowning out the messages from the reality outside.

Understanding verbal messages involves the ability to form abstract ideas and concepts. People with schizophrenia often have great difficulty with abstraction and using words that are reality oriented. Transmitting messages is a problem for many depressed clients; messages that identify and verbalize they feel are commonly stated in one or two words.

Although verbal communication is the most overt form of interaction, it actually represents only a small part of an entire communication. Words are only symbols; they do not have the same meaning to all people. To complicate matters, the differences intensify as words become more abstract. Emotions are an excellent example of abstractions that cannot be easily communicated on the verbal level. This is an important point for caregivers to remember. If communications are to be effective, you must understand the client's **meanings** of his or her words.

NONVERBAL COMMUNICATION

Messages sent and received without the use of words define nonverbal communication. Messages sent at the nonverbal level are expressed in at least one of four ways: **appearance, body motions, use of space,** and **nonlanguage sounds** (verbalizations without words). One's appearance can convey strong nonverbal messages. Hygiene and personal grooming habits, choice of clothing and accessories, hairstyle, and jewelry all send messages. Facial expressions, gestures, posture, and use of the body can communicate one's emotions more easily than words. Caregivers who are aware of this are careful to use their nonverbal behaviors therapeutically. To illustrate, note the position of your body when you are interacting with someone you find unpleasant. Are your arms crossed? Is your body position open and inviting communication or closed with crossed legs or an angled stance? The use of space and distance (see Chapter 4) communicates concepts such as authority and intimacy.

In short, the nonverbal level of communication includes everything outside the realm of speaking, writing, or singing. It is a subtle world, rich in variation. The more caregivers are able to recognize and use nonverbal levels, the more effective their interventions will become. Each level of communication, verbal and nonverbal, sends and receives messages during every interaction. If messages are successfully sent and received, the results are interactions rich in variety and complexity.

INTERCULTURAL COMMUNICATION

Communicating with people from other cultures requires special considerations. How people communicate is based on cultural backgrounds, language systems, and social patterns. Cultures are transmitted through communication, and cultures define how

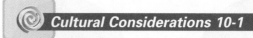

Cultural Considerations 10-1

Sidney Jourard (1971) studied the cultural differences relating to the use of touch by observing the behaviors of pairs of people in coffee shops throughout the world. Observations revealed that more touch occurred in certain cities.

CITY	COUPLES TOUCHED (TIMES/HR)
San Juan, Puerto Rico	180
Paris, France	110
Gainesville, Florida	2
London, England	0

emotions are expressed and shared. The use of touch and other nonverbal forms of communication varies considerably with different cultures (see Cultural Considerations 10-1).

Cultures, and the social groups within them, vary in their use of verbal and nonverbal communications. Caregivers who work with clients from culturally different backgrounds should resist the tendency to stereotype people and work to learn the most culturally appropriate methods for communication.

INTERCULTURAL DIFFERENCES

To fulfill basic needs, people must interact and communicate with each other. For people of differing cultures, this interacting with others can be a difficult process. Communication styles, nonverbal behaviors and values, as well as the use of the language, are areas in which cultural communications basically differ.

Communication style refers to the rituals connected with greeting and departure, the lines of conversation, and the directness of communication (Giger and Davidhizar, 2008). Assess greeting rituals by observing the greeting interaction, including the use of compliments and physical behaviors such as touching, handshaking, or kissing. Case Study 10-1 demonstrates this point.

Are lines of communication linear or circular? **Linear communication styles** come directly to the point. To illustrate, most Anglo-American men use an open and frank conversation style, whereas Thai Americans favor a more circular line of communication known as **kreng jai,** a consideration for the feelings and needs of others. **Circular communication styles** direct the conversation around the main point. Often, the main point is left unstated. Once the important information has been communicated, it is assumed that the receiver got the point. This style is often found in Asian and far Eastern cultures. "There's a fire in the wastebasket" is an example of a linear message, whereas "I saw someone drop a match in the wastebasket earlier; now it appears to be smoking" illustrates a circular style of communication.

Case Study 10-1

Sarah had been working with clients on a reservation for almost 6 months. During her interviews with clients, she had great difficulty in obtaining information, although she knew she was practicing good interviewing skills and attending behaviors.

One morning, she was discussing her problem with the reservation physician, who had been working with her clients for several years. He asked, "How is your eye contact?" "Good," she replied. "I always look clients in the eye when interviewing and express interest in what they say—when I can get them to talk to me." "That is your problem, then," the physician replied. "These people believe that it is an invasion of privacy to give direct eye contact, especially if you are not a member of their group. Try looking at their feet. It will convey respect, and they may be more likely to communicate with you."

Sarah followed the suggestion, and soon her clients began sharing important health information.
- How could Sarah have prevented this situation from occurring?

The directness and openness with which people solve their problems influence communications. Are problems communicated directly, communicated in a circular manner, or denied and ignored? How appropriate is it to state an opinion or offer help?

Cultural differences affect the nonverbal tone of the receiver. Body language, such as eye contact, gestures, and distance, is culturally determined. Much of the message is lost when one does not understand the communications of the body.

Values guide many communications within cultures. They help determine whether the individual or the group is more important and how individuals of various statuses should be treated. How individuals from various cultures use time is an example of a cultural value that affects communications. Religious beliefs and practices can also affect communications. For example, followers of Buddhism may not share that they are in pain because they believe their suffering is due to a failure of righteousness.

Cultures that place a high value on nonverbal communications practice **"high-context"** communications, in which nonverbal cues and sensitivity play a larger role than the actual verbal message. Cultures that practice **"low-context"** communications tend to focus more on the words rather than the emotional tones of the message.

Another major cultural communication difference is the use of a society's language. **Language** use includes a culture's use of names and titles; the structure of grammar; the use of vocabulary, jargon, and slang; and vocal qualities such as tones, pronunciation, rhythm, and speed of communications. The meaning of silence also varies from culture to culture. Caregivers need

---

Box 10-3 | *Improving Intercultural Communication*

To improve your intercultural communications:
1. Recognize what is different from your own cultural style.
2. Adapt your behavior to accommodate the difference.
3. Call attention to the difference to explain the confusion in communication (Bennett, 1994).
4. Accept the client as a person with a willingness to work toward therapeutic goals of care.

---

to be aware of the meanings of culturally different communications. The effectiveness of the therapeutic relationship depends on it. Box 10-3 offers suggestions for improving intercultural communications.

THERAPEUTIC COMMUNICATION SKILLS

The goals of therapeutic communications are to focus on the client and foster the therapeutic relationship. Therapeutic communication techniques are abilities that assist care providers in effectively interacting with clients. Each therapeutic communication skill is based on eight principles (Table 10-1) that serve as guidelines for effective interactions. Refer to them often because they will help you cope with the complexities of human communications.

Therapeutic communication techniques are divided into two equally important areas: listening skills and interacting skills. Each is vital if communications are to be clearly understood and therapeutic actions are to be successful.

LISTENING SKILLS

In our fast-paced world, people are so intent on sending their messages that they seldom take the time to listen—to truly hear what the other person is trying to communicate. The art of listening is a necessary ingredient for every health care provider, not just those who work in psychiatry. Effective listening improves one's abilities to meet clients' needs. In addition, effective listening can identify hidden messages and agendas, minimize misunderstandings, and clarify messages. Although it may require time and practice to perfect your therapeutic listening skills, the rewards are worth the efforts (Box 10-4).

To polish your listening skills, first **concentrate on the speaker.** Next, **listen objectively.** Use appropriate eye contact and body language. Remember the speaker's cultural background. Maintaining a relaxed body position at eye level with the speaker communicates acceptance and interest. Make sure that your **nonverbal messages match the verbal messages.** Do not interrupt. Let the speaker be fully expressive. If you must interrupt, explain that the conversation is

Table 10-1 | *Principles of Therapeutic Communication*

PRINCIPLE	ILLUSTRATION	EXAMPLE
Acceptance	Communicate a favorable reception by implying, "You have a right to exist, to live your life, to have somebody care about you." One does not have to approve of another's behavior to be accepting. It is only when people feel accepted for what they are that they will consider changing.	*Client:* "I know it's been destructive for me to live with my parents, and I get irresponsible living there, but I feel like that's where I need to go after I leave the hospital." *Caregiver:* "I may not agree with your decision about where to live, but I accept your choice to do that and will work with you to evaluate how it works."
Interest	Communicate interest by expressing a desire to know another person. Interest is conveyed by asking about those aspects of a person's life that others often reject. Caregivers communicate by their attitude that "everything can be talked about here."	*Client:* "I'm so ashamed of what I've done, I can't tell you about it. You won't ever talk to me again!" *Caregiver:* "Sandy, I'm interested in everything about you, the good, the bad, the sad, the happy. This is not just a "good times only" relationship. You and I have committed to working on a number of issues of importance, and I have a feeling that this is one of them. So why not go ahead and begin?"
Respect	Show consideration for another by communicating a willingness to work with the client. Accept the client's ideas, feelings, and rights. Listen attentively, express belief in the client's ability to solve personal problems and assume responsibility for his or her own life, collaborate on shared goals, arrive and leave on time, and keep your word. False reassurance and critical judgment are to be avoided.	*Client:* "I know it's silly for me to feel so frightened about living alone, but I'm terrified." *Caregiver:* "I could tell you that you have nothing to worry about, that you'll do just fine. But, I hear your terror, your voice is shaking, and you're all perspired. It must be hard to imagine being able to survive on your own after being married for 30 years."
Honesty	Demonstrate honesty by being consistent, open, and frank. Communicate with the client as an authentic person. Use tact and timing in judging the use of honesty so that clients are not burdened with information or feedback they are not ready to hear. Be honest and nondefensive about thoughts and feelings discovered through self-assessment.	*Client:* "I hate the way he treats me; he takes me for granted, leaving and not telling me when he's coming home. It will never change." *Caregiver:* "Carol, we've discussed this pattern before and the alternative ways for dealing with the situation. Quite honestly, I think a major reason for Lou's not changing his behavior is that you allow him to continue it." *Client:* "What do you mean?" *Caregiver:* "I mean that unless or until you let him know that his behavior is unacceptable, why should he change? This way he doesn't have to be accountable to anyone, even his wife."
Concreteness	Be specific, to the point, and clear. Use understandable language, and avoid the use of jargon. Clients who speak in vague, general, unfocused ways are helped to be more specific and focused.	*Client:* "I feel sort of uneasy, I get a feeling like ... that every so often ..." (perspiring, wringing hands, tapping feet) *Caregiver:* "Describe the feeling for me."
Assistance	Commit time and energy to therapeutic relationships. Convey that you are present and available and have tangible aid to offer that will help clients choose and develop more functional ways of living.	*Caregiver:* "While you're in the hospital, you and I will be meeting every day at 2 PM for 45 minutes. I am available to you to help you work out the problems that are bothering you. I'll also see you lots of other times since I work on the unit. I hope you'll feel free to approach me if you need something."
Permission	Communicate permission by conveying the message that it is acceptable to try new ways of behaving. Often clients are afraid to choose freely and act autonomously. They often need to be given permission and encouragement to see and do things in new ways.	*Client:* "How can I suddenly trust people when I've been hurt so badly in the past?" *Caregiver:* "Clarify for me who hurt you." *Client:* "Well, my brother, you know how he hurt me." *Caregiver:* "Yes, I do know that. What about other people? Can you tell me about them?" *Client:* "Well, I can't tell you any others specifically. It's just the way I feel about people." *Caregiver:* "I think you may be looking at other people and seeing your brother in them. You might be bringing the past into the present."
Protection	Protect clients by ensuring safety. Work with clients to anticipate trouble spots with new behavior and develop effective ways of dealing with anticipated or actual problems, thus maximizing the possibility of success.	*Caregiver:* "I hear that you're scared, and that's very natural for you to feel. Let's work together to try to anticipate what will happen over the weekend and see if, together, you and I can come up with some strategies for dealing with those hot spots."

From Haber J and others: *Comprehensive psychiatric nursing*, ed 5, St. Louis, 1997, Mosby.

Box 10-4 *Therapeutic Listening Skills*

- Concentrate on the speaker and the message.
- Keep distractions and interruptions to a minimum.
- Change the setting (environment) if necessary.
- Assess nonverbal communications and metacommunications.
- Listen objectively.
- Discover which words trigger emotional responses in you.
- Use eye contact and body language that is culturally appropriate.
- Do not interrupt. Let the speaker finish delivering the message.
- Jot down notes if needed.
- Do not assume that you have understood another person's thoughts.
- Clarify any message about which you are unsure.

important but your time is limited. **Follow up** with telling the speaker when you will return to finish the conversation. The last and most important guideline for becoming an effective listener is to **clarify.** If you are uncertain about what was communicated, ask for clarification. Clarification is a primary therapeutic communication technique that, when used in combination with good listening skills, enhances every caregiver's abilities to successfully interact with clients.

INTERACTING SKILLS

Therapeutic techniques that relate to the care provider's actions while communicating are called **responding strategies** or interaction skills. These are verbal and nonverbal responses that encourage clients to communicate in a way that encourages growth. To practice therapeutic interactions, use words that have meaning to the client. Communicate directly, and relate to the situation. Messages with a clear meaning are more easily understood. Allow enough time for a response. Do not use the word *why* in a question because it requires a response that justifies one's actions or opinions.

Twelve commonly used therapeutic communication techniques (Stuart and Laraia, 2005) encourage clients to continue communicating. Carefully study the information in Box 10-5. Practice these techniques, and note the results. With patience and repeated use, these techniques will become important tools for effectively interacting with all clients.

NONTHERAPEUTIC COMMUNICATION

Messages that hinder effective communication are called **nontherapeutic communications** because they are interactions that slow or halt the development of a helping relationship. Nontherapeutic communications include barriers that arise within the environment, the caregiver, or the client and the responses that block further communications.

BARRIERS TO COMMUNICATION

Barriers can arise during each step of the communication process. They are protective behaviors used when one feels threatened. The problem is that their use can increase the client's insecurity and helplessness. If allowed to go unchecked, the use of barriers will smother the therapeutic relationship and prevent the client from reaching the treatment goals.

Because the environment is difficult to control, it can often have a negative effect on communications. It may be too noisy or crowded for the sharing of personal information. Sometimes the client will attempt to send an important message in an inappropriate setting. For example, while waiting in line at the lunchroom your client announces that he is leaving his wife. In this instance, the environment acts as a barrier to further exploration because of the noise level and lack of privacy.

Problems with the individuals involved in the communication can arise. The caregiver may be physically tired or would prefer not to interact with the client. Such feelings may lead to **incongruent communications**, in which the verbal messages do not match the nonverbal communications. Incongruent communications can be sent by either the client or the caregiver, but it is the caregiver's responsibility to match the communication with the message.

On occasion, a client will refuse to communicate or cooperate. This lack of cooperation erects a large barrier and prevents other people from attempting to interact. Such a client requires extra patience and repeated messages of acceptance. With time and persistence, clients usually become more willing to interact because no person likes to be cut off from his or her fellow human beings.

The following are methods for coping with the barriers to communications:

1. Recognize that a problem exists.
2. Identify what purpose or need the problem is filling.
3. Explore appropriate alternative behaviors.
4. Implement the alternative behaviors when interacting.
5. Evaluate whether communications have improved. If they have not, reassess and try another approach. Being aware of communication barriers allows you to intervene early and effectively.

NONTHERAPEUTIC MESSAGES

According to Sundeen and others (1998), nontherapeutic communications are problems of omission or commission. Nontherapeutic communication techniques

Box 10-5 *Therapeutic Communication Techniques*

LISTENING

Definition: Active process of receiving information and examining reactions to messages received

Example: Maintaining eye contact and receptive nonverbal communication

Therapeutic value: Nonverbally communicates caregiver's interest and acceptance

Nontherapeutic threat: Failure to listen

BROAD OPENINGS

Definition: Encouraging client to select topics for discussion

Example: "What are you thinking about?"

Therapeutic value: Indicates acceptance by caregiver and value of client's initiative

Nontherapeutic threat: Caregiver dominates interaction; rejecting responses

RESTATING

Definition: Repeating main thought expressed by client

Example: "You say that your mother left you when you were 5 years old?"

Therapeutic value: Indicates that caregiver is listening and validates, reinforces, or calls attention to something important that has been said

Nontherapeutic threat: Lack of validation of caregiver's interpretation of message; being judgmental; reassuring; defending

CLARIFICATION

Definition: Attempting to put into words vague ideas or unclear thoughts of client; asking client to explain what he or she means

Example: "I'm not sure what you mean. Could you tell me about that again?"

Therapeutic value: Helps to clarify feelings, ideas, and perceptions of client and provides explicit correlation between them and client's actions

Nontherapeutic threat: Failure to probe; assumed understanding

REFLECTION

Definition: Directing back client's ideas, feelings, questions, and content

Example: "You're feeling tense and anxious, and it's related to a conversation you had with your husband last night?"

Therapeutic value: Validates caregiver's understanding of what client is saying and signifies empathy, interest, and respect for client

Nontherapeutic threat: Stereotyping client's responses; inappropriate timing of reflections; inappropriate depth of reflections; inappropriate responses to cultural experience and educational level of client

HUMOR

Definition: Discharge of energy through comic enjoyment

Example: "That gives a whole new meaning to the word *nervous*," said with shared kidding between caregiver and client

Therapeutic value: Can promote insight by making conscious repressed material, resolving paradoxes, tempering aggression, and revealing new options; is socially acceptable form of sublimation

Nontherapeutic threat: Indiscriminate use; belittling client; screen to avoid therapeutic intimacy

INFORMING

Definition: Skill of information giving

Example: "I think you need to know more about how your medication works."

Therapeutic value: Helpful in client education about relevant aspects of well-being and self-care

Nontherapeutic threat: Giving advice

FOCUSING

Definition: Questions or statements that help client expand topic

Example: "I think that we should talk more about your relationship with your father."

Therapeutic value: Allows client to discuss central issues; keeps communication process goal directed

Nontherapeutic threat: Allowing abstractions and generalizations; changing topics

SHARING PERCEPTIONS

Definition: Asking client to verify caregiver's understanding of client's message

Example: "You're smiling, but I sense that you are really very angry with me."

Therapeutic value: Conveys understanding to client and can clear up confusing communication

Nontherapeutic threat: Challenging client; accepting literal responses; reassuring; testing; defending

THEME IDENTIFICATION

Definition: Underlying client issues or problems that emerge repeatedly during caregiver-client relationship

Example: "I've noticed that in all of the relationships that you have described, you've been hurt or rejected by a man. Do you think this is an underlying issue?"

Therapeutic value: Allows caregiver to promote client's exploration and understanding of important problems

Nontherapeutic threat: Giving advice; reassuring; disapproving

SILENCE

Definition: Lack of verbal communication for therapeutic reason

Example: Sitting with client and nonverbally communicating interest and involvement

Therapeutic value: Allows client time to think and gain insights; slows pace of interaction and encourages client to initiate conversation while conveying support, understanding, and acceptance

Nontherapeutic threat: Questioning client; failure to break nontherapeutic silence

SUGGESTING

Definition: Presenting alternative ideas for client's consideration relative to problem solving

Example: "Have you thought about responding to your boss in a different way when he raises that issue with you? For example, you could ask him if a specific problem has occurred."

Therapeutic value: Increases client's perceived options or choices

Nontherapeutic threat: Giving advice; inappropriate timing; being judgmental

Modified from Stuart GW, Laraia MT: *Principles and practice of psychiatric nursing*, ed 7, St Louis, 2001, Mosby.

Table 10-2 | *Nontherapeutic Communications*

NONTHERAPEUTIC TECHNIQUE	DESCRIPTION	EXAMPLE
Failure to listen	Placing own thoughts above client, not being involved in communication	Yawning when client is speaking, looking at watch frequently, missing client's messages
Failure to explore client's point of view	Does not ask client to describe abstract words such as *pain, angry, sick*	*Client:* "My head hurts." *Caregiver:* "You're just getting used to your new medication." *Better:* "Tell me more."
Failure to probe	Does not seek clarification or validation from client	*Client:* "I've had bad experiences with doctors." *Caregiver:* "That's too bad." *Better:* "Would you like to explain?"
Eliciting vague descriptions	Does not encourage client to explain or expand on message	*Client:* "I keep hearing voices." *Caregiver:* "O.K." *Better:* "What do they say?"
Giving inadequate answers	Does not collect enough data to answer client's question accurately	Instructs client about medication and then finds out he is allergic to it
Parroting	Continuous repeating of client's words	*Client:* "I haven't slept in 2 nights." *Caregiver:* "You haven't slept in 2 nights?" *Better:* "What do you think is causing this?"
Following standard forms too closely	Using a question-and-answer format to elicit specific information	*Caregiver:* "Do you have any problems chewing?" *Client:* "No, but I have this pain in my jaw at night." *Caregiver:* "Do you have any problems with indigestion or constipation?" *Better:* "Tell me about your jaw pain."
Being judgmental: giving approval or disapproval, agreeing or disagreeing	Many responses that tell clients that they must think as you do	*Client:* "I saw my wife today." *Caregiver:* "You should be nicer to her." *Better:* "How did it go?"
Giving advice	Telling clients what to do; gives message that they are inferior and not able to make good decisions	*Client:* "I'm nervous about meeting Dr. Dow." *Caregiver:* "You just march in there and say what you want, but don't raise your voice." *Better:* "I can understand that."
Being defensive	An attempt to protect something or someone; prevents clients from communicating	*Client:* "That last nurse is a dope." *Caregiver:* "All of our nurses here are highly trained." *Better:* "What makes you think that?"
Challenging	Inviting or daring client to explain, act, or compete	*Client:* "I'm really dead, you know." *Caregiver:* "If you are really dead, then why is your heart still beating?" *Better:* "You're dead?"
Giving reassurance	Messages that negate feelings of client	*Client:* "I'll never get out of here." *Caregiver:* "Everything will turn out for the best." *Better:* "You feel that you have been here a long time?"
Rejecting	Refusal to discuss feelings or areas of concern	*Client:* "You know that I raped my sister." *Caregiver:* "Let's not talk about that." *Better:* "Would you like to talk about it?"
Using stereotyped responses	Using clichés, popular sayings, or trite expressions	*Client:* "I feel so depressed today." *Caregiver:* "Everyone gets the blues now and then." *Better:* "What's making you feel so blue?"

Modified from Sundeen SJ and others: *Nurse-client interactions: implementing the nursing process,* ed 6, St. Louis, 1998, Mosby.

of **omission** relate to the caregiver's failure to do something (e.g., to use a therapeutic technique) when the moment is right. Examples of communication acts of omission include failure to listen, probe, or explore the client's point of view. Eliciting vague descriptions, giving inadequate answers, parroting, and following standard forms too closely are also in this category.

Those nontherapeutic techniques in which the caregiver communicates in an undesirable manner fall into nontherapeutic communications of commission. They include giving advice or disapproval, being defensive, making judgments, challenging, making stereotyped responses, reassuring, or rejecting client messages.

Table 10-2 lists several nontherapeutic communication techniques. Become an observer of your own communications. See if your verbal and nonverbal communications send the same message. Evaluate your use of different techniques, and work to enhance your ability to effectively communicate.

PROBLEMS WITH COMMUNICATION

For many people, communicating with others can be a difficult process. Sensory-impaired clients have difficulty receiving or sending messages because of problems with sight, hearing, or understanding. Some people may have problems with sending messages. Persons with aphasia (inability to speak), dyslexia (impaired ability to read sometimes accompanied by a mixing of letters or syllables in a word when speaking), and speech cluttering (rapid, confused delivery of unrhythmic speech patterns) cannot focus on verbal communications as their main form of human interaction.

The first step in interacting is to achieve a successful introduction. If the client knows your name and purpose, cooperation is more likely. If possible, learn how the client communicates (signing, writing, touch) and then encourage him or her to become actively involved in the communication process. Maintain good eye contact (when appropriate) and attentive nonverbal behaviors. Tune in to the client's nonverbal behaviors, and become extra alert for the messages being sent. Communicate directly with the client. Do not try to finish the client's sentence or fill in words. Allow extra time for the client to think and form responses. Last, do not forget the importance of the use of touch. For people who have diminished sight or hearing, touch is a powerful communication tool. In addition, the speech therapist can be a valuable member of the multidisciplinary treatment team for clients with communication problems.

Developing communication systems for people with language problems is the goal of several research projects. Computer devices, such as TouchSpeak and TalksBack, allow users to communicate "by producing pre-prepared conversation 'chunks' via a voice synthesizer at the touch of a button" (University of Dundee Press Release, 1999).

COMMUNICATING WITH MENTALLY TROUBLED CLIENTS

Problems with communication are a common feature in many forms of mental illness. People with mental-emotional difficulties find it difficult to develop trust in other people. Loneliness is the companion of mental illness. Sincere, respectful caring of another person can help remove barriers that isolate the mentally ill individual from the world.

To communicate effectively with mentally and emotionally troubled clients, realize that **every interaction is a part of the total therapeutic process.** A climate of trust and respect must be established before clients feel safe enough to honestly share themselves. Establishing this trusting climate requires patience, persistence, and consistency. Mental health clients need **routine,** the security of a dependable environment, and care providers with calm, reliable temperaments. This consistency satisfies basic needs and allows clients to focus on communicating.

Begin your interactions with mental health clients by introducing yourself and explaining your purpose. Then introduce a neutral subject, such as weather, sports, or entertainment events. Wait quietly for the client to comment, using the opportunity to assess nonverbal behaviors or barriers to communication. Once the client is communicating, avoid a verbal assault of questions. Data may need to be obtained but not at the expense of threatening the fragile communication line so recently established. As long as the client is interacting, necessary data will eventually be revealed.

One of the most important tools for communicating with mentally ill clients is therapeutic listening. Attentive listening alone communicates acceptance and respect, messages not often received by mental health clients. Once the client believes that you sincerely care about him or her as a person, a flow of communications will come easily. Sample Client Care Plan 10-1, based on the use of therapeutic communication principles, is presented on p. 107.

ASSESSING COMMUNICATION

Because the flow of information between people occurs naturally, we seldom take the time to assess a client's abilities to communicate. However, a communication assessment is an important component of the mental health workup.

First, assess the client's ability to hear and speak. Then note the content, quality, and pace of the client's speech. Is speech coherent, logical, or easy to follow? Is the pace fast or slow? Is the volume loud, too soft, or whispered? Are there any physical speech problems, such as stuttering? Are the number of words used excessive or few? How much time lapses before the client responds to your message? Can the client read or write? Is a cultural communication assessment necessary? The answers to these questions provide a solid database and offer valuable information for the multidisciplinary treatment team in establishing appropriate therapeutic goals. Table 10-3 describes some of the more common abnormal speech patterns seen in clients with psychiatric problems.

The ability to therapeutically communicate is an important skill. Good communication techniques must be practiced daily and evaluated frequently. Assess each communication and evaluate your effectiveness by asking yourself, "Was the interaction appropriate to the goals of care? Was there enough communication and feedback to meet the goals? Was the interaction flexible enough to allow for a balance between spontaneity and control? Was the communication effective?" Practice, patience, and a continual willingness to evaluate your interactions are the keys to developing effective communication skills. Work hard to become a good communicator. Your clients' well-being depends on it, no matter what the diagnosis.

SAMPLE CLIENT CARE PLAN 10-1

Communication

ASSESSMENT *History.* Amy, a 30-year-old married woman, is suffering from depression. Currently, she refuses to speak or acknowledge anyone, including her husband and children. Today she is being admitted for evaluation and treatment of her depression.

Current Findings. An untidy woman who stares at the floor and does not respond to staff members' questions. Sighs frequently. Sits immobile in chair for long periods.

Multidisciplinary Diagnosis	Planning/Goals
Impaired verbal communications related to emotional state	Amy will communicate her wishes and feelings with at least one staff member by April 22.

Therapeutic Interventions

Interventions	Rationale	Team Member
1. Present a calm, patient attitude rather than attempting to make Amy speak.	Helps decrease fears and anxieties; demonstrates respect and acceptance.	All
2. Actively listen, observe for verbal and nonverbal cues and behaviors.	Helps piece together communication methods in an effort to understand Amy's messages.	All
3. Encourage other ways of communicating, such as drawing or writing.	Demonstrates empathy, helps develop trust, and encourages communication.	All
4. Anticipate needs until Amy can communicate them.	Provides safety, comfort, and support; helps develop trust.	Nsg
5. Spend time (at least 15 minutes twice each day) with Amy in a private, quiet setting.	Promotes trust and interest; helps promote self-esteem.	Nsg
6. Praise any attempt to communicate.	Encourages communication and demonstrates interest.	All

Evaluation

The second day after admission, Amy began to draw. By the fourth day of hospitalization, she answered "yes" or "no" questions. On April 17, Amy was able to discuss her feelings with one nurse.

？ CRITICAL THINKING QUESTIONS

1. Amy began to draw pictures on her second day of admission. How could the caregiver encourage her to verbally communicate based on her drawings?

2. How do you think you would feel sitting in silence with another person for 10 minutes?

A complete client care plan includes several other diagnoses and interventions.
Nsg, Nursing staff.

Table 10-3 | *Speech Patterns Associated With Psychiatric Problems*

SPEECH PATTERN	DESCRIPTION	EXAMPLE
Blocking	Loses train of thought, stops speaking because of unconscious block	"Then my father ... what was I saying?"
Circumstantiality	Describes in too much detail, cannot be selective	When asked "How are you?" replies, "My left hand aches a bit, my nose has been leaking, my hair won't stay in place ...."
Echolalia	Repeats last word heard	"Please wait here" is responded to with "Here, here, here ..."
Flight of ideas	Shifts rapidly between unrelated topics	"My cat is gray. The food here is good."
Loose associations	Speaks constantly, shifting between loosely related topics	"Martha married Jim, who is a cook. I can cook. Cows are something that we can cook."
Mutism	Able to speak but remains silent	
Neologism	Coins new words and definitions	"Zargleves are good to eat," referring to any candy snack.
Perseveration	Repeats single activity, cannot shift from one topic to another	Answers new question with previous question's answer.
Pressured speech	Speech becomes fast, loud, rushed, and emphatic	Persons with mania often move and speak very rapidly with great urgency.
Verbigeration	Repeats words, phrases, sentences several times over	*Nurse:* "It's time to take your pill." *Client:* "Take your pill, take your pill, take your pill ...."

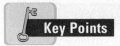

Key Points

- Communication is the exchange of information between two persons or among a group of persons.
- In the 1960s, Dr. Eric Berne coined the term *transactional analysis* to describe the process of investigating what people do and say to each other.
- Neurolinguistic programming focuses on patterns of an individual's communications, which include eye-accessing clues, different language patterns, and the pace and rhythm of speech.
- For communication to occur there must be a sender, a message, a receiver, feedback, and a context.
- The process of communicating involves perception, evaluation, and transmission.
- Communications occur on both verbal and nonverbal levels at the same time.
- Health care providers who work with clients from culturally different backgrounds need to learn culturally appropriate methods for communication by recognizing different communication styles, adapting their own communications, and accepting the client as a person.
- Therapeutic communication techniques are skills that assist in effectively interacting with clients.
- Principles of therapeutic communication include acceptance, interest, respect, honesty, concreteness, assistance, permission, and protection.

- The goals of therapeutic communications are to focus on the client and foster the therapeutic relationship.
- The art of listening is a necessary ingredient for every health care provider.
- Therapeutic communication techniques (responding strategies) are verbal and nonverbal responses that encourage clients to communicate. They include listening, offering broad openings, restating, clarification, reflection, humor, offering information, focusing, sharing perceptions, identifying themes, suggesting, and silence.
- Messages that hinder effective communications are called nontherapeutic communications.
- Problems with communication are a common feature of many forms of mental illness.
- To communicate effectively with psychiatric clients, remember that every interaction is a part of the total therapeutic process.
- A communication assessment focuses on the client's ability to communicate, actual speech, and current or potential communication problems.

evolve Be sure to visit the companion Evolve site at http://evolve.elsevier.com/Morrison-Valfre/ for additional online resources.

11 The Therapeutic Relationship

Objectives

Upon completion of this chapter, the student will be able to:

1. Describe the difference between a social relationship and a therapeutic relationship.
2. Illustrate the five dynamics of the therapeutic relationship.
3. List three ways to establish therapeutic rapport.
4. Describe the four characteristics of the therapeutic relationship.
5. Explain the meaning of "therapeutic use of self."
6. Identify the four phases of the therapeutic relationship.
7. Describe four roles of the caregiver in the therapeutic relationship.
8. Discuss three problems that may be encountered in the therapeutic relationship.

Key Terms

autonomy (aw-TŎN-ə-mē) (p. 110)
countertransference (KOUN-tĕr-trăns-FĔR-ĕns) (p. 117)
dynamics (p. 109)
empathy (p. 110)
genuineness (p. 112)
hope (p. 111)
limit setting (p. 114)
mutuality (MŬ-tū-ə-ĂL-ə-tē) (p. 110)
noncompliance (p. 117)
rapport (răh-PŎR) (p. 112)
resistance (p. 117)
secondary gain (p. 117)
therapeutic relationship (p. 109)
transference (trăns-FĔR-ĕns) (p. 117)
trust (p. 109)

The **therapeutic relationship** is a directed energy exchange between two people, a flow that moves clients toward more constructive ways of thinking and effective ways of coping. Caregivers use their abundant energies to first balance or stabilize clients. Then they assist clients to mobilize and direct their own energies into more life-fulfilling directions.

The art of helping others involves a dynamic energy exchange that takes place every time caregivers interact with their clients. This chapter focuses on how health care providers use their energies to establish and direct the therapeutic relationship.

DYNAMICS OF THE THERAPEUTIC RELATIONSHIP

The term **dynamics** refers to the interactions that occur among various forces. A **social relationship** includes dynamics such as having fun together, supporting each other through difficult times, and enjoying each other's company. A social relationship is a two-way energy exchange based on the sharing of personal opinions, attitudes, and tastes.

A **work relationship** has the purpose of achieving certain goals. It includes the dynamics of motivation, performance, and evaluation. People within a work relationship are there to achieve a goal, produce a product, make a profit, or deliver a service.

The **therapeutic relationship** differs from other relationships. First, the focus of energies is primarily on the client. Second, the therapeutic relationship is consciously directed. Friendships and other social relationships just happen. In therapeutic relationships, care providers consciously establish a connection with clients to help them cope with their life demands.

The dynamic components of the therapeutic relationship include the concepts of trust, empathy, autonomy, caring, and hope. Use these concepts as a framework to develop the skills and sensitivity necessary to direct your energies toward effective helping relationships.

TRUST

Trust is defined as "a risk-taking process whereby an individual's situation depends on the future behavior of another person" (Anderson, Anderson, and Glanze, 2006). Attitudes regarding trust are based on experiences, which have the power to influence the present and future. Without trust, individuals become isolated and incapable of relying on other people. Within the therapeutic relationship, trust is "the assured belief that other individuals are capable of assisting in times of distress and will probably do so" (Travelbee, 1971). Trust is an important part of any therapeutic relationship. Every person for whom we care needs to be able to trust that we will act in his or her best interests.

Illness or dysfunction of any kind requires energy. When clients arrive for care, their energies are usually very low. The role of "receiver of care" fosters a dependency on caregivers and feelings of vulnerability. Learn to recognize this situation, and work to establish a sense of trust in each client.

Caregivers direct their energies toward establishing trust with clients in several ways. They first **assess the client's ability to trust** others. Each therapeutic behavior is then designed to promote trust. For example, a caregiver who says she will return in 10 minutes arrives at the appointed time. One simple action reassures clients that caregivers will follow through on their verbal statements.

Second, care providers must **be honest** with their clients. To tell a child, for example, that the injection will not hurt makes him or her less likely to believe the next health care provider's explanations. If these experiences are repeated often enough, people develop a mistrust of the entire medical care system (see Think About 11-1).

The third focus in the establishment of trust is **clear communication.** Give information to clients slowly, using terms that can be understood by the average person. Clients cannot learn to trust if they cannot understand. Offer clients the time to share their feelings and apprehensions. "Without the establishment of trust, the helping relationship will not progress beyond the level of mechanical provision for tending to superficial needs" (Sundeen and others, 1998).

EMPATHY

Empathy is the ability to understand the emotions, viewpoints, and situations of another. Empathy allows one to walk a mile in another person's shoes. It enables caregivers to enter into the life of an individual and share important emotions, meanings, and attitudes. Empathy is demonstrated verbally, nonverbally, and behaviorally. It is the **connection** between caregiver and client that increases the effectiveness of the therapeutic relationship. In short, empathy is the ability to share in the client's world.

? Think About 11-1

Mary J. is a 42-year-old woman who has been treated for severe depression for 21 years. She has received several electroconvulsive therapy treatments that she was told would relieve her depression; they did not. Various psychotropic medications have had little success. Currently, you, as one of the staff at the community mental health center, have been following Mary's care.

Although Mary is required to return to the clinic weekly for medication monitoring, she keeps her appointments only when she wants more medication. When questioned about her refusal to keep her appointments, she tells you that no one really cares about her so why go through the motions. "Just fill the prescription, keep your mouth shut, and let me go," she replies to your statement of concern.

• How could Mary be encouraged to return to treatment?

Unfortunately, there are no specific directions for developing empathy. However, you can become more empathetic by focusing your attention (energies) on what clients are trying to communicate. Learn to listen with more than just your ears. Concentrate on the speaker and listen objectively, without passing judgment. Accept what is being said. You do not have to agree with what the client says, but you need to demonstrate acceptance of the communications.

The development of empathy can also be nurtured by becoming secure in your therapeutic actions. When care providers are confident with their abilities, their energies can be devoted to clients and their situations, instead of being concerned about performance. The caregiver's confidence sends a message that encourages clients to share more of themselves.

Last, learn to consciously focus on your client. Enter into each interaction expecting to learn something new. Become aware of the entire message the client is sending. Observe body motions, gestures, eye movement, facial expressions, and vocal tones. Together, these small cues send powerful messages.

AUTONOMY

The concept of **autonomy** relates to the ability to direct and control one's activities and destiny. When people seek health care they risk losing their autonomy because health care delivery is a specialized, complex world, full of the unknown.

People with mental health difficulties have problems with autonomy because the nature of their illness often results in their making inappropriate decisions. However, autonomy is just as important for these individuals. Frequently, care providers think that clients are incapable of making good health care decisions. They assume an attitude of paternalism and become the judge of what is best for the client. This attitude limits the client's ability to make decisions and increases dependency on others. Autonomy is encouraged by the caregiver through use of the concept of mutuality.

The concept of **mutuality** relates to the process of sharing with another person. When a therapeutic relationship has mutuality, both client and caregiver focus their unique strengths on fulfilling health care needs. The care provider has theoretical knowledge that can assist the client in identifying specific problems and possible solutions, and the client has the knowledge of self and the needs that are important to him or her. Both contribute to the plan of care.

Because clients are unique individuals, therapeutic interventions are modified to meet each person's needs. For example, clients who are unable to remember their appointments are reminded. Mutuality also helps both clients and care providers meet goals. When goals are based on the client's needs, they are more apt to be achieved because clients have a role in establishing them.

CARING

Caring is a vital part of the therapeutic relationship; its thread is interwoven through every aspect and interaction. Caring is the energy that allows caregivers to unconditionally accept all people, even when they are most unlovable.

Clients will often question caregivers about their sincerity. Statements such as "You are just doing this because it's your job" or "You don't really care—you're getting paid to be nice to me" express the need to be accepted, cared for, and valued. People who have had negative experiences with the health care delivery system become cautious and suspicious of the intentions of their care providers. They can tell when someone is sincere or merely concerned with the diagnosis, test, or function rather than the person. Caregivers who demonstrate high levels of caring are able to enjoy the uniqueness of each individual. They are able to give of themselves without losing their own identity. To develop and nurture your caring abilities, practice the behaviors listed in Box 11-1. Caring behaviors communicate concern, sensitivity, and compassion. Cherish and nurture your ability to care because it is the connection that enhances the therapeutic relationship.

HOPE

The concept of hope involves the future. For many people, especially those who are ill or distressed, the future can appear bleak. Hope is not easily defined, but, from a therapeutic point of view, we can say that hope is "a multidimensional dynamic life force characterized by a confident yet uncertain expectation of achieving a future good" (Dufault and Martocchio, 1985). For hope to be achievable, it must be realistic, possible, and personally significant. Hope is a highly personal concept, and it serves as an energy that motivates people toward health.

For caregivers, hope is a therapeutic energy tool that can have a powerful effect on client care outcomes. The emotions and behaviors relating to hope are many, ranging from feelings of despair to inspiration and determination. They are illustrated on a continuum or range (Figure 11-1), with the behaviors of despair on one end and great hope on the other.

Dufault and Martocchio (1985) have described six dimensions related to the concept of hope. The first is the **affective dimension.** It includes all the feelings that one has about hope, such as anticipation, the desirability attached to the outcome, and dread. It is the emotional aspect of hope.

The second area, the **affiliative dimension,** focuses on how hope is related or interwoven. It includes spirituality—how one relates to life and other people. Behaviors in this dimension include the seeking or receiving of help, using others as a source of hope, and seeking support and encouragement.

Third is the **behavioral dimension,** which consists of the actions or behaviors that may make the hoped-for situation come true. For example, people who begin an exercise program hoping that they will prevent heart problems are operating in the behavioral dimension.

Fourth is the **cognitive dimension,** or the thinking area. It is the process of thinking through and analyzing the hope. Some people operate within this dimension by defining what their hopes are. Others explore all the factors that relate to the hoped-for situation, whereas some compile facts to encourage a successful outcome. Acts associated with problem solving are in the cognitive dimension.

Fifth is the **temporal dimension** of hope, the experience of time as it relates to hope. Because hope is accompanied by time, one's past, present, and future interact. One may hope to repeat the pleasant experiences of the past and use them as a frame of reference to avoid problems in the future.

Last is the **contextual dimension** of hope, which includes one's personal life situation as it relates to hope. It becomes much easier to have hope if one's environment is stable. Inadequate resources (physical, financial, emotional) provide a context in which hope may be difficult to muster. Hope conforms to an individual's point of view.

There are several therapeutic interventions relating to hope. Table 11-1 lists an intervention for each dimension of hope. The concept of hope is a basic component of the therapeutic relationship because without it, no progress toward a goal is real.

The dynamics of the therapeutic relationship are not overt. They lie quietly, waiting to be energized by the therapeutic agent. Trust, empathy, autonomy, caring,

Box 11-1 *Developing Caring Abilities*

To develop and nurture your ability to care, do the following:
1. Become aware of the client as an individual.
2. Learn to respect the uniqueness of each person.
3. Increase your knowledge of the client's needs.
4. Develop mutual sharing.

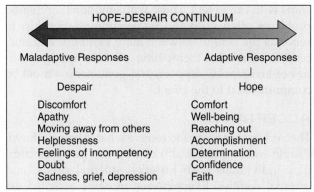

HOPE-DESPAIR CONTINUUM

Maladaptive Responses   Adaptive Responses

Despair   Hope

Despair	Hope
Discomfort	Comfort
Apathy	Well-being
Moving away from others	Reaching out
Helplessness	Accomplishment
Feelings of incompetency	Determination
Doubt	Confidence
Sadness, grief, depression	Faith

FIGURE **11-1** The hope-despair continuum.

Table 11-1 *Interventions Related to Hope*

DIMENSION	THERAPEUTIC INTERVENTIONS
Affective	Provide an opportunity for expression of feelings
	Respond empathically
	Assist in coping with feelings
Affiliative	Support helpful relationships
Behavioral	Encourage appropriate actions
	Enhance self-esteem to decrease feelings of helplessness
Cognitive	Clarification
	Provide information
Temporal	Help to see the relationship between past experiences and hope
Contextual	Help to create a supportive, hopeful environment

Modified from Dufault K, Martocchio BC: Symposium on compassionate care and the dying experience, *Nurs Clin North Am* 20:379, 1985.

Box 11-2 *Components of the Therapeutic Relationship*

T = Trust
E = Empathy
A = Autonomy
C = Caring
H = Hope

and hope are the techniques with which caregivers build the foundation of the therapeutic relationship. Look closely at the first letters of each word, which, when aligned together, spell the word **teach.** With these tools, caregivers can guide the therapeutic relationship and move (teach) their clients toward their highest levels of wellness (Box 11-2).

CHARACTERISTICS OF THE THERAPEUTIC RELATIONSHIP

Therapeutic relationships vary in importance to clients. For clients who are hospitalized or institutionalized, the therapeutic relationship assumes a greater importance. People with chronic conditions usually place a high degree of importance on their relationships with caregivers. Those with emotional or mental problems often need the therapeutic relationship to serve as the bridge between mere existence and success. To establish a therapeutic relationship, the qualities of acceptance, rapport, and genuineness must be communicated to the client.

ACCEPTANCE

The verb **accept** means to receive what is being offered. People entering the health care system arrive as complex individuals with histories, internal needs, and external realities. Every person must be accepted exactly as he or she is. Most people are cooperative and interested in working toward relieving the problems for which they sought care. However, some people are more difficult to accept, especially when their behaviors are unusual or not socially appropriate. "It is difficult to fully understand the overwhelming experience of having to live with mental illness" (Vellenga and Christenson, 1994), but the importance of accepting these individuals cannot be stressed enough in the therapeutic relationship.

Whereas care providers may be concerned with the long-term aspects of a client's mental illness, distressed individuals are more concerned with their present pain and the need for relief.

They must not only cope with the discomforts of their illness but also deal with the alienation forced on them by others. The stigma of being mentally ill follows them into home and workplace and results in the loss of emotional relationships and vocational opportunities. Many individuals experience **distress,** which is described as feelings of hopelessness, fright, and an inability to function. "Clients believed that acceptance lent them a sense of strength and value and made them feel more normal" (Vellenga and Christenson, 1994). For people with mental-emotional problems, acceptance is of prime importance.

Caregivers can develop acceptance by remembering that it is the person (the individual) who must be accepted, not the behaviors or the attitudes. The very purpose of mental health care is to replace inappropriate behaviors with more effective actions. However, if the client feels accepted for who he or she is, then treatment strategies will be far more effective.

RAPPORT

The second ingredient for an effective therapeutic relationship is **rapport**—the ability to establish a meaningful connection with clients. Rapport is a dynamic process, an energy exchange between caregiver and client that provides the background for all therapeutic actions. Rapport is a personal concept—the person of the caregiver therapeutically interacting with the person of the client.

Rapport is developed through a concern for others and an active interest in the well-being of one's clients. A belief in the worth and dignity of each individual, along with an accepting attitude, is essential for forming rapport. Every care provider has a certain degree of skill in establishing rapport with clients. Actively work to improve your abilities to establish meaningful connections with clients. Rapport is not a scientific tool but an application of our willingness to care.

GENUINENESS

Something that is genuine is real. **Genuineness** "implies that the nurse (caregiver) is an open, honest, sincere person who is actively involved in the relationship" (Stuart and Laraia, 2005). The quality of honesty is a part of being genuine. However, the goal of the therapeutic relationship is to move the client toward wellness. Sharing yourself must be done while remembering that the client is the primary focus. In this way, you can be genuinely involved without using the therapeutic relationship to meet your own needs.

THERAPEUTIC USE OF SELF

The most therapeutic tool of any care provider is the **self:** the ways in which we interact with, attend to, and encourage clients. Caregivers are role models for health and coping, especially with people who are mentally or emotionally troubled. Our behaviors set examples for successful actions.

Caregivers direct themselves therapeutically by focusing energies on the client. Sometimes they share small bits of personal information, but that sharing always has a purpose that benefits the client. For example, a client asks how many children the caregiver has. The care provider answers the question and then focuses on the client by asking him how many children he has. This technique allows you to maintain the focus on the client.

To improve your skills in using "self" therapeutically, remember two important points. First, **feel good about yourself.** You cannot be therapeutically effective when your personal life is in turmoil. Clients can sense a caregiver's emotional discomfort. Work to become aware of your own feelings and attitudes and how they affect your therapeutic relationships.

Second, work to develop an awareness of **how your actions,** gestures, and expressions **affect other people.** During each interaction, "step out" of the situation and consider how the client may be reacting. With experience and effort, the majority of your actions will be therapeutic, no matter what the practice setting or client you encounter.

PHASES OF THE THERAPEUTIC RELATIONSHIP

The therapeutic relationship is a time-limited, purposeful series of interactions. Every therapeutic relationship moves through four phases, and each phase has identifiable tasks and goals (Table 11-2). As these tasks are accomplished, a readiness to move on to the next phase is experienced. Interventions are guided by the therapeutic goals of the client's treatment plan throughout the relationship. The four stages or phases of the therapeutic relationship are called the preparation, orientation, working, and termination phases.

PREPARATION PHASE

The preparation phase is the data-gathering stage in which the caregiver prepares for the relationship. Complete information about the client is usually not available, but it is very important to learn as much as possible about the client before the first meeting. The therapeutic goals for this phase are to establish a client database and assess your own feelings regarding the client.

| Table 11-2 | *Client-Caregiver Relationship* |

PHASE	GOALS	CAREGIVER BEHAVIORS
Preparation	Gather data	Reviews information and considers own reactions
Orientation	Develop mutual trust	Establishes mutually acceptable contract
	Establish caregiver as significant other to client	Responds to testing behavior of client by adhering strictly to terms of contract
Maintenance	Identify and address client's problems	Highly individualized to nature of client's problems
		Empathic, nonpunishing limit setting
Termination	Assist client to review what was learned and to transfer this learning to interactions with others	Understands client's sense of loss
		Helps client express and cope with feelings
		Encourages client to channel feelings into constructive activity, such as farewell party
		Recognizes own feelings of loss

Modified from Taylor CM: *Essentials of psychiatric nursing*, ed 14, St. Louis, 1994, Mosby.

To establish a database, **review all possible information** relating to the client. Past medical records, current records, and interactions with significant others in the client's life are excellent sources of information. Once information is gathered, look for the recurring patterns of behavior to develop a picture of the client. You can now begin to form ideas about the relationship and forecast possible problems. A word of caution: Do not accept labels as fact. Keep an open mind. Because a client is labeled as psychotic, do not expect him or her to behave as other people with the same label. People are individuals with their own unique behaviors.

Because caregivers are also unique individuals with attitudes and behaviors that affect the therapeutic relationship, the next step is to **look** inward **to your own reactions.** Identify your initial reactions to the client. Is there anything that may block your ability to help? For example, a caregiver's attendance at a support group for the spouses of alcoholics may have an influence on his or her ability to help a client being treated for alcoholism.

Next, assess for **stereotyping:** If the client is a member of a particular group or culture, will he or she behave in a certain way? The belief that people with mental illness cannot behave responsibly is a stereotype that can affect the therapeutic relationship. Be aware of any preconceived ideas or attitudes about the client.

Finally, **recognize the anxiety** that is generally present in the caregiver during this phase. Mild anxiety is common and sharpens the senses. High anxiety levels can affect one's judgment, so seeking assistance from a supervisor is advised when anxiety may affect the therapeutic relationship.

During this phase caregivers also begin to think about the termination phase. Because the therapeutic relationship is based on helping clients with their problems, it is time limited and caregivers reinforce this throughout each phase of interaction.

The last step in the preparatory phase is to make plans for the first interaction with the client. Find a quiet **setting**—free from interruptions. Plan for sufficient **time,** and identify what **information** must be obtained during the first interaction. Make a mental outline, and your preparations are complete.

ORIENTATION PHASE

During the orientation phase, caregiver and client become acquainted, agree to work with each other, and establish the purpose for the relationship. The first meeting establishes the tone and forms the impressions that both people will carry with them throughout the entire relationship. The basic goals for this phase are to build trust and establish the caregiver as significant in the life of the client.

The most important step at this time is to identify each other. Introduce yourself by name and position. Establish how the client wishes to be addressed. When the client responds, an exchange begins. Next, explain your role as it relates to the client. This gives the client an idea of what may be expected in the relationship. Once client and caregiver are comfortable, an agreement to work with each other is established.

Establishing a working agreement (caregiver-client contract) is the next step in the orientation phase of the therapeutic relationship. Both client and care provider discuss their expectations and then agree on the goals they want to meet. The contract, which includes a description of each person's roles and responsibilities, is then established in writing or verbally. The word **contract** may provoke anxiety in some persons, so it is seldom used when interacting with clients. The term is less important than actually gaining the client's agreement. Once arrangements are made, it is extremely important for the nurse to keep his or her end of the bargain or, as Taylor (1994) states, "to respond to the client's behavior with meticulous consistency."

During the orientation phase, both the client and the caregiver carry out assessments or "size up" each other. The care provider learns about the client as a real person, unique and individual. Work to keep a nonjudgmental attitude. The label of "client" will soon be replaced with a genuine person-to-person exchange that begins to evolve into a therapeutic relationship.

Clients will often test the reliability of their caregivers. **Testing** is an important step in establishing trust in the therapeutic relationship. Although clients may not appear for scheduled appointments, use profane language, or resist sharing their feelings, the caregiver must demonstrate a willingness to continue the therapeutic relationship by doing what was promised in the contract. This **reliability** is important because many troubled people have never had a consistent relationship. When the care provider has established reliability and the client has gained enough trust to no longer test, the therapeutic relationship is ready for the next stage.

WORKING PHASE

The focus of the working phase is to achieve the goals in the client-caregiver agreement. This is the time for solving problems and trying out new behaviors. During this phase, care providers are guided by their knowledge of human behavior, the client's plan of care, and the agreed-on goals.

The working phase consists of periods of growth and resistance. If the relationship is moving toward its goals, behavioral changes are seen in the client. At this time, it is important to explore the meaning of the change with the client and mutually decide if the change is meeting the agreed-on goals. Periods of growth are accompanied by episodes of resistance. Changing one's behavior is very hard work. It requires energy and self-disclosure. Clients often feel self-conscious, shameful, and vulnerable during this time. The caregiver's gentle acceptance and reliability help clients move through their periods of resistance.

An important technique for care providers is knowing when to set limits. **Limit setting** is an intervention designed to prevent clients from harming themselves or others. The necessity for setting limits often occurs during the working phase because the client may be experiencing many painful emotions. Setting limits requires a calm, nonthreatening manner. The client is not being punished, just protected until self-control can be regained. Clients often feel a sense of relief and trust when they know that someone cares enough to protect them, even if the threat is from themselves.

Client and caregiver continue to work on meeting the goals of the relationship. Other members of the treatment team may also be involved in specific areas of the client's therapy. Therefore it is important to understand how each member of the team functions and shares responsibility in relation to the client. During the working stage, caregivers frequently assess for behaviors that indicate the goals are being met. Clients are educated about exploring community resources. Preparations for terminating the relationship are made. The time finally arrives when the goals are accomplished or one of the people is no longer able to maintain the relationship. It is the signal for the final phase, termination.

TERMINATION PHASE

When the goals of the therapeutic relationship are achieved, both the client and caregiver share a sense of accomplishment. However, this is balanced by the loss of a meaningful person in the client's life. When the mutual goals have not been met, termination can be difficult. This is a major reason why it is important to set realistic goals at the beginning and frequently monitor the client's progress.

Steps toward termination should begin before the last meeting. Both parties need time to prepare the client for independence. During this phase, the caregiver reviews the steps taken toward achieving the goals. Clients feel a sense of pride and accomplishment when they can review their progress. This is also an opportunity to encourage clients to apply their new and more effective behaviors to other situations.

People respond to the loss of a therapeutic relationship as they would to any loss. Some may show signs of regression or withdrawal or engage in behaviors to continue the relationship (Table 11-3). The feelings underlying these behaviors should be identified and shared. Looking toward the future and reminding clients of their progress help to ease the transition to independence. Saying goodbye is never easy, but a client who is able to function more effectively as a result of your interventions is the reward of a successful therapeutic relationship.

ROLES OF THE CAREGIVER

Throughout the course of the therapeutic relationship, caregivers play several roles, each designed to assist clients in meeting specific therapeutic goals. Care providers who work with mental health clients assume the roles of therapeutic change agents, teachers, technicians, and therapists. Together, these roles help move clients toward more successful and adaptive coping behaviors.

CHANGE AGENT

The therapeutic environment is more than a physical space. The psychological atmosphere created by caregivers is one of the major contributions toward successful recovery. Caregivers provide an accepting atmosphere that values the contributions of each individual. They accept the fact that some client behaviors may not be appropriate, but they never discredit the person. Individuals are encouraged to exchange their unsuccessful actions for more effective behaviors. Caregivers' attitudes foster a climate that anticipates, expects, and promotes positive change. Each staff member acts as a role model for successful living, thus demonstrating to clients that there are other ways of behaving. When the atmosphere promotes change and provides the security to practice those changes, clients are more likely to improve.

Care providers also function as socializing agents. They assist clients in participating in group activities and various social interactions. They introduce clients to each other, encourage conversations, and help clients focus on the healthy aspects of their lives. Interactions with others are seen as opportunities to encourage successful social experiences for their clients.

TEACHER

Members of the mental health care team are constantly alert for opportunities to teach. In the mental health care setting, teaching opportunities range from instructions about daily living activities to major lifestyle changes (Table 11-4).

All clients must be taught about areas such as their medications and diet, but equally important opportunities for instruction exist with every client interaction. Through these interactions, you are able to assess and monitor existing problems, plan for corrective learning opportunities, and forecast possible difficulties. Clients and their families trust caregivers, and they often confide in them. Times of sharing become great teaching opportunities. Teaching is an important part of care because it provides a solid bridge for the passage to effective adaptation.

TECHNICIAN

The technical roles of the mental health team members focus on holistic care. Attention is paid to the whole client. Too many times providers involved with the client's care focus on the mental-emotional status of the client and exclude the physical realm. For this reason, caregivers must remain alert to the physical problems that may be present with mental health clients. Remember Maslow's hierarchy of needs—physical needs are satisfied first. Many mental health clients experience physical problems, just as many medical clients experience psychological problems. The technical role for nurses in

---

Table 11-3	*Client Responses to Termination*

REGRESSION	WITHDRAWAL	CONTINUATION
Return to previous maladaptive behavior	Denial of caregiver's help	Tries to continue relationship
Increased anxiety	Demands to stop relationship now	Brings up new problems
Tardiness or absence from appointments	Absence from appointments	Becomes helpless
Expresses doubts about value of relationship	Superficially interacts with caregiver	Wants caregiver to solve his or her problems

Modified from Sundeen SJ and others: *Nurse-client interaction*, ed 6, St. Louis, 1998, Mosby.

Table 11-4 *Teaching Opportunities for Caregivers*

TOPIC	HEALTH TEAM MEMBER
Activities of daily living	All members
Mental illness and its treatments	Nursing, therapists
Effects, side effects, adverse reactions of medications	Nursing
Early signs and symptoms of return to maladaptive functioning	All members
How to cope with stressors of daily living	All members
What to say to others about their mental illness	Nursing, therapists
Teaching the public about mental health and illness	All members

Case Study 11-1

It took 3 weeks for Marguerite's client to engage in a meaningful conversation with her. Today, as the discussion progressed, Marguerite could see that her client was about to share something important. Suddenly three people entered the room and began to demand that the client join them for coffee. The moment was lost; the client mumbled something about later and left.

• How could Marguerite have prevented this interruption from happening?

---

the mental health setting includes administering, monitoring, and evaluating medications; managing medical problems within the mental health environment; assessing the difference between physical and psychiatric conditions; maintaining safety; and managing environmental factors. Other team members have technical roles related to their specialties.

THERAPIST

All care providers use every opportunity to assist their clients in developing more effective behaviors, and, in this sense, all caregivers are mental health therapists. However, some caregivers are specifically trained as therapists. Nurses who function as mental health therapists, for example, are usually educated at the master's level in the principles of psychotherapy.

Caregivers function in many roles when working with mental health clients. Through "practiced awareness," they are able to use a variety of roles to assist clients toward their goals. The therapeutic use of self is applied each time caregivers interact with their clients, and every interaction is seen as a learning opportunity.

PROBLEMS ENCOUNTERED IN THE THERAPEUTIC RELATIONSHIP

Throughout the therapeutic relationship, caregivers continually assist their clients toward more effective functioning. However, problems or barriers arise and challenge us to devise creative solutions. The most common problems fall into three broad areas: the environment, the care provider, and the client. By remaining alert for these potential areas of difficulty, caregivers are able to prevent larger problems and increase their therapeutic effectiveness.

ENVIRONMENTAL PROBLEMS

Problems with the environment include things such as a lack of privacy, an inappropriate meeting place, or uncomfortable furniture, lighting, or temperature. Noise

and frequent interruptions disrupt interactions and become troublesome, especially if clients are attempting to share personal information. See Case Study 11-1 for an example of this situation.

To minimize environmental problems, make appropriate arrangements for interactions with the client. Find an area where interruptions and distractions will be minimal. Being interrupted stops the communication flow between caregiver and client and does little to foster the relationship. Be alert to how the environment affects the therapeutic relationship, and problems will be easier to prevent.

PROBLEMS WITH CARE PROVIDERS

The barriers relating to care providers in the therapeutic relationship include difficulties with attitude, setting helping boundaries, and countertransference.

Care providers are human beings with attitudes, opinions, and problems of their own. Working within a therapeutic relationship requires energy, time, and persistence. If the caregiver is expending energies in coping with personal difficulties, there is little left for the client. Historically, health care providers were taught to leave their personal lives at the door and to ignore them during working hours. Now we know that it is not possible to separate the caregiver from the person. They are one, and it is the "person" aspect of the caregiver that is so effective in helping clients.

Personal health (physical and mental) is a primary ingredient of effective client care. A study by the National Survey on Drug Use and Health (2007) found that workers in the personal care and service category had high rates of depression. To prevent this, caregivers must renew themselves routinely if they are to be effective with their clients.

Attitude is also important in how the caregiver views the client. Care providers who are skeptical about the client's willingness or ability to change are already dooming the relationship to failure. Discomfort with the feelings expressed by the client can also slow the relationship. To be effective, one must know oneself.

| Box 11-3 | *Self-Assessment of Helping Boundaries* |

1. Have you ever felt too involved with a client?
2. Have you ever received feedback that you are overly intrusive or involved with clients or their families?
3. Do you have difficulty setting and enforcing limits?
4. Do you spend more than the allotted time with the client or arrive early or stay late for appointments?
5. Do you relate to clients as you do family members?
6. Do you feel that you are the only one who "really understands" the client?
7. Do you feel that other staff members are too critical of "your" client or jealous of the relationship you have with the client?
8. Do you find it difficult to handle the client's unreasonable requests or behaviors?
9. Do you look forward to the client's praise, appreciation, or affection?

A "yes" answer to any question indicates a need to identify the behaviors that are blurring the boundaries of the therapeutic relationship.

Modified from Pilette PC, Berck CB, Achber LC: Therapeutic management of helping boundaries, *J Psychosoc Nurs Ment Health Serv* 33:40, 1995.

Compassion is a key quality, but when that compassion leads one to "rescue" clients, the caregiver is becoming too involved. "Owning" client problems wears the caregiver out and does nothing to promote the client's abilities to cope. To prevent this situation, establish your own professional boundaries that define the limits of the client-caregiver relationship. The focus of the therapeutic relationship is the client. Clients must be allowed to own their problems, or the therapeutic relationship loses its effectiveness. Caregivers' actions are designed to move clients toward the goals of therapy. Box 11-3 offers a tool for assessing your helping boundaries.

Countertransference is a barrier in the therapeutic relationship based on the caregiver's inappropriate emotional responses to the client. The caregiver's personal needs or reactions begin to inhibit the effectiveness of the therapeutic relationship. Common responses include intense feelings of caring, involvement, disgust, hostility, or anxiety. To prevent countertransference, remember that the focus of the relationship is the client's needs. Recognizing when one's personal needs are beginning to overshadow the client's needs is a good way to prevent countertransference.

PROBLEMS WITH CLIENTS

Progress in the therapeutic relationship can also be slowed or blocked by the client. Frequently clients engage in various behaviors to stall the effectiveness of therapeutic actions. Client behaviors that block progress fall into three basic categories: resistance, transference, and noncompliance.

Resistance was first defined by Freud as a client's attempts to avoid recognizing or exploring anxiety-provoking material. Behaviors are classified into primary and secondary types of resistance. Clients who demonstrate primary resistance are unwilling to change even when they are aware of the need for change. Behaviors include attempts to thwart the therapeutic process, a refusal to work toward the therapeutic goals, and attempts to manipulate the situation. Clients may also resist in reaction to the caregiver's interventions. In addition, if the caregiver is not an appropriate role model for therapeutic behavior, primary resistance may occur.

Secondary resistance is encountered when the client is motivated by drives other than the need to regain health. Many times the payoff for remaining ill outweighs the advantages of recovery. **Secondary gain** occurs when clients profit or avoid unpleasant situations by remaining ill. For example, the client who is facing legal problems on discharge attempts to remain in the therapeutic environment because he does not want to go to jail. Secondary gain can be a powerful motivation for resisting the treatment team's therapeutic efforts.

Transference is a client's emotional response, based on earlier relationships, to the caregiver. The most outstanding characteristic of transference is the inappropriateness of the client's responses. Because the client is transferring emotions associated with one person to another (the caregiver), little opportunity for self-awareness exists. Clients may become hostile, express their feelings by demanding an end to the relationship, or show no interest in therapeutic interventions. Other clients can become dependent, submissive, and passive or overvalue the caregiver's characteristics and place unreachable expectations on the relationship.

To prevent or cope with transference, first listen. Hear what the client is trying to communicate. Recognize areas of resistance, and then clarify them with the client. Explore behaviors and try to identify possible reasons for their use. With time and experience, you will become adept when working with the unique behaviors of transference.

Noncompliance is not following the prescribed treatment regimen. For individuals with mental-emotional problems, noncompliance is very high. According to Forman (1993), the main reasons for noncompliance are a lack of knowledge, medication side effects, and the caregiver-client relationship. Throughout the therapeutic relationship, caregivers are continually assessing and monitoring the progress of their clients. Identifying and sharing problems of compliance with the client help to remove another barrier from recovery.

When clients are prescribed medications for the control of their symptoms, every caregiver must

---

SAMPLE CLIENT CARE PLAN 11-1

Therapeutic Relationship

ASSESSMENT   *History.* Heather is a 14-year-old girl who is being treated for an eating disorder. She and the members of the treatment team have set a goal for a weight gain of 2 pounds per month. Sue, the treatment team's nurse, has assumed responsibility for seeing Heather weekly and monitoring her weight gain.

Current Findings. Heather keeps her appointments but tends to display negative reactions to every suggestion offered by the treatment team. Discussions with other care providers are superficial with little meaning. When interacting, Heather assumes a challenging attitude. Her weight has remained stable for the past 3 weeks.

Multidisciplinary Diagnosis	*Planning/Goals*
Ineffective coping related to a disturbance in self-concept	Heather will establish a trusting relationship with a member of the treatment team by September 23.

Therapeutic Interventions

Intervention	Rationale	Team Member
1. Prepare for first meeting by researching data about Heather, her family, and her past history.	Helps define the client as an individual with particular strengths and problems.	All
2. Plan time, setting, and outline of goals for each meeting.	Helps to define and focus on the goals of the relationship.	All
3. Establish an atmosphere of warmth and acceptance during first meeting.	Communicates respect and a willingness to become involved with Heather.	All
4. Help Heather define her problems.	Helps reduce emotional reactions and break her problems into smaller, more manageable units.	Psy, Nsg
5. Develop a contract (working agreement) for a self-motivated weight gain of 6 pounds per month.	Defines limits, expectations of goals; helps to plan steps for meeting goals.	Psy, Nsg
6. Assist Heather in learning positive thinking techniques.	Helps replace self-defeating thoughts and actions with more effective ways of coping.	All

Evaluation

Heather remained silent during the first two interactions with Sue. By September 10, she was willing to talk to Sue. By September 19, Heather began the interaction and stated that she would be willing to work on gaining weight and discussing her problems.

? CRITICAL THINKING QUESTIONS

1. How does a working agreement (contract) allow Heather to retain some control over her situation?

2. What would Sue (the nurse) do to encourage the relationship when Heather begins to initiate conversation?

A complete client care plan includes several other diagnoses and interventions.
Psy, Psychologist; *Nsg,* nursing staff.

---

remain especially alert for side effects. Many clients stop taking their psychotropic medications because of distressing side effects. Others simply feel that they do not need their medications. Whatever the reasons, caregivers are in excellent positions to monitor and encourage their clients' compliance during the therapeutic relationship.

Health care providers have a powerful tool for client care within the therapeutic relationship. Throughout each phase, clients are encouraged to focus their energies toward more effective and adaptive ways of living. Sample Client Care Plan 11-1 describes several interventions for establishing a therapeutic relationship. Learn to work with the dynamics of the therapeutic relationship. It is a tool that promotes the client's movement toward self-awareness and independent functioning.

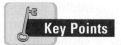 **Key Points**

- The therapeutic relationship is a directed energy exchange between two people that guides clients toward more effective behaviors. A social relationship is an energy exchange based on the sharing of personal opinions, attitudes, and tastes.
- The dynamic components of the therapeutic relationship include trust, empathy, autonomy, caring, and hope.
- Characteristics of rapport include a concern for others, an active interest in the well-being of the client, a belief in the worth and dignity of each individual, and an accepting attitude.
- Therapeutic use of self relates to the ways in which we interact with, attend to, and encourage clients. Caregivers act as role models for health and coping

by using behaviors that set examples for successful actions.

- Caregivers direct themselves therapeutically by focusing energies on the client.
- To use the "self" therapeutically, feel good about yourself and work to develop an awareness of how your actions, gestures, and expressions affect other people.
- The four stages or phases of the therapeutic relationship are the preparation, orientation, working, and termination phases.
- To successfully establish a therapeutic relationship, the care provider communicates the qualities of acceptance, rapport, and genuineness to the client.

- Care providers who work with mental health clients function as therapeutic change agents, teachers, technicians, and therapists.
- The most common problems in the therapeutic relationship relate to the environment, the caregiver, and the client.

evolve   Be sure to visit the companion Evolve site at http://evolve.elsevier.com/Morrison-Valfre/ for additional online resources.

Objectives

Upon completion of this chapter, the student will be able to:

1. List two situations that indicate a need for hospitalization.
2. Describe three types of clients treated in the inpatient therapeutic environment.
3. State two goals of the therapeutic environment.
4. Discuss five environmental factors that are assessed daily.
5. Explain the importance of setting limits on clients' behaviors.
6. Identify three ways the therapeutic environment helps clients meet their needs for love and belonging.
7. Examine how care providers' expectations influence clients' behaviors.
8. List three techniques to improve client compliance.

Key Terms

acceptance (p. 126)
chronicity (krō-NĬS-ĭ-tē) (p. 121)
involvement (p. 126)
limit setting (p. 125)
noncompliance (p. 127)
recidivism (rē-SĬD-ĭ-vĭz-əm) (p. 121)
therapeutic environment (milieu) (p. 120)

The history of treating mentally troubled people has not been kind. By the 1900s, the U.S. government established a state hospital system of large, custodial care institutions designed for treating the mentally ill. Once people were admitted, they usually stayed for months or years regardless of their ability to function in the community. Today, publicly financed mental health services are available in community hospitals and clinics, but they have been burdened "with ineffective service-delivery programs and stagnant bureaucracies" (Editors, *Mental Health Weekly*, 2002). In addition, with state hospital systems no longer in place, communities have been forced to provide increased emergency psychiatric services and short-term inpatient care for an expanding number of acutely ill psychiatric clients. Although many people are treated on an outpatient basis, the therapeutic environment remains an important component of psychiatric care.

In 1953, Maxwell Jones published a small book in England that described the value of the environment as a therapeutic tool. It was later published in the United States with the title *The Therapeutic Community*. The publication soon sparked the development of treatment settings that promoted personal worth and dignity (Jones, 1953). The therapeutic environment has become an important part of clients' treatment plans.

The term therapeutic environment (milieu) describes certain settings or environments designed to help clients replace inappropriate behaviors with more effective personal and psychosocial skills (Stuart and Laraia, 2005). Principles of treatment are based on the concept that every interaction within the client's environment has therapeutic potential. Physical surroundings are pleasant but safe. Activities are structured, and clients are expected to participate in their treatments. Therapeutic milieus can exist within hospital, home, or community settings. Because most therapeutic environments require certain limits and controls, they are most often located in inpatient settings, as part of a community hospital, for example. The Joint Commission has developed standards describing the therapeutic milieu and several tools for assessing the therapeutic environment are available.

Most people with mental-emotional problems manage within their communities. However, there are times when a more secure and stable environment is required. Admission to an inpatient facility can be on a voluntary or involuntary basis. Box 12-1 lists the most common reasons for admission. Once clients are in the facility, treatment plans are designed to return them to their communities as soon as possible.

Caregivers who work in therapeutic inpatient settings provide the framework for the quality of the environment. Without a staff who possesses insight, understanding, personal warmth, and skill, the concept of a therapeutic community could not be a reality. The ways in which mental health caregivers communicate, interact, behave, and use therapeutic techniques require study and practice to learn. Therapeutic tools include the use of eye contact, facial expressions, body movement, and other nonverbal behaviors. Other techniques are developed through experience and interactions with people from various cultures and backgrounds.

Psychiatric nursing practice has moved from custodial care to the management of complex therapeutic environments. Nurses are now required to manage

Box 12-1 *Criteria for Inpatient Admission*

Admission to a psychiatric inpatient facility occurs when the following are true:
1. A person's behavior becomes a threat to the safety of self or others.
2. People within the environment are not able or willing to support the mentally troubled person.
3. The person perceives himself or herself as unable to cope or maintain behavioral control.

clients' environments, implement therapeutic interventions, coordinate and integrate multidisciplinary care delivery, and evaluate the outcomes of treatment for each client with whom they work.

USE OF THE INPATIENT SETTING

Today's psychiatric facilities offer shorter stays, more intensive therapies, and support during the transition from institution to community. Inpatient services are provided for three main groups of people: those experiencing crises, those with acute mental or emotional problems, and those with chronic mental illness.

CRISIS STABILIZATION

People experiencing a crisis seek help when their discomfort becomes greater than their need to solve their problems privately. In many cases, **crisis stabilization** interventions are provided by placing clients in 1- or 2-day treatment settings where balance (homeostasis) can be reestablished. Clients undergo intensive counseling designed to solve their immediate problems. Medications, such as antidepressants or sedatives, may be prescribed. Basic stress management techniques are taught to help modify stressful behaviors. Cognitive, relaxation, and behavioral therapies are often used to assist clients. The goal of inpatient crisis therapy is to help clients successfully cope with crisis. After clients are discharged from the crisis stabilization unit, they may be referred for assertiveness training; time, anger, or conflict management; or problem-solving education.

ACUTE CARE AND TREATMENT

The inpatient environment is also necessary when people cannot function sufficiently to satisfy their basic needs. By the time people seek voluntary admission to a treatment facility, they usually feel weakened and hopeless (Cohen, 1994). Clients may be drug impaired or intoxicated. Some have experienced severe stress, such as a job layoff, illness, or loss of support systems.

Admission to an inpatient psychiatric unit is a highly emotional experience for most people. Those who are admitted involuntarily experience an intense discomfort during their first hospital experience and a sense of failure on subsequent admissions. Hospitalization can

"dehumanize" an individual: personal items are taken away, and staff members often remember the diagnosis before the name. Care providers should try to "humanize" the hospital experience because the foundation of the client's success or failure lies with the first experiences in the therapeutic environment. Most people with acute psychiatric problems can be successfully treated if interventions are vigorous and well coordinated. Even with the best of therapies, however, some individuals progress to chronic maladaptive responses and cycles of repeated admissions.

THE CHRONICALLY MENTALLY ILL POPULATION

Many mental health problems are associated with a degree of chronicity, with problems that tend to persist for a long time. People with chronic mental disorders may have periods of relative comfort and then fall rapidly into acute psychiatric states. For these people, life evolves into a seesaw existence between two worlds.

Often, people with chronic mental health problems know when they are beginning to decompensate (or "lose it" as some clients say) and will voluntarily admit themselves to an inpatient facility. Many more, however, do not have the insight or judgment to know when they are acting in maladaptive ways. Others are paranoid (suspicious, afraid of others) and do not seek help or refuse treatment when it is offered. Last, there is the growing number of mentally troubled individuals who have never sought assistance or received treatment. They live with their distresses the best they can.

The inpatient therapeutic environment fills many needs for troubled individuals. The physical necessities of clean water, wholesome food, clean clothing, and a comfortable bed are available (see Think About 12-1). It also provides protection, safety, and security from a harsh world, along with a staff of mental health care providers who offer individual attention and emotional support. From the chronically troubled person's point of view, life in the inpatient facility may actually be better than lonely existence in the community.

Recidivism (repeated inpatient admissions) has become a way of life for many chronically mentally troubled individuals. This is especially true for clients with cycles of assaultive behaviors. Recidivism is a frustrating aspect of inpatient mental health care for both clients and care providers. Clients feel like failures, and caregivers become frustrated that their efforts during past admissions were not successful. Several suggestions for managing feelings associated with return clients are listed in Box 12-2. Recidivism, also called the **revolving-door syndrome,** continues to be a problem, especially for individuals with schizophrenia and those who use chemicals. The primary reason clients return to the inpatient environment is refusal to take their prescribed psychotropic medications (noncompliance).

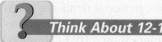

Think About 12-1

Many clients with chronic mental problems will admit themselves to an inpatient unit because they are looking for "three hots and a cot."
- What is the meaning of the statement?
- How does this statement relate to Maslow's hierarchy of needs theory? (Hint: see Chapter 5.)
- How do you think it affects the client's attitude toward the therapeutic treatment plan?

Box 12-2 | *Coping With Recidivism*

RELATING TO CLIENTS
Accept clients for themselves. They are doing the best they can at this time.
Learn about their lives outside the inpatient setting.
Explore after-discharge resources in the community.
Maintain a positive attitude. Clients do better when they are encouraged, rather than discouraged.

RELATING TO CAREGIVERS
Remember who "owns" the problem. Caregiver roles are to support, educate, and assist.
Attend a support group regularly. Discuss ways to stay positive.
Keep client problems "at the office."

One of the most important factors in preventing recidivism is adequate community resources. Delaney (1998) recommends psychosocial rehabilitation clubhouses where clients receive support and educational and vocational opportunities. With the focus on the "least restrictive environment," many chronically mentally ill clients now live in small, homelike, sheltered group settings within the community, but many others are homeless and continually involved in the revolving-door syndrome of admission and discharge.

GOALS OF A THERAPEUTIC ENVIRONMENT

Dr. Peter Breggin, author of *Toxic Psychiatry* (1991), defines mental illness as "overwhelm" and believes that people should be offered mental health care in small, local "sanctuaries" (rather than in psychiatric institutions) until they are able to cope with the demands of everyday life once again. Effective therapeutic environments provide the safety, security, and time to cope with difficulties. Members of the health care team offer therapeutic human contact designed to assist clients in learning about themselves and how they relate to others.

The goals of a therapeutic environment (milieu) are to provide protection, support, and education. A treatment team, composed of several specialists, is assigned to work with each client. On admission, a thorough

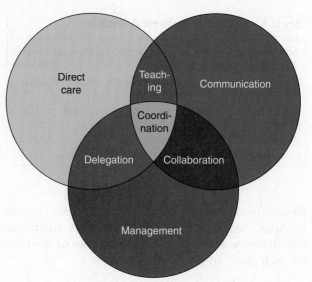

FIGURE **12-1** Mental health practice.

assessment is performed and a therapeutic plan of care is developed with the client. Figure 12-1 illustrates the roles of the mental health team members. Nurses are more involved with direct care and management; however, all care team members communicate, collaborate, and teach.

HELP CLIENTS MEET NEEDS

People are admitted to therapeutic environments because they are unable to maintain their activities of daily living. Care providers assist inpatient clients in meeting their most basic needs first. Food, shelter, safety, and security are provided. Socialization needs are met during therapy and interactions with staff and other clients. Treatment plans provide opportunities for satisfying self-esteem needs through vocational training.

TEACH PSYCHOSOCIAL (ADAPTIVE) SKILLS

People use behaviors that tend to work. When actions result in success, behaviors are more likely to be repeated, whether or not they are socially acceptable. Admission to an inpatient therapeutic treatment environment allows people with maladaptive behaviors the opportunity to learn more acceptable ways of behaving. With the help of the treatment team, clients can learn to replace their usual ways of behaving with more effective and adaptive actions.

THE THERAPEUTIC ENVIRONMENT AND CLIENT NEEDS

Maslow's theory of a hierarchy of needs (see Figure 5-1) states that if a basic physical need goes unmet, it will be fulfilled before other, higher level needs. People who are experiencing mental and emotional troubles frequently are unable to obtain even the most basic of life's requirements.

We all feel hunger and thirst, but the person with a mental illness may not be able to recognize or act on the body's signals. Sometimes that person's reality makes no provisions for the care of the body. For example, some people may believe that it is inappropriate to eat or practice good hygiene, some do not care about the condition of their bodies, and others are just not aware of their bodies. The therapeutic environment offers a constructive setting for people to learn how to meet their own needs, as well as the support and encouragement to practice effective physical care behaviors.

Remember that a change in one area of functioning brings about a response within the whole person. Therefore assisting clients in satisfying their more basic needs prepares the way for changes in other areas of life. Using Maslow's hierarchy as a guide, let's consider how the therapeutic environment relates to meeting human needs.

PHYSIOLOGICAL NEEDS

The first and most basic need is to breathe. Without **air** or the ability to exchange it, a person will not survive for more than a few minutes. For most people, breathing is not a problem, but for those with lung disease, for example, the simple act of exchanging air can be their first and major priority throughout each day.

The second basic need is for **nourishment.** Many clients have had little to eat before admission and welcome the opportunity to receive wholesome food and clean drinking water. Others may require special diets because of their medical conditions or medications. Frequently, clients who are experiencing hallucinations or paranoid (suspicious) thoughts will refuse to eat or drink for fear of being poisoned, drugged, or controlled by the use of food. Drug Alert 12-1 is a reminder of the importance of monitoring diets.

The act of eating and sharing food is a social event in many cultures. Numerous customs have evolved around obtaining, preparing, and consuming food and drink. Learn about clients' perceptions associated with food. How does the cultural background influence the foods they consume? What are their food preferences? How do their mental health problems involve food? Assessing client behaviors associated with food allows caregivers to intervene at a basic level, prevent further problems, and evaluate the effectiveness of therapeutic actions. Table 12-1 lists several client problems and therapeutic actions related to food.

Hygiene needs are important in the therapeutic environment. Clients are frequently admitted in various states of cleanliness ranging from obsessively tidy to extreme neglect. People who are experiencing acute episodes of schizophrenia, for example, seldom relate to their state of hygiene. Some individuals will dress

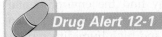
Drug Alert 12-1

Remember that clients who are taking monoamine oxidase inhibitors (MAOIs) are not allowed to eat certain meats (bologna, liver), dairy products (aged cheeses, sour cream, yogurt), vegetables (fava beans, avocados), fruits (bananas, figs), and alcoholic beverages (beer, ale, red wines, sherry). Clients should eat no chocolate and should avoid caffeine in large amounts.

Monitor clients' food and fluid intake daily. Also routinely monitor vital signs, especially the pulse and blood pressure. Report any complaints of chest tightness, stiff neck, or throbbing headache to the physician immediately because these symptoms may herald the onset of hypertensive crisis.

Table 12-1 **Mental Health Problems and Interventions Associated With Food**

PROBLEM	NURSING INTERVENTION
Client believes food is poisoned or tainted.	Serve each food item in single-serving, disposable containers. Allow client to casually observe other people eating same food items.
Client has no interest in food or eating.	Serve meals at regular intervals. Leave food within easy reach of client. Offer frequent snacks. Use odors of certain foods to encourage client to eat.
Client uses food as emotional substitute.	Provide opportunities for interaction with people who do not relate to eating. Work with client to discover which needs are being met through use of food.

inappropriately, putting on several shirts at one time or wearing undergarments over their coats.

Encourage good hygiene habits. Discover if the client has a preference or ritual for bathing or dressing. Compliment clients on their appearance when efforts have been made. Good hygiene practices help fill more than one basic physical need; they also communicate a willingness for social contact.

The **physical surroundings** of the therapeutic environment are important. Today, the architecture of the old asylum has been replaced by environments that include provisions for personal space and privacy. Physical properties of an environment have an effect on the people who live within that space. The physical properties of a therapeutic environment include temperature, lighting, sound, cleanliness, and aesthetics. Nurses are responsible for monitoring how each aspect of the physical environment affects clients.

The **temperature, air circulation, and humidity** of the unit all have an effect on clients. People respond in highly individual ways. For example, an agitated or hyperactive individual may find the environmental temperature too high and react by becoming even more distressed. Hot days and high humidity can increase aggressiveness or make clients lethargic. People who are depressed and hypoactive may be more affected by cooler temperatures. Caregivers must be aware that the environmental temperatures and humidity levels have an impact on behavior. Therefore the daily assessment of the therapeutic environment should include temperature and humidity.

Next, the environment's **lighting** needs to be assessed. Lighting includes the "amount of light, its diffusion, and the reflection of light waves off environmental surfaces combined with the impact of surface colors" (Haber and others, 1997). Lighting should be constant and of the right intensity. Flickering lights can trigger delusions or hallucinations, whereas lighting that is too bright can result in overstimulation and aggressive behaviors. Lighting that is too low can present inaccurate stimuli, resulting in misperceptions of actual objects. For example, it becomes easier to perceive an animal where a chair is located when the room's lighting distorts environmental cues. Sunlight has an effect on clients who are receiving psychotherapeutic medications. When outdoors, these people must wear protective clothing, sunscreen lotion, and a large-brimmed hat. They also require extra fluids.

Some clients experience hypersensitivity to color, especially if they are confused, agitated, or hyperactive. Colors are very symbolic. Bright colors are stimulating, whereas dark colors are depressing. Neutral colors tend to calm emotions and behaviors. Certain colors hold meaning for some clients. Care providers should assess the impact of color and lighting for each client and observe client behaviors in various settings.

The acoustical or **sound** environment is composed of noises generated by people and equipment. Walls, floors, and objects within the environment have sound-absorbing or acoustical qualities. Floors with carpeting, for example, absorb sound waves and quiet the environment, whereas hard tile floors tend to magnify sounds. Upholstered furniture absorbs more sound than wooden or plastic furniture.

Environmental noise can have a calming or agitating effect on clients. High noise levels can lead to distorted perceptions, altered thinking, and sensory overload. High noise levels in inpatient environments are common and result in "negative physical effects because of increased physiological stress on the body. Excessive sound also interferes with cognitive functioning" (Holmberg, 1999). Calm music, the sound of ocean waves, or a light rain can produce relaxation.

People experiencing mental illness are commonly hypersensitive to sounds. When noise levels become too intense, clients tend to become distracted and agitated. This does not imply, however, that each staff member must walk around in silence, but it does alert you to the important role that sound plays in the therapeutic environment (Table 12-2).

The hygiene associated with the environment refers to the state of **cleanliness** of the physical space and the objects within it. Because many clients live close to one another, the likelihood of infection is increased. The stresses of mental illness can also decrease resistance to infection. In addition, the potential for nuisances such as mice, cockroaches, and other vermin is increased if the physical surroundings are not kept clean.

People with mental or emotional difficulties can have little regard for the cleanliness of their surroundings. Sometimes people with lice, scabies, or crabs are admitted to the therapeutic environment, and if these problems are allowed to continue unchecked, every client within the area will require treatment. Nurses and direct care providers assess the state of the unit's cleanliness on a daily basis. Clients should be protected from communicable health problems. Small assessments today prevent large problems from developing tomorrow.

Last is the issue of **aesthetics.** Does the environment make one want to stay and relax or leave quickly? Is the space pleasing to the eye? The condition of the furniture and other objects within a setting leaves people with a certain impression. An environment that is tidy and in good condition sends a message of caring and pride in appearance. The careful use of color and texture can also produce an environment that communicates a sense of hospitality and belonging.

It is important for health care providers to remember that we go home every night to our own homes. Clients who are living within the therapeutic setting do not. They are there 24 hours of every day. If you were in this situation, you would appreciate the efforts of others to make the physical environment as pleasant as possible.

SAFETY AND SECURITY NEEDS

The safety and security of the therapeutic environment is one of the most important factors in mental health care. Safety and security needs within the therapeutic environment include the feeling of physical safety, the security of a limited setting, and the ability to feel

Table 12-2 *A "Sound" Exercise*

ACTION	EVALUATION
Listen to a short composition of classical music.	Record how you felt as soon as the piece was finished.
Listen to a hard rock musical selection.	Record your feelings as soon as the song is finished.
Compare your immediate feelings associated with both musical selections.	Did one composition make you feel more excited, calmer? How do you think different types of music affect your mental health clients?

secure with others. For clients who are depressed or suicidal, the therapeutic environment offers special protection from self-harm. Clients with aggressive behaviors are protected from themselves and assured that limits will be placed on their actions.

Safety also includes a freedom from hazards. Objects that have the potential for harm are removed from the environment, and the design of electrical fixtures, doors, and other equipment helps to promote safety. Paging systems with identification codes allow help to be summoned quickly when needed. Often, a client will "act out" or behave impulsively. When this occurs, members of the treatment team set limits on the maladaptive actions and then attempt to identify the feelings that motivated the behaviors.

People also need to feel secure within their environments. The inpatient therapeutic environment provides the comfort of order and organization in the form of a daily routine, a set of rules, schedules, and activities. For many psychiatric clients, knowing what is going to happen tomorrow adds to their sense of security today.

The use of **space** is important in maintaining a therapeutic environment. The design of the building has an influence on how space is used for daily activities. Factors such as the location of the recreation room, medication area, and clients' sleeping areas define how physical space is used. Caregivers are also concerned with the concepts of space that relate directly to client care: territory and distance.

Chapter 4 discusses distance and territory in detail, but the importance of these two concepts to the therapeutic environment is emphasized here. Each person needs personal space with defined boundaries (Goren and Orion, 1994). Mental health clients in an inpatient setting establish a territory that "belongs to them." Usually clients claim their rooms, dressers, and sleeping areas as their own. Every person who works with clients or their environments (e.g., housekeepers) must be aware of invading clients' territories. Behaviors such as knocking or announcing oneself before entering a client's room demonstrate respect for personal space.

The physical **distance** between people affects clients. People with suspicious feelings usually feel more comfortable when caregivers are outside their intimate space. Depressed persons may need touch and physical contact—an excellent opportunity for therapeutic touch. Aggressive clients may interpret the close presence of a caregiver as threatening. Touch must be used cautiously as a therapeutic tool and with the client's best interest in mind. Inappropriate use of touch can lead to charges of sexual harassment and possible litigation (legal proceedings). When clients are observed carefully, it is usually possible to tell which distances are most comfortable for interacting.

Limit setting allows the therapeutic environment to be consistent and predictable. Every human being must function within certain limits established by one's culture, social group, and laws. Many clients with mental problems have difficulty behaving within these limits. Clients know that care providers will enforce the external controls that keep everyone within the environment safe. Knowing that aggressive actions will be contained fosters a sense of safety and security. Two important therapeutic interventions for setting limits are to reinforce the established structure (rules, routine) of the therapeutic setting and to be consistent. When the environment is controlled, clients have an opportunity to safely explore their feelings and learn new, more effective behaviors (see Case Study 12-1).

The concept of **time** is impaired for many psychiatric clients. This causes various degrees of disorientation and insecurity about the environment. The perception of the passage of time may be altered, and time may pass very quickly or too slowly. Some individuals do not pay attention to time. As a result, clients have problems with appointments, scheduled events, and tasks— anything that involves the concept of time (Table 12-3). Interventions focus on routinely orienting clients to time with clocks, written schedules, and diaries.

LOVE AND BELONGING NEEDS

The fact that a person is struggling with a mental health problem does not dismiss the need to be accepted and find one's place within a group. Life in the community can be a lonely existence with no friends, few acquaintances, and fewer resources. The isolation of mental illness is intense. Sometimes, the lack of human contact, combined with an existing psychiatric problem and the roadblocks created by stigmas, overwhelms the individual and results in more intense or frequent psychotic episodes. The therapeutic environment offers clients many opportunities to appropriately meet their needs for companionship and group identification. Clients' love and

 Case Study 12-1

Ned was admitted 4 days ago and proved to be quite a manipulator. When other clients were involved with therapy or other group activities, Ned would be found lying on his bed reading comic books. He often offered the excuse that another caregiver had given him permission to be in his room. The staff agreed to limit his behavior by keeping him involved in physical activities. By 10:00 AM, Ned was complaining of a headache and wanted to lie down. He pleaded with three different caregivers, and they all tried to refocus him into an activity. His request to the fourth staff member was feeble, and by noon he was no longer complaining of a headache.

- What message(s) did the staff's behavior toward Ned send?
- How did Ned react to the situation?

Table 12-3 *Examples of Impaired Time Concepts*

DISORDER	CHANGE IN CONCEPT OF TIME
Organic mental disorders (Alzheimer's disease and others)	Difficulty understanding passage of time *Example:* Clients ask frequently about date, day, schedules. Clients think they were just admitted when they have been there for several days. Clients are poor historians.
Substance abuse Hallucinogenics	Time passes quickly, space is smaller. *Example:* Clients arrive early, write larger than usual.
Tranquilizers	Time passes slowly, space is larger. *Example:* Clients arrive late, writing is small, cramped. Ignore past, focus on present, and are unrealistic about future.
Depression	Time passes slowly. Clients tend to focus on past, ignore present, and show little interest in future.

Modified from Haber J and others: *Comprehensive psychiatric nursing,* ed 5, St. Louis, 1997, Mosby.

belonging needs are fulfilled within the therapeutic setting through use of communication, social interactions, and relationships.

Communication takes place on several levels, and not all aspects of every communication are obvious. In the inpatient setting, clients are respected as individuals who have the right to express themselves as long as their behaviors are appropriate. Caregivers communicate respect by encouraging clients to interact. Through caring, sensitive communications and interest in each person, care providers help their clients fill their needs for human companionship.

Love and belonging needs are also met through the social group to which one belongs. Whenever people are together, they tend to form groups. Clients with mental health problems are no different in this respect. Clients will attempt to form relationships with others. Activities as simple as walking together to an appointment help clients meet their belonging needs.

Social relationships can contribute greatly to meeting clients' needs for belonging, but the potential for abuse does exist. Caregivers need to be alert to the social relationships that are forming within the therapeutic environment. They must observe, monitor, and evaluate the appropriateness of certain relationships and discuss their concerns with the treatment team. Social relationships within the therapeutic environment have the same potential for positive or negative outcomes as any other relationship, and clients can become too dependent on other clients for social support. Many inpatient units have visiting regulations

for clients after they are discharged. Caregivers must protect the more vulnerable and easily led clients from becoming dependent on more aggressive or manipulative people.

The caregiver-client relationship is another major tool for meeting clients' love and belonging needs. All members of the treatment team interact therapeutically with clients, but the direct caregivers assist clients with the activities of daily living. They are in the special position of always being there, demonstrating consistency, reliability, and acceptance. It is the energy exchange of the therapeutic relationship that helps clients move from the overwhelming aspect of their illness to the dependency of the therapeutic environment and then to the independence of autonomy.

SELF-ESTEEM NEEDS

Respect, esteem, and recognition must first be granted to oneself. Self-respect, self-esteem, and self-recognition must be realized first. To state it simply: You must love and respect yourself before others can love and respect you. In the therapeutic setting, caregivers assist clients in meeting self-esteem needs through acceptance, expectations, and involvement.

Acceptance, in the mental health context, means that caregivers acknowledge clients as human beings worthy of respect and dignity. Although clients may behave in maladaptive or unacceptable ways, they are still worthy of respect. It is very important to **separate the behavior from the person.** You may not approve of the client's actions, behaviors, or attitudes, but you do accept the person. If a client is to be corrected or reminded, focus on the behavior rather than on the person. For example, the statement "I have trouble following your thoughts when you speak so loudly" communicates more acceptance than "Stop yelling." Correcting or refocusing the behavior instead of the person spares self-esteem.

Expectations play a role in the development of clients' abilities to meet self-esteem needs. When caregivers communicate what is expected, clients commonly meet those expectations. This can work both ways. There is a valuable lesson here: Do not limit clients with your own expectations. Assume that they will succeed, but keep observations and assessments based in reality. You may be surprised at what clients are capable of achieving.

Clients also need involvement to meet their self-esteem needs. Involvement is the process of actively interacting with the environment and those persons within it. When clients are involved, they are actively sharing. These experiences foster ego strength and feelings of worth and importance. Involvement also offers opportunities to modify ineffective behaviors and try out new ones. Therapeutic settings that focus on involvement use cooperation, compromise, and confrontation to bring about behavioral control, effective social interactions, and a sense of self-worth in clients.

SELF-ACTUALIZATION NEEDS

The need to achieve one's full potential lies within us all. However, not all people will become self-actualized. Remember Maslow's basic point: Lower-order needs must be fulfilled before the person can take steps to meet higher-order needs. Consequently, people who cannot meet their basic physical needs will have little success in addressing self-esteem or self-actualization needs.

As clients in the therapeutic environment begin to stabilize, they become better able to cope. With the treatment team's assistance, new ways of behaving are developed and tried. The process of trying and of becoming actively engaged leads clients in the direction of self-actualization. Living up to one's full potential means being the best one can be. People with mental-emotional problems deserve the opportunity to strive for this goal no less than the rest of us.

VARIABLES OF THE THERAPEUTIC ENVIRONMENT

Psychiatric hospitalization is a traumatic experience. Before admission, people often experience intense discomfort with the activities and details of their lives. Individuals who are being admitted for the first time report a sense of panic and lack of control over their situation. Those clients who are facing readmission most often express a sense of failure and worthlessness (Joseph-Kinzelman and others, 1994). Health care providers can do much to relieve the discomforts faced by clients. The mental health treatment team develops the therapeutic treatment plan, and each member has a special role in caring for the client. However, every staff member assists clients with the activities of daily living and monitors each step made toward the treatment goals.

ADMISSION AND DISCHARGE

The process of admitting a client to a health care facility is detailed but straightforward. However, when clients are admitted to a psychiatric setting their emotional state plays a large role in the actual admission process. Caregivers try to explain the rules, routines, and rituals of the unit, but clients are almost always too anxious to understand or remember anything in detail. They are then expected to follow the rules and engage in the appropriate activities, even though the memory of the first few days at the facility is absent or blurred.

People with high anxiety levels seldom remember what was said, especially when they are in unfamiliar settings. Approach clients in a calm and respectful manner. Give simple but clear explanations, and repeat them as necessary. Provide simple written instructions

that allow clients to read about the rules after their anxiety decreases. Answer any questions the client may have. Make sure that the client is more important than the admission form you must complete. Take the time to behaviorally communicate that you are concerned for his or her welfare. Make efforts to support the client in becoming familiar with the therapeutic environment.

Most inpatient facilities have an established procedure for admitting clients and standard forms for data collection. Refer to the admission assessment in Box 12-3 for an example. During the admission process a person may be interviewed by several members of the treatment team, all of them asking the same questions. This situation causes unnecessary anxiety for clients and is a poor use of the therapist's time. Having one person perform the initial admission interview prevents confusion and added stress for the client. Once the client is emotionally stabilized, additional information is easily obtained. The admission process establishes the tone for the client's entire stay. This experience with the therapeutic environment often leaves long-lasting impressions.

The process of preparing for discharge begins on admission. The length of stay for mental health clients has decreased dramatically. Because of this, discharge planning has assumed an important role in treatment as the bridge from the sheltered therapeutic environment to the reality of life in the community. Little research has been done to discover how well clients reintegrate into their communities. Care providers are in excellent positions to assist clients in applying the new behaviors learned within the therapeutic setting to the less predictable world of the community.

By the time most clients are ready for discharge, they are actively participating in their treatment program. Decisions about housing, employment, treatment, and management of their mental health problems are made with the treatment team's assistance. A multidisciplinary discharge care plan is developed. Appropriate referrals to various agencies are arranged, and follow-up care in the community is planned. Clients are assigned a case manager to work with them after discharge.

Returning to the community is a hopeful but demanding time. The support of the treatment team, as well as family and friends, helps to ease the transition. As one researcher stated, the mentally ill "have no formal ceremonies to transform them back to 'normal' status" (Herman, 1993). The activities of the treatment team are vital in reinforcing and strengthening clients' adaptive abilities throughout the discharge process.

COMPLIANCE

Clients who follow prescribed treatments are said to be "in compliance." The term noncompliance refers to not cooperating with the treatment plan. Assisting clients in complying can be caregivers' biggest challenge, especially when working with troubled people.

Box 12-3 *Admission Assessment*

DEMOGRAPHIC DATA: Full name, gender, age, date of birth, address, marital status, family members' names and ages, and (sometimes) religious preference.

ADMISSION DATA: Date and time of admission, type of admission (voluntary or committed).

REASON FOR ADMISSION: Current problems as perceived by the patient. These include stressors, difficulty with coping, and "emergency behaviors" (suicidal or homicidal ideas/attempts, aggression, destructive behaviors, risk of escape).

PREVIOUS PSYCHIATRIC HISTORY: Dates, inpatient/outpatient, reasons for and types of treatment, and their effectiveness.

DRUG AND ALCOHOL USE/ABUSE: Amount, frequency, duration of past and present use of legal/illegal substances, date and time of last use.

DISTURBANCES IN PATTERNS OF DAILY LIVING: Sleep, intake, elimination, sexual activity, work, leisure, self-care, and hygiene.

SUPPORT SYSTEMS: Amount of contact, nature/quality of relationships, and availability of support.

GENERAL APPEARANCE: Type and condition of clothing, cleanliness, physical condition, and posture.

BEHAVIORS DURING THE INTERVIEW:
Expression of anger: Covert, overt, verbal, or physical.
Degree of cooperation, resistance, or evasiveness.
Social skills: Positive/unpleasant habits, shyness, withdrawal.
Amount/type of motor activity: Psychomotor retardation, agitation, restlessness, tics, tremors, hypervigilance, lack of activity.

Speech patterns: Amount, rate, volume, pressure, mutism, slurring, or stuttering.
Degree of concentration and attention span.

ORIENTATION: To time, place, and person; level of consciousness.

MEMORY: Recent/remote, amnesia, blackouts, confabulation.

THOUGHT PROCESSES REFLECTED IN SPEECH: Blocking, circumstantiality, loose associations, flight of ideas, perseveration, tangential ideas, ambivalence, neologisms, or "word salad."

THOUGHT CONTENT: Helplessness, hopelessness, worthlessness, guilt, suicidal ideas/plans, homicidal ideas/plans, suspiciousness, phobias, obsessions, compulsions, preoccupations, antisocial attitudes, blaming of others, poverty of content, or denial.

HALLUCINATIONS: Visual, auditory, or other.

DELUSIONS: Of reference, influence, persecution, grandeur, religious, or somatic.

INTELLECTUAL FUNCTIONING: Use of language and knowledge, abstract vs. concrete thinking (proverbs), or calculations.

AFFECT/MOOD: Anxiety level; elevated or depressed mood; labile, blunted, or flat affect; or inappropriate affect.

INSIGHT: Degree of awareness of problems and their causes.

JUDGMENT: Soundness of problem solving and decisions.

MOTIVATION: Degree of motivation for treatment.

Modified from Keltner NL, Schwecke LH, Bostrom CE: *Psychiatric nursing,* ed 5, St. Louis, 2007, Mosby.

Estimates indicate that "40% to 80% of patients don't comply with their prescribed therapeutic course" (Wichowski and Kubsch, 1995). To improve clients' compliance, care providers must understand the reasons for clients' unwillingness to follow the treatment plan (Table 12-4).

A complete assessment of clients, their daily activities, their attitudes toward treatment, and their coping resources will help identify the overt (outward) causes of noncompliance. However, many times the reasons for noncompliance lie within clients' negative attitudes toward treatment and recovery. Alert caregivers can help their clients recognize and change many self-defeating attitudes that bind them to their problems.

Challenging clients' expectations is one technique for increasing compliance. Helping clients to remove self-imposed boundaries offers them the hope that improvement is possible or even attainable. Other techniques involve using a positive outlook and redirecting negative attitudes into more constructive ones. A genuine concern is a powerful tool. These techniques are designed to help your clients

Table 12-4 *Reasons for Noncompliance*

PROBLEM	INTERVENTION
LACK OF ONE OR MORE:	
Understanding	Education, support
Finances to pay for treatment	Refer to Social Services
Access to treatment services	Refer to Social Services
Support from family and significant others	Involve family, support groups
Ability to understand or follow treatment plan	Education, involve family
CLIENT SUFFERING FROM:	
Physical side effects	Refer to physician; monitor client's response to medication
Mental-emotional side effects	Communication, therapy, support

improve their outlooks on life. When one believes that success is attainable, it becomes easier to comply with the therapies and medications prescribed in the plan of care. Sample Client Care Plan 12-1 offers some specific interventions to improve compliance.

SAMPLE CLIENT CARE PLAN 12-1

Noncompliance

ASSESSMENT *History.* Tom is a 24-year-old man with a history of paranoid schizophrenia and several admissions to the unit. Following his last discharge, he refused to take his medications or seek follow-up therapy and, consequently, began to hallucinate and behave inappropriately. He is being admitted today to adjust his medications and devise a plan of treatment.

Current Findings. A disheveled young adult who refuses to eat or drink because people "are trying to poison my brain."

Multidisciplinary Diagnosis	*Planning/Goals*
Noncompliance related to suspiciousness	Tom will eat three meals per day by June 22.

Therapeutic Interventions

Intervention	Rationale	Team Member
1. Offer prepackaged foods every 3 hours while awake.	Tom may think there is less likelihood that food is poisoned.	Nsg, Diet
2. Monitor food and fluid intake.	Prevents malnutrition; to find which foods and fluids Tom is willing to consume.	Nsg
3. Offer fluids (prepackaged) every 2 hours.	Prevents fluid imbalance; to gain trust.	Nsg, Diet
4. Leave snacks within reach.	Tom may eat when he thinks that he is not being watched.	Nsg, Diet
5. Allow Tom to see what other clients are eating and drinking.	Helps lessen suspiciousness.	Nsg

Evaluation

By the fifth day of hospitalization, Tom was drinking 1000 mL of prepackaged liquids. He was still refusing to eat but would occasionally take a bite of bread if someone else started eating it first.

❓ **CRITICAL THINKING** QUESTION

1. How can care providers structure (change) the environment to encourage Tom to eat solid food?

A complete client care plan includes several other diagnoses and interventions.
Diet, Dietitian; *Nsg*, nursing staff.

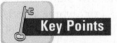

Key Points

- The therapeutic milieu is an environment structured to assist clients in controlling inappropriate behaviors and learning effective coping skills.
- Therapeutic environments provide services for people experiencing crises, those with acute mental or emotional problems, and individuals with chronic mental illnesses.
- The basic goals of a therapeutic environment are to protect the client and others during periods of maladaptive behaviors, help individuals develop self-worth and confidence, and teach more effective adaptive skills.
- The physical properties of a therapeutic environment should be assessed daily; they include temperature, lighting, sound, cleanliness, and aesthetics.
- Setting limits allows the therapeutic environment to be consistent and predictable because clients know that external controls will be enforced.
- Clients' love and belonging needs are fulfilled within the therapeutic setting through communication, social interactions, and caregiver-client relationships.

- In the therapeutic setting, caregivers assist clients in meeting their self-esteem needs through acceptance, expectations, and involvement.
- When caregivers communicate what is expected, clients usually live up to those expectations.
- To improve clients' compliance, understand the reasons for their unwillingness to follow the treatment plan; perform a complete assessment; challenge their expectations; help remove self-imposed boundaries; offer a positive outlook; redirect negative behaviors or attitudes into more constructive ones; and offer a genuine concern.
- Discharge planning is the bridge from the sheltered therapeutic environment to life in the community.
- An important responsibility of the inpatient staff is to educate and encourage clients to play an active and responsible role in their own care.

13 Problems of Childhood

Objectives

Upon completion of this chapter, the student will be able to:

1. Identify three common problems of childhood and list two therapeutic interventions for each.
2. Describe the impact of homelessness, abuse, and neglect on children.
3. Identify two therapeutic interventions for the child with anxiety.
4. Name four behaviors that are seen in children with attention-deficit/hyperactivity disorder.
5. Explain the importance of early diagnosis of disruptive behavioral (conduct) disorders.
6. State three therapeutic actions for children with mental retardation.
7. Identify three types of learning disorders.
8. Describe the behaviors seen in children with pervasive developmental disorders.
9. List three general interventions for children with mental health problems.

Key Terms

abuse (p. 134)
anxiety (p. 135)
attention-deficit/hyperactivity disorder (p. 137)
autism (p. 144)
bullying (p. 137)
cephalocaudal (SĔF-ă-lō-KAW-dəl) (p. 130)
communication disorders (p. 140)
conduct disorders (p. 138)
development (p. 130)
dyslexia (dĭs-LĔK-sē-ə) (p. 140)
encopresis (ĕn-kō-PRĒ-sĭs) (p. 139)
enuresis (ĕn-ū-RĒ-sĭs) (p. 139)
growth (p. 130)
homelessness (p. 133)
learning disorder (p. 140)
mental retardation (p. 139)
neglect (p. 134)
pervasive developmental disorders (p. 141)
pica (PĪ-kə) (p. 139)
posttraumatic stress disorder (PTSD) (p. 136)
proximal-distal (PRŎK-sĭ-məl DĬS təl) (p. 130)
schizophrenia (SKĬ-sō-FRĒ-nē-ə) (p. 141)
somatoform (sō-MĂT-ō-form) **disorder** (p. 136)
victimization (VĬK-tĭ-mī-ZĀ-shən) (p. 134)

rowth and development are a vital part of life. We are all involved in a lifelong process of learning and mastering life's tasks. Children grow with great speed and constantly changing mental, social, and emotional abilities. Each child develops at an individual rate and may master the skills in one area of development while lagging in another. Behaviors considered normal in one age-group become worrisome when they occur at another age. Health care providers who work with children must have an understanding of normal growth and development as well as an awareness of each child's individual pace.

This chapter presents an overview of normal developmental patterns for children, the mental health problems that can arise during childhood, and therapeutic actions for the care of mentally, emotionally, and developmentally troubled children.

Many theories about the growth and development of children exist. Table 13-1 lists the most common theories of childhood development. Chapter 5 provides a more thorough explanation of each theory.

Maslow's hierarchy of needs, although not a developmental theory, is also important to consider when working with children. Basically, Maslow states that a child's most basic physical needs (air, water, food, elimination, sleep) must be met before higher-level needs (e.g., security, love, belonging, esteem) are considered. Children must master skills that move them from complete dependence to independent functioning in only a few short years. Health care providers have a responsibility to nurture and foster the development of our youngest clients—our children.

NORMAL CHILDHOOD DEVELOPMENT

Growth is the increase in physical size. It is measured in pounds, inches, kilograms, or centimeters. **Development** refers to the increased ability in skills or functions. Although each child moves at an individual pace, all follow organized and orderly patterns throughout the growth process. Children grow in a **cephalocaudal** direction, where growth occurs from head to tail. Infants learn to control head movements before those of the trunk and arms. Growth also occurs in a **proximal-distal** (near-far) pattern. For example,

Table 13-1 *Theories of Childhood Growth and Development*

THEORY	EXPLANATION
Freud—psychosexual development	Individuals grow and develop by taming their primitive libidinal (sexual, pleasurable) energies as they move through the stages of childhood.
Piaget—intellectual (cognitive) development	Growth is the ability to organize and integrate experiences.
Erikson—psychosocial development	Each person has a core task or problem that must be resolved before he or she can successfully move on to the next stage.

the child's central nervous system develops before the peripheral nervous system. Last, growth moves from simple to complex (**differentiation**). Children learn to control the body's large muscle groups, such as walking, before mastering the fine motor skills of writing or building.

Growth is a continuing process. Recognizing the general patterns and principles of growth and development allows us to accurately assess, assist, and guide young clients (Box 13-1).

Development is the result of growth, learning, and the ability to combine the two. Children with growth or learning problems often mature later than other children. Development proceeds from simple to complex, from gross to fine, and from large to small. To illustrate, a child's reasoning is simple and uncomplicated until the nervous system develops the more complex organization required for abstract thinking.

Social and emotional development also move from simple to complex. Younger children have simpler emotions and communication abilities. The emotional development of children is an ongoing process. During each stage, the child must learn to solve a central problem or task, which lays the basis for the next stage of development. If the child is unable to cope with the task or central problem, then mental health difficulties may arise (Table 13-2).

The process of growth includes **sensitive periods**— certain times in which children are more affected by influences (positive or negative) within the environment. For example, according to Erikson, without a consistent adult caregiver during infancy, the child could develop problems trusting other people. Without nurturing, a child is ripe for developing mental health problems that may last a lifetime. Children who were raised in institutional settings often have difficulties bonding with significant others as adults. Nurses and other caregivers often provide the only consistency in these children's young lives.

Box 13-1 *Developmental Periods*

PRENATAL PERIOD: CONCEPTION TO BIRTH
Germinal: Conception to approximately 2 weeks
Embryonic: 2 to 8 weeks
Fetal: 8 to 40 weeks (birth)
A rapid growth rate and total dependency make this one of the most crucial periods in the developmental process.
Adequate prenatal care is extremely important for a healthy child.

INFANCY PERIOD: BIRTH TO 12 MONTHS
Neonatal: Birth to 28 days
Infancy: 1 to approximately 12 months
The infancy period is one of rapid motor, cognitive, and social development. Through bonding with the caregiver (parent), the infant establishes a basic trust in the world and the foundation for future interpersonal relationships. The critical first month of life is filled with major physical adjustments to life outside the womb and psychological adjustment of the parents.

EARLY CHILDHOOD: 1 TO 6 YEARS
Toddler: 1 to 3 years
Preschool: 3 to 6 years
This period, which extends from the time the child attains upright locomotion until he or she enters school, is characterized by intense activity and discovery. It is a time of marked physical and personality development, while motor development advances steadily. Children acquire language and social relationships, learn role standards, gain self-control, develop increasing awareness of dependence and independence, and begin to develop a self-concept.

MIDDLE CHILDHOOD: 6 TO 10 YEARS
Frequently referred to as the "school age," this period is one in which the child is directed away from the family group and is centered on the wider world of peer relationships. There is steady advancement in physical, mental, and social development with emphasis on developing skill competencies. Social cooperation and moral development take on more importance. This is a critical period in the development of a self-concept as peers' and teachers' evaluations become part of the child's self-assessments.

LATER CHILDHOOD: 10 TO 19 YEARS
Prepubertal: 10 to 13 years
Adolescence: 13 to approximately 19 years
The period of rapid maturation and change known as adolescence is considered to be a transitional period that begins at the onset of puberty and extends to the point of entry into the adult world. Biological and personality maturation are accompanied by physical and emotional turmoil, and there is a redefining of the self-concept. In the late adolescent period, the child begins to internalize all previously learned values and begins to focus on an individual identity.

From Hockenberry MJ and others: *Wong's nursing care of infants and children,* ed 8, St. Louis, 2007, Mosby.

Table 13-2 | *Emotional Developmental Tasks of Childhood*

STAGE	AGE	CORE TASK
Infancy	Birth-1 yr	Trust vs. mistrust
Early childhood	1-3 yr	Autonomy vs. shame and doubt
Preschool years	3-6 yr	Initiative vs. guilt
School age	6-12 yr	Industry vs. inferiority
Puberty	12-18 yr	Identity vs. diffusion

COMMON BEHAVIORAL PROBLEMS OF CHILDHOOD

Most children experience problems during each developmental stage. Some of the most common behavioral difficulties during the early years of childhood are colic, problems with feeding and sleeping, temper tantrums, and breath-holding spells.

Colic is a set of behaviors most commonly seen in middle-class infants. Severe periods of late-afternoon crying begin when the infant is about 2 weeks old. The infant cries with clenched fists and pained looks and refuses attempts to soothe him or her. Behaviors usually peak around 2 or 3 months, but they can persist until the infant is 4 or 5 months old. A colicky infant is defined as a healthy and well-fed child who cries for more than 3 hours every day for more than 3 weeks (Hockenberry and others, 2008). Interventions that are designed to calm both parents and child appear to help. Teach parents to manage colic by helping them learn about the normal characteristics of crying and recognize their infant's cues. Changing feeding procedures and allowing adequate time for burping and cuddling help control symptoms. Other effective measures include creating a quiet, restful environment, aromatherapy with lavender, and avoiding overhandling the infant. Massage can soothe, relax, and calm some infants. Most children outgrow colicky behavior by 5 months, but parents need a great deal of emotional support and encouragement during this stressful time.

Feeding disorders range from overeating (which leads to obesity) to undereating (which leads to malnutrition). The number of children in the United States who are overweight has nearly **tripled** since 1980 (Ogden and Tabak, 2005). Early intervention and education are needed to prevent the long-term complications that result from childhood obesity.

Infants may not feed if the experience is not satisfying. Young children may refuse to eat if they have had an unpleasant experience with food (being force-fed or choking) or are engaged in a conflict (power play) with caregivers. Physical problems, such as poor oral motor control or swallowing problems, can cause unpleasant experiences with food. Children suffering from depression often refuse to eat, and adolescents may engage in self-destructive behaviors such as anorexia or bulimia.

Problems with sleep are common to many children. They include night terrors, problems falling asleep, and nighttime awakenings. In the past, the usual course of action was for the parents to let children "cry it out" until they fell asleep. Today, each child's sleeping characteristics are assessed and parents' expectations and fears are addressed. Treatments are then designed to assist both parents and child in establishing restful sleep patterns. Following bedtime rituals, such as reading a book or limiting television viewing, is often helpful.

Temper tantrums are a common expression of anger and frustration for children between 1 and 4 years of age. In fact, temper tantrums occur in 50% to 80% of children in this age-group (Hagerman, 2001). In the young child, temper tantrums are seen as normal behavior. Children are attempting to master their environments and become frustrated when they are unable to achieve control. Temper tantrums are the result of a **loss of control.** Most children feel a blow to their self-image, and some children are quite upset about the experience. Tantrums only become a problem when children use them to express more emotions than just frustration or when they occur so frequently that they disturb family functioning. Adults in the environment should remain calm during the tantrum. Therapeutic interventions for temper tantrums are listed in Box 13-2.

Breath-holding spells rarely occur before 6 months of age and can last until the child is about 5 years of age. Typically the child becomes frustrated or upset in some way and begins to cry, but no sound emerges. He or she stops breathing, begins to turn blue, goes limp, and becomes unresponsive. Seizurelike behaviors, where the child arches the back and jerks uncontrollably, may occur. Fortunately, the spell resolves within 30 to 60 seconds when the child catches his or her breath and begins to cry or scream. A physician should examine the child after the first episode to rule out any medical problems. Thereafter, the treatment is to not reinforce the breath-holding behaviors. This must be done consistently. After ensuring that the child has not choked on something, parents should ensure that the child is in a safe place and then ignore the behaviors. Behaviors that are not rewarded or reinforced soon fade because they are no longer useful to the child.

MENTAL HEALTH PROBLEMS OF CHILDHOOD

Each stage of life flows into the other. In reality, there are no clear divisions in the process of development. Many mental-emotional problems diagnosed in adulthood find their roots in the experiences of childhood. Health care providers play an important role in the recognition and treatment of children's mental health problems because without love and assistance, many children are doomed to an adulthood of failure. The major mental health problems of childhood are grouped into seven categories (Table 13-3). Clients may be

Interventions for Temper Tantrums

PREVENT TANTRUMS

1. Childproof the environment: Remove anything that the child is not allowed to touch. Fewer restrictions lessen the chances for conflict.
2. Present choices and options: Allow the child to choose (within acceptable limits). Offer the opportunity to practice autonomy and mastery skills.

CONTROL TANTRUMS

1. When frustration increases, use distraction. Focus the child's attention on calmer activities, and reward positive behaviors.
2. Protect the child during the tantrum. Do not allow a child to hurt himself or herself or others.
3. Do not abandon the child during the tantrum. Stay close, but do not intrude on his or her space.
4. Point out to the child that he or she is out of control. Do not react negatively or try to discipline the child. Praise when control is regained.
5. Fight only those battles that must be won. The conflicts that serve no important purpose should be avoided. However, do not give into the demands that led to the tantrum.

AFTER THE TANTRUM

1. Do not hold a grudge or hold on to negative emotions. Recognize that the child probably feels worse than you do.
2. Praise the child for gaining control.
3. Keep reinforcing desired behaviors. Do not overreact to undesirable actions.

Table 13-3 | *Mental Health Problems in Childhood*

CATEGORY	EXAMPLES
Environmental problems	Poverty, homelessness, child abuse, child neglect, violence
Problems with parent-child interactions	Primary caregiver dysfunction, parent-child conflict
Emotional problems	Anxiety, depression, somatoform disorders (physical signs or symptoms with psychological causes), posttraumatic stress disorder
Behavioral problems	Attention-deficit/hyperactivity disorder, disruptive behavior (conduct) disorder, antisocial disorder, oppositional defiant disorder
Eating or elimination problems	Anorexia, bulimia, enuresis, encopresis
Developmental problems	Mental retardation, learning disorders, communication disorders
Pervasive developmental disorders	Autism, childhood disintegrative disorder, schizophrenia

labeled with one diagnosis yet engage in behaviors that belong to another category. Remember, each child is an individual. The diagnosis is less important than the person.

Many children have "mental health problems" sometime during the journey from infant to adult. Emotional difficulties arise more frequently during periods of change. The birth of a sibling or moving to a new city can disrupt a routine, create new demands, or make children more vulnerable. Stresses can push children to behave in worrisome ways. Peers can have influences that are not always desirable. How do parents know when their children's problems are a part of the normal process of growing up and when they are serious enough to require professional assistance? When a child demonstrates an absence of growth, an inability or refusal to change, or a failure to achieve the developmental tasks of his or her age-group, mental health assistance should be sought.

ENVIRONMENTAL PROBLEMS

Many children must cope with more than just developmental tasks. Growing up is a difficult process for children who are poor, homeless, abused, or neglected.

Problems associated with the environment can have a strong impact on mental health. Poverty, for example, influences the growth and development of children more than one would expect. In 2001, the U.S. Census Bureau reported that more than 16.9% of the nation's children live in poverty-stricken families (U.S. Census Bureau, 2001a). The rate of poverty for children in the United States is greater than the rates in Canada and Western Europe.

Poverty and mental health problems go hand in hand. By age 5 years, poor children scored much lower on IQ tests and demonstrated higher rates of anxiety, unhappiness, and fearfulness. Programs such as Head Start help prepare children for school and work to improve thinking, communication, and social skills. However, more remains to be done if we are to prevent the many mental health problems that accompany the lack of an adequate income.

HOMELESSNESS

The lack of a permanent residence (homelessness) affects children in many ways (Figure 13-1). Studies (Rafferty and Shinn, 1991) revealed that homeless children had very high infant mortality rates, twice the normal incidence of illness and disease, and elevated lead levels in the blood. They also experienced hunger; behavioral problems, developmental delays, speech delays, sleep disorders, and immature motor actions; short attention spans, withdrawal, aggression, and return to toddler behaviors; inappropriate social interactions with adults; and immature peer interactions. The problem described in Case Study 13-1 is unfortunately all too common.

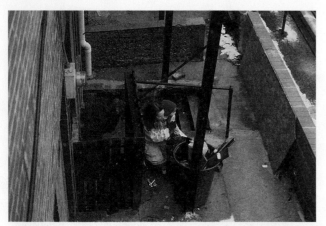

FIGURE **13-1** Many of the homeless are young mothers with young children.

Case Study 13-1

Carol had come to us as a very lost, exhausted, young girl, dressed in tattered jeans and with sad, red eyes that seemed to cry every time she opened her mouth to talk to us.

For her first few weeks at Covenant House, we could not really get her to talk about herself ... who she was, why she was here, where she came from, how we could help her. The only words she spoke were cried out unconsciously in her nightmares, which crept up on her while she was vulnerable and alone at night, unable to run away.

"You don't want to know about me." "It hurts too much," she would say. "I ... I can't talk about it."

Finally, one night after another nightmare, her lonely pain became unbearable and she began to open up. She was born in South Carolina but ran away because her parents beat her. "They were on drugs," she shrugged. "I guess they couldn't help it," she said. Frightened for her life and unable to stand the abuse any longer, she had run away to the city. Penniless and alone, she soon began to sell the only worldly possession she had—her body.

Then one night she met "him." He was 70, like a grandfather. "He said he would take care of me. I was so alone. And those first few days were great. He gave me everything—money, clothes. He made me feel good. Then he started crawling in bed with me at night ... and doing terrible things. He began to give me cocaine and stuff to make it easier. He ... I had no place to go. And then he started to hit me for no reason. I ran away, but I am so afraid he will find me...."

- In which behaviors did Carol engage to fulfill her basic needs?
- How do you think Carol can be helped?

Modified from McGeady MR: *"Does God still love me?": letters from the street,* New York, 1995, Sr Mary Rose McGeady.

Care providers must learn about the lifestyles of their clients and families. Practice good communication skills, and remain nonjudgmental. Table 13-4 offers other special guidelines for care providers who work with homeless clients of all ages.

Table **13-4** | *Therapeutic Actions for Homeless Clients*

TOPIC	NURSING ACTIONS
Psychological	Know your own feelings about homeless people.
	Approach clients with a positive attitude.
	Greet clients and communicate that they will be treated with care and respect.
Client interview	Delay asking questions about occupation, address, next of kin, educational level until later in the interview.
	Promise that information is confidential.
	Ask simple, concrete questions:
	Where do you get your money?
	When did you have your last drink?
	Relate to homelessness in a matter-of-fact way.
Health assessment	Educate as you assess.
	Assess children for signs of malnutrition, abuse, or neglect.
Discharge planning	Ask these questions:
	Do you understand what your problem is?
	How will you get your prescriptions filled?
	Where will you sleep tonight?
	Help client to keep follow-up appointments.
	Write down all instructions.

Modified from Hunter JK: Making a difference for homeless patients, *RN* 55:48, 1992.

ABUSE AND NEGLECT

Victimization is the process of causing harm. **Abuse** is defined as causing harm to or maltreating another. **Neglect** is not meeting a child's basic needs for food, clothing, shelter, love, and belonging. Child abuse and neglect are reaching crisis levels. The problems of abuse and neglect are becoming threats to the lives of infants and small children throughout our world.

The victimization of children comes in many forms. Physical abuse is commonly associated with burns, bruises, fractures, and head and abdominal injuries. Sexually abused children have been violated with inappropriate sexual activities. Emotional or psychological abuse erodes children's self-esteem through rejection, criticism, isolation, or terrorism. Children also suffer from neglect—the failure to provide for their physical, emotional, and medical needs. According to the U.S. Census Bureau (2001b), over 51% of documented maltreatment cases are due to neglect.

Childhood abuse and neglect also have long-term effects. Today a wide variety of behavioral and physical disorders seen in adulthood, such as chronic anxiety and depression, are thought to be associated with childhood abuse.

Factors that influence the potential for abuse and neglect include parental characteristics, such as social isolation, teenage motherhood, and difficulty controlling aggressive impulses. Children who are unwanted or disabled are at a higher risk for abuse and neglect.

Environments filled with chronic stress may lead to child mistreatment. Researchers have found that family or parental stress is a significant precipitating factor in child maltreatment, especially physical abuse and chronic neglect (Cowen, 2001). By recognizing these problems and referring families to appropriate services, health care providers may prevent abuse and neglect from occurring.

Preventing and treating child abuse and neglect are the responsibility of every health care provider, no matter what training or title. Education is a powerful first step. Programs such as "Don't Shake the Baby" (Showers, 1992) and materials from the National Clearinghouse on Child Abuse and Neglect (800-394-3366) are increasing awareness of this international tragedy.

Helping the victims of child abuse also requires caregivers to look at their own feelings about abuse. Being objective and supportive can be difficult in these situations, but it is important. Health care providers are in positions to recognize abuse and help provide early intervention. The problems of our children are the problems of us all.

PROBLEMS WITH PARENT-CHILD INTERACTION

A healthy family is able to cope with most of its emotional problems and knows when to seek help. Every child faces difficult emotional adjustments throughout childhood as change creates many new demands for children and their parents. One of the most common parent-child problems is conflict.

PARENT-CHILD CONFLICTS

Children require consistent guidance and unconditional acceptance. Relationships with their caregivers serve as a testing ground for learning right from wrong and which behaviors result in reward or punishment. Parents who **set limits** and **enforce** them **consistently** provide the stability for children to test their limits in healthy ways. Conflicts between children and parents frequently occur and can take the form of verbal arguments or silent power struggles. No child or parent escapes childhood without conflict; however, when conflicts are constant and worsen over time, mental health assistance should be sought.

Primary Caregiver Dysfunction

When a parent is unable to meet the needs of a child, a disturbance in the parent-child interaction exists. The parent is often a person who has had difficult times in the past with personal relationships, psychiatric disorders, or behavioral problems. Perhaps the pregnancy was unwanted, or the child seems unresponsive. In these situations, the child is frequently described by the caretaker as difficult, defective, or disappointing.

The signs and symptoms seen in the child that suggest primary caregiver dysfunction include feeding and sleeping problems, delays in development, failure to thrive, signs of inadequate physical care or abuse, frequent visits to the physician, and excessive parental worry. Treatment focuses on supporting and educating the parents and helping them develop more effective and appropriate child care skills. With aggressive intervention, the long-term outlook for the children of these parents improves.

EMOTIONAL PROBLEMS

Emotional problems occur in children when they cannot successfully cope with their situations. They can range from anxiety to severe depression and suicide. Fortunately, most children are able to cope successfully with life's anxieties when they are nurtured and supported. This section focuses on the emotional problems of children that are most likely to be encountered in everyday treatment settings: anxiety, depression, somatoform disorders, and posttraumatic stress disorders.

ANXIETY

Anxiety is a vague, uneasy feeling that occurs in response to a threat. Most children experience fear and anxiety as a part of growing up. One of the most frequent anxieties of infants and toddlers, **separation anxiety,** is a fear of being apart from their parents. Eventually, the fear decreases as children broaden their worlds to include others. However, if a child older than 4 years has separation anxieties lasting for more than a few weeks, a problem may exist. Severe levels of anxiety in children may result in obsessive-compulsive behavior, a condition that is discussed in Chapter 18.

Anxiety-based school refusal or **school avoidance** is a behavioral pattern in which the child refuses to attend school. Causes include anxiety or fear of leaving home (separation anxiety). Fear of being ridiculed or embarrassed at school (social phobia) or great concern about some aspect of school (school phobia) can also result in avoidance behaviors. The main goals of treatment are to help the child identify the source of the anxiety. Then the child is assisted in confronting and overcoming the anxiety so he or she can return to school. Many times, health care providers work with school personnel and parents to develop a plan for returning the child to school in a supportive manner. Antidepressants may be prescribed for severe symptoms of anxiety or depression (see Drug Alert 13-1).

Most children's bouts of anxiety are relieved when they receive reassurance and emotional support. If anxiety does not interfere with family, friends, or school, the child is coping effectively. However, when the anxiety is so pronounced that it is impossible for the child to function, then help should be sought (see Think About 13-1).

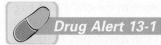

Drug Alert 13-1

When children are prescribed antidepressant medications, the child and family should be taught to do the following:
1. Drink plenty of fluids, especially water
2. Eat foods that are high in fiber to prevent constipation
3. Exercise regularly to help prevent constipation
4. Ensure the child's safety because he or she may experience dizziness

Think About 13-1

Bullying is becoming a problem in many countries. In Great Britain "eight out of ten children with a learning disability are bullied or scared to go out due to fear of being bullied" (Community Care, 2007).

The Finnish study "From a Boy to a Man" revealed that bullying behaviors in childhood predicted antisocial personality, substance abuse, and depressive and anxiety disorders. Victim behaviors "predicted anxiety disorders, and mixed bully victim status predicted antisocial personality and anxiety disorder" (Sourander and others, 2007).

In the United States, studies reveal that "6 out of every 10 students witness bullying in school at least once a day" (Curriculum Review, 2007).

DEPRESSION

Mood disorders, such as depression, are increasing in children. The term *depression* describes a symptom, an emotional state, and a clinical syndrome. Depression occurs in children and adolescents, but symptoms often go unnoticed and untreated. Children who have one or more depressed parents are more likely to be depressed themselves. Depression is seen more frequently as children grow older, and it occurs equally in boys and girls.

The clinical findings of depression arise from a persistent state of unhappiness that interferes with pleasure or productivity. "Children with depressive disorders lack interest in activities they previously enjoyed, criticize themselves, and are pessimistic or hopeless about the future" (Hazel, 2002). School-age children often "act out" their depression by becoming disruptive or failing academically. Older children and adolescents may become withdrawn. The clinical signs and symptoms of depression are discussed in Chapter 21. Treatment is designed to relieve the child's discomforting symptoms and help those in the environment to respond to the child's needs. Therapeutic interventions focus on reducing the problems that are causing the depression and providing the child with the emotional support to cope effectively.

SOMATOFORM DISORDERS

A somatoform disorder is one in which the child (or adult) has the signs or symptoms of illness without a traceable physical cause. The individual does not consciously take on the signs or symptoms, but he or she truly feels ill. Children often complain of headaches, upset stomachs, or pain.

Somatic symptoms are common in school-age children. They are thought to be expressions of stress, anxiety, or underlying conflict. Sometimes the child's signs or symptoms resemble those seen in another family member. In most cases, when the stress is relieved, the child returns to a healthy level of functioning. Somatoform disorders are covered in greater depth in Chapter 22. Here it is important to remember that children with somatoform disorders need understanding and reassurance.

POSTTRAUMATIC STRESS DISORDER

When children are repeatedly exposed to or participate in acts of violence, their psyches take steps to emotionally protect them. Posttraumatic stress disorder (PTSD) usually develops following an extremely traumatic event that involves injury or threat to the child. Examples include experiencing a fire or witnessing a shooting death. The child feels intense helplessness, fear, and horror. In younger children, behaviors become agitated and disorganized. Traumatic events are relived repeatedly, and the child goes to great lengths to avoid anything associated with the trauma. Eventually, the traumatic event becomes generalized into nightmares of monsters or threats to the self. The past is relived through playing out of events related to the trauma. Somatic complaints, such as upset stomachs and other discomforts, may occur. Treatment focuses on early recognition and emotionally supportive care.

BEHAVIORAL PROBLEMS

Children experiment with various behaviors to test the limits of their environments and the people within them. Every child goes through periods of misconduct: refusing to do as told, lying, cheating, stealing, or bullying others. Most often, these behaviors decrease with time and consistent guidance. However, we all need to become aware of the influence that everyday violence has on our children.

CHILDREN AND VIOLENCE

"American children watch an average of three to four hours of television daily" (AACAP Facts for Families, 1999), and studies reveal that greater aggressiveness and less sensitivity to others are seen in children who view TV violence. Acts of aggression are common in schools, where children may be bullied or intimidated. Children may witness violence in the home and adopt it as a method for solving problems or resolving conflict.

Box 13-3	*Warning Signs of Violence*

Loss of temper on a daily basis
Frequent physical fighting
Vandalism or damage to property
Carries a weapon
Announces threats or plans to hurt others
Use of drugs and/or alcohol
Enjoys hurting animals
Engages in risk-taking behaviors
Details plans to commit acts of violence

Box 13-4	*Attention-deficit/hyperactivity disorder*

A. A disturbance of at least 6 months during which at least eight of the following are present:
   1. Often fidgets with hands or feet or squirms in seat (feelings of restlessness in adolescents)
   2. Has difficulty remaining seated when required to do so
   3. Is easily distracted by outside stimuli
   4. Has difficulty awaiting his or her turn in games or group situations
   5. Often blurts out answers to questions before they have been completed
   6. Has difficulty following through on instructions from others (e.g., fails to finish chores)
   7. Has difficulty sustaining attention in tasks or play activities
   8. Often shifts from one uncompleted activity to another
   9. Has difficulty playing quietly
   10. Often talks excessively
   11. Often interrupts or intrudes on others (e.g., butts into other children's games)
   12. Often does not seem to listen to what is being said to him or her
   13. Often loses things necessary for tasks or activities at school or at home (e.g., toys, pencils, books, assignments)
   14. Often engages in physically dangerous activities without considering possible consequences (e.g., runs into street without looking)
B. Onset before the age of 7 years
C. Does not meet the criteria for a pervasive developmental disorder

Modified from Hockenberry MJ and others: *Wong's nursing care of infants and children*, ed 8, St. Louis, 2007, Mosby.

Young children engage in violent behavior, but it is often dismissed as just a "phase" the child is going through. "Violent behavior in a child at any age always needs to be taken seriously" (AACAP Facts for Families, 2001). Children can engage in a wide range of aggressive behaviors ranging from explosive temper tantrums to bullying, cruelty, and destruction of property. **Bullying**, which is the repeated use of aggressive behaviors to intentionally intimidate another, is very common in schools today. Children who bully others often behave aggressively toward parents, teachers, and other authorities. They have strong self-esteem and little ability to relate to the emotions of others. Bullies use violence, manipulation, and intimidation to achieve control over their victims.

The victims of bullying tend to be smaller, quieter, and more sensitive than their peers. Often they are different, physically or behaviorally. All have poor self-worth, believing they are stupid, ugly, or unwanted. If allowed to continue, bullying can result in serious academic, behavioral, legal, and social problems for both bullies and their victims.

As behaviors become more difficult to manage, these children clash with friends and classmates. They may develop a reputation for being unruly bullies or, worse yet, dangerous. The American Psychological Association has developed a checklist for the warning signs of violence (Box 13-3). Children who demonstrate these behaviors are at risk for engaging in violent behaviors.

When a child's conduct becomes inappropriate over time, a **disruptive behavioral disorder** is usually diagnosed. Sometimes behavioral problems are linked to a physical cause, such as a lack of neurotransmitter production in the brain. The two disruptive behavioral disorders most commonly encountered by nurses are attention-deficit/hyperactivity disorder and conduct disorder.

ATTENTION-DEFICIT/HYPERACTIVITY DISORDER

During the 1850s, a German nursery rhyme told the story of "Phillip," a bad boy who could not sit down. A century later, the children who exhibit Phillip's behaviors are diagnosed as having **attention-deficit/ hyperactivity disorder**, commonly called ADHD, which is now the most commonly diagnosed mental health problem in childhood. It affects about 3% of American children, and its symptoms can persist into adulthood. ADHD occurs more frequently in boys, with a ratio of about seven boys to one girl. Although ADHD was thought to be primarily a problem of childhood, it is often seen in adolescents and adults. It is a syndrome—a cluster of behaviors relating to inattention and impulsive actions. Within the ADHD category, a variety of subgroups exist: ADHD with learning disabilities, ADHD without hyperactivity, ADHD with speech disorders, ADHD with other psychiatric disorders, and ADHD with disorders of brain function. Box 13-4 lists the diagnostic criteria for ADHD.

There are two common clinical histories for children with ADHD. The first is the child who has been "fussy" or "a difficult child" from birth. As infants, they were difficult to soothe, and they have behaved impulsively as far back as family members can recollect. They are remembered as being "a handful." The second type of child is referred to as an immature child who displays silliness, distractibility (short attention span), restlessness, and clumsiness. Both types of children have problems with self-control, hyperactivity, relating to others, and focusing their attention. On entry into school, children with ADHD have difficulty in completing their schoolwork because they are easily distracted. They are usually academic underachievers, although they may have normal or above-average intelligence. They may also have problems making friends because of their excitable and impulsive behaviors. Almost half the children with ADHD show symptoms of anxiety, aggression, depression, and resistance to any authority.

Treatment for children with ADHD requires a multidisciplinary approach. Families are educated about the problem, and many children receive special education. Positive reinforcement programs help children choose more socially appropriate behaviors and reduce impulsive actions. Therapeutic interventions for children with ADHD focus on providing a consistent and structured therapeutic approach. Caregivers must be prepared to set limits on clients' behaviors and then be consistently willing to enforce them. They should also strive to acknowledge and reward the child for appropriate behaviors. In cases in which the child is receiving drug therapy (i.e., methylphenidate [Ritalin], antidepressants [e.g., imipramine, desipramine], clonidine), nurses must carefully monitor each child's response to the medications (see Drug Alert 13-2).

DISRUPTIVE BEHAVIORAL (CONDUCT) DISORDER

Misconduct is common in every child, but when a persistent pattern of unacceptable behaviors is present, a conduct or disruptive behavioral disorder is established. Children with conduct disorders are defiant of authority. They engage in aggressive actions toward other people, refuse to follow society's rules and norms, and violate the rights of others. Many come from broken homes and backgrounds of violence, drug abuse, alcoholism, poverty, and lack of consistent caregivers.

The typical picture of a child with a conduct disorder is a boy with social and academic problems, truancy, and failure in school. He is defiant of authority and often engages in temper tantrums, running away, and fighting. Treatment focuses on providing a stable environment and consistently enforced limits. Associated neurological, educational, or psychiatric problems are also treated. The long-term outlook for children with conduct disorders is poor if the problems are present before the child is 10 years old or if the adults in the environment engage in antisocial behaviors. Nearly half these children grow up to have antisocial or conduct disorders in adulthood. This makes early diagnosis and treatment very important if these children are to become productive members of society.

Oppositional Defiant Disorder

A recurring pattern of disobedient, hostile behavior toward authority figures describes the problem of oppositional defiant disorder. Children with this problem frequently lose their tempers, argue with adults, deliberately annoy other people, and refuse to compromise. They blame others for their misbehaviors and continually test their limits by arguing, ignoring, or becoming aggressive. Treatment includes family therapy that stresses limit setting and consistency.

PROBLEMS WITH EATING AND ELIMINATION

The most common mental health problems seen in children that relate to eating are feeding disorders, pica, anorexia nervosa, and bulimia. Disorders of elimination include encopresis and enuresis. Eating disorders are most often encountered in adolescents, but young children can also use food inappropriately to cope with their emotions. Early recognition and treatment help prevent greater problems later in life. Anorexia nervosa (a severe disturbance in eating behavior that results in a body that is much lower than its ideal weight) and bulimia (uncontrolled ingestion of large amounts of food followed by inappropriate methods to prevent weight gain) are discussed in Chapter 14.

EATING DISORDERS

Children with eating disorders either do not eat enough or eat the wrong things. The diagnostic category of **feeding and eating disorders of infancy or early childhood** describes children who routinely fail to eat adequately. Weight loss or a failure to gain weight for at least 1 month in a child with no gastrointestinal tract problems is the most significant sign. Food is available, but the child does not eat. Most feeding disorders occur in children under 1 year, but they occur in some 2- and 3-year-olds. The long-term complications are malnutrition and delays in development.

Feeding disorders can result from repeated unsuccessful attempts to feed an irritable infant. Infants

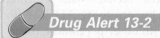
Drug Alert 13-2

Psychotherapeutic medications are powerful chemicals. When these medications are prescribed for children, parents must be taught to routinely monitor for side effects, adverse reactions, any unwanted effect, and interactions with over-the-counter medications, such as cold medications (see Chapter 7). Nurses have an important responsibility to provide parents with written information about the medication(s) the child is receiving, how to monitor the child's response to the drug, and what side effects to report. They should be willing to monitor the child throughout the period he or she is receiving psychotherapeutic drugs.

may be difficult to console, apathetic, or withdrawn during feedings. Some infants may have difficulty regulating their nervous systems, resulting in altered periods of alertness. Other factors associated with feeding disorders are parental mental health problems, abuse, and neglect. Treatment focuses on ruling out a physical cause, teaching parents appropriate feeding techniques, and monitoring the child's weight and developmental gains. In some cases, family therapy is helpful.

Pica is the term used to describe persistent eating of nonfood items for more than 1 month. The nonfood items chosen seem to vary with age. Infants and younger children will typically eat paint, hair, string, plaster, or cloth. Older children may eat sand, pebbles, insects, animal droppings, or leaves; adults may consume clay, soil, or laundry starch. Pica is often seen in children with mental retardation and pervasive developmental disorders (e.g., autism). Treatment includes ruling out any physical problems, such as vitamin or mineral deficiencies, removing the item from the child, and helping the child to replace the unacceptable item with more acceptable foods.

Rumination disorder is an uncommon feeding disorder in which the infant regurgitates (brings up) and rechews food. It is most often seen in infants from 3 to 12 months old but may occur in older children or adults with mental retardation. Characteristically, the infant will arch the back, hold the head back, make sucking movements with the tongue, and give the impression of receiving satisfaction when the food is regurgitated. Malnutrition may occur because the food is brought back to the mouth soon after it is eaten. The disorder often disappears as the child grows older, but if the behaviors continue, erosion of the esophagus from exposure to stomach acids may result.

ELIMINATION DISORDERS

The two most common elimination problems of childhood are enuresis and encopresis. Enuresis is the involuntary urinary incontinence of a child 5 years or older. It often has a tendency to occur in families. Enuresis is divided into three categories: primary nocturnal enuresis (wetting the bed at night), diurnal enuresis (daytime wetting), and secondary enuresis (develops after child has achieved bladder control).

Primary nocturnal enuresis is common in children. It occurs three times more frequently in boys and often disappears without intervention. The actual cause of nighttime wetting is not known, but it is believed that a developmental delay in the sleep-wake mechanism or bladder capacity of the child may be a factor. Daytime wetting **(diurnal enuresis)** is less common. It is usually seen in shy children or those with ADHD. Daytime wetting occurs equally in boys and girls. Approximately 60% to 80% also wet the bed at night.

Secondary enuresis develops when a bladder-trained child becomes incontinent. Usually it follows a stressful event, such as the birth of a sibling or a divorce. Both diurnal enuresis and secondary enuresis are associated with high levels of emotional stress and anxiety.

Treatment for children with enuresis ranges from simple reassurance to various mental health therapies. Medications (desmopressin, imipramine) may be prescribed. Nurses can help parents cope by obtaining an accurate history of the child's problems, helping parents to establish a bedtime routine for the child, and providing emotional support. When mental health therapy is required, the focus is on helping the child verbally express the feelings associated with the symptoms.

Encopresis is defined as the repeated, usually voluntary, passage of feces in inappropriate places in a child over 4 years of age with no physical abnormalities. It affects boys four times more frequently than girls and is rarely seen in adolescence. After any physical problems are ruled out, treatment focuses on establishing a routine bowel care program. Praising the child for continent periods and having him or her assume the responsibility for rinsing the soiled clothing are often effective. Children who show little concern or distress about their incontinence are more difficult to treat.

DEVELOPMENTAL PROBLEMS

Children develop by mastering increasingly more difficult and complex tasks. Because each child is unique, some lags in certain areas of development are common and to be expected. However, if the child persistently falls behind in a developmental area, a disorder of intellectual functioning, learning, or communication is suspected. The developmental problems most often seen by health care providers include mental retardation, various learning disorders, and several types of communication disorders.

MENTAL RETARDATION

Children who function significantly below the average intellectual level for their age-group and are limited in their abilities to function are said to be mentally retarded. The diagnosis of mental retardation is a powerful label and too often applied in haste. For a child to be considered retarded, he or she must have problems in general intellectual and adaptive functioning.

The degree of intellectual functioning is established by having the child complete one or more standard intelligence (IQ) tests. Children who repeatedly score lower than 70 are defined as retarded. The more important measure is the child's adaptive functioning: how well the child copes with the demands of life. It includes the skill areas relating to self-care, home living,

Table **13-5** *Classification of Mental Retardation Levels*

MILD (85% INCIDENCE)	MODERATE (10% INCIDENCE)	SEVERE (3%-4% INCIDENCE)	PROFOUND (2% INCIDENCE)
Develops social and communication skills; has academic skills to sixth-grade level; has skills adequate for self-support; may need supervision and guidance but is able to successfully live in community	Develops communication skills; has academic skills to second-grade level; profits from vocational training; can attend to personal care with supervision; can work in sheltered setting or work in community under supervision; adapts well to community life in supervised environments	May learn to talk and do basic self-care skills; can learn key "survival" words (e.g., stop, bus, police); performs simple tasks with close supervision; adapts well to life with families or group homes	Exhibits associated neurological conditions, delays in development; has impaired sensorimotor function; is unable to care for self independently; may improve in highly structured environment; will always require sheltered environment with close supervision

Modified from American Psychiatric Association: *Diagnostic and statistical manual of mental disorders*, ed 4, text revision, Washington, DC, 2000, The Association.

communication, social skills, use of community resources, academic skills, self-direction, and the child's work, leisure, safety, and health activities. Table 13-5 describes the various levels of retardation.

Fetal alcohol syndrome is the leading known cause of retardation in children. Inborn errors of metabolism, Down syndrome, birth injuries, shaken baby syndrome, high fevers, hormonal imbalances, poisonings, accidents, and falls are known causes of retardation. Heredity, problems with fetal development, pregnancy, or infancy, and environmental influences are thought to be related factors. However, no clear cause of mental retardation can be found for 30% to 40% of all occurrences. Treatment is individually developed and focuses on encouraging the child to function at the highest levels possible. Therapeutic actions focus on meeting the child's basic needs, providing a safe environment, and encouraging the development of life skills.

LEARNING DISORDERS

Formally called academic skills disorders, the category for problems with learning is broad. A **learning disorder** is diagnosed when a child with normal intelligence routinely falls below the results of other children in the same age and grade groups on standard reading, mathematics, or written tests. Learning disorders can affect the child's thinking, reading, writing, calculation, spelling, and listening abilities. Approximately 5% of children in the U.S. public school system have learning disabilities (American Psychiatric Association, 2000).

Children with learning disabilities often feel low self-esteem and lack the social skills of other children. Many become discouraged and drop out of school early. Although no specific cause has been found for learning disorders, they have been associated with conditions such as fetal alcohol syndrome, lead poisoning, and fragile X syndrome (a genetic problem). Learning disorders are diagnosed only after physical disorders, such as hearing, speech, and visual problems, are ruled

out. Cultural influences are also considered. A child is said to have a learning disorder only if the specific problem interferes with academic achievement or the activities of daily living.

Children with a reading disorder may have problems reading, understanding the written word, reading aloud, or writing. Individuals with **dyslexia** have problems with reading because although they can see and recognize letters, they have difficulty integrating visual information and thus tend to twist, substitute, distort, or omit many words. Children are seldom diagnosed before they have received several years of reading instruction in school. Early intervention is important because special education often results in great improvement. Reading disorders, if not addressed, may follow the child into adult life.

Many learning disorders are seen in children with ADHD. Other children with learning disabilities are quiet, with low activity levels. They are frequently overlooked because of their quiet manners or are mistaken for being retarded. Most children with learning disabilities respond well to special education classes and encouragement.

COMMUNICATION DISORDERS

In children, the most common **communication disorders** are problems with expression, receiving messages, the pronunciation of words, and stuttering. Communication disorders may be the result of neurological or other medical conditions, but the cause is often unknown.

Problems with language usually begin in children around age 3 years. The child may fail to use expected speech sounds for his or her age-group **(phonological disorder);** speak at a rapid or slow rate, with strange rhythms and word use **(expressive language disorder);** or have a disturbance in the pattern of speech in which sounds are frequently repeated **(stuttering).** Each is considered a disorder only if the problem interferes with the child's activities of daily living or ability to academically achieve.

Children with developmental problems must struggle for their learning more than other children. They need love, patience, and encouragement on a daily basis. Too often, adults fall into the "label trap" and condemn these children to performing at levels far below their actual abilities. Caregivers must remember that working with developmentally different children comes with a commitment to help them achieve to the best of their abilities.

PERVASIVE DEVELOPMENTAL DISORDERS

The word *pervasive* is defined as a tendency to spread throughout. When applied to mental health, the word means that a problem is severe enough to affect several areas of functioning. Children with pervasive developmental disorders have difficulty with social interaction skills, communication skills, and learning. Their behavior is definitely different from that of other children of the same age and developmental level. Actual causes for these disorders remain unknown, but they are often seen with mental retardation, congenital infections, and abnormal central nervous system functions.

Pervasive developmental disorders include the following:
- Autism: A disorder of communication, social interactions, and behavior
- **Rett syndrome:** The development of motor, language, and social problems and loss of previous skills that occurs between 5 months and 4 years of age; head growth declines, hand movements resemble hand wringing, and loss of social interest and severe speech impairments occur
- **Asperger's syndrome:** Severe and long-lasting impairments in social interactions with repeated patterns of behavior, interest, and activities
- **Childhood disintegrative disorder:** A period of severe regression in many areas following 2 years of normal development

Rett syndrome and childhood disintegrative disorder appear after a period of normal functioning, whereas autism and Asperger's syndrome are present in infancy. Autism is the most often encountered pervasive developmental disorder of childhood. It shares many of the same characteristics with the other listed disorders and serves as an example for learning about the behaviors of children with pervasive developmental disorders.

AUTISM

Autism is not a disease but a syndrome of associated behaviors. It results from some condition that affects the development of the nervous system, and it can remain with the individual throughout life. Autism is diagnosed when the child has serious problems with social interactions, communication, and use of imagination and demonstrates a markedly restricted scope of activities and interests.

The onset of autistic signs and symptoms begins in infancy or early childhood. Autistic disorders affect children from all classes and groups. Typically, autism is seen four times more frequently in boys. The majority of autistic children measure low on IQ tests. Motor skill development may be good, but the child's use of motor skills is inappropriate. Many autistic children become functioning adults, whereas others are totally dependent for care. Children who are able to develop language skills before the age of 5 years have better outcomes. If the child has seizures around puberty, the outlook for improvement is generally poor.

No single behavior or symptom is diagnostic of autism. Behaviors must be considered in relation to the whole child and his or her functioning. Monitoring children's early social responses, communication skills, and behaviors allows health care providers to intervene early when a problem is suspected.

The outstanding feature of autism is its **different behaviors.** Autistic children tend to use people in the environment like objects; they are unable to imitate others or make social contact. Other characteristics of autistic disorder include abnormal speech and communications, abnormal play activities, preoccupation with certain objects and routines, restricted body movements, and a very narrow range of interests.

Caregivers who work with children must become keen observers and careful history takers. Parents are questioned about the child's birth, developmental history, social responses, and communications. The picture of an autistic child begins to emerge when it is learned that the child does not act appropriately for his or her mental age, even with family members and other familiar people. Once the disorder is suspected, the child receives a complete physical examination to rule out central nervous system problems. The child is then referred to a treatment team that specializes in children with autistic problems. Parents are encouraged to work with physicians, nurses, therapists, and special educators. Programs are designed to meet the individual child's unique needs. Then the parents, child, and treatment team work together for each small gain in functioning.

SCHIZOPHRENIA

Schizophrenia is a condition associated with disturbing thought patterns and a distorted reality. Considerable disagreement exists concerning the onset of schizophrenia in childhood. Schizophrenia usually develops during late adolescence or early adulthood, but it has been seen in children. Recent research has demonstrated that schizophrenic children may have attention and memory problems that interfere with their ability to carry information into the short-term or working memory. As a result, many are unable to monitor the responses of other people or they interact and respond with illogical or disconnected statements (Frazier and others, 2007).

The signs, symptoms, and behaviors of children with schizophrenia vary widely, but the core disturbance lies in a lack of contact with reality and the child's retreat into his or her own world. Common behaviors include bizarre movements; alternating periods of hypoactivity and hyperactivity; inappropriate emotions, language, and use of the body; distorted sense of time; treating self and others as nonhuman; compulsions; phobias; and temper tantrums. Early recognition and treatment are important because schizophrenia is often a long-term disorder.

THERAPEUTIC ACTIONS

Therapeutic interventions for children with mental health problems are first directed toward early identification and treatment. Health care providers fill a valuable role by performing health screening and routine examinations for healthy children in a variety of settings (Table 13-6).

Once a disorder is diagnosed, special treatment programs and specific goals are developed for each child. Nurses routinely assess and monitor the child's progress toward meeting each goal. All caregivers provide the emotional support and encouragement

Table 13-6 *Pediatric Mental Health Screening Tool*

ASSESSMENT	SUBJECT
Childhood history	Ambulation, behavior problems, bowel and bladder training/habits, communication (problems in speech or learning), discipline, eating habits, playmates (social interactions), psychiatric history (treatments, medications, suicide potential), school (reactions, experiences), sleep habits, unusual illnesses or injuries, current problem (with description of events that led to current situation)
Family history	Current household (members, relationship to child), mother and father, type of family (birth, blended, adopted, foster), mental health history of family (e.g., drug, alcohol use; arguments; violence; suicide attempts)
Mental status examination	General appearance, communication, emotion (mood, affect), intellectual level, orientation, thought processes

that are much needed by the parents and other family members.

The care for each child is special and based on individual needs. Nursing diagnoses for children with mental health problems are listed in Box 13-5. Therapeutic actions are focused on providing holistic care within an environment that fosters growth and development. Sample Client Care Plan 13-1 offers an example of a care plan for a child with mental retardation. General interventions are focused on meeting basic needs, providing opportunities, and encouraging self-care activities.

MEET BASIC NEEDS

Meeting the child's basic physical needs can range from a gentle reminder to providing total personal care. Caregivers are responsible for making sure the child adequately eats, sleeps, eliminates, and maintains personal cleanliness. Helping a child to meet basic needs includes the provision of love and acceptance, no matter how unusual or odd the behaviors. Many children with mental health problems have a special need to be nurtured. Often, the child's caregivers are the only persons in the environment who provide that energy.

Box 13-5 *Mental Health Nursing Diagnoses for Children*

Anxiety
Behavior, risk-prone health
Body image, disturbed
Communication, impaired verbal
Coping, defensive
Coping, compromised family
Coping, ineffective
Denial, ineffective
Environment, impaired environmental interpretation syndrome
Family process, interrupted
Fear
Growth and development, delayed
Health maintenance, ineffective
Hopelessness
Infant behavior, disorganized
Infant feeding pattern, ineffective
Injury, risk for
Knowledge, deficient
Loneliness, risk for
Nutrition, imbalanced: more than body requirements, less than body requirements
Parent/child attachment, impaired
Parental role conflict
Parenting, impaired, risk for
Personal identity, disturbed
Post-trauma syndrome
Powerlessness
Protection, ineffective
Rape-trauma syndrome
Self-care deficit

PROVIDE OPPORTUNITIES

Even the most profoundly retarded or mentally troubled child will achieve something if given the opportunity, instruction, and support. Assessment tools, such as those listed in Table 13-7, allow care providers to screen for developmental levels, school readiness, and potential problems.

Each child is capable of something. Encourage young clients to grow and to reach for higher levels of function. Provide opportunities for small successes, which encourage everyone (especially the child) to strive for more.

ENCOURAGE SELF-CARE AND INDEPENDENCE

Mentally troubled children grow and develop just as ordinary children do. Despite their problems, many become productive adults who live successfully within their communities. Health care providers who work with these children help them learn the important skills of daily living. Daily hygiene skills, such as how to dress, bathe, brush teeth, and comb hair, are taught and reinforced. Caregivers coordinate with teachers, occupational therapists, and physical therapists to help teach the more complex skills of living, such as how to take a bus, spend money, or pay bills. Many will not be able to engage in the more complicated activities of daily life, but each child deserves the encouragement to function as independently as possible.

Caring for children with mental health problems is challenging work, but the rewards are many and worth the efforts. Our children are our priceless gifts to the future, and even the most troubled deserve our best efforts.

SAMPLE CLIENT CARE PLAN 13-1

Mental Retardation

ASSESSMENT *History.* BJ is a 6-year-old boy with moderate mental retardation. His birth and the first 6 months of life were uneventful. At 7 months, BJ contracted "a virus" and since then has shown little developmental progress.

Current Findings. A slightly overweight 6-year-old boy who is screaming uncontrollably at the time of interview. Mother reports that BJ is able to speak but prefers to communicate by pointing at the desired object and grunting. When needs are not immediately met, BJ begins to scream in a shrill voice. He feeds himself finger foods and refuses to use a spoon. He is not bowel or bladder trained and follows no daily routine at home. He has no eating and sleeping routines.

Multidisciplinary Diagnosis	*Planning/Goals*
Altered growth and development related to physical dysfunctions as evidenced by impaired developmental abilities	BJ will develop a daily routine for eating, sleeping, and activities by October 2.

Therapeutic Interventions

Intervention	Rationale	Team Member
1. Supervise closely for first 7 days on unit.	To assess strengths, abilities, and needed interventions.	All
2. Approach BJ in a calm, peaceful manner.	Promotes self-esteem, decreases anxieties.	All
3. Introduce no more than two new people into the environment per week.	Decreases anxiety, provides security.	All
4. Establish a daily routine for food, naps, activity.	Prevents anxiety, provides security.	Nsg
5. Name each object that BJ points to, and encourage him to repeat the name.	Encourages the use of speech and control over environment.	All
6. Assist with personal care as needed; praise any attempt at self-care.	Promotes comfort, acceptance. Praise encourages further attempts at self-care.	Nsg, OT

Evaluation

By the tenth day in the unit, BJ was able to follow a simple daily routine with frequent coaching. Sleep at night progressed from 3-hour periods to 9-hour periods.

? CRITICAL THINKING QUESTIONS

1. How can the health care team ensure that BJ will maintain his new routine at home?

2. What information should be included in the family teaching plan?

A complete client care plan includes several other diagnoses and interventions.
Nsg, Nursing staff; *OT,* occupational therapist.

Table 13-7 *Assessment Tools for Children*

TOOL	AGES	FOCUS
Denver II	Birth-6 yr	Gross and fine motor skills; language; social skills
Preschool Readiness Screening Scale	4-5 yr	Maturation; school readiness
Early Language Milestone Scale	Birth-36 mo	Speech and language development
Infant Temperament Questionnaire	1-2 mo	Temperament
Toddler Development Scale	1-3 yr	Temperament
Behavioral Style Questionnaire	3-7 yr	Temperament
Middle Childhood Questionnaire	8-12 yr	Temperament

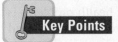

Key Points

- Health care providers who work with children must have an understanding of normal development and an awareness of the child's individual pace of growth and development.
- Common behavioral difficulties during the early years of childhood are colic, problems with feeding and sleeping, temper tantrums, and breath-holding spells.
- Many children must cope with the mental health problems that are a result of poverty, homelessness, abuse, or neglect.
- Behavioral problems, developmental delays, speech delays, sleep disorders, immature motor actions, and short attention spans are common in homeless children.
- The most common emotional problems of children include anxiety, depression, somatoform disorders, and posttraumatic stress disorders.
- Most children's anxieties are relieved when they receive reassurance and emotional support from significant others.
- The two disruptive behavioral disorders most commonly encountered by caregivers are attention-deficit/hyperactivity disorder (ADHD) and conduct disorder.
- Children with ADHD have problems with behavioral self-control, hyperactivity, relating to others, and focusing their attention.
- The long-term outlook for children with conduct disorders is poor if the problems are present before the child is 10 years old. This makes early diagnosis and treatment very important to prevent antisocial or conduct disorders in adulthood.

- The most common pediatric mental health problems that relate to eating are feeding disorders, pica, anorexia nervosa, and bulimia.
- Disorders of elimination include encopresis and enuresis.
- The developmental problems most often seen include mental retardation, various learning disorders, and several types of communication disorders.
- Interventions for mentally retarded children focus on meeting the child's basic needs, providing a safe environment, and encouraging the development of life skills.
- Children with pervasive developmental disorders have serious problems with social interaction skills, communication skills, and learning.
- Autism is characterized by few social interactions, a lack of communication, no use of imagination, and a restricted scope of activities and interests.
- The signs, symptoms, and behaviors of children with schizophrenia vary widely, but the core disturbance is a lack of contact with reality and the child's retreat into his or her own world.
- General interventions include meeting basic physical and emotional needs, providing opportunities for each child to grow and develop, and encouraging self-care activities.

evolve Be sure to visit the companion Evolve site at http://evolve.elsevier.com/Morrison-Valfre/ for additional online resources.

evolve http://evolve.elsevier.com/Morrison-Valfre/

Objectives

Upon completion of this chapter, the student will be able to:

1. Describe three common problems of adolescence.
2. Discuss three problems faced by adolescents with troubled family lives.
3. Identify the diagnostic criteria for behavioral disorders.
4. Explain how the signs and symptoms of adolescent depression differ from those seen in adult depression.
5. Define two eating disorders and describe the associated signs and symptoms and behaviors.
6. Describe the stages of chemical dependency in adolescence.
7. List four signs or symptoms indicating a potentially suicidal teen.
8. Identify four therapeutic interventions designed specifically for adolescent clients.
9. Explain how health care providers help adolescents develop effective coping skills.

Key Terms

adolescence (p. 145)
adolescent suicide (p. 155)
anorexia nervosa (ăn-ō-RĔK-sē-ə nĕr-VŌ-sə) (p. 152)
bulimia (p. 152)
chemical dependency (p. 153)
gangs (p. 149)
maturation (MĂCH-ū-RĀ-shən) (p. 145)
obesity (p. 152)
peer groups (p. 149)
personality disorder (p. 154)
puberty (p. 145)
sexual disorder (p. 154)
surveillance (p. 157)

Adolescence is a time of great change. Generally, adolescence begins at age 11 to 12 years and ends between ages 18 and 21 years. Physical and sexual growth are usually complete by age 16 to 18 years, but in Western societies "the adolescence period is prolonged to allow for further psychosocial development before the young person assumes adult responsibilities" (Kaplan and Mammel, 2001). Adolescents are also called teenagers or teens. All adolescents share the same growth and developmental processes, but each person's society and culture strongly influence that process of "growing up" (see Cultural Considerations 14-1).

ADOLESCENT GROWTH AND DEVELOPMENT

The journey from child to adult is a time of physical and psychosocial growth. Adolescents undergo great changes in the physical, intellectual, emotional, social, and spiritual areas of their lives. Care providers should understand how adolescents grow and change if they are to assist them through this important developmental stage. Many adult problems find their roots in adolescence.

PHYSICAL DEVELOPMENT

Changes in the body during adolescence occur in two general areas: physical maturation and sexual development. Maturation is the process of attaining complete development (Hockenberry and others, 2007). Physical maturation is the process of developing an adult body. Many physical changes occur during adolescence. Weight and height increase, and muscles grow. The major organs of the body double in size, and one's voice and appearance change.

Adolescence is also a time for sexual development. As changing bodies begin to secrete certain hormones called gonadotropins, the process of puberty begins. Puberty is defined as the stage during which an individual becomes physically capable of reproduction. With girls, puberty begins between 8 and 14 years of age. Today the average girl in the United States experiences the 24-month to 36-month puberty growth spurt around 9 years of age and begins to menstruate (menarche) at about 12 years and 9 months. Menarche begins as early as 10 years or as late as 16 years of age. Breast development, body fat distribution, and the other physical changes that prepare the teen's body for adulthood are usually complete by age 16 to 18 years.

Boys develop more slowly. The first signs of puberty in boys occur around age 10 to 12 years. The testicles enlarge, pubic hair develops, and the penis increases in length and width. The male growth spurt begins at age 11 years and continues until about 14 years. Puberty lasts until about 18 years of age, but most male adolescents as young as 12 years old are capable of fathering

Researchers at the University of Michigan studied the frequency of stressed and anxious feelings in more than 4000 U.S., Taiwanese, and Japanese teenagers. They found some interesting results. Japanese adolescents were found to have the fewest reports of physical problems and depressed moods, whereas Taiwanese teens displayed more physical complaints and depressed moods. Students in the United States and Taiwan thought of school as a source of stress, but only U.S. teens mentioned out-of-school activities and sports as sources of stress. Japanese teens felt that peers were a greater source of stress.

Parents in the United States expected lower academic performance of their teens than the parents of Japanese and Taiwanese adolescents. Doing well in school was more supported and encouraged by the families of Asian teenagers. High achievers in the United States reported that they were frequently torn between their desires to put extra time into their studies and to follow other activities, such as dating, working, playing sports, and socializing.

children. Puberty is a time of change for both boys and girls. For a more thorough review of the growth and development of adolescents, you are encouraged to consult a text on pediatric nursing.

PSYCHOSOCIAL DEVELOPMENT

The term **psychosocial** refers to the nonphysical realms of functioning. There are periods in teens' lives when they feel awkward, inadequate, and unworthy. Adults who are aware of these changes are better able to offer the emotional support and acceptance so needed by an adolescent. This section briefly explores the major developmental tasks for each psychosocial area of functioning.

Intellectual changes **(cognitive development)** involve learning to use abstract thinking. Children's thinking is concrete, based on what is observed or experienced in the present time. Young adolescents (10 to 13 years) have trouble thinking realistically about the future. As teens mature, thinking moves from the present and concrete to the future and what is possible. To illustrate, an 8-year-old makes a judgment based on what he or she sees; a 17-year-old makes a judgment based on reasoning. Teens begin to look at the world in new and exciting ways, to think beyond the present time, to consider a sequence of events or relationships, and to solve problems through scientific reasoning and logic.

By the middle teens (14 to 17 years), **abstract thinking** (adaptable, flexible thinking that uses concepts, generalizations, and problem solving) is well entrenched, along with a feeling of power and self-centeredness. Many believe that they can change the world by just thinking about it. At about 17 years of age, teens' abstract thinking becomes more realistic

and they are able to plan reachable actions, goals, and careers.

Emotional development during adolescence is marked by rapid periods of change and adjustment. By 10 to 13 years of age, the emotional stability of childhood is replaced with a preoccupation about body changes. This brings about changes in self-esteem, body image, and self-concept. Coping with all these changes becomes confusing to the adolescent. Behaviors swing rapidly from the pleasant, cooperative child to the moody, unpredictable, emotional teen. Early adolescence is marked by rapid shifts between disturbed behavior and relative calm. Moods swing from upbeat and happy to withdrawn and depressed. Reactions to small events can trigger outbursts and aggressive behaviors.

Adolescents also **daydream** much of the time. Daydreaming is important for adolescents because it allows them to try out new roles and place themselves in "what if" situations. Because of this, they often miss many messages from other people and become labeled as sullen or withdrawn.

The emotions and mood swings of puberty become intense when teens are between 14 and 17 years old. At this age, they tend to stay alone, looking within themselves and at how they fit into the world. For many teens, this is a troubled, lonely time. By about 18 years of age, most adolescents are in control of their emotions and have an established self-concept.

Social development is an important area for adolescents. Younger teens struggle to establish a group identity as well as a personal identity. Most teenagers feel the need to belong to a group. At this age, many needs are fulfilled by peer groups. The most important function of the group is to help adolescents define the differences between themselves and their parents. Dress, music, dancing, and language are all designed to display differences and to show how unique the group really is. Unless the standards set by the peer group place teens in danger, these standards should be tolerated by adults. Belonging to a group serves as a stepping-stone in the process of establishing an individual identity and separating from the family.

Middle teens establish their identities by experimenting with different images of themselves. By this time, the peer group determines new standards for dress, behavior, and activities. Teens at this stage begin to see themselves as others might see them. The social relationships of 14 to 16 year olds are usually self-centered. Sexuality becomes more important, and by age 18 years, the majority of adolescents have engaged in sexual intercourse. Social relationships for adolescents over 17 years shift from the group to the individual. Caring more about others than oneself begins, and dating becomes more personal and intimate.

Spiritual development for adolescents begins with questioning family values and beliefs. Some teens cling furiously to family values during periods of conflict, whereas others completely disregard them. Adolescents also use their new abstract thinking abilities to question their childhood religious and spiritual practices. Often they will stop attending church services, change churches, or choose to worship within the privacy of their rooms or other special space. Many teens are attracted to new religious sects or movements that suggest promises of unconditional acceptance and love during a time when adults are seen as critical and intolerant. Most teenagers experience great inner emotional turmoil. Because teens fear that nobody will understand, they may become extremely private. Most adolescents have deep spiritual concerns and require acceptance, understanding, and patience as they struggle to find the spiritual rock that will anchor them in adulthood.

Adolescence is a time of rapid and uncontrollable change. Between the ages of 10 and 20 years, adolescents grow, develop, and mature within each area of functioning. Table 14-1 offers a brief explanation of the major changes experienced throughout adolescence. As adolescents mature, they begin to move away from the family and function independently. Society welcomes them as adults, with all the rewards and obligations of the adult role.

COMMON PROBLEMS OF ADOLESCENCE

The world is large and complex. Even the most successful people feel overwhelmed by the sheer amount of information and experiences that are currently available. Adolescents, who are just beginning to emerge from the security of childhood, must gain understanding and control of themselves. At the same time, they must learn to cope with living in an uncertain world. Most of the common problems of adolescence fall into two categories: problems that arise from within oneself (internal sources) and those that are rooted outside the teen's sphere of control (external sources).

INTERNAL (DEVELOPMENTAL) PROBLEMS

Most difficulties of early adolescence arise from within the individual. Physical changes are taking place, and new sensations are experienced. One's own body ceases to cooperate at times, and floods of intense emotions bring on dramatic, emotional ups and downs. An important developmental problem of adolescence is defining oneself—establishing an identity separate from one's family. At this stage, teens begin to look into themselves. They engage in **introspection** (the process of examining one's own thoughts, emotions, reactions, attitudes, opinions, values, and behaviors by looking at the inner self). They consider who they are, how they see themselves, how they think others may see them, and how relationships with various people affect them. This process of looking inward helps teens to define

themselves, but it also brings about many changes in mood, attitude, and behavior. Problems that threaten self-esteem or confidence routinely arise during the journey to adulthood. It is important for teens to feel secure and emotionally supported by adults during these confusing periods. Just knowing that someone accepts and cares goes a long way toward helping teens through troubled times.

EXTERNAL (ENVIRONMENTAL) PROBLEMS

Problems that arise outside the teen are called external problems. They fall into three basic areas: family, social, and environmental. Even teens who are blessed with the best of everything experience difficulties in these areas of functioning.

Family problems change as the adolescent develops independence. During early adolescence (11 to 14 years), teens experience the pull between wanting to stay dependent and moving toward independence. They begin to seek their freedom but still require the emotional ties provided by the family structure.

By midadolescence (age 14 to 17 years), the push for independence is in full swing, and major conflicts over control motivate the teen to detach from the family. Conflicts slowly fade as the adolescent matures into an independently functioning adult. Separating from the family and establishing independence are problems faced by every teen, but difficulties often arise from within the family that are not related to the adolescent's developmental stage. Families can range from the overprotective parents who limit their children's experiences and do not allow them to make decisions to those whose children grow up on the streets with little or no sense of belonging.

Children have no control over the child-rearing methods chosen by their parents, living conditions, or the environment in which they must grow. Many adolescents must cope with physical violence, sexual abuse, neglect, or parents who abuse alcohol or drugs. About 7 million children and adolescents have a parent in jail or on parole (Inmates' Kids, 1999). These types of problems cannot be solved by just waiting for the adolescent to outgrow them. They are faced every day, and they require energy that should be spent in self-discovery.

Adolescents who are not fortunate enough to have a caring, supportive family are at risk because the conditions to which they are currently exposed may threaten further development (see Case Study 14-1). Every adolescent has some family problems because that is the nature of the maturing process. Those teens who are not blessed with a nurturing family face problems that would test the strongest adult.

Adolescents are also challenged with numerous social problems. Early teens seek out their peers and form intense bonds with certain groups. Peer groups are important for the social growth of adolescents.

Table 14-1 *Growth and Development During Adolescence*

EARLY ADOLESCENCE (11-14 YR)	MIDDLE ADOLESCENCE (14-17 YR)	LATE ADOLESCENCE (17-20 YR)
GROWTH		
Rapid growth	Growth slowing in girls	Physically mature
Reaches peak	Reaches 95% of adult height	Structure and reproductive growth
Sexual growth begins	Sexual growth well advanced	almost complete
COGNITION (INTELLECT)		
Explores ability for limited abstract thought	Developing abstract thinking	Established abstract thought
Groping for new values and energies	Enjoys intellectual powers, often in idealistic terms	Can perceive and act on long-range operations
Compares "normal" with peers of same gender	Concern with philosophical, political, and social problems	Able to view problems comprehensively
		Intellectual and functional identity established
IDENTITY		
Preoccupied with rapid body changes	Modifies body image	Body image and gender role definition
Trying out of various roles	Very self-centered	nearly secured
Measures attractiveness by acceptance or rejection of peers	Tendency toward inner experience and self-discovery	Mature sexual identity
Conformity to group norms	Has rich fantasy life	Brings together identity
	Idealistic	Stability of self-esteem
	Able to perceive future implications of current behavior and decisions	Comfortable with physical growth
		Social roles defined
RELATIONSHIPS WITH PARENTS		
Defining independence-dependence boundaries	Major conflicts over independence and control	Emotional and physical separation from parents completed
Strong desire to remain dependent on parents while trying to detach	Low point in parent-child relationship	Independence from family with less conflict
No major conflicts over parental control	Greatest push for emancipation; disengagement	Emancipation nearly secured
	Final and irreversible emotional detachment from parents; mourning	
RELATIONSHIPS WITH PEERS		
Seeks peers to counter instability generated by rapid change	Strong need for identity; self-image	Peer group fades in importance in favor of individual friendships
Close idealized friendships with members of the same gender	Behavioral standards set by peer group	Testing of male-female relationships; possibility of permanent alliance
Struggles for mastery within peer group	Acceptance by peers extremely important—fear of rejection	Relationships characterized by giving and sharing
	Explores ability to attract opposite gender	
SEXUALITY		
Self-exploration and evaluation	Multiple relationships	Forms stable relationships and
Limited dating, usually group	Decisive turn toward heterosexuality (if is homosexual, knows by this time)	attachments
Limited intimacy	Exploration of "self appeal"	Able to give and take
	Feeling of "being in love"	Dating as a male-female pair
	Begins to establish relationships	Intimacy involves commitment rather than exploration and romanticism
PSYCHOLOGICAL HEALTH		
Wide mood swings	Tendency toward inner experiences; more introspective	More constant with emotions
Intense daydreaming	Tendency to withdraw when upset	Anger more apt to be concealed
Anger outwardly expressed with moodiness, temper outburst, verbal insults, and name-calling	Wide emotion swings in time and range	
	Feelings of inadequacy common; difficulty in asking for help	

Modified from Hockenberry M and others: *Wong's nursing care of infants and children,* ed 8, St. Louis, 2007, Mosby.

Carol was a bright, energetic 5 year old when her parents divorced, forcing her mother to live on a welfare income. Between the ages of 6 and 13 years, Carol experienced a series of "fathers" who lived with them for various periods of time. Some were kind to Carol, but one physically and sexually abused her. Her mother was usually away from home or with other adults, and Carol soon learned to fend for herself. By age 12, Carol had already experimented with different drugs and found alcohol most to her liking. By the time she was 14 years old, Carol was uncontrollable. She had learned to drive and would often steal her mother's car after her mother was asleep for the night. Unprotected sex happened frequently. Soon Carol dropped out of school because "it really doesn't matter."

- List the factors in Carol's life that put her at risk.
- Identify two of her problems.
- What do you think could help Carol?

They serve many purposes and help teens cope with their life changes (Table 14-2).

Peer groups and gangs both consist of adolescents of about the same age and circumstances. The difference between the two groups lies in the behaviors or actions of the members. **Gangs** are usually associated with negative behaviors or destructive actions. **Peer groups** focus their energies in constructive ways, such as volunteer work and projects that benefit their communities. Peer groups are often influenced by adults. Examples include coaches for sports teams or leaders for youth church groups. Adolescents choose to join groups. Concerned parents should support their teen's choices but remain aware of the powerful influences groups exert on a developing individual.

Other social problems encountered by most adolescents relate to establishing their sexuality. Intimacy (emotional closeness) is limited in early adolescence. Same-gender friends are still of primary importance. As time passes, interest in people of the opposite gender begins to increase. By age 14 years, teens explore the concepts of "sex appeal" and "being in love." More than 50% of them have experienced sexual intercourse by this age. Dating may be limited to one person at a time, but many relationships are experienced as adolescents struggle to define themselves, both socially and sexually. Around 20 years of age, people begin to form stable, attached relationships based on a sense of giving rather than receiving.

Finally, environmental conditions have an impact on adolescent development because problems in the environment can threaten basic needs. The dirty air of so many cities, the quality and quantity of foods eaten, and the purity of the water have an impact, however subtle, on developing human beings. Exposures to drugs, crime, prostitution, corruption, and violence are very real environmental problems for many teens.

Activities that glamorize sex and violence through music, television, and the movies have a strong impact on the developing teen psyche. Adults who push children into becoming adults too soon are also environmental influences with which teens must cope.

Most adolescents, however, are concerned with more immediate problems of learning to function effectively within their physical and social environments—the problems that "come with the territory" and are a part of daily life. Environments that foster growth offer fewer problems than surroundings that require a constant state of awareness just to live through the day. Health caregivers must recognize the environmental conditions and problems that accompany our teens if we are to provide our teenagers with the tools for a successful transition to adulthood.

MENTAL HEALTH PROBLEMS OF ADOLESCENCE

Adolescence is the time for teens to develop the personal strengths and social skills that promote effective functioning in the adult world. It is a period involving great emotional swings, focus on oneself, and increasingly active sexual and aggressive drives. In an effort to cope with these changes, adolescents engage in a wide variety of behaviors. Some actions help teens to successfully adapt, whereas others result in negative outcomes. This is a period of "trying out" new behaviors, and adults need to consider this fact.

Adolescent mental health also includes the concept of well-being, the inner strengths that promote optimal functioning. Well-being includes the ability to function well socially (social competence), have positive interactions with others, cope with stress and troubled times, and become involved in activities and relationships with others.

The word **dysfunction** is defined as an impairment in everyday life. It means that the problems faced by the teen are so severe that he or she cannot or will not partake in the activities of daily living. When an adolescent's problems or emotions impair performance (school, social, or work) or threaten physical well-being, a mental health problem exists. Table 14-3 lists several categories of mental health disorders that affect adolescents.

Mental health services for adolescents focus on promoting positive life skills, prevention, and treatment of dysfunctions. Nursing interventions focus on health education, assisting with group and individual therapy, medication management, setting limits, and providing emotional support.

BEHAVIORAL DISORDERS

Every child goes through periods of misconduct, of refusing to do as told, of "being bad." However, for some teens the misconduct continues to occur. Behaviors

Table 14-2 *Peer Groups and Adolescents*

FUNCTIONS OF PEER GROUPS

Help to loosen family ties

Provide stability during times of change

Help adolescents define present and future social roles; test their views of themselves; learn to trust their own choices; learn to make and stand by their commitments

Establish behavioral and dress standards

POSITIVE ASPECTS	**NEGATIVE ASPECTS**
Provide emotional support, a sense of belonging	Rules and standards of the group may be too rigid
Help teens establish values and behavioral standards	Values and behaviors may not be in keeping with society's definition
Provide protection, safety	May encourage self-destructive behaviors and disregard for others
Allow teens to test and try out new behaviors	outside the group

Table 14-3 *Adolescent Mental Health Disorders*

CLASSIFICATION OF DISORDERS	EXAMPLES
Behavioral disorders	Conduct disorder, attention-deficit/hyperactivity disorder
Emotional disorders	Anxiety disorder, mood disorders (e.g., depression, posttraumatic stress disorder, suicidal thoughts and attempts)
Eating disorders	Anorexia nervosa, bulimia
Chemical dependency	Abuse of alcohol, amphetamines (speed), caffeine, cocaine, marijuana, nicotine, hallucinogens, inhalants, opiates, prescription drugs
Personality disorders	Antisocial disorder, borderline personality disorder, dependent disorder, obsessive-compulsive disorder, paranoid personality disorder
Schizophrenia	Paranoid-type schizophrenia, disorganized-type schizophrenia, delusional disorder
Sexual disorders	Gender identity disorder, inappropriate sexual behaviors
Other disorders of adolescence	Adjustment disorder, impulse-control disorders, problems related to abuse or neglect

begin to disrupt their families, social interactions, and performance at school. These teens may clash with classmates, developing a reputation for being unruly, mean, or even dangerous. When a persistent pattern of disruptive behaviors is present, mental health interventions are usually necessary. Disruptive behavioral disorders consist of two basic diagnoses: attention-deficit/hyperactivity disorder and conduct disorders.

Attention-deficit/hyperactivity disorder (ADHD) is usually diagnosed earlier in childhood, but its impact lasts through adolescence and into adulthood (Box 14-1). The key features of ADHD are inattention and impulsivity. Teens with ADHD experience problems in focusing their attention, behavioral self-controls, and relating to others. Because of these difficulties, many teens become chronically unhappy. They may begin to abuse chemicals or go on to develop conduct disorders.

Treatment for adolescents with ADHD requires a multidisciplinary approach. Small, structured classes and firm, but nonjudgmental, teachers are needed in the school environment. Positive reinforcement programs that reward appropriate behaviors are helpful at home and school. Behavioral therapy assists both teens and their parents. Parents are taught how to structure and enforce limits on the teen's behaviors without becoming overly harsh, inconsistent, or angry. If the adolescent has specific learning disabilities, special

Box 14-1 *Adolescents With ADHD*

"Only about one-third of children with ADHD reach mid-adolescence with no diagnosable psychiatric disorder" (Clark, 2001). Teens with ADHD often have low self-esteem and poor socialization skills. Impulse control is usually a problem.

ADHD, Attention-deficit/hyperactivity disorder.

education may be necessary. Medications to treat ADHD include stimulants, tricyclic antidepressants, and antipsychotics (Table 14-4 and Drug Alert 14-1). Adolescents who are taking prescribed medications may also be using various other substances. Serious drug interactions can occur when street and pharmaceutical drugs are mixed. Do not judge the teen, but be sure to obtain a complete history of past and current use of chemically active substances.

Conduct disorders are characterized by a defiance of authority and aggressive behaviors toward others. Often teens with conduct disorders violate the rights of other people or defy society's norms and standards. A common factor in the development of conduct disorders appears to be harsh parental discipline with physical punishment. Early harsh discipline tends to foster aggressive behaviors later in a child's life.

Table 14-4 *Medications for Teens With ADHD*

DRUG EXAMPLES	DOSE	CLIENT TEACHING
STIMULANTS		
Dextroamphetamine (Adderall)	5-60 mg/day, divided dosed	Avoid caffeine, alcohol, OTC drugs.
Methylphenidate (Ritalin, Concerta)	0.3-1.5 mg/kg, 1-3 doses daily	Watch for effects on growth; behavior deteriorates
Pemoline (Cylert)	0.5-3.0 mg/kg/day	when drugs are stopped abruptly.
ANTIDEPRESSANTS		
Imipramine (Tofranil)	No more than 5 mg/kg/day	May cause dry mouth, blurred vision, constipation,
Clomipramine (Anafranil)	No more than 5 mg/kg/day	insomnia.
ANTIPSYCHOTICS		
Chlorpromazine (Thorazine)	6-8 mg/kg/day	May cause dry mouth, blurred vision, weight gain,
Haloperidol (Haldol)	0.05-0.15 mg/kg/day	low blood pressure. Report any abnormal muscle
		and body movements to physician.

ADHD, Attention-deficit/hyperactivity disorder; *OTC,* over-the-counter.

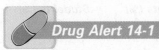

Drug Alert 14-1

Be sure to obtain a complete history of all drugs, herbs, medicines, or tonics taken. Write the names of each substance as they are given by the client. Many different names are used for the same item. Remember to ask about over-the-counter items too. Assess the teen's understanding of the prescribed drug, especially the side effects.

The typical adolescent with a conduct disorder is a boy with a history of social and academic problems. Common symptoms include fighting, temper tantrums, running away from home, destroying property, problems with authorities, and failure in school. Stealing and fire setting may occur. Truancy, vandalism, and substance abuse are frequently encountered. Many teens with conduct disorders, especially those with violent histories, also have various physical and mental health problems, such as anxiety disorders and depression.

Treatment for adolescents with conduct disorders focuses on first stabilizing the teen's home environment and then working to improve family interactions and disciplinary techniques. Individual therapy and family therapy help the family learn to communicate and problem solve effectively. A combination of behavioral, emotional, and cognitive therapies helps the teen learn self-control. Success hinges on including the family, teachers, and other adults who are involved with the teen. Efforts are made to treat the adolescent within the home environment; however, residential (inpatient) treatment may be necessary when the teen becomes a danger to himself or herself or others.

The outlook for adolescents with conduct disorders is poor. Nearly half the children with antisocial behaviors or conduct disorders become antisocial as adults (Clark, 2001). These teens need care providers with patience, a willingness to set limits, and the courage to enforce them.

EMOTIONAL DISORDERS

Disturbed feelings or moods are a normal part of everyday living. Adolescents, because of their many developmental tasks, experience frequent emotional changes. Periods of feeling "down" or "blue" are common with teens. However, when moods or feelings disrupt the teen's daily activities, mental health care may be needed.

Problems that affect the emotional realm of human functioning include anxiety disorders and mood disorders. A more detailed discussion is presented in later chapters, but a brief description of how these problems affect adolescents is important here.

Anxiety disorders result when an adolescent's ability to adapt is overwhelmed. When teens are overstressed, anxiety may balloon into an ever-present emotional state that triggers physical changes as the body attempts to adapt. The combination of physical and emotional symptoms can result in problems such as panic disorder, phobias, obsessive-compulsive disorders, and posttraumatic stress disorder. Anxiety is also associated with the development of depression and substance abuse problems. It is important to recognize and treat anxiety in children as early as possible because long-standing problems become difficult to change.

Mood Disorders

Adolescents with **affective or mood disorders** display a wide range of behaviors from profound depression to racing hyperactivity. Mood is the ever-present emotional state that colors one's perception of the world. Moods change rapidly as adolescents struggle with issues of self-image and confidence. Most teens have short periods of "the blues," but when sad moods are prolonged or the teen's behavior alternates between extreme highs and lows, an emotional disorder is suspected.

The number of depressed adolescents is growing. As many as one in eight teens may experience depression (Center for Mental Health Services, 2003). Many will exhibit the primary signs and symptoms of

---

Box 14-2 | *Signs and Symptoms of Depression in Adolescents*

Moodiness: irritable moods, acting-out behaviors, gloomy, sad
Decreased social activity
Decreased school performance
Hopelessness
Difficulty in thinking
Inability to concentrate, make decisions, or solve problems
Physical complaints: loss of energy, headache, stomachache, eating and sleeping problems

---

depression listed in Box 14-2. Many, however, will suffer in silence, with their symptoms going unnoticed (Hazell, 2002).

Other interpersonal difficulties are often present, such as problems with parents and siblings, drug use, and fighting. Acting out depression through antisocial behaviors, such as theft, vandalism, and truancy, may result in involvement with the law and its criminal justice system. Sexual acting out is also common. Depression in adolescence is "characterized by irritable moods and acting-out behaviors, in contrast to the classic 'depressed mood' and 'loss of interest' characteristic of adults" (Hogarth, 1991). In short, depressed adults lose interest; depressed teens act out.

Severe anxiety and depression are not average adolescent conditions. The majority of teens negotiate this developmental period without major problems. They develop positive personal identities, manage healthy peer relationships, and maintain close family ties. The best prevention for emotional disorders in teens is early recognition. Emotional problems left untreated in adolescence frequently develop into serious mental health disorders in adulthood.

EATING DISORDERS

Teens' eating patterns and food behaviors may follow the latest trend or change to reflect the preferences of the peer group, but as long as the teen is well nourished there is little cause for concern. Eating disorders are "severe disturbances in eating behavior" (American Psychiatric Association, 2000) that can result in a body that is far below or above its ideal weight.

The weight control practices of adolescents have been a cause for concern in today's society. "Each year, eating disorders affect millions of Americans, 85% to 90% of whom are teen and young adult women" (National Institute of Mental Health, 2007). The message of "slim equals attractive" bombards individuals throughout childhood, and weight control becomes an important concern. Think About 14-1 describes a research study that demonstrates this concern.

Obesity is defined as a body weight that is 20% or more above the average weight for a person of the

Think About 14-1

Self-assessment surveys were administered to more than 11,000 high school students and 60,000 adults. The results were as follows:
  44% of female students were actively trying to lose weight
  26% of female students were trying to prevent weight gain
  15% of male students were trying to lose weight
  15% of male students were trying to prevent weight gain
  Further, high school students reported using the following weight control methods within the past 7 days before the survey:

Method	Female Students (%)	Male Students (%)
Exercise	15	30
Skipping meals	49	18
Using diet pills	4	2
Vomiting	3	1

• Discuss how this information could be used to plan care for an adolescent client with an eating disorder.

Modified from Serdula MK and others: Weight control practice of U.S. adolescents and adults, *Ann Intern Med* 119(7 pt 2):667, 1993.

---

same height and build. Because the eating patterns of obese teens do not pose an immediate threat, chronic overeating is not considered a mental health disorder. However, many overweight teens use food to help them through troubled times. In these cases, mental health interventions may help individuals find more effective ways of satisfying their needs. Eating disorders are on the rise. About 90% to 95% of teens with eating disorders are girls, but eating disorders do occur in male teenagers, usually athletes. The mortality rate for eating disorders is about 9%—a mental health problem that can lead to death.

Common eating disorders in adolescence are anorexia nervosa and bulimia. **Anorexia nervosa** is a prolonged refusal to eat to keep body weight at a minimum. It is characterized by an intense fear of becoming fat and a relentless pursuit of thinness. **Bulimia** is a cycle of binge eating followed by purging. Anorexia is seen from about 12 years old, with peaks around 13 to 14 years and again at 17 to 18 years. Bulimia often may not occur until 17 years or so. Both disorders also occur in adults, but the incidence decreases sharply after the mid-30s.

The typical picture of an anorectic teen is one of an overly cooperative, achievement-oriented girl who sees herself as overweight and begins to diet. There may be a history of eating or mood disorders in the family. Over a period of months, her concern with dieting evolves into an obsessive need to be thin. All her behaviors soon center around remaining thin. She may restrict calories, exercise excessively, induce vomiting,

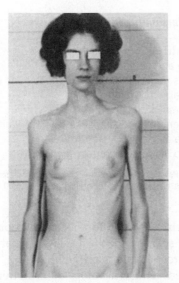

FIGURE **14-1** Adolescent with anorexia nervosa.

or use laxatives, diuretics, diet pills, or street drugs to prevent even the smallest weight gain.

As the disorder progresses, the teen cuts back on her social activities and begins to avoid friends. She becomes increasingly anxious, irritable, and depressed. Now all her thoughts focus on food and weight loss. Although it is glaringly apparent to everyone who sees her, the anorectic teen will deny that a problem even exists. Soon the physical and psychological effects of starvation begin to appear (Figure 14-1). Long-term, even life-threatening complications can result unless medical and mental health interventions are undertaken.

Bulimia is more difficult to detect because of the secretive nature of the problem. However, it is estimated that as many as 20% of college-age women are bulimic. The road to bulimia begins with an intense interest in dieting. Struggles with food result in secret binge-eating episodes in which the person consumes 5,000 to 20,000 calories of high-carbohydrate foods. Feelings of intense guilt or depression follow bingeing. The teen then makes extreme attempts to control weight gain through vomiting, exercise, or the use of drugs. Self-imposed starvation may occur between binges. Some weight loss may occur, but body weight usually remains within 20% of normal. The medical complications of bulimia include erosion of tooth enamel, gastric dilation, inflammation of the pancreas, and electrolyte abnormalities. Most people with bulimia are aware of their behavior, but they are ashamed and afraid to admit that they are out of control. Binge episodes frequently follow a stressful life event.

Treatment for eating disorders has three goals: to manage the medical dangers, such as metabolic disturbances, cardiac problems, and dehydration; to restore normal nutrition and eating patterns; and to meet the psychiatric treatment needs of the client and the family.

Nursing (care team) diagnoses for eating disorders include activity intolerance, imbalanced nutrition (more or less than body requirements), disturbed thought processes, disturbed body image, chronic low self-esteem, defensive coping, denial, and disabled family coping. Attempts are made to treat the teen within the family setting, but if the condition is severe, the teen is hospitalized. A plan to gradually improve the teen's nutritional intake (a refeeding program) is developed by the dietitian and other team members. Therapeutic interventions are designed to stabilize the client's physical condition. Force feeding is discouraged because the goal is to help the teen choose to eat.

As the teen begins to feel better, she is encouraged to express her feelings. With both types of eating disorders, the primary issue is one of control, not food. Psychotherapy helps the teen recognize underlying depression that is often present and develop more effective coping skills.

CHEMICAL DEPENDENCY

For adolescents, the temptation to "find out what it is like" is a strong motivator. Most teens who experiment with alcohol and drugs do not become dependent or addicted. However, for a growing number of teens, the use of chemicals is becoming a way of coping with the difficulties of life. The problems associated with substance abuse are many: accidents caused by lack of judgment, interpersonal violence, depression, and worsening relationships with others. Young adolescents who use chemical substances usually become sexually active at an earlier age. Perhaps the most critical fact is that the use of chemicals interferes with normal adolescent growth and development.

All adolescents are at risk for developing substance abuse problems, especially those who were abused as young children. Teens from families who approve of, use, or promote the use of chemicals and teens with other mental health problems are also at high risk. **Chemical dependency** is a state in which one physically and psychologically requires a drug. Identifying teens with substance abuse or chemical dependency problems is difficult. Many of the signs and symptoms of long-term abuse are absent.

Teens who become chemically dependent progress through four general stages: experimentation, active seeking, preoccupation, and burnout (Box 14-3). Frequently, the most important clues to substance abuse in teens are small ones. A change in habits, mood, or personality often hints of a problem. Sometimes a teen will suddenly become rebellious. The adolescent will disappear with friends and avoid contact with family members. The teen who becomes chemically dependent needs mental health intervention. Underneath a hardened exterior there lies an individual who has few friends and little or no self-esteem.

Treatment focuses on helping the teen replace the use of chemicals with more effective coping skills. Many

| Box 14-3 | *Stages of Chemical Dependency* |

1. *Experimentation:* Pleasant moods and social belonging associated with drugs are experienced; drugs are used for the first time within the comfort of the peer or other social group.
2. *Actively seeking:* Teen looks forward to and actively seeks out the mood changes brought about by the chemicals; becomes expert in the use of chemicals to regulate moods; schoolwork and relationships with family erode; friends become limited to other teens who "use."
3. *Preoccupation:* Teen believes that he or she cannot cope without chemicals; has lost control over the use of the drug; develops a tolerance, and may begin to use other substances; chemical is now used to prevent withdrawal symptoms; psychosocial functioning begins to fail; friends are lost and may be replaced with antisocial, illegal, or violent behaviors.
4. *Burnout:* Focus of drug use now is to prevent negative feelings; if the teen attempts to stop using the chemical, withdrawal symptoms appear; those who progress to this level of addiction are usually no longer able to function productively in society; most are late adolescents or young adults.

| Box 14-4 | *Personality Disorders* |

A **personality disorder** is "an enduring pattern of inner experience and behavior that:
1. Deviates markedly from the expectations of the individual's culture
2. Is universal and inflexible
3. Has an onset in adolescence or early adulthood
4. Is stable over time
5. Leads to distress or impairment"

From American Psychiatric Association: *Diagnostic and statistical manual of mental disorders*, ed 4, text revision, Washington, DC, 2000, The Association.

treatment programs in the United States, Canada, and Great Britain are modeled on the principles of Alcoholics Anonymous, whose goal is a chemical-free lifestyle. Settings for treating teens range from outpatient counseling to residential treatment programs and therapeutic communities. Individual psychotherapy and group psychotherapy are often combined with behavioral and cognitive therapies. Therapeutic inpatient care provides a safe environment because many of these teens are suicidal.

Drug and alcohol abuse is a complex problem affecting all aspects of an adolescent's life. Few teens seek treatment, and therapies for chemical dependency vary in their effectiveness. Prevention and early recognition remain the most effective tools for coping with adolescent substance abuse.

PERSONALITY DISORDERS

Personality is the combination of behavioral patterns that each of us develops to cope with living. Our personalities are important parts of our identities. They characterize us as unique individuals and allow us to function effectively within society. However, adolescents who have long histories of inappropriate or maladaptive behaviors may be diagnosed with a personality disorder. Box 14-4 lists the common behaviors associated with these problems.

A major characteristic of a personality disorder is **impulsivity**—the temptation to engage in acts harmful to oneself or others. Spur-of-the-moment decisions lead to inappropriate actions, such as overeating, casual sexual practices, shoplifting, and thrill seeking. Intense

emotional changes lead to anger and depression. Self-esteem and self-confidence are low. The ability to look inward (introspection) is minimal.

These teens tend to develop "all-or-nothing" relationships, in which others are either idealized or considered worthless. They flip between distance and closeness within their relationships and harbor deep fears of being abandoned. Some become suspicious. Many attempt suicide. Frequently a personality disorder will coexist with another mental health diagnosis.

Treatment for teens with personality disorders involves the use of psychotherapy and various medications. Recent studies have shown that personality disorders may be related to problems with the neurotransmitter serotonin. Treatment with selective serotonin reuptake inhibitors (SSRIs), such as fluoxetine hydrochloride (Prozac), has been successful. Long-term individual therapy, in combination with selective medications, provides a promising outlook for teens with personality disorders.

SEXUAL DISORDERS

One of the tasks during adolescence is to establish a sexual identity and role. To do this, many teens experiment with various sexual attitudes, outlooks, and behaviors. Attitudes about sexuality change as societies evolve; therefore the definition of a sexual disorder is characterized by significant distress and impaired ability to function.

Adolescents with sexual disorders relating to gender identity are still struggling with conflicts that began in childhood. Individuals with **gender identity disorders** have a continual discomfort with their assigned gender. There is a strong and persistent need to identify with the other gender. The individual often insists on wearing clothing designed for the other gender. During play, he or she identifies with or role-plays the opposite gender. Playmates and activities are limited to those associated with the desired gender. For example, a boy might like to wear dresses, play house acting as the mother, and choose only girls as friends.

As these teens grow older, they become preoccupied with ridding themselves of their sexual characteristics and assuming those of the desired gender. They

Think About 14-2

Neurotic behaviors are recognized by the person as unacceptable, recurring, and persistent. Behaviors may be odd or unusual, but they are within socially acceptable limits. The individual is in contact with reality and able to carry out the activities of daily living.

Psychotic behaviors are characterized by personality disintegration, reduced awareness, and an inability to function within socially acceptable limits. The individual is not in contact with reality and is unable to carry out the activities of daily living.

• When do neurotic behaviors become psychotic?

Box 14-5 | *Warning Signs of Teen Suicide*

Change in grades at school
Loss of interest, initiative
Rapidly changing emotional highs and lows
Defies rules, regulations; pushes limits
May become secretive
Withdraws from family interactions
Changes in personal hygiene
Isolates self from others
Discusses suicide with peers, close friends
Gives away prized possessions
Hints about intentions (e.g., "After I'm gone …")

---

may request hormonal therapy, surgery, or other procedures that may produce characteristics of the desired gender. Treatment consists of medical and mental health therapies to relieve distress and help teens solve their problems.

Sexually acting out is common for teens. However, if their behaviors result in discomfort or harm to themselves or others, society defines the behaviors as inappropriate. Many sexual problems faced by adolescents can be solved with good communication skills. Replacing ignorance with accurate knowledge can assist a teen along the road toward healthy sexual maturity.

PSYCHOSIS

The defining feature of **schizophrenia** and other psychoses is a grossly impaired ability to function because of not being in touch with reality. Psychotic disorders are discussed in detail in Chapter 31, but here it is important to know that the onset of schizophrenia usually takes place in adolescence. The adolescent who suffers from schizophrenia is typically a good child who begins to develop a whole new set of (sometimes bizarre) behaviors and activities (see Think About 14-2).

The major characteristic of adolescent psychosis is **loss of contact with reality.** The teen may have hallucinations, delusions, and feelings of paranoia. He or she lacks judgment, behaves impulsively, and shows little insight. Behaviors may become inappropriate, ritualistic, or repetitive. Disordered thought patterns lead to communication problems and difficulties with relationships. As a result of this loss of contact with reality, personal hygiene (even eating and drinking) may be neglected. The teen usually requires hospitalization and close supervision.

Treatment for psychosis includes a combination of psychotherapy and medications. Antipsychotics, antidepressants, and lithium may be ordered. Care is focused on providing basic physical needs, including feeding, bathing, and exercise; providing a safe environment; and developing skills for successful living. As the

adolescent begins to respond to treatment, education about the nature and control of the disorder is begun. Schizophrenia is lifelong, and the major problem with management is poor compliance in taking the prescribed medications. Both adolescents and their families need ongoing support. Family members are often encouraged to join a support group for the emotional assistance needed to cope with a teen who has a psychosis.

SUICIDE

The number of adolescents who take their own lives is growing at an alarming rate. From 1960 to 2000, the rate of adolescent suicide more than doubled (U.S. Bureau of the Census, 2001). In 2004 alone, suicide rates for teens increased by 18% (Ash, 2007). Adolescent girls attempt suicide three times more often than their male counterparts, but boys are more successful in their attempts because they choose more lethal methods. Teens who are hospitalized for injuries or motor vehicle (especially single-car) accidents may actually be attempting suicide.

A suicide attempt by an adolescent is a call for help. Today's society is complex and has many stresses on a developing adolescent. Factors that may influence suicidal behavior include more competition for fewer resources, exposure to abuse and neglect, instability within the family, the presence of depression or other illness, the availability of handguns or other weapons, and an increased use of alcohol and drugs. Box 14-5 lists the warning signs of suicide.

Teenagers who attempt suicide usually fall into one of three groups: the teen with depression, the teen who is trying to influence others, and the teen with a serious mental health problem. When a teen cannot keep up with school and social activities, withdraws from others, has problems eating or sleeping, and feels hopeless, then he or she is at risk for suicide resulting from depression.

The teen who uses a suicidal gesture as a way to get back at someone (usually a parent, boyfriend, or girlfriend) is attempting to influence someone. Often there is little or no depression and no real wish to die.

SAMPLE CLIENT CARE PLAN 14-1
Suicidal Adolescent

ASSESSMENT *History.* Rita is a 15-year-old girl admitted to the medical unit of the local hospital for suicidal attempts. About 4 hours ago, she consumed approximately 35 tablets of diazepam (Valium) and had her stomach pumped in the emergency department. Three earlier suicidal attempts have involved drug overdoses and slashed wrists. *Current Findings.* A sleepy teenage girl in no acute distress. Answers questions with one-word statements. States she attempted suicide to "get everyone off my back." Skin on wrists and forearms has numerous jagged scars. Rita refused further physical assessment.

Multidisciplinary Diagnosis	*Planning/Goals*
Risk for self-directed violence related to family behaviors, developmental conflict	Rita will contract with staff for no suicidal attempts. Rita will verbalize an awareness of her pattern of self-harm by May 7.

Therapeutic Interventions

Intervention	Rationale	Team Member
1. Assess potential for self-harm.	Helps prevent harm or injury; helps determine level of surveillance needed.	All
2. Ensure safety; place on suicidal precautions.	Prevents impulsive reactions to stressful situations.	Nsg
3. Monitor activities continually for first 24 hours.	Helps assess level of suicidal intention, effectiveness of behaviors.	Nsg
4. Establish a verbal or written contract not to harm self; renew every 24 hours.	Prevents suicidal behaviors, demonstrates respect.	Nsg
5. Establish rapport; offer support; be available to listen; ensure confidentiality.	Acceptance of Rita's feelings shows respect and encourages self-worth even though her behavior is unacceptable.	All
6. Encourage Rita to keep a diary and write in it daily.	Helps Rita identify her reactions and behaviors.	Psy

Evaluation

Rita willingly contracted each day for no self-harm. By May 1, Rita was seeking Mary P., a nurse, for interaction. By May 7, Rita was able to identify one area in which she was having problems.

❓ **CRITICAL THINKING** QUESTIONS.

1. Given her history of past suicide attempts, what can be done to change Rita's harmful coping behaviors?

2. How important is therapeutic rapport in this case?

A complete client care plan includes several other diagnoses and interventions.
Nsg, Nursing staff; *Psy,* psychologist.

The teen is angry, and the gesture has the goal of gaining attention or scaring another person. Teenage girls engage in this type of suicidal behavior more often than boys.

Adolescents who attempt suicide in the third group are seriously ill. They can see no other way out of their discomfort and actually welcome the relief they expect death to bring.

The highest group at risk for suicide is white adolescent males who have expressed their intention to die. Previous attempts, written plans, and available tools for committing suicide all heighten the risk for future attempts. Increases in suicidal attempts are often seen after a schoolmate has committed suicide. Health care providers who work with adolescents must assess every teen for his or her suicidal risk. Chapter 27 takes a more in-depth look at this problem.

The goals of treatment for suicidal adolescents are to protect them from harm, build trusting therapeutic relationships, and assist them in developing self-awareness and alternate coping skills. Sample Client Care Plan 14-1 illustrates a client care plan designed for a suicidal adolescent.

THERAPEUTIC INTERVENTIONS

Adolescents require special care because they are developing and maturing at the same time they are experiencing mental health problems. Although each adolescent is unique, several therapeutic interventions can serve as strategies for all teens. The relationship between client and caregiver serves as an instrument for understanding and helping each teen. Therapeutic communication skills help adolescents define their problems and then develop new and more effective ways of solving them. Specific interventions for adolescents center around five basic strategies (Box 14-6).

Box 14-6   *Therapeutic Interventions for Suicidal Teens*

Surveillance
Limit setting
Building self-esteem and confidence
Role modeling
Skill development

SURVEILLANCE AND LIMIT SETTING

Surveillance is the process of watching over clients to determine if they are safe, are following their rules, are making good decisions, or need adult intervention. The degree of the problem determines the amount of surveillance. Some adolescents need only minimal supervision, whereas others may require 24 hour/day observation. The goal of surveillance is to assist teens in developing new skills and coping methods, as well as to protect them from harm. The alert caregiver can turn a potential crisis situation into an opportunity for growth.

Setting limits is also essential for adolescents. Part of the process of growing up is to test the limits of authority. Teens are struggling with learning to control their emotions. Care providers work to change the focus of control from external to internal (self-control). Situations in which the teen attempts to exceed the limits are treated as learning experiences. When limits are set on behaviors, it is important that the teen understand what is acceptable behavior and the consequences of inappropriate behaviors. The goal of setting limits is to encourage responsibility.

Quite often, adolescents do well with the problem-solving approach. Here the teen is asked what he or she is feeling and doing. The teen is encouraged to see if the behavior is helping to get what he or she wants. The teen then develops a plan for meeting the goal or coping with the feelings and follows it through. This process helps adolescents learn to solve problems and gain some control over their situations. Positive actions are praised and reinforced, and the teen is encouraged to apply the process to other situations.

BUILDING SELF-ESTEEM

Adolescents, even the best-adjusted ones, experience the discomfort of low self-esteem at some time or another; but for the teen with mental health problems, this discomfort can be great. Teenagers are masters at reading nonverbal behaviors. Caregivers who use eye contact, address each teen by name, and actively listen make them feel accepted and valued. Do not lecture or give advice. Instead, direct teens toward problem solving and assuming responsibility for their feelings. Convey respect by requesting rather than ordering, and thank them for their help. Praise each small effort, and point out the adolescent's progress (Box 14-7). If limits must be enforced, then do so without anger or embarrassment for the teen.

Box 14-7   *Interventions to Build Self-Esteem*

Use **eye contact** (consider the cultural background).
Address each individual by his or her **name.**
Actively **listen** (use the therapeutic communications in Chapter 10).
Convey **respect**—ask, do not order.
Help teens to assume **responsibility** for their behaviors and their consequences.
Praise each effort at changing behaviors, and point out their progress and successes.
Teach **problem solving,** and help them apply it to their own behaviors and problems.
Enforce limits respectfully; focus on the behaviors that need to be changed.
The goal is to **encourage responsibility** for one's own actions and self-development.

Self-esteem is also fostered through **role models.** The impression caregivers present will have an impact on the effectiveness of therapeutic actions. Adolescents watch how their therapists and care providers interact with each other and solve problems. It is important to remember that caregivers are always being watched and evaluated. If teens feel that your behaviors are effective, they will often adopt them for use in similar situations. Acting as a role model for healthy behavior requires a lot of energy, but it is a highly effective way of helping teens learn to cope.

SKILL DEVELOPMENT

One of the most important therapeutic interventions involves assisting adolescents in developing the skills that are essential for functional living. Caregivers help their teen clients with cognitive (intellectual) skills, such as applying the problem-solving process to actual problems. They help young clients practice appropriate social skills. Working cooperatively within a group, learning how to listen to other people, and exploring new methods for controlling anger or aggression are other therapeutic actions designed to help adolescents develop **effective living skills.** Working with adolescent clients is demanding and rewarding. Effective mental health interventions at this stage of life are extremely important if we are to prevent future problems.

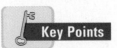

Key Points

- The passage from child to adult is a time of physical, sexual, and psychosocial growth.
- Many common problems of adolescence arise from internal sources and external sources.
- A mental health problem exists when an adolescent's problems impair performance or threaten physical well-being.

- The category of disruptive behavioral disorders is divided into attention-deficit/hyperactivity disorder (ADHD) and conduct disorders.
- Emotional ups and downs are a normal part of adolescence, but many teens suffer from anxiety and mood disorders, such as depression.
- Anorexia nervosa and bulimia are eating disorders characterized by severe disturbances in eating behavior, which can result in a body that is far below its ideal weight.
- Teens who become chemically dependent or addicted move through four general stages: experimentation, active seeking, preoccupation, and burnout.
- Adolescents with long histories of inappropriate or maladaptive behaviors may be diagnosed with a personality disorder.
- A sexual disorder is diagnosed when problems cause the teen significant distress and impair his or her ability to function.

- The major characteristic of adolescent psychosis, such as schizophrenia, is a loss of contact with reality.
- Teenagers who attempt suicide are usually depressed, are trying to influence others, or suffer from a serious mental health problem.
- In addition to the use of therapeutic relationships and communications, interventions for adolescents center around five basic strategies: surveillance, limit setting, building self-esteem and confidence, role modeling, and skill development.

evolve Be sure to visit the companion Evolve site at http://evolve.elsevier.com/Morrison-Valfre/ for additional online resources.

15 Problems of Adulthood

evolve http://evolve.elsevier.com/Morrison-Valfre/

Objectives

Upon completion of this chapter, the student will be able to:

1. List two developmental tasks of young adults.
2. Explain the importance of having a strong sense of personal identity.
3. Identify three characteristics of a successful adult.
4. Discuss three internal (developmental) problems faced by most adults.
5. Name four stresses associated with parenting or guiding the next generation.
6. Describe how environmental problems can limit an adult's ability to function effectively.
7. Identify two effects of a lack of social support for adults.
8. Explain how the fear of human immunodeficiency virus (HIV) and acquired immunodeficiency syndrome (AIDS) is affecting young adults.
9. Name three therapeutic interventions to help the psychosocial functioning of adults with problems.

Key Terms

acquired immunodeficiency syndrome (AIDS) (p. 164)
adulthood (p. 159)
marriage (p. 162)
maturity (mə-CHOOR-ĭ-tē) (p. 159)
mortality (mŏr-TĂL-ĭ-tē) (p. 161)
poverty (PŎV-ĕr-tē) (p. 163)
social isolation (p. 164)
spiritual dimension (p. 161)

For many years, adulthood was thought of as the end of growth and development. Once adolescents reached the age of 21 years or so, they were viewed as adults, completely mature and ready to assume their full places in society. Adulthood was once considered a time of stability with little or no change. Today, however, we see adulthood as dynamic, filled with learning, struggle, rewards, and change. Adulthood is a time of personal, professional, and social development. It is the time to nurture and guide the next generation and for individuals to move beyond themselves and direct their energies for the benefit of others.

The period of life labeled **adulthood** includes ages (approximately) 18 to 65 years. **Maturity** is the ability to accept responsibility for one's actions, delay gratification, and make priorities. Remember, these

divisions are for the sake of discussion. In reality, each adult is an individual who ages at his or her own particular pace.

Adulthood, like every other age, is filled with tasks, problems, and opportunities for learning. Refer back to Chapter 5, and review Erikson's developmental theory and Maslow's hierarchy of needs. All young adults are faced with the developmental tasks of establishing their careers, their identities, and the relationships that will emotionally support them throughout their lives. As they age, adults must learn to cope with changes in families, careers, and relationships. All this is accomplished within a society so complex that no single person is able to understand its workings.

ADULT GROWTH AND DEVELOPMENT

Physical growth for men is complete by about 21 years of age. Women mature earlier, reaching their full growth around 17 years of age. Physical abilities are at their peak efficiency in young adulthood. Body systems have a remarkable ability to compensate, so the young adult is able to maintain a healthy state with little interruption, even during periods of illness (Edelman and Mandle, 2006). Because of this remarkable ability, young adults usually have few if any health concerns. Although many adults begin to show signs of aging after 30 years old, a healthy lifestyle and the absence of any chronic conditions usually allow them to enjoy good health well into later life.

Physical growth may be complete, but adults continue to develop in other dimensions. The emotional, intellectual, sociocultural, and spiritual areas of one's character begin to receive attention. The developmental tasks of young adulthood are to establish oneself as fully functional and capable of living independently. Other core tasks include choosing a career or vocation, establishing long-term goals, and committing oneself to personal relationships.

For many, adulthood is also a time of change, marriage, family, and parenting. Middle adulthood sees the growth and maturity of one's family and profession. As individuals encounter each life change, they rely on previously learned behaviors to help them cope. If one has learned to solve problems effectively as a child, then adulthood will pose fewer crises.

However, problems of childhood, if not resolved, can follow one through life.

Emotional development of young adults centers on learning to function within a stressful environment. Work and school offer many opportunities to cope with stress. When used positively, stress motivates young adults to achieve their goals, some of which are long term. When ignored, stress can lead to many problems. Young adults still have occasional emotional outbursts, but they attempt to find new ways of coping with the many feelings experienced during this time. Those who care for young adults must be willing to explore inappropriate or troublesome feelings with them. Assessments of the emotional status for all adults should include "the client's perception of how his emotions affect his ability to develop satisfactory relationships or achieve professional goals" (Rawlins, Williams, and Beck, 1993).

Later in adulthood, emotional development deals with the struggle of seeing oneself age. Individuals who have successfully coped with life's problems gracefully accept and adapt to the fact that they are growing older. The anxiety generated by the prospect of a limited time on this earth motivates many middle adults to make the best of the benefits of middle age.

Fear of poor health, death, and loss of financial security causes anxiety in many adults, which can result in stress-related illness and behavioral problems. Feelings of anger can arise when interactions with work and family members are not as expected. Guilt over parents, children, and the failure to meet personal goals is often experienced. Health care providers should always assess their adult clients for signs of stress, anxiety, and depression. About 15% of adults in the United States experience a major depressive problem at some time, but less than one third receive treatment (U.S. Surgeon General, 2002).

Intellectual development focuses on the young adult's ability to solve intellectual and abstract problems. Young adults must process large amounts of information and learn many new skills to become successful in education or employment. As young adults effectively cope with their situations, their horizons broaden and they develop flexibility—the ability to adapt to change. This flexibility, combined with the willingness to take risks, encourages them to respond to available personal and career opportunities.

Adults continue to grow intellectually if they use their abilities to think. People who exercise their intellects have few losses of mental ability. Those who do not engage in productive mental activities may experience a decline in intellectual performance as they age. The "use it or lose it" principle also applies to the use of intellectual abilities.

Social development for young adults focuses on interactions and relationships with others (Box 15-1). If the sense of personal identity is strong and well established, individuals learn to form close personal

Box 15-1	*Social Tasks of Adults*

Commitment—to significant other, to career
Communications—with significant other, with children, with co-workers
Compromise—with significant other, with children, with co-workers

relationships and become willing to make lasting commitments. Habits learned in childhood are likely to become lifelong. Patterns of communicating and interacting with others help to establish young adults' interactional styles, which have a strong impact on employment, relationships, and choice of goals. For example, low self-esteem and withdrawal from social situations may result from an ineffective interactional style with inadequate social or communication skills.

Establishing intimacy is an important task for young adults. Those who have strong senses of personal identity are able to merge themselves with another in marriage or a long-term relationship. Individuals still struggling with their identities may seek serial relationships to fill their unmet psychosocial needs.

Parenting is a major challenge for most adults. The responsibilities of parenthood force an individual to shift energies from self to caring for others. Parenthood is a 24 hours per day career. Its demands can create anxiety, feelings of inadequacy, and a sense of isolation and helplessness. Women who manage both parenting and working outside the home are especially vulnerable. As the family unit gradually stabilizes and children begin to gain independence, parents often expand their focus beyond the immediate family or work situation and become involved in community activities.

Social tasks for adults also relate to the change from parent back to the role of partner. As children prepare for their careers and move out of the home, the middle-age couple has the opportunity to redefine their marriage relationship. With the responsibilities of parenting over, the couple begins to reexplore the communication, commitment, and compromise aspects of their relationship.

Marriages that have weathered the challenges of career and parenting are based on a solid foundation. Each partner recognizes the individuality of the other and the other's need to achieve personal growth. Couples who have **effective communications** can freely share their attitudes, opinions, and emotions. They reaffirm their commitment to each other and the relationship. Couples who are unable to communicate are frequently faced with the possibility of divorce or separation.

Compromise involves a willingness to negotiate and enter into interactions in which neither person wins or loses. Conflicts are resolved by defining and solving the problem. The focus is kept on the issue. Couples who compromise, communicate openly, listen carefully, and try to understand their partner's point of view find that their relationship is respected and cherished.

Development within the spiritual dimension focuses on defining one's value system and belief system. Young adults often challenge their current religious practices by changing churches or refusing to attend services. A reexamination of values occurs as individuals become established within the community and begin to raise families. Children offer many opportunities for parents to reflect on their values, beliefs, and ethics.

The spiritual tasks of adults are also concerned with finding meaning in life. Religious and spiritual beliefs are reexamined in light of one's own mortality (eventually having to die). Religious, social, and community activities become important. Volunteering to help others enriches adults' lives and provides many opportunities for socialization.

Frequently, middle-age adults will dramatically change their lifestyles. The 40-year-old wealthy businessperson who sells everything and volunteers at a homeless shelter and the mother who begins to study for a college degree are examples. Adults who do not or cannot find meaning in their lives become stagnant, self-absorbed, and isolated. The potential for serious mental health problems is greater for the unhappy, self-focused adult, no matter what the age.

To summarize, adults with good mental health are able to adapt to life's changes. Once their personal identities have been established, they are capable of using life experiences as lessons in personal growth. They develop the abilities to solve problems, set priorities, and identify reasonable expectations for themselves. They form bonds with other people and become willing to devote their energies to guiding the next generation or making the world a better place in which to live. They are able to give of themselves in both intimate and social situations, and their self-confidence remains unaffected by the opinions of others. There is a balance between give and take. In short, successful adults have developed the inner strength to carry them through the joys, sorrows, and everyday activities of daily living (Box 15-2).

COMMON PROBLEMS OF ADULTHOOD

Diagnosable mental health disorders that affect adults are described in detail in later chapters. Here we consider some of the risk factors and difficulties faced by adults in today's society.

All adults are faced with situations that produce anxiety. The stresses that accompany everyday life are many. Physical and psychological stress-related problems can develop when individuals become too anxious. Common difficulties that challenge adults are divided into internal and external types of problems. One's personal outlook (internal) defines stressful or

Box 15-2 *Characteristics of a Successful Adult*

Accepts self
Adapts to changes, is flexible
Establishes priorities
Sets realistic goals and expectations
Learns from past experiences
Functions in stressful circumstances
Has achieved emotional control
Solves problems and thinks abstractly
Makes sound decisions
Establishes and maintains intimate and social relationships
Guides next generation
Finds meaning in life
Finds balance between give and take
Has inner strength to effectively adapt to new situations

anxious situations, whereas the environment (external) plays an important role in determining the opportunities for jobs, education, and living conditions.

INTERNAL (DEVELOPMENTAL) PROBLEMS

Because life is a dynamic process, everyone must cope with change. As we do, we learn and, hopefully, develop more effective ways of living. As children, our developmental problems are clear. As adolescents, we discover that we are unique individuals within a seemingly ever-changing body. Adults experience developmental problems too, but theirs are not so obvious. They must cope with decisions about themselves and about relationships, education, occupation, marriage, and family. Choices made affect one's life. When adults feel they have made the right choices, they develop the inner strength to weather future storms. When they allow anxiety, anger, or other emotions to be the focus, effective adaptation does not occur as easily. Those who provide health care for adults should be aware of clients' problems and coping skills. Intervening early is a good form of preventive mental health care.

Personal Identity

Problems with establishing a strong personal identity begin in childhood. People who were not guided, nurtured, or accepted in childhood find it more difficult to feel good about themselves as adults. Overcoming a childhood filled with negative examples is a difficult task. It requires the willingness to look at one's behaviors and learn new methods of handling complex situations. With the support and examples of effectively functioning people, many adults are able to overcome the difficulties of their pasts. They mature into capable individuals with strong senses of personal identity and self-worth.

Care providers have many opportunities to assist individuals by offering the emotional support and encouragement to problem solve. They can act as valued resources, directing their clients to support groups and other community resources. Helping a young adult develop a positive personal identity will lessen the possibility of future mental health problems. Box 15-3 lists several interventions designed to help young adults establish a positive personal identity.

Problems of personal identity can also relate to a person's intellectual abilities: how one solves problems, makes decisions, and interprets stress. When an individual's ability to solve problems in effective ways is limited, behavioral and personality difficulties are much more common.

Emotional problems plague all adults, but those who are able to put things into perspective cope with fewer stress-related effects. Mentally healthy adults can identify and accept their emotions without acting inappropriately on them. Unfortunately, anger-control problems plague many adults, especially those who were exposed to aggressive acts as children. Drug and alcohol abuse may also result from a person's need to deal with emotional problems, such as feelings of inadequacy, anxiety, or depression.

Interpersonal Relationships

Human beings are always changing and adapting. Young adults, who are still discovering their unique natures, also search for relationships that will fulfill their needs and encourage their personal growth. Adulthood is a time for commitment to others, be it through marriage or career. The need for intimacy and belonging is great throughout life, and adults usually form many relationships. Young adults often seek relationships in an attempt to fill a personal void or escape an unhappy situation. Sometimes errors in judgment have enormous consequences for their future.

Many adults commit themselves solely to another in marriage. In U.S. society, marriage is a legal state that bonds two people as a family unit. Most often, children are produced and the responsibilities of life focus on nurturing and providing for the offspring. As children mature and leave home, the marriage relationship is reevaluated and decisions are made to continue or end the relationship. Other adults choose to cohabitate (live together) in opposite-gender or same-gender relationships. Homosexual families fill the same needs and engage in the same tasks as traditional families, but they are at greater risk for mental health problems because of the stigma and discrimination that still exist.

Many adults (especially women) are caught in the cycle of violence that comes with abusive relationships. Despite more frequent health care visits, most women still are not screened for intimate partner violence (Bauer, 2002). Chapters 25 and 26 discuss these problems in depth.

Caring for one's aging parents is fast becoming a problem for many adults. Today members of the "sandwich generation" face the dual responsibilities of caring for their children and their aging parents at the same time. Providing care for both adds many new stresses to the family as adults work to balance the requirements of career, children, and parents.

Conflict relating to gender roles and their stereotypes can arise when adults wish to engage in activities, behaviors, or career choices that traditionally belong to one gender. To illustrate, a woman who wants to become a heavy equipment operator faces greater social resistance than a woman who works as a beautician.

Problems with interpersonal relationships can extend to work and social environments. Individuals who have little or no ability to see how their attitudes and behaviors affect other people often have difficulties with long-term relationships. They become superficial and unwilling to consider the feelings of others. Small problems with social relationships can balloon into serious mental health problems. Learning effective communication and interpersonal skills can spell the difference between a functional adult and an unhappy, unfulfilled adult. Nurses and other caregivers can play an important role in preventing mental illness by identifying those clients with interpersonal problems and offering them support, education, and resources.

Guiding the Next Generation

Most adults have children, and children are not isolated events. They arrive as package deals, along with responsibility, fatigue, self-doubt, love, and joy. If pregnancies are planned, children are eagerly anticipated. Unplanned pregnancies, however, are stressful and sometimes unwanted. Choices about terminating the pregnancy, single parenting, or marrying for the sake of the child are decisions faced by unmarried adults that will have an impact on the rest of their lives.

The child-rearing practices of adults vary considerably. Most parents raise their offspring based on how they were treated as children. Parents who were

---

| Box 15-3 | *Therapeutic Interventions for a Positive Personal Identity* |

Assist the individual to:
Define a life dream
Develop occupational choices and goals
Differentiate self from the nuclear family by sorting through the beliefs and values of childhood to establish a belief system that is one's own
Decide about relationship choices and levels of commitment, such as marriage, cohabitation, remaining single
Assess how one's emotions influence the ability to achieve professional goals and develop healthy interpersonal relationships

Data from Haber J and others: *Comprehensive psychiatric nursing*, ed 5, St. Louis, 1997, Mosby.

strongly disciplined as children tend to use physical discipline when correcting their children. Likewise, adults who were disciplined in nonphysical ways continue the practices with their offspring. Other factors, such as money, family relationships, safety, housing, health practices, and spiritual beliefs, all affect the family, parenting practices, and children. For example, relationships between individuals and with extended family members, as well as social interactions, can support or discourage certain child-rearing habits. Box 15-4 lists several factors that influence child-rearing practices.

The rise of single-parent families needs consideration. Today it is estimated that more than 8% of all households in the United States are headed by women alone (U.S. Census Bureau, 2002). In these families, the single parent must function as father, mother, and provider. The joys of children can be overshadowed by the work and stress of providing for them. Without support and intervention, these families have a high potential for developing several mental health problems.

Single parenthood can also be a positive experience. The conflict of different outlooks about child-rearing practices is not present. Providing the guidance that allows children to experience life in positive ways and securing environments free from adult conflicts are other rewards of single parenthood.

With remarriages (blended families) and adoptive families, children and adults who were once strangers instantly become relatives "without the shared experience of developing their parent-child relationship over time" (Stanhope and Lancaster, 2004). These families must establish new relationships, roles, and family boundaries. Sometimes they must cope with a natural parent living outside the family.

Childless adults contribute to the next generation through devotion to a career or volunteer activities. The need to share and leave one's mark increases by middle adulthood.

Economics

One of the greatest stressors for adults of all ages is financial security. Young adults must choose a vocation or profession that offers an opportunity to provide the necessities of life. Food, shelter, and clothing

cost money—a fact that many young adults fail to learn until they leave the security of the family. Decisions about education and training, made young in life, will affect the quality of living far into the future.

Unemployment is a multisided problem. A parent who does not work becomes unable to financially provide for the children. Loss of self-esteem and self-worth accompanies loss of employment. This absence of a regular income and its associated stresses begin the family on a downward spiral that may include poverty, physical illness, and psychosocial disorders. A stressful family environment with an unemployed head of household is associated with child neglect, maltreatment, and abuse. Care providers can play an important role in assisting families in finding support and retraining services.

Although adults experience many challenges, most learn to cope with each problem and apply lessons learned to the next difficulty. As time passes, the inner strength built through experience becomes a part of who we are. This inner strength provides encouragement to grow and expand beyond the limits of who we are today.

EXTERNAL (ENVIRONMENTAL) PROBLEMS

The environment plays a strong role in the development of an individual during childhood. In adulthood, one's environment can limit or encourage further development. Some of the major environmental problems affecting adults today include a lack of education, poverty, homelessness, substance abuse, human immunodeficiency virus (HIV)/acquired immunodeficiency syndrome (AIDS), and lack of social support. Each of these problems can have a strong impact on the mental health of adults. Health care providers should be aware of these problems.

Education

An individual's training or education is closely associated with his or her economic status. Less educated people tend to be poorer, with few savings or financial reserves. Many families live from paycheck to paycheck, where one small demand (e.g., the car breaking down or a sick child) can throw the family into financial turmoil. Adults who are vocationally trained or educated tend to have more financial and health care resources and are better able to cope with everyday problems. Encourage your clients to seek further education or training by referring them to various community agencies that offer help or training. A lack of education limits abilities and fosters disabilities.

The result of unemployment (or underemployment) is poverty. **Poverty** is the lack of resources necessary for reasonable and comfortable living. Poverty means unstable housing, poor educational opportunities, work problems, and an increased risk for becoming a victim. Adults who survive below the poverty line

---

Box 15-4	*Factors That Influence Child-Rearing Practices*

Family relationships
Financial status
Health practices
Housing, living environment, safety
Parenting styles
Socialization with others
Spiritual beliefs
Type of discipline

often have children who suffer because of their parents' misfortune. Poverty, homelessness, and a lack of education go hand in hand. Adults who must cope with this three-pronged dilemma usually need support and intervention.

The **homeless** are a diverse group. Many are single men, but one third are homeless women and children. Many chronically mentally ill people inhabit the streets because they are unable to use their resources wisely. Discouraged by their prospects, homeless individuals run a much greater risk for depression, drug abuse, and other mental health disorders. Homeless people have special health care needs. Health care interventions must consider each individual's situation and lifestyle. Therapeutic actions are effective when they are realistic and attainable (see Case Study 15-1).

Lack of Social Support

Perhaps one of the most distressing problems for adults is social isolation—a lack of meaningful interactions with others. Before the time of rapid transportation, families tended to remain in one geographical area for generations. Small communities were often composed of relatives and extended family members who could provide strong emotional

Case Study 15-1

Joan is a nurse in a center for homeless people located in a large U.S. city. She describes the qualifications necessary for her position: patience, persistence, and the ability to apply creative approaches to client care problems. Her role is one of facilitator and advocate who helps clients gain access to other services in the community. She ensures that each person is clean and presentable when requesting services. Although the shelter provides shower and laundry facilities, Joan makes sure everyone uses the toothbrushes, deodorant, soap, and razors.

She reschedules missed appointments for her homeless clients, providing for transportation if necessary. Clarifying instructions from other agencies and helping clients with job applications are also on her list of caregiving interventions. Every opportunity to provide client education is taken. Joan instructs her homeless clients on the importance of good nutrition, safe sexual practices, communicable diseases, and other health-related subjects. She works with each individual to set and reach realistic goals. She sees every person as worthy of respect and dignity. Although her successes may be small, "hearing someone express that since he was able to get help for his problems, he now feels better about himself and is motivated to change his lifestyle provides this nurse's personal reward and professional satisfaction in working with the homeless" (Foster, 1992).
- According to Maslow, what needs is Joan helping her clients fulfill? (Refer to Chapter 5.)
- What resources are available for the homeless in your community?

and social support during difficult times. People shared their anxieties, hopes, and difficulties with each other and received the emotional support and energy to cope with their problems.

Today, families live physically apart from each other—surviving as isolated, single units. The social interconnectedness that bonded people together is no longer intact. Adults must establish new connections, new relationships, and new support systems each time they move to a different community. This results in people feeling socially isolated and disconnected from their fellow human beings.

Social support is the friendship from others that helps carry individuals through life's more difficult moments. With trusted friends, adults can share their problems, concerns, and stresses. These interactions can make the difference between mental health and illness. Be sure to assess clients' social support systems (ask about friendships, and help them identify possible support people, such as neighbors or coworkers). Refer them to various support or community groups as needed. Remember that social isolation is not healthy for human beings. Acknowledging this fact can help prevent many future mental health difficulties.

Acquired Immunodeficiency Syndrome

Acquired immunodeficiency syndrome (AIDS) was first recognized in the United States in 1981. Since then, millions of people, especially adolescents and young adults, have been exposed to this devastating disease. It is spread through sexual activities, the sharing of needles, or exposure to blood and body fluids. AIDS prevents the body from fighting off infectious diseases, and its signs and symptoms are not apparent for many years in some cases.

People with AIDS often have vague physical complaints, such as night sweats, cough, weight loss, or fever. Other problems can include ear, nose, throat, or stomach complaints or skin changes. About one third suffer from anxiety, depression, or lapses in memory.

AIDS has an impact on all members of society, but it is especially felt among sexually active young adults. People this age are more vulnerable to contracting the disease because they lack the emotional maturity and judgment to make sound decisions and feel the invulnerability of youth—the attitude that "it will never happen to me." Only when a friend or loved one contracts the disease does its reality strike home. Adults who can appreciate the seriousness of the disease have made changes in their lifestyles or suffer the anxieties associated with high-risk behaviors.

Fear of AIDS has spread to persons whose lifestyles offer little likelihood of contracting the disease. The acronym AFRAIDS (acute fear regarding AIDS) has been coined to describe an anxiety-related condition caused by a fear of AIDS. Individuals with poor or marginal coping skills may find it difficult to deal with the emotional aspects of this epidemic.

Every health care provider has a responsibility to educate clients about AIDS. The most important tool for the prevention of this devastating disease is education. Knowledge can be a powerful weapon if it leads individuals toward making health-promoting decisions. Knowledge can decrease fear and anxiety. Knowledge can help in detecting the need for diagnosis and treatment. AIDS has many physical consequences, but its psychosocial and emotional effects can be equally devastating.

There are many potential health problems, both physical and mental, in the adult world. Decisions made regarding oneself and one's environment have greater consequences than they did during earlier years. Health care providers working with adult clients can find many opportunities to encourage and teach healthy living practices, which in turn can prevent future problems from developing.

MENTAL HEALTH PROBLEMS OF ADULTS

A great number of the mental health disorders experienced by adults have their roots in childhood. Adults who were diagnosed with attention-deficit/ hyperactivity disorder (ADHD), conduct disorders, or learning disorders in childhood must now learn to cope with the responsibilities of adulthood. Many become substance abusers, others become members of the prison system, and a few progress toward successful adulthood.

It is sobering to think that 22% of the adult population in the United States has some diagnosable mental disorder or that 5.4 million people meet the criteria for severe mental illness (Kessler and others, 1999). Millions of adults are struggling with depression or addictions (alcohol, gambling, shopping). All must cope with the problems and crises of everyday living. Health care providers have countless opportunities to provide the psychosocial care so needed by so many.

According to the **Diagnostic and Statistical Manual of Mental Disorders (DSM-IV-TR)** (see Appendix B), there are 16 categories of mental disorders. Box 15-5 lists adult categories. Remember, however, that beyond the diagnostic label lies an individual. If caregivers are willing to put aside their biases and values, they will do much to encourage higher levels of functioning in each client.

THERAPEUTIC INTERVENTIONS

Although specific interventions for each mental health disorder are described in later chapters, a look at the interventions available in every practice setting may be helpful. The focus of most therapeutic mental health interventions relates to prevention and assisting clients to cope.

HEALTH CARE INTERVENTIONS

When working with adults, nurses can use their assessment skills to uncover clients' descriptions of their difficulties. Frequently the physician or nurse will actively intervene with a problem that is not as important to a client as it is to the health care provider. Make sure clients define their problems. Therapeutic actions will have greater results if the goals of care are as important to the client as they are to the health care provider. Sample Client Care Plan 15-1 for an adult with situational problems offers some suggestions for interventions.

Work within the client's reality. Learn about the client's living conditions. Assess the cultural influences relating to the client (see Cultural Considerations 15-1). It does no good to instruct a client to take medication four times daily if he or she has no watch or means of telling time. Too many therapeutic interventions fail because the client's total situation is not considered.

Give clients written instructions if you expect educational efforts to be effective. Everyone experiences anxiety when interacting with the health care system. People do not remember information when they are under stress. Written instructions allow them to refer back to the information when they are less anxious and more willing to follow instructions.

PREVENTING MENTAL ILLNESS

Health care providers in every setting can do much to prevent mental-emotional disorders. Always remember that it is the whole person who receives our care.

Box 15-5   *DSM-IV-TR Classification of Adult Mental Health Disorders*

Adjustment disorders
Anxiety disorders
Cognitive disorders: delirium, dementia, amnesia
Dissociative disorders
Eating disorders
Factitious disorders
Impulse-control disorders
Mental disorders resulting from a general medical condition
Mood disorders
Personality disorders
Schizophrenia and other psychotic disorders
Sexual and gender identity disorders
Sleep disorders
Somatoform disorders
Substance-related disorders

Data from American Psychiatric Association: *Diagnostic and statistical manual of mental disorders,* ed 4, text revision, Washington, DC, 2000, The Association.

SAMPLE CLIENT CARE PLAN 15-1

Ineffective Coping

ASSESSMENT *History.* Jed is a 33-year-old man who has recently lost his job and his wife and is now being sued. Last night he had several drinks before driving home. His car ran off an embankment and rolled into an irrigation ditch. Jed was found uninjured, sleeping in the car early this morning. He has been referred to the clinic for evaluation. *Current Findings.* In no acute distress; several bruises on arms and face; odor of alcohol. Jed states that 6 months ago his business as a roofer failed. After 4 months of trying to find employment, Jed began to drink. One evening he and his wife had an argument. When he returned later that night, she had moved her personal belongings out of the house and left a note saying that his drinking was becoming more than she could tolerate. For the past 2 months Jed has been spending his time "getting drunk."

Multidisciplinary Diagnosis	*Planning/Goals*
Ineffective coping related to loss of support systems	Jed will remain sober throughout treatment. Jed will attend Alcoholics Anonymous meetings every evening. Jed will recognize his maladaptive behaviors and take action to solve his identified problems by July 10.

Therapeutic Interventions

Intervention	Rationale	Team Member
1. Establish a trusting relationship with Jed.	Trust must be present if problems are to be solved.	All
2. Assess for degree of anxiety, depression, intent to do self-harm.	To determine interventions needed; to understand Jed's viewpoint.	All
3. Help Jed identify each of his problems and current coping mechanisms.	Problems must be defined before they can be solved.	Psy, Nsg
4. Have Jed make a list of his available resources and support systems.	Use of previously successful coping mechanism helps develop multiple skills	Soc Svc
5. Replace the use of alcohol with crisis support person and phone number to call at any time.	Jed knows his drinking is an excuse to forget about his problems and is willing to call his support person when he wants a drink.	Nsg, Soc Svc
6. Help Jed devise new, more effective coping responses.	Builds on Jed's current abilities to solve problems.	All
7. Refer to Social Services for placement in the employment program.	Provides new resources for exploring job availability and opportunities.	

Evaluation

During the first 3 weeks of clinic visits, Jed had been drinking. By the fourth week, he had decided to quit drinking so that he could concentrate on "getting (his) life back together." By the sixth week, Jed was able to identify two of his most pressing problems.

? CRITICAL THINKING QUESTIONS

1. What strategies should Jed and his care providers devise to keep him from using alcohol as a coping mechanism?

2. How does establishing a trusting relationship with Jed help him solve his problems?

A complete client care plan includes several other diagnoses and interventions.
Nsg, Nursing staff; *Psy,* psychologist; *Soc Svc,* social services.

We may separate the human being into parts, but we must consider and treat the entire person.

Each physical illness has emotional components, and each mental disorder is accompanied by physical changes. Therapeutic interventions need to include all aspects of the client's problems. A positive step toward preventing mental illness is to recognize the need for making mental health interventions available for all individuals, not just those people who are "diagnosed" with a mental disorder.

 Cultural Considerations 15-1

Culture has a powerful influence on one's outlook relating to health and illness, especially mental illness. Some Appalachians, for example, have a general mistrust of health care organizations and seek help only in extreme situations. People in Burundi define illness as having insufficient food and poor hygiene. In the Dominican Republic, it is believed that people with "the evil eye" can cause illness in others, especially children. Health care providers must consider each client's cultural beliefs if treatment is to be effective.

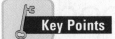

Key Points

- Adults continue to develop the emotional, intellectual, sociocultural, and spiritual dimensions of their characters long after physical growth is completed.
- Developmental tasks of young adults include choosing a career or vocation, establishing long-term goals, and committing to personal relationships with others.
- Parenting provides many challenges for most adults.
- Adults who are responsible for their behavior, use effective communications, are willing to make commitments, and cooperate with others successfully adapt to life's changes.
- If an individual's sense of personal identity is strong and well established, he or she learns to form close personal relationships.
- Developmental problems faced by most adults include decisions about themselves, their relationships, education, occupation, marriage, and family.
- The family, parenting practices, and children are affected by factors such as money, family relationships, safety, housing, health practices, and spiritual beliefs.

- Some of the major environmental problems affecting adults today include a lack of education, poverty, homelessness, substance abuse, and minimal social support.
- People feel socially isolated and disconnected without social support. Without trusted friends, adults cannot share their problems, concerns, and stresses.
- The acronym AFRAIDS (acute fear regarding AIDS) has been coined to describe an anxiety-related condition caused by fear of AIDS.
- Each physical illness has emotional components, and each mental disorder is accompanied by physical changes.
- Basic therapeutic interventions allow caregivers to elicit the client's definitions of his or her problems, work within the client's reality, and provide written instructions during educational efforts.
- Health care providers must recognize the need for making mental health interventions available for all clients.

evolve Be sure to visit the companion Evolve site at http://evolve.elsevier.com/Morrison-Valfre/ for additional online resources.

16 Problems of Late Adulthood

Objectives

Upon completion of this chapter, the student will be able to:

1. Examine the facts relating to three myths associated with aging.
2. Identify three mental and behavioral changes seen in older adults.
3. Explain how a lack of finances or access to health care affects the mental health of older adults.
4. Describe the drug misuse (abuse) patterns of older adults.
5. Define the term *elder abuse*, and describe a typical victim.
6. Explain how depression can affect older adults' abilities to function.
7. Discuss how the standards of geriatric nursing care are used in other health care practices and vocations.
8. Identify three interventions that help older adults learn.
9. Identify three therapeutic interventions that promote mental health in older adults.

Key Terms

ageism (ĀJ-ĭsm) (p. 169)
aging (p. 168)
elder abuse (p. 175)
functional assessment (p. 176)
gerontophobia (GĔR-ŏn-tō-FŌ-bē-ə) (p. 169)
hoarding (p. 172)
integrity (ĭn-TĔG-rə-tē) (p. 169)
memory loss (p. 176)

Aging is the process of growing older. Older adulthood, or **maturity,** is the period in life from 65 years of age until death. Until recently, people older than 65 years were seen as "old," but our ideas of aging have changed. We now consider more than the number of years an individual has been alive. There are several theories or ideas about the aging process. Biological theories attempt to explain why we age physically, whereas psychosocial theories consider the mental health aspects of aging. This chapter focuses on the psychosocial adaptations made by older adults and the mental health disorders that commonly affect this age-group.

OVERVIEW OF AGING

The aging process begins at birth, but few signs are noted until well into middle age. With the passage of time, however, changes become apparent. Physical maturity is replaced by the aging process. These are the senior citizen, geriatric, or elderly years—a time where outlooks range from deep satisfaction and happiness to despair and sadness (Figure 16-1).

The number of people 65 years of age and older is growing dramatically. "As of the year 2000, 13% of the people in the United States reached age 65—a figure that will double in just 30 years" (Burggraf and Barry, 2001). Older adults are an important segment of the population. In the United States, the number of people over 55 years entering or remaining in the workforce is growing (Box 16-1). Many older adults become active members of their communities. Organizations such as the Gray Panthers and the American Association of Retired Persons (AARP) have strong economic and political influences. Today, because of scientific, medical, and technological advances, we are living longer and enjoying better health than our ancestors (Figure 16-2).

FACTS AND MYTHS OF AGING

Many people carry mental pictures or myths of older adults as people who are wearing out, biding their time until the inescapable end arrives. These are myths—beliefs based on little or no fact. In reality, the majority of older adults are dynamic individuals, living within their homes and functioning successfully within their communities (Edelman and Mandle, 2006).

Another myth is that elders live in nursing homes. In reality, the majority of seniors live outside institutions. More than half of adults over 65 years are still living at home with a spouse. Many maintain their households alone.

"The majority of the elderly are poor" and "the majority of the elderly are rich" are two myths that explode on further examination. The economic status of older adults is as varied as that of any other age-group. Income for the majority of people over 65 years falls between the 500,000 millionaires and the 12% of older adults who are living in poverty.

Perhaps the cruelest myth, however, is that young and attractive are "good," whereas old and imperfect are

MENTAL HEALTH CONTINUUM IN AGING

Maladaptive Responses   Adaptive Responses

Maladaptive Responses	Adaptive Responses
Ignores or neglects health and hygiene	Practices good health habits
Views life with despair; becomes embittered, depressed; blames others	Adapts to aging process
	Enjoys each day
	Keeps mind active
Refuses to learn; refuses to change or adapt	Pursues social activities
	Has strong relationships with others
Becomes socially isolated; interacts only when necessary	Has comforting spiritual beliefs
Has no relationships; does not seek out others	
Has no spiritual beliefs or may be angry with God	

FIGURE **16-1** Mental health continuum in aging.

Box 16-1 | *Changing Statistics for Older Adults*

The number of older Americans has increased by almost four times since the early 1900s.
In 1980 there were about 24 million adults over the age of 65 years in the United States.
In 1998 there were more than 34 million older Americans. Nearly one of every eight adults in the United States is 65 years or older.

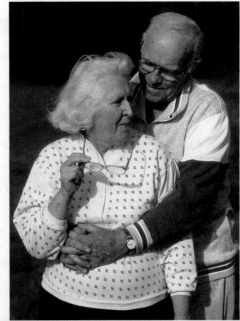

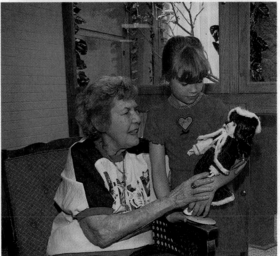

FIGURE **16-2** Older adulthood can be a rewarding time.

"bad." Today's modern society places little value on its elders. Other cultures hold older adults in high esteem and value their wisdom and experience (Giger and Davidhizar, 2004) (see Cultural Considerations 16-1).

It is difficult for young people to imagine growing old. As they mature, adults and children alike are routinely exposed to the negative aspects of aging. Through the years, a fear of growing old develops and anything associated with aging is avoided. "The fear of aging and refusal to accept the elderly into the mainstream of society is known as **gerontophobia**" (Wold, 2008). This attitude leads to **ageism**, a practice of stereotyping older persons as feeble, dependent, and nonproductive. It is important for health care providers to look at their attitudes and values about aging. The journey through life is (for the most part) taken as an adult, swimming through the currents of change.

PHYSICAL HEALTH CHANGES

As an individual ages, so does every body system. The physical changes of aging are not noticeable until the late 30s. By the 50s, one cannot deny the effects of time. Signs of aging continue to show themselves until around 85 years. After that, people appear to age little.

The physical aging process varies greatly. It is affected by genetics, early physical and mental health care, current lifestyle practices, and attitude. Refer to a basic text for a discussion of the physical changes that are associated with normal aging. Figure 16-3 shows one effect of decreasing sensory abilities in an elderly woman.

MENTAL HEALTH CHANGES

Older adulthood is a time for adjusting to change, or adaptation. Developmental tasks at this stage are challenging. According to Erikson, older adults who have developed a sense of personal **integrity** (state of wholeness) accept the worth and uniqueness of their lifestyles. They are able to find order and meaning in their lives. A sense of the flow of time (past, present, future) allows them to face life's challenges with grace and inner strength. They know they will survive because they have so many times in the past. If relationships with their children have been positive, they experience love and respect from their offspring. In short, the elder is able to accept his or her life (as it actually was and is) and value the contributions that he or she has made.

For older adults who have not reached a sense of wholeness, life is filled with despair. Individuals become unhappy and feel that life has been a waste. They focus

Cultural Considerations 16-1

In traditional Korean families, elders hold a high place of honor. The responsibility of caring for them in old age falls to the first-born son, who inherits the family leadership and most of the property.

The Japanese have close ties between the generations. Care of elderly individuals traditionally falls to the oldest son or an unmarried adult in the family. Until recently there were few long-term care facilities for aged people in Japan.

American Indians value the wisdom of their older adults. Historically most of their tribal leaders had attained much experience and knowledge before assuming leadership positions. American Indian families are large, extended groups, and the care of elderly people is shared by every family member.

The Chinese value the family and consider it their responsibility to care for their elders. Older Chinese family members are respected and obeyed. Decisions are made through agreement of family members.

African Americans have large support groups that offer help and comfort for their elderly members.

Hispanic American elderly individuals live with their married children when they are no longer self-sufficient. Cultural and folk medicine beliefs are passed down by older family members.

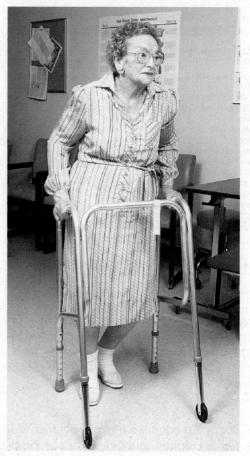

FIGURE **16-3** Decreased sensory abilities and function.

on what might have been. They blame others for life's misfortunes. A sense of loss and contempt for other people leads these elders to a sad and lonely lifestyle.

Recently, mental health changes in older adults have been the subject of much study. The popular belief was that mental abilities decrease slowly with advancing age. The truth, we are learning, is not so simple. Some mental functions peak in childhood and others in adolescence. Although short-term memory and speed begin to decline in the 40s, mental capabilities, such as judgment and wisdom, continue to improve as one grows older. Research over the past decades shows that the mind constantly adjusts its way of doing things and compensates nicely for any losses in efficiency. Table 16-1 lists several mental changes associated with aging and their resultant behaviors.

COMMON PROBLEMS OF OLDER ADULTS

Older adults cope with many changes. They must adjust to physical changes that accompany the passage of time. They learn to cope with losses through the deaths of spouse, family, and friends. Retirement brings a loss of income and opportunities for socialization. Living arrangements may need to be changed, and relationships with adult children are often redefined. Sometimes, several losses occur at the same time. For example, the individual who has just suffered a stroke (CVA) faces losses of function, physical health, mobility, body image, and independence at the same time.

Losses that occur at the same time seriously decrease the older person's ability to cope effectively. For some older adults, adaptation to change comes easily and without discomfort. For others, however, each life change is stormy and produces major stresses.

Health care providers, especially those in the nursing profession, play a major role in caring for older adults. The problems of elderly clients challenge and test our resources. As the population ages, health care providers will be called on to assist many clients in coping with the changes of growing older.

PHYSICAL ADAPTATIONS

Because of normal changes associated with aging, many people believe that an inability to perform physical activity is the natural result of growing older. However, much research has pointed to the importance of remaining physically active throughout life. Aerobic and muscle-strengthening exercises can prevent many of the physical problems associated with aging. Although a 70-year-old man cannot perform the same amount of physical labor in the same time a 30-year-old man does, he can perform the same amount if given extra time. The task will be done—it just takes longer. It is important to encourage daily physical activity in every client. A sound physical body has a better chance of housing a sound psychosocial "body."

Table 16-1	*Mental Changes of Aging*

AREA OF FUNCTION	BEHAVIORS ASSOCIATED WITH AGING
Attention: Alertness, maintaining focus, noticing	Attention declines slowly after age 70 yr; becomes easy to distract
Cognitive style: Ability to adapt, to roll with punches	Mental decline is more rapid in people who are rigid; flexibility in midlife reduces risk for mental decline
Crystallized intelligence: Specialized accumulated knowledge (nursing, engineering, technical skills)	Remains intact until 75 yr or older; may possibly remain intact until death
Episodic memory: Ability to register and store memories of events in time and space, to retrieve memories	Retains memories of recent events when able to anchor them to own experiences, knowledge base; long-term memory better than short-term memory
Information processing: Ability to relate to, store, and retrieve information	Processing speed decreases with age; may take longer to retrieve information; needs time to process information
Learning new tasks	Learning enhances many mental functions; people who do not continue to learn experience slowing and decline in many areas (which is reversible when one resumes learning)
Memory: Names and faces	Decreases fairly rapidly in middle age; often considered worse than truly is; like people of all ages, older adults must process information by associating it to related data
Metamemory: Judgment of one's ability to monitor and control one's own mental processes	After 40 yr, older adults make conscious efforts to learn, manage, store, and remember new information; metamemory remains active in older adults who use their intelligence and lead active lives
Mood: Emotions, feelings	People with frequent negative emotions have higher incidence of depression; depression caused by loss is common in older adults
Perceptual speed: Ability to become alert and respond	Perceptual speed slows after age 50 yr but may not be noticed; elderly people score lower on timed tests but better on others
Personality: Behavioral traits that make one a unique individual	Personality is established in childhood and remains stable throughout life; if one was a happy child, one is usually a happy older adult
Reasoning: Ability to solve problems and make choices, comparisons, and judgments	Great individual differences between 60 and 80 yr; after 80 yr, some loss noticed; people with active mental lives decline more slowly
Retrieval of information: Ability to bring stored information into active consciousness	Takes longer after 50 yr; more errors in retrieving; as persons age, there are more data to match up; slower information retrieval is sign of rich, well-stocked memory
Working memory: Random access memory; memory to which one refers	Increases through childhood and peaks during early adulthood; strengthens with use through connecting of neurons that occurs with learning

Modified from White K: Aging and mental changes, *Psychol Today* 26:38, 1993. Reprinted with permission from *Psychology Today* magazine. Copyright © 1993 Sussex Publishers, Inc.

Besides changes in endurance and the ability to do physical work, older adults must cope with a body that wants to adjust itself to a new routine. Changes in eating and sleeping patterns take place as one ages. Once, one was able to sleep through the night. Now some need or another often awakens the older adult. One used to be able to eat anything, and now antacids are placed at strategic locations throughout the house. The volume on the television creeps up; lights are adjusted to decrease the glare, and the odors drifting from the kitchen while awaiting dinner seem to be less inviting. Even without the problems of a chronic illness, older adults must adjust to the small, everyday physical changes of aging.

Older adults face many alterations in their lifestyles that may affect them physically. Individuals who live alone, for example, tend to neglect their nutritional needs. They may eat too much or not enough. Too often, they use their limited finances to buy costly, empty-calorie foods. Many elders are not physically able to prepare their meals. Others suffer from sensory, dental, or digestive problems. Over time, the lack of adequate food intake results in chronic malnutrition. Resistance to the effects of stress and disease drops,

and the risk for serious health problems increases. Case Study 16-1 presents a typical experience.

Sexuality remains important for many older adults. The focus shifts from having children to an expression of caring, intimate communication, and sharing. Adaptations may be needed in the expression of sexuality because of physical limits or chronic health problems. A decrease in hormone levels leads to physical changes in the reproductive systems of older adults, but both men and women are capable of remaining sexually active well into their 90s.

Physical adaptations to aging include the loss of ability to move about freely. Losing a driver's license has a strong impact on one's independence and ability to provide for the necessities of living. Without private or public transportation, many elderly people are severely restricted in their abilities to move freely about the community.

Adapting to the physical changes of aging can pose many problems that place an individual at higher risk for mental health disorders. Physical problems can lead to changes in mental status. Older adults commonly have vague, nonspecific physical signs and symptoms that may mask a mental health disorder.

Case Study 16-1

Ned was 70 years old when he lost his beloved Molly, his wife of 52 years. They met while they were still in high school, married soon after the war, and vowed never to be apart again. Four children filled the years with joy and hard work, and retirement was packed with new friends and experiences. But once Molly was gone, life for Ned became filled with gloom. He no longer sought out his longtime friends and stopped playing golf or horseshoes. He sold the motor home and retired into his darkened living room. Well-meaning friends often stopped by, but by the time they departed, they had taken on Ned's gloom instead of cheering him.

Soon Ned stopped eating. Molly had always prepared his meals, and he felt lost and unhappy every time he walked into the kitchen where Molly had spent so many hours. By the time his daughter visited Ned, he was confused and unable to care for himself. Assuming he had suffered a stroke, Ned's children admitted him to a long-term care facility.

• Describe early interventions that could have prevented Ned from being removed from his home.

Drug-drug interactions, food-drug interactions, or drug side effects can cause both physical and psychological problems. Every health care provider who works with older adults must be alert for the existence of physical problems. Early assessment and intervention are key for keeping older adults' minor problems from becoming major ones.

Health Care

The availability of health care is an important factor in maintaining the health of older adults. In the United States, people 65 years and older are covered by a national health program called **Medicare.** Canadian and British citizens have national health insurance for people of all ages. Medicaid programs are state-administered programs designed to help "defray expenses for those who could not meet the cost of Medicare contributions or who exhausted their Medicare benefits" (Ebersole and Hess, 2007). Most older Americans receive benefits from Medicare or Medicaid.

Older adults in the United States must pay premiums for their medical insurance. In addition, they are required to cover other out-of-pocket expenses, such as medication costs and associated deductible and coinsurance costs. Many elderly individuals place their health care needs in the background when they are unable to afford the costs.

Health services may be available and affordable, but without transportation, visits to health care providers are few. Older adults who live alone or have sensory problems find it difficult to obtain health services because of the obstacles they must overcome. Periods of confusion and forgetfulness may cloud an elder's ability to follow therapeutic instructions, and many confused people attempt to disguise their problem by being cooperative and voicing understanding.

A concern about human immunodeficiency virus (HIV)/acquired immunodeficiency syndrome (AIDS) is emerging with older adults. "In fact, the number of deaths related to AIDS in the elderly population more than doubled between 1987 and 1993" (Burke and Laramie, 2004). Good health care is especially important for these seniors.

PSYCHOSOCIAL ADAPTATIONS

Before the 1920s, it was common for individuals to grow up, marry, raise a family, and grow old within one community. People were cared for in their homes as they aged, with relatives or friends attending to their well-being. If they became confused or forgetful, friends and surroundings were a source of comfort and familiarity.

Today, growing old has become more impersonal. The comforts of family and friends may be miles away. Older adults may have problems relating to money, adequate food and housing, or health care. The loss of loved ones, social status, and earning power withers social support systems, and decreasing sensory abilities leave many elders questioning the soundness of their judgments.

The majority of older adults benefit from health care interventions. Nurses, because of their focus on the activities of daily living, are able to help elderly people fill many of their needs. Health care providers who work with older adults also help to fill the gap for missing family members by providing emotional and social support. The following section discusses a few of the most important problems faced by the elderly population and some basic therapeutic interventions.

Economics

The financial outlook of older adults differs greatly from that of young adults. People in their 80s were born before the Great Depression of the 1930s. They are old enough to recall the pangs of hunger when food was scarce. They remember men selling apples on street corners. They have experienced the uncertainty of wondering how they were going to survive tomorrow. Many even raised children during the Depression, sacrificing food from their own mouths to feed their offspring. The Depression years of the 1930s forged an indelible memory in our older adults. Many of their seemingly strange behaviors, such as hoarding (the act of collecting and saving assorted, seemingly useless items), are the result of attitudes learned during those difficult years. The 90-year-old who takes doggie bags from the restaurant to wither in the refrigerator remembers the Great Depression and cannot bear to waste food. The collections of newspaper, clothing, string, old magazines, and other assorted odds and ends are protection for leaner days that may lie ahead.

Because of inflation, the value of a country's currency (e.g., dollar, pound, mark) changes, sometimes dramatically. During this time, many elderly people have followed savings plans or invested for their later years. Some are now financially comfortable. Others, not having realized the change in the actual value of a currency, are coping with fewer resources than they had expected. People who made no preparations for later life often find themselves at the mercy of an impersonal system, living on meager resources with a poor quality of life.

Elderly individuals are also faced with the problem of being financially vulnerable. Older adults trust other people to take them "at their word." This background, combined with diminishing senses or understanding, leaves older adults vulnerable to the scams, deceptions, and threats of con artists and criminals. Many older adults have lost their life's savings because they could not understand the language on a contract. Many allowed themselves to be charmed or intimidated out of their money.

Interventions relating to money are usually provided by social workers. Other caregivers can assess for indications of financial problems and refer clients to the appropriate resource. Remember to monitor elderly clients because worries about money can lead to mental health problems such as depression, anxiety, or paranoia. Box 16-2 describes a financial assessment for older adults.

Housing

Problems with housing for older adults range from having "too much house" to having none at all. The majority of older adults in the United States live in their own homes with their spouses. The numbers do not account for elderly individuals who have no homes, because homeless people are difficult to count.

The problems of "too much house" usually arise when one spouse passes away and the remaining person is unable to care for the property. Because women tend to outlive men, the most common scenario is that of a newly widowed woman faced with the care of a house about whose maintenance she knows nothing. She may live there for many years of widowhood, but eventually she will be forced to move to a safer environment with less responsibility and upkeep.

The problems of "too little house" (inadequate housing) include homelessness and despair. Many homeless elderly individuals are mentally ill and are "usually sicker and have more needs for health services than the younger homeless" (Hogstel, 1995). Others have been forced out of their homes because they were unable to afford the expenses associated with them.

As the elder population increases, new arrangements in housing are being developed. Inventive new plans and living arrangements for older adults are evolving. Independent living centers, life contract facilities, foster homes, subsidized housing, and assisted living situations are all being explored as housing options for elderly people.

Box 16-2 | *Financial Assessment for Older Adults*

Demonstrate respect during questioning, but ask about the following:
Sources of income
Housing and food costs
If they have money left for health costs
How they obtain their medications and whether they share medications
Money remaining (after paying expenses) for clothing and recreation

---

Loss and Death

We travel life's paths with companions, friends, relatives, and people who have become important in our lives. With the passage of time, many older adults lose the individuals who are important for their emotional support and well-being. When a spouse of many years is lost, the remaining partner is left to cope alone. Depression often becomes one's companion after the death of a spouse or significant other. Frequently, couples who have been together for many years will die within months of each other. It seems the will to carry on without the loved one is lost, and death becomes an opportunity to be reunited.

Losses during the older years also arrive in various other forms. The loss of physical stamina and endurance and the loss of sharp senses with which to enjoy the world present challenges for older adults. Although the concept of loss is described in Chapter 20, it is important to remember that coping with loss is one of the most difficult problems of older adults. Compassion, understanding, and support help them reestablish the psychosocial connections that bind us together (see Think About 16-1).

Substance Abuse

The misuse or abuse of medications is a complex issue for older adults. Elderly people have a great number of prescription drugs to treat multiple and chronic health problems (Box 16-3).

Older adults also metabolize and excrete drugs more slowly. Their decreased tolerance for most drugs can result in overdoses and severe interactions with other medications and foods. Problems with sight and memory also contribute to the misuse of medications by older adults.

Elders with several health problems may visit many specialists, with each one prescribing a different medication. In a recent study, only 15% of older adults on medications "could recall the drug names, dosages, or reasons for taking them" (Editors, 2002). The purchase of over-the-counter drugs compounds the situation by increasing the potential for adverse reactions. In addition, many elderly people use several pharmacies, share their prescriptions with friends, and follow the recommendations of anyone offering relief from their discomfort. Hoarding drugs is common because of the expense and possible need for them in the future. Many individuals will underdose themselves to save money and make medications last longer. Outdated medications are seldom thrown away.

Think About 16-1

- How do you picture yourself at 80 years of age?
- How physically active do you expect to be?
- Have you thought about or made any plans for retirement?
- At what age do you feel a person should think about retirement?

Box 16-3 *People Older Than 45 Years*

Seventy-five percent use some kind of medication.
More than 30% of those medications are over-the-counter drugs.
Twenty-five percent of all prescriptions are written for persons over age 65 years.
Many older adults share medications or skip their medications to help keep costs down.
Few elderly individuals have knowledge of side effects or drug interactions.

Nurses have a special responsibility to ensure that their older clients are using their medications correctly. This responsibility includes a thorough assessment of a client's drug history, current drug use (prescribed, over-the-counter, and recreational), and an understanding of the medications currently being taken. Drug Alert 16-1 offers a tool for assessing an older adult's drug and substance use.

Although the use of recreational or street drugs decreases with age, some drugs, especially alcohol, still cause problems for many older adults. Alcohol use helps provide a substitute for social interactions. Many elderly people drink to dull the discomforts associated with isolation. Older adults who were heavy drinkers in the past often show the results of long-term alcohol abuse.

The use of opiates (heroin, opium) is even more invisible than the use of alcohol. Older Asian Americans with opium addictions or retired white-collar workers addicted to cocaine seldom reach the attention of health care providers unless their habits result in serious medical complications.

All health care providers need to assess older adults for signs of substance abuse, especially when an unusual accident or event occurs. Often a history of minor accidents and injuries signals a problem with drugs. If problems with drug or alcohol use are suspected, the client is referred to a physician for a medical assessment.

 Drug Alert 16-1

NURSING PROCESS

Assessment

1. Obtain a complete drug history: name of drug, reason prescribed, amount taken, how often taken. Is drug taken with other medications, on an empty or full stomach, at a certain time? What is your client's knowledge about the drug's side effects, drug-food interactions?
2. Instruct the client to put every medication he or she has into a paper bag and bring them to you. Check each medication for its expiration date. Be alert for several bottles of the same medication. Include all over-the-counter products, vitamins, and herbal or natural remedies.
3. Assess client's ability to follow verbal and written instructions and willingness to learn about each medication.

Planning

1. Based on the client's abilities to understand and cooperate, develop a plan for teaching and monitoring the client's use of each drug.
2. Arrange for the client to show you the steps in identifying and taking the medication if necessary. Include family members in the teaching process when possible.

Nursing Diagnoses

Possible nursing diagnoses include the following:
  Deficient knowledge related to use, administration, and monitoring of prescribed medications

Ineffective therapeutic regimen management because of sensory loss
Noncompliance related to altered thought processes

Therapeutic Interventions

1. Teach the client and significant others about the proper use and dosage of each medication, side effects and what to do about them, and expected therapeutic actions.
2. Devise a system for taking daily medications. Pill dispensers are available at most pharmacies. These multiboxed units can hold up to 1 week's medications. They usually consist of a series of small compartments, which are filled with all the drugs that must be taken at a certain time. The client opens the compartment at the prescribed time and takes every medication in the box. Having the client return weekly with his or her medications and pill dispenser allows the nurse and other caregivers to monitor the medications taken.

Evaluation

1. Assess the client's therapeutic response to the medications. Did the drug do what it was intended to do?
2. Evaluate the client's willingness and ability to cooperate. Has there been any change in the client's alertness, level of understanding, or memory?

MENTAL HEALTH PROBLEMS OF OLDER ADULTS

People over age 65 years experience the same mental health disorders as adolescents and younger adults. They also face the problems of vulnerability, abuse, memory loss, dementia, and Alzheimer's disease (discussed in Chapter 17). Mental health difficulties can result from physical or biochemical disorders, such as diabetes or medication imbalances. Many mental health threats arise from loneliness and social isolation. Psychological problems with which individuals have struggled throughout their lives follow them into old age. Although all major mental health disorders can occur in older adults, by far the most common disorders relate to loss, depression, abuse, and dementia.

ELDER ABUSE

Older adults view the world from a different point of view than younger people. Many are lonely and easily trust someone who is kind or shows interest in them. Older adults without adequate support are a vulnerable population—open to assault or attack by others. They are the abused elderly.

Elder abuse is defined as any action that takes advantage of an older person, his or her emotional well-being, or property. The three basic categories of elder abuse are domestic abuse, where the abuser has a special relationship with the elder; institutional abuse, where caregivers who are legally obligated to provide protective care fail to do so; and self-neglect or self-abuse. Acts of elder abuse appear in various forms, ranging from physical neglect to stealing money and exploiting the older person's resources. Table 16-2 lists several ways in which elder abuse occurs.

The victims of elder abuse are divided into those in which the elder has physical or mental impairment and depends on the family for daily care needs and those whose care needs are overshadowed by the abusive behavior of the caregiver. The typical abused elder is a woman, at least 75 years of age, with physical or mental problems who is living with a relative. Often the responsibilities of care can lead even well-intentioned family members or caregivers to lose their tempers when they feel stressed or pressured. However, losing control assists neither the victim nor the caregiver.

Abuse of elderly people is not new, but it has just begun to receive public attention. The actual numbers of abused elderly individuals are unknown. Surveys by the National Commission on Elder Abuse (2006) indicate a 19% increase in reported abuse incidents. Experts agree that current statistics show only the tip of the iceberg and the actual numbers are far greater. Every care provider must be alert for the indications of abuse in every older client. Chapter 26 focuses on the recognition, prevention, and treatment of this problem.

DEPRESSION

Along with the losses experienced through death, retirement, and relocation, many older adults are faced with losing their social supports. As stresses mount and resources are lost, many older individuals become saddened. This emotional state continues, and unless it is interrupted by the attentions of others, their outlook is bleak and hopeless. A dark mood becomes overpowering and reaches into every aspect of one's life. Individuals feel hopeless and powerless to do anything about it. The future holds no joy, only the possibility of suffering more tomorrow than today. This is the face of depression in older adults (see Chapter 21).

Depression is probably the most common mental health disorder of late adulthood. It is estimated that more than 15% of older adults in the community have depressive signs and symptoms. Elders in long-term care institutions or hospitals have even higher rates. Depression is commonly underdiagnosed and undertreated. Sometimes vague complaints are the only clue. Other times, depression will mask itself as a physical illness. Knowing clients' lifestyles, preferences, social

Table 16-2 *Forms of Elder Abuse*

TYPE OF ABUSE	DESCRIPTION AND EXAMPLES
Exploitation	Improper use of a person for one's own profit. *Examples:* theft of objects, diversion of elder's money, use of legal power assigned by the older adult for own gain. An estimated 10% of elderly people are exploited.
Neglect	Refusing to meet basic physical and mental health needs. *Examples:* depriving food, drink, clothing, shelter, hygiene, corrective and remedial devices (e.g., glasses, hearing aids); refusal to seek medical care, even when urgently needed; refusing to interact, to provide for love, belonging, social needs. About 65% of abused elderly people are neglected.
Physical abuse	Physical harm caused by the actions of another person. *Examples:* beating, whipping, scalding, cigarette burns, bruises, fractures.
Psychological abuse	Threats to mental health caused by another person. *Examples:* poor personal hygiene, grooming, environmental conditions; threats of nursing home placement; being humiliated, threatened, or socially isolated; verbal assaults, name calling; being treated like a child; being placed in seclusion.
Violation of rights	The refusal to allow another the exercise of individual rights, including the right to consent for medical treatment or surgery, to refuse treatment, to live in a safe environment of choice, to privacy, and to use personal financial resources as desired.

Modified from Hogstel MO: *Geropsychiatric nursing*, ed 2, St. Louis, 1995, Mosby.

habits, and attitudes toward life is important. With this knowledge, nurses can assess for the behaviors that signal the onset of depression. Box 16-4 lists several signs and symptoms of elder depression.

Frequently the signs and symptoms of depression can mimic dementia (loss of multiple abilities, including memory, language, and understanding). Careful assessments are required to distinguish the difference. Many medications, such as cardiovascular drugs, anticancer drugs, psychotropic drugs, hormones, and antiinflammatory agents, are associated with elder depression.

Depression is treated with individual and group therapy and medications. Reminiscence therapy and validation therapy have proved effective in improving confusion and lifting spirits. Box 16-5 explains the basics of validation therapy. Antidepressant drugs have mixed effects because clients may experience unwanted reactions or toxic accumulations. The selective serotonin reuptake inhibitor (SSRI) antidepressants have fewer side effects in the elderly population than other medications. Clients must be monitored for orthostatic hypotension (rapid drop in blood pressure on arising) and gastrointestinal (GI) symptoms. Offering emotional support and interest helps prevent depression by reestablishing the human connection that elders so often need. Remember that one person can make a difference in the quality of an elderly individual's life.

Box 16-4 | *Signs and Symptoms of Depression in Older Adults*

PHYSICAL
Muscle aches
Abdominal pain, nausea/vomiting
Dry mouth
Headache

COGNITIVE (INTELLECTUAL)
Decreased or slowed memory
Slowing intellectual functions
Agitation
Paranoia
Focus on the past
Thoughts of death and suicide

EMOTIONAL
Fatigue
Lack of interest
Increased anxiety or dependence
Inability to experience pleasure or laughter
Feels useless, hopeless, helpless

BEHAVIORAL
Activities of daily living become difficult
Changes in appetite
Changes in sleeping patterns
Lowered energy levels
Poor grooming
Withdrawal from people and activities

THERAPEUTIC INTERVENTIONS

Therapeutic care for older adults is not effectively accomplished unless a special ingredient is present. That special ingredient is respect: the courtesy, consideration, and esteem due each individual who has reached this stage of life. Every older adult, alert or not, cooperative or not, deserves respect. Respect is demonstrated by each action and each interaction we perform. Treat clients as you would like to be treated if you were in their situation.

When assessing an older adult client, remember to perform a functional assessment, which is an analysis of the client's ability to perform the activities of daily living. The environment in which the client lives, as well as cultural and social patterns, should also be assessed.

STANDARDS OF GERIATRIC CARE

The American Nurses Association (ANA) has developed guidelines (standards) for nurses who work with older adults. These standards offer nurses a means for providing and measuring the nursing care they deliver to older adults. Every nurse who works with older adults is responsible for following the standards of geriatric nursing practice. Other caregivers have the responsibility to care for older adults with respect, kindness, and sensitivity. Box 16-6 lists each standard.

AGE-RELATED INTERVENTIONS

Therapeutic interventions for older adults differ from those for younger people in several ways. The normal process of aging slows the older adult's mental functions. Memory loss is a natural part of the aging process relating to the inability to recall certain details or events. Therapeutic interventions need to account for this by allowing more time for completion of tasks. More time is also needed to recover from physical exertion.

The "capacity of the brain to process, store, and retrieve information begins to function less efficiently" (Burke and Laramie, 2004) in older adults, so finding the right word in conversation becomes difficult. Allow extra time for the elder to communicate, and listen

---

Box 16-5 | *Validation Therapy*

Older individuals must justify having lived, resolve old conflicts, and make peace with themselves. **Validation therapy** acknowledges the truth of clients' feelings by using a combination of the following:
- Eye contact
- Touch
- Mirroring the client's body movement
- Matching the client's voice and rhythm patterns
- Empathy
- Putting the client's cues about feelings into words
- Accepting the client without passing judgment
- Genuine, total listening

carefully. Face the client, and speak slowly and clearly. Use nonverbal communications to help convey your message. It is best not to overload the client with information. One simple yet understood message is more effective than a lengthy discourse.

Music therapy is proving to be "a powerful tool for maintaining and restoring health and is particularly suited to elder care" (Kramer, 2001). Music can alter moods and provide relaxation or distraction. For older adults, music provides an opportunity to remember and enjoy.

When teaching elderly people, there are several things to keep in mind. First, assess for any physical or sensory changes that may interfere with their learning (and your teaching). Clients with cataracts usually

cannot make out the different colors of their pills, especially blue, green, and violet (Ruholl, 2003). When teaching clients about their medications, refer to the medications by name and shape rather than color. If clients are hard of hearing, be sure their hearing aids are working at the proper settings. Face clients. Speak slowly and clearly in lower tones. Ask them to repeat your message.

Draw on clients' wisdom and knowledge. Find out what they already know. Break a complex task into small, key steps. Be patient and respectful. Write out important points. Your clients' willingness and ability to learn will greatly improve.

MENTALLY ILL OLDER ADULTS

With a stable environment and daily routine, adults with serious mental illness can continue to function well into old age. However, many will be coping with the complications of long-term antipsychotic medications. The most common complications are movement disorders, such as tardive dyskinesia, and cognitive deficits. Cognitive deficits can also significantly impair activities of daily living. These clients may require assistance with grooming and other activities of daily living.

A decrease in intellectual function (cognitive impairment) is common in older adults with a long history of mental illness. Clients should be assessed for their level of impairment so that therapeutic interventions can be individually tailored to promote the highest level of functioning.

MENTAL HEALTH PROMOTION AND PREVENTION

Many problems of older adults can be prevented or minimized if they are discovered early. Health care providers must work together and grasp every opportunity to promote healthful practices in their older clients. They should assess clients for changes in social, emotional, behavioral, and physical functioning and intervene early. Caregivers should not hesitate to help satisfy clients' needs, even though it may take some creative planning. Newer interventions, such as using dolls and stuffed animals to provide comfort (doll therapy) and life review (reminiscence therapy), are proving effective with many older adults. Sample Client Care Plan 16-1 focuses on an older adult who is having trouble recovering from a significant loss.

Caregivers play a major role in the mental health care of elderly individuals. Interventions often require the services of several specialists, such as nurses, physical therapists, social workers, and homemakers. Sharing information and coordinating care promote quality in the lives of older adults. Health care providers also have the opportunity to make a significant difference in public policies regarding older adults, as well as in the lives of all the persons they touch.

Box 16-6 *Standards of Geriatric Nursing Practice*

I. Organization of Geriatric Nursing Services
Services are directed by a baccalaureate- or masters-prepared nurse with geriatric experience.
II. Theory
Nurses participate in developing new theories and use concepts to guide their practice.
III. Data Collection
Clients are routinely assessed, and the results are shared with clients, family, and multidisciplinary team members.
IV. Nursing Diagnosis
Nurses use assessments to develop nursing diagnoses (nursing process).
V. Planning and Continuity of Care
Nurses collaborate to develop a plan of care to help clients achieve the highest level of health, well-being, and quality of life possible, including a peaceful death.
VI. Intervention
Nurses provide care to maintain or restore abilities and prevent complications.
VII. Evaluation
Nurses continually evaluate client and family responses to determine progress toward goals and care plan revisions.
VIII. Interdisciplinary Collaboration
Nurses plan and meet regularly with other members of the health care team to evaluate and adjust the plan of care.
IX. Research
Nurses participate in, share, and use research knowledge.
X. Ethics
Nurses use the ANA code of ethics to guide decision making in practice.
XI. Professional Development
Nurses assume responsibility for professional growth through peer review and evaluations of the quality of nursing practice. Nurses contribute to the professional growth of other health care team members.

ANA, American Nurses Association.

SAMPLE CLIENT CARE PLAN 16-1

Complicated Grieving

ASSESSMENT *History.* Moe and Mary were married for over 40 years when Mary died last month. Since her death, Moe has refused to leave his home. His days are spent in front of the television, eating snack food. Friends no longer visit because Moe refuses to turn off the TV, and it is too difficult to converse above the noise. For the past week, Moe has not bathed or changed his clothes.

Current Findings. A sad-looking man, untidy, with a strong body odor. Speech is slow, answers with one word. When asked, states that "life is no longer worth living without Mary."

Multidisciplinary Diagnosis	*Planning/Goals*
Complicated grieving related to loss of long-time spouse	Moe will acknowledge his loss and express emotions appropriate to the grief process.

Therapeutic Interventions

Intervention	Rationale	Team Member
1. Identify which task of mourning must be accomplished (acknowledge loss, work with pain, adjustment to loss).	Helps client begin grief work and reintegration into life.	Psy, Nsg
2. Help Moe express his feelings about Mary's death.	To prevent unexpressed emotions from being directed inward.	All
3. Assure Moe that his emotions are normal expressions of grief.	Provides reassurance, acceptance of feelings.	All
4. Encourage Moe to talk about both positive and negative sides of their relationship.	Realistic appraisal of loss gives clearer perspective and promotes acceptance of current situation.	All
5. Engage Moe in social activities and refer to senior support group.	Decreases isolation and withdrawal; helps regain trust that "life will go on."	Soc Svc

Evaluation

After 3 weeks, Moe was able to discuss his feelings of loss, anger, and hopelessness associated with Mary's death.

❓ CRITICAL THINKING QUESTIONS

1. How important is interacting with others (socialization) to Moe at this time?

2. Does Moe need to be referred to home care services? Why or why not?

A complete client care plan includes several other diagnoses and interventions.
Nsg, Nursing staff; *Psy,* psychologist; *Soc Svc,* social services.

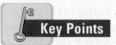

Key Points

- Older adulthood, or maturity, is the period of life from 65 years of age until death.
- According to the theorist Erikson, older adults with a well-developed sense of personal integrity accept the worth and uniqueness of their own lifestyles.
- Although short-term memory and speed begin to decline in the 40s, mental capabilities such as judgment and wisdom continue to improve as one grows older.
- Physical problems can lead to changes in mental status.
- Older adults experience several physical and social losses.
- Problems with elder housing range from having too much house to having none at all.
- The availability of health care for the elderly population is an important factor in maintaining both physical and mental health.

- One of the greatest mental health challenges is coping with the loss of loved ones and friends.
- The misuse or abuse of drugs and alcohol is a complex issue for older adults who receive a great number of prescription drugs to treat multiple and chronic health problems.
- Elder abuse is defined as any action on the part of a caregiver to take advantage of an older person, his or her emotional well-being, or property.
- Depression is one of the most common mental health disorders of late adulthood.
- Care for older adults cannot be effective without respect, courtesy, consideration, and the esteem due each individual who has reached this stage of life.

---

evolve Be sure to visit the companion Evolve site at http://evolve.elsevier.com/Morrison-Valfre/ for additional online resources.

17 Cognitive Impairment, Alzheimer's Disease, and Dementia

evolve http://evolve.elsevier.com/Morrison-Valfre/

Objectives

Upon completion of this chapter, the student will be able to:

1. Describe two normal age-related changes in cognition.
2. Identify five main categories of confusion.
3. Explain why medication use can lead to confusion in older adults.
4. Describe at least three signs or symptoms of delirium.
5. Identify five symptoms of dementia.
6. Describe the signs and symptoms seen during the progression of Alzheimer's disease.
7. List three mental health care goals for clients with Alzheimer's disease.
8. Describe the need-driven dementia-compromised behavior model.
9. Identify two types of support groups for the caregivers of clients with Alzheimer's disease.

Key Terms

affective loss (p. 183)
Alzheimer's (AWLTZ-hī-měrz) **disease (AD)** (p. 183)
catastrophic (KĂT-ə-STRŎF-ĭk) **reactions** (p. 184)
cognition (p. 179)
conative (KŎN-ə-tĭv) **loss** (p. 184)
confusion (p. 179)
delirium (də-LĬR-ē-ŭm) (p. 180)
dementia (də-MĔN-shə) (p. 181)
functional assessment (p. 186)
memory loss (p. 180)
sundown syndrome (p. 182)

CONFUSION HAS MANY FACES

The words cognition and **cognitive** describe activities of the mind involved in thinking and thought processes. Cognition refers to intelligence, learning, judgment, reasoning, knowledge, understanding, and memory—all higher brain functions. A **cognitive impairment** is a disruption in higher brain functions that results in confusion. The client's ways of knowing and understanding the world have changed. This chapter focuses on confusion, its causes, and its treatments.

NORMAL CHANGES IN COGNITION

Changes in brain chemistry and function occur as we age. Neurons are lost, the production of neurotransmitters decreases, and the brain shrinks in size. However, "the brain has a remarkable ability to compensate for these losses" (Lang, 2001). The most significant losses are slower response times and short-term memory. More time is needed to process, store, and retrieve information.

Several other factors influence how one ages mentally. Culture, education, general health, genetics, and living conditions all have an influence on one's cognitive (intellectual) abilities. We all age individually, but one thing is certain: **confusion is not normal.** Although it most often occurs in older adults, individuals of any age can become confused. No matter what the age, **confusion demands investigation.**

THE FIVE "Ds" OF CONFUSION

The word **confusion** is a very general term that is difficult to define. Commonly, it means mixed-up, bewildered, or uncertain. For health care providers, confusion is a symptom of an underlying problem that requires immediate attention. Confusion can be traced to physical, biochemical, social, or cultural sources. It can be acute, subacute, chronic, reversible, or irreversible. Sources of confusion are grouped into five broad categories. To help you remember the causes of confusion, use the five "Ds": damage, delirium, dementia, depression, and deprivation. See Figure 17-1 for examples of each group.

Damage from head injuries or conditions that cause a lack of oxygen **(hypoxia)** to the brain can lead to confusion. Exposure to certain chemicals, toxic substances, or diseases can cause brain damage and confusion. Anything that interrupts or alters the blood supply or nerve pathways in the brain can result in acute or lasting confusion.

People who suffer great losses can experience confusion caused by **depression.** When one's focus is inner sadness, outside stimuli can be misinterpreted or misunderstood. The individual becomes labeled "confused," and the depression is ignored. Certain medications can cause depression. Chapter 21 offers a more thorough discussion of depression. Here, remember

Delirium
- Acute onset
- Causes: metabolic disorders, diseases: infections, fever, dehydration, pain, drug reactions, lack of oxygen to the brain
- Reversible if treated early

Damage
- Acute onset
- Causes: stroke, head injury, disease, exposure to chemicals
- Sometimes reversible

Dementia
- Slow onset
- Causes: cardiovascular disease, HIV, metabolic problems, Alzheimer's disease; more than 60 causes
- Usually not reversible

Depression
- Causes: loss, drugs, inner sadness, metabolic imbalances
- Subacute onset
- Usually reversible

Deprivation
- Variable onset
- Causes: sensory impairments, poor hearing, poor vision, loss of touch, lack of social interaction
- Sometimes reversible

FIGURE **17-1** The five "Ds" of confusion.

that confusion (especially in older adults) can be caused by depression and other mood disorders.

Commonly, confusion in older adults is related to **sensory deprivation.** We all use our senses to gain an accurate picture of our world and the people in it. When hearing is poor or eyesight diminished, it becomes difficult to understand one's environment. Visual clues are missing. Sounds become distorted. The world evolves into a blur for people with cataracts and other eye diseases. Those with hearing problems miss the richness of sound and speech. Messages become garbled or go unheard. Caregivers should be sure their clients' hearing aids and glasses are in good working order and appropriately used. When was the last eye and hearing examination? It is easy to become confused when the messages are unclear.

MEDICATIONS AND THE ELDERLY POPULATION

Many medications and drugs cause confusion, especially in elderly people. Metabolism is slower in older adults. This means that drugs are eliminated more slowly and can reach toxic levels if not closely monitored. People who take several medications are at risk for confusion resulting from drug interactions. Over-the-counter drugs, especially those with anticholinergic side effects, can cause confusion, disorientation, and memory loss. Drug Alert 17-1 lists several drug classes that have confusion as a side effect.

"Since the 1990s, the use of psychotropic drugs has increased in the nursing home setting" (Higginbottom, 2003). Most often, their use is appropriate and helps improve behaviors that pose a risk to self or others. However, these powerful medications can cause sedation and confusion, so clients must be carefully

monitored for effectiveness, side effects, and adverse reactions. Confusion is often the first sign of a drug reaction.

CLIENTS WITH DELIRIUM

Memory loss is the inability to recall a certain detail or event. It is a natural part of the aging process and affects most people older than 70 years. **Delirium** is a change of consciousness that **occurs quickly.** The signs and symptoms of delirium include "disorganized thinking, a decreased attention span, lowered or fluctuating level of consciousness, disturbances in the sleep-wake cycle, disorientation, and changes in psychomotor activity" (Henry, 2002). Individuals may have **delusions** (false ideas that resist change) or **hallucinations** (seeing things that are not in reality). They are usually agitated and hyperactive. However, hypoactive behaviors, such as lethargy and reduced activity, are common but often overlooked behaviors.

The onset of delirium is rapid (acute), occurring in hours to days. **Delirium is reversible if treated early.** Once the underlying cause is found and treated, full recovery of mental functions occurs. It is important for health care providers to recognize the signs of delirium. Box 17-1 lists a method for assessing delirium.

FINDING THE CAUSE

Delirium is caused by various medical conditions, a variety of drugs and their interactions, or other problems. Infections, fevers, and dehydration are common causes of delirium. Metabolic and endocrine conditions, such as diabetes, thyroid problems, and kidney or liver disease, may all result in delirium. Reactions to

Drug Alert 17-1

DRUGS THAT CAN CAUSE CONFUSION

Medications used to Treat:	Over-the-Counter Drugs used to Treat:
Allergies	Cold and flu
Arthritis	Diarrhea
High blood pressure	Hay fever
Irritable bowel syndrome	Insomnia
Migraine headaches	
Pain	
Parkinson's disease	

Antipsychotics
Sedatives
Hypnotics

Box 17-1 *Assessing Delirium*

Obtain information from a family member or someone who knows the client and his or her usual behaviors.

ONSET AND COURSE

Questions to ask: Has there been an acute change in mental status? How long ago was the change first noticed? Do the behaviors fluctuate (come and go) during the day? Are behaviors worse at night?
A positive (yes) answer to any question indicates delirium.

ATTENTION

Questions to ask: Does he or she have trouble paying attention? Can he or she keep track of what is being said? Is he or she easy to distract?
A positive (yes) answer to any question indicates delirium.

THINKING

Questions to ask: Is thinking unorganized? Is there an illogical or unclear flow of ideas? Does he or she switch from subject to subject? Does his or her conversation ramble?
A positive (yes) answer to any question indicates delirium.

LEVEL OF CONSCIOUSNESS

Questions to ask: Overall, how would you rate his or her level of alertness (consciousness) compared with usual levels? Is he or she alert? Vigilant? Hyperalert? Drowsy but arousable? Difficult to arouse?
Any answer other than "alert" indicates delirium.

Modified from Henry M: Descending into delirium, *Am J Nurs* 102:49, 2002.

certain drugs are common causes in elderly individuals. Delirium can also occur when people abruptly stop their medications. It can occur after surgery, especially in older adults. Pain, constipation, extremely high or low body temperatures, alcohol use, a lack of oxygen to the brain, and malnutrition can all trigger delirium.

Case Study 17-1

Mr. J. is an alert, outgoing 80-year-old man who lives with his cat in a senior citizens' complex. Despite several chronic conditions, he remains active and volunteers at the senior center. His daughter visits weekly.

Today she was called by another volunteer at the senior center and told that Mr. J. has not been there for 3 days. Although she had visited only 2 days before and found her father "his usual cheery self," she rushed to her father's home. On her arrival, she finds that he does not know who she is. He tells her that he is afraid she has come to steal his late wife's jewelry. He is inattentive and drowsy. The daughter calls his physician and takes him to the emergency room.

The medical workup shows continuing confusion and a slight fever. Blood and urine tests indicate an infection. The physician diagnoses acute delirium related to a urinary tract infection. Orders are given for intravenous (IV) antibiotics and fluids. After a few days' hospitalization, Mr. J.'s confusion is completely gone and he is ready to return home.

The causes of delirium, sometimes called **acute confusion,** are many. "In order to identify delirium, clinicians must be familiar with the client's baseline mental status and the characteristics of any changes" (Henry, 2002). Delirium is a frightening experience that can last from hours to days. Case Study 17-1 gives an example of a client with delirium.

TREATING DELIRIUM

The treatment of delirium depends on its cause. The first priority is to **treat the source.** Antibiotics are given for infections. Older adults lose their sense of thirst, and delusions often subside quickly as water and minerals are replaced. If medications are the culprit, they are withdrawn (gradually in some cases) and the client is monitored closely.

The second focus of care is supportive. Providing an environment that has low stimuli helps clients remain calm. Have clients wear their hearing aids and glasses. Encourage fluids to prevent dehydration. Use clocks and calendars to help orient clients. Allow clients to be involved with their care. Ambulate clients frequently if allowed, and balance rest with activity. Always protect the client from injury.

Do not attempt to talk clients out of their delusions or convince them that they are false. Their reality is different at this time, but it is real to them. Use a low, calm voice, and maintain eye contact. Project a calm, unhurried manner. Use simple orienting statements, such as "It is warm for June" or "Isn't it a nice evening?" Clients with delusions require close monitoring and supervision. As the cause of the confusion is corrected, clients will become more oriented and cooperative.

Dementia is a loss of multiple abilities, including memory, language, and the ability to think and understand (judgment and abstract thought). It is a broad term that describes a group of symptoms relating to a severe loss of intellectual functions. Personality and behavioral changes may also be present. The losses are severe enough to interfere with daily living activities and social and work functioning. Unlike delirium, with dementia there is no change in one's level of consciousness.

CAUSES OF DEMENTIA

Dementia can be primary, as with Alzheimer's disease (AD), or it may occur as a result of disease, such as human immunodeficiency virus (HIV; secondary). Cardiovascular disease, strokes, and problems with circulation in the brain are also linked to dementia. There are more than 60 causes associated with dementia, including metabolic problems, hormonal abnormalities, infections, brain traumas, and tumors. Pain; sensory deprivations; toxic alcohol reactions; anemia; chemical intoxication; drug interactions; and nutritional deficiencies, such as vitamin B_{12}, folic acid, or niacin, can all result in dementia. Refer to Box 17-2 for an easy way to remember the causes of dementia.

The two most common types of dementia are **vascular dementia** and **Alzheimer's disease.** Vascular dementia occurs as a complication of cardiovascular disease. Not enough blood is nourishing the brain to keep it functioning properly. Unlike AD, "the course of vascular dementia may not be smoothly progressive but rather may be characterized by plateaus" (Watari and Gatz, 2002).

People with dementia are found in every culture, but researchers have found that the types of dementia vary among cultures. Cultural Considerations 17-1 points out a few of these differences. No matter what the cause or culture, early diagnosis is important. Dementia, excluding AD, may be reversible if discovered and treated early. However, the longer the wait before diagnosis, the more likely dementia will be permanent.

SYMPTOMS OF DEMENTIA

With elderly clients, dementia is classified as Alzheimer's or non-Alzheimer's type. In the early stages, dementia is difficult to differentiate from **age-associated memory impairment.** Persons with age-associated memory impairment tend to learn and recall things more slowly. Yet, if given extra time, they are able to function. Individuals with dementia are increasingly unable to process new information. At the same time, they are losing the ability

to retrieve and use the information accumulated through their lifetimes.

Each person is unique, and no two people react the same way or follow the same course. One's general health, intelligence, personality, and social situation all influence the behaviors seen in dementia. However, all people with dementia have progressive problems with memory, judgment, and abstract thinking.

Dementia has a **slow, gradual onset.** In the beginning, only small changes are noticeable. Individuals often attempt to hide their impairments. There is often an associated depression at this stage. The most common early symptom is a declining memory. For example, the client may ask the same question repeatedly and then promptly forget the answer. Problems with abstract thinking follow. For example, an accountant becomes unable to balance his checkbook because he forgets what numbers are and how to use them. A homemaker can no longer plan meals or put together a shopping list. Problem-solving skills are lost. Things are misplaced and then forgotten. Familiar routines and tasks are no longer performed. Behaviors that demonstrate poor judgment become common. Communication problems and personality changes follow.

Sundown syndrome describes a group of behaviors characterized by confusion, agitation, and disruptive actions that occur in the late afternoon or evening. The cause is unknown, but sundowning is associated with dementia, loss of cognitive functions, and physical or social stressors. As visual cues and social interactions decrease with the onset of nighttime, individuals become more confused, irritable, and agitated. The signs and symptoms and interventions for clients with sundown syndrome are listed in Box 17-3.

Cultural Considerations 17-1

ALZHEIMER'S DISEASE	VASCULAR DEMENTIA
More Common in United States and northern Europe	More common in China and Japan
Higher rates in African Americans	
Higher rates in women	No gender differences
Rates increased for Japanese who immigrated to the United States	Rates declined for Japanese who immigrated to the United States

---

Box 17-2 | *Possible Causes of Dementia*

Remember: MEND A MIND

Metabolic disorders	**A**rterial disease	**M**echanical disorders
Electrical disorders		**I**nfectious disease
Neoplastic disease (cancer)		**N**utritional disorders
Degenerative disease		**D**rug toxicity

Remember to assess older clients thoroughly and routinely. To do this you must know the client's baseline or usual behavior. Family members and significant others become a valuable resource for gathering information. The minor observations of one caregiver can make a difference. The label **dementia** should never be applied until after clients and their abilities have been thoroughly investigated.

The incidence of dementia increases with age. Alzheimer's dementia is the most common severe cognitive impairment in the United States. It accounts for "the majority of patients with dementia who are older than 55 years (50% to 90%)" (Gerstein, 2002). AD is often called "the long good-bye" because it slowly robs the individual of his or her memory, intellect, and personality.

ALZHEIMER'S DISEASE

Dementia of the Alzheimer's type presents special challenges. Alzheimer's disease (AD) is a progressive, degenerative disorder that affects brain cells and results in impaired **memory, thinking,** and **behavior.** In 1907, Alois Alzheimer, a German psychiatrist, first described the unique characteristics of this condition. He related the case of a 51-year-old woman who had a severely impaired ability to encode information, compromised language functions, and delusions. When she died from this severe form of progressive dementia, an autopsy of her brain revealed that it was shrunken, contained abnormal tangles of nerve fibers, and was filled with clusters of degenerated nerve endings. Since this first description the pathological findings of AD have been the subject of intense study and research.

Scientists divide AD into early onset and late onset. "People younger than 65 who develop Alzheimer's have the early-onset form. Although this group is

Box 17-3 | *Care for Clients With Sundown Syndrome*

ASSESS FOR:
Hunger, thirst, pain, the need to eliminate
Feelings of fear, insecurity
Isolation, little contact with other people
Recent move or change in routine

THERAPEUTIC (NURSING) INTERVENTIONS
Maintain comfort, toilet as necessary, keep dry.
Control pain with nondrug interventions (back rub, massage, touch, distraction).
Reduce environmental stimulation during late afternoon and evening.
Maintain daily routine.
Provide environmental cues, turn on lights before dusk, provide night-light.
Provide soothing music.
Provide reassurance and companionship during evening hours.

relatively small in number, it spans a wide age range. There are rare instances where people in their 30s have developed Alzheimer's" (Peterson, 2002).

Scientists now believe that "as many as 4.5 million Americans suffer from AD. The disease usually begins after age 60, and risk goes up with age. While younger people also may get AD, it is much less common. About 5 percent of men and women ages 65 to 74 have AD, and nearly half of those age 85 and older may have the disease. It is important to note, however, that AD is not a normal part of aging" (National Institute on Aging, 2007).

The cause of AD is unknown. Each year more than 250,000 new cases of AD are diagnosed. Because people with AD can live more than 20 years after diagnosis, many elderly people need extensive care. Caregivers need to be knowledgeable about the effects and treatment of AD and other dementias.

SYMPTOMS AND COURSE

The diagnosis of AD is not clear-cut. Therefore a diagnosis is made by exploring and ruling out all other causes of dementia. A client's confusion or dementia may be the result of a drug interaction or reaction. Other times, dementia occurs as the result of a medical condition. Careful and thorough history, physical examination, and mental status examinations are performed. The diagnosis of AD is made only after all the findings are considered. Today, researchers are working intensively to develop a diagnostic test for AD. Promising results have been seen with a type of skin testing, brain imaging techniques, and genetic studies.

AD involves a gradual, progressive death of one's brain and its functions. The incidence increases as age advances. The signs and symptoms of AD are listed in Table 17-1. AD progresses slowly and involves a loss in every area of functioning. In normal aging, cognitive (intellectual) and psychomotor (physical) changes are to be expected. Reaction times slow, and lapses of memory commonly occur. Learning new skills requires more time and practice, but intelligence and understanding remain intact. People with AD, however, lose their cognitive abilities and experience many intellectual losses.

Losses of Alzheimer's Disease

AD slowly robs an individual of his or her "personhood," and each decline is accompanied by a loss. Individuals with AD become unable to make even the simplest decisions or choices. Following a conversation becomes impossible because speech becomes disjointed, simplified, and empty. The intellectual losses of AD are accompanied by the slow drain of one's own personality (affective loss). Emotional control declines as the individual fades into childlike, antisocial, or emotionally labile behaviors. As the disease progresses and the ability to process information fades, people with AD become lost and absorbed in themselves. Some may even experience delusions, hallucinations, and feelings of paranoia.

Table 17-1 *Assessment of Alzheimer's Disease*

SIGNS AND SYMPTOMS	EXAMPLE
Memory loss	Especially short term; forgets and never remembers; trouble with associations
Difficulty performing familiar tasks	Forgets what order to put clothes on; prepares meal but then never serves it; leaves the car running
Problems with language	Forgets simple words; substitutes the wrong word; uses unusual words; hard to understand what is wanted because of word usage
Poor judgment	Inappropriate dress; buys unneeded items; forgets to watch child and leaves house for the day
Problems with abstract thinking	Stops paying bills; cannot balance checkbook; stops reading; has difficulty following a conversation
Misplaces things	Puts things in unusual places, such as a sandwich in the underwear drawer, milk in the oven, a watch in the freezer
Disoriented to time and place	Gets lost on one's own street; forgets where he or she is or how he or she got there
Loss of initiative	May become passive; sits in front of TV for hours; does not want to go places or see other people; loses interest in hobbies; sleeps more than usual
Changes in mood or behavior	May have rapid mood swings; may show less emotion than usual
Changes in personality	May become anxious, angry, apathetic, depressed, fearful, irritable, suspicious; may become agitated in situations where memory problems are causing difficulties

Another loss for people with AD relates to the ability to make and carry out plans (conative loss) even for the simplest activities. The everyday tasks of living, such as dressing, grooming, and bathing, become overwhelming challenges. The harder they concentrate on the activity, the more difficult the activity becomes to perform. Stress, anger, and frustration increase fatigue levels because everything requires so much energy. Short-term memory fades, and everything seems to be happening for the first time.

Finally, there is the loss of the ability to withstand stress. People with AD become less and less able to cope with stress as the disease progresses. Minor anxieties cascade into full catastrophic reactions, in which the person becomes increasingly confused, agitated, and fearful. They may wander, become noisy, act compulsively, or behave violently. Because of the lowered stress threshold, it takes fewer and fewer stimuli to produce these overwhelming behavioral reactions. For this reason, care for clients with AD centers around providing a low-stimuli environment with as few stress-provoking situations as possible.

Stages of Alzheimer's Disease

The progression of AD is divided into three stages. Disease progression, however, is not orderly because each individual is unique. Sometimes, symptoms seem to plateau for a time, but slow, progressive decline is the usual course.

The **early stage** begins with the loss of recent memory. An inability to learn, to process, and to retain information, followed by language problems, occurs. Judgment and abstract thinking decline. Individuals in the early stage forget where they put things and begin to have difficulty performing the activities of daily living. Many individuals react to their loss of memory and control with irritability, agitation, or hostility. Individuals are still social at this time, but family members begin to report strange behaviors and mood swings.

In the **intermediate stage,** clients cannot recall any recent events or process new information. Remote memory is affected but not totally lost. As the disease progresses, they usually develop **aphasia** (loss of language), **apraxia** (loss of ability to perform everyday actions, activities), and **visual agnosia** (loss of recognition of previously known or familiar people and objects). Individuals become increasingly forgetful and may require assistance with toileting, bathing, dressing, and eating. Behavior becomes further disorganized, and wandering, agitation, and physical aggression often occur. By now, individuals have lost all sense of time and place. However, they are still ambulatory and at high risk for falls and other accidents.

The **severe stage** of AD is characterized by an inability to do anything. Clients are usually incontinent, unable to walk, and entirely dependent on others for care. Memory, both recent and remote, is completely lost. An inability to swallow increases their risk for developing pneumonia and malnutrition. Many develop **mutism** (inability to speak) or communicate only in grunts.

In the **end stage,** clients slip into a coma and death from pneumonia or other infection occurs.

AFTER THE DIAGNOSIS

On hearing the diagnosis of AD, most clients and their loved ones experience shock and denial (the beginning of the grieving process). People with AD may live from 2 to 20 years after diagnosis. The average is about 8 years. Although they are in great emotional turmoil, family members must cope with the reality of the disease and begin planning for the future.

Some day care facilities are available to care for AD clients while family members work or attend to other obligations. Most people with AD are cared for in the

Table 17-2 *Alzheimer's Disease In-Home Caregiver Skills and Responsibilities*

SKILLS	RESPONSIBILITIES
Good organization—tracking medical, legal, financial records, medication schedules, physician appointments, and other caregivers' schedules **Physical stamina**—coping with custodial duties, lifting, carrying the person; going without a regular eating and sleeping schedule yourself **Emotional stamina**—coping with your own feelings, the feelings of the person with AD, feelings of other family members and friends; distancing yourself from the intense emotional responses of others **Ability to cope with repetitive, distasteful tasks**—in early stages exercises to slow mental and speech decline; continual supervision is necessary; most work in the middle and late stages is focused on feeding, elimination, personal hygiene, and ensuring safety while still ambulatory **The need to manage your life**—protecting your own health and well-being; making peace with death and dying; shifting focus to your own life and future	**Early stage**—being alert to any changes; helping with memory and communication problems; being attentive to the person's needs; providing a stable, routine environment; financial and estate planning, if possible **Middle stage**—adapting home for safety and convenience; making legal and financial decisions; managing medication schedules; managing hygiene, elimination, feeding, and exercise needs; coping with the changing personality and behaviors of the loved one **Severe stage**—being attentive to needs that can no longer be expressed; arranging for nursing home care; maintaining medication schedules; preparing for eventual death **Final stage**—complete physical care required; saying good-bye in your own way; preparing for the future

Data from Larkin M: *Alzheimer's outreach* at www.zarcrom.com/users/alzheimers.

home by family members until placement becomes necessary. Table 17-2 lists the skills and responsibilities of in-home care providers. As you can see, there are many challenges in caring for a loved one with AD.

In the early stages, responsibilities for care are to supervise and protect the person's safety. As the disease progresses, assistance is required with dressing, bathing, or other activities of daily living. When the demands of care become too great or the individual's safety is threatened (e.g., wandering, smoking, combative behavior), most are admitted to long-term care facilities. Some arrive earlier if family support is unavailable because people with AD cannot be left alone for any length of time.

Once the client adjusts to the new surroundings, the quality of life often improves. Family members are frequently relieved because the tremendous responsibility of constantly providing every need of their loved one (without recognition or thanks) is lifted from their shoulders.

PRINCIPLES OF MANAGEMENT

Treatments for AD are presently limited to providing physical and emotional support. Drug therapy is showing promise with medications that "improve cognition, behavior, and functioning in some patients" (Gray-Vickery, 2002) (Box 17-4). Alternative therapies, such as ginkgo biloba, vitamin E, and coenzyme Q-10, are currently under investigation.

Institutional long-term care is necessary for the majority of individuals with AD. As a result, the therapeutic environment has become an important aspect of treatment. Some long-term care facilities have 1950s-style surroundings, and residents seem

Box 17-4 *Drug Treatment for Alzheimer's Disease*

GENERIC NAME	BRAND NAME EXAMPLES
tacrine	Cognex
donepezil	Aricept
rivastigmine	Exelon
galantamine	Reminyl
Certain antiinflammatory drugs (may slow the rate of decline)	Advil, Naprosyn

comforted by an environment with memories of younger times. Others employ music therapy and audiotapes of family members to calm agitated clients. Regardless of the environment, the daily management of people with AD is focused on providing the highest quality of life possible during the slow progression of the disease.

THERAPEUTIC INTERVENTIONS

Therapeutic care for clients with AD has three major goals:
1. To provide for clients' safety and well-being
2. To manage clients' behaviors therapeutically
3. To provide support for family, relatives, and caregivers

People with AD are unable to care for themselves, even in the most basic ways. Bathing, grooming, eating, and physical activity for persons with AD all require interventions tailored to the individual. Elders with AD have no sense of safety or idea of danger. When they wander they may walk in the street, step out in front of moving vehicles, or sit on railroad tracks. Because of this absent sense, many facilities that care for AD clients have restricted or locked environments. Here clients are safe from the threats of both physical harm and overstimulation.

Several interventions help manage client behaviors therapeutically. When behaving inappropriately, clients are gently redirected to less stressful activities. Music therapy, validation therapy, and exercise have all been used successfully to reduce stress and quell agitated behaviors.

ASSESSMENT

On admission to a long-term care facility or health care service, a client undergoes a functional assessment—an analysis of each client's abilities to perform the activities of daily living. Areas of assessment are listed in Box 17-5. How does the client eat, bathe, move, and provide for his or her hygiene? What are the cognitive patterns, communication patterns, and sensory deficits? Are there any psychotic symptoms or signs of depression? What are the current medications and treatments? In short, how is the client's physical, intellectual, psychosocial, and emotional level of function? This information helps to establish an important baseline for comparisons later as the client deteriorates. The Medicare-required Minimum Data Set (MDS) is an example of one tool for gathering these data.

The assessment should also include the client's "support system, identify the primary caregiver and the patient's decision-making capacity. The family and caregivers are an important source of information" (Alzheimer's Association of Los Angeles, 2007). They should be included in the planning and care process whenever possible.

Box 17-5 *A Functional Assessment*

Conduct and document initial and ongoing assessments of the following client areas:

Daily Functions: Eating and drinking, personal hygiene, bathing, dressing, mobility, toileting, continence, ability to manage own medications, finances

Cognitive Status: Mental status examination, memory, orientation, judgment, abstract thinking, intellectual functioning, state of consciousness

Medical Conditions: Current medical problems, high blood pressure, diabetes, heart disease, etc.

Behavioral Problems: Agitation, anger, fear of being alone, frustration, insensitivity to others, irritability, loss of inhibitions, jealousy, paranoia, suspicion

Psychological Status: Personality changes, mood swings, flat emotional responses, psychotic symptoms, depression

Psychosocial Status: An initial psychosocial history and ongoing assessments of communications, interactions with others, spiritual needs

---

Nurses usually perform functional assessments. In many facilities, a dietitian, physiotherapist, occupational therapist, and an activity therapist also assess the client. The multidisciplinary team then meets. Information from each specialty is shared, and goals for care are developed.

INTERVENTIONS WITH ALZHEIMER'S DISEASE

Care for the individual with AD involves gradually increasing services for both client and family. The **case management** process allows for continual monitoring and modification of services as needed. Cultural beliefs are taken into account as care is planned. Specific interventions for each client are developed based on current abilities.

Care for the person with AD takes place in the home, a day care center, a long-term care facility, or an acute care agency. The main goal of care is to preserve as much function as possible by promoting good caregiver-client relationships within a safe and supportive environment. Treatment goals change as the client's functional abilities decline. Box 17-6 lists several basic interventions for clients at all stages of this devastating disease.

Early Stage

Therapeutic interventions in the early stage focus on preserving mental abilities. Scientists have found that the neurotransmitter **acetylcholine** is greatly decreased in people with AD. Researchers then developed a class of drugs, called **cholinesterase inhibitors,** that help prevent the breakdown of acetylcholine and thus preserve cognitive functions. "Currently, cholinesterase inhibitors are used only in the mild to moderate stages of Alzheimer's—generally 3 to 6 years after diagnosis" (Peterson, 2002). Drug Alert 17-2 lists the most common cholinesterase inhibitors and their side effects.

Cognitive training, which focuses on preserving learning and memory, may be started. Frequent orientation to time, place, and person is needed. A calendar with large letters and a clock with large numbers are helpful. Monitor personal hygiene and daily activities. Keep a daily routine. Be sure the environment is safe, and monitor for falls and other accidents.

Box 17-6 *Interventions for Clients With Alzheimer's Disease*

1. Treat the person, not the condition.
2. Support the relationship between client and caregiver.
3. Treat each person as an individual.
4. Establish and maintain communications.
5. Provide physical care, rest, and exercise.
6. Maintain a safe and supportive environment.
7. Maintain routine and consistency.
8. Manage difficult behaviors without reacting.

Establish good communications in the early stages. Know the client's personal history, and link present behaviors to past events. Do not react to inappropriate behaviors. Work with the person to discover what the negative behaviors are attempting to communicate. Box 17-7 offers several specific techniques for communicating with individuals with AD.

Maintaining a supportive environment is an important goal of care. Individuals who are cared for in the home need an environment that is simple, free of clutter and other safety hazards, and familiar. Orienting cues help individuals remember where they are and decrease agitation. Box 17-8 offers several interventions that help keep clients oriented to their environments.

A simple daily routine is soothing to people with AD. Daily activities, such as eating, toileting, bathing, and exercise, should follow a consistent schedule. Individuals with AD depend on their routines and structure. They do not adapt well to change, and the consistency of a stable environment helps keep stress levels more manageable.

Simple physical exercises and activities are included in the daily routine for as long as the client is ambulatory. Exercise helps maintain balance, induce fatigue and restful sleep, prevent constipation, and reduce wandering. Sports, card games, musical activities, painting, and gardening can be enjoyed by individuals well into the moderate stage of AD.

Middle and Late Stages

Physical care is increasingly necessary as behavior gradually becomes more disorganized. Personal hygiene, eating, and elimination are totally neglected without caregivers (see Sample Client Care Plan 17-1). All sense of time and place is lost by the middle stage. Behavioral disorganization is seen with behaviors such as agitation, hostility, physical aggression, uncooperativeness, and

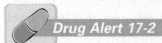

Drug Alert 17-2

COMMON CHOLINESTERASE INHIBITORS
Used during the early stages of Alzheimer's disease to improve cognition, memory, and behavior

Generic Name	Brand Name	Side Effects
donepezil	Aricept	Generally mild; include nausea, vomiting, diarrhea, dizziness, headache, insomnia, high or low blood pressure, urinary problems, cough, rash, seizures
rivastigmine	Exelon	Tremors, confusion, insomnia, depression, anxiety, headache, sleepiness, fatigue, dizziness, nausea, vomiting, anorexia, diarrhea, constipation, increased sweating, urinary tract infection, weight changes
galantamine	Reminyl	Tremors, insomnia, depression, dizziness, headache, sleepiness, fatigue, anemia, slow heart rate, blood in urine, nausea, vomiting, anorexia, gas, diarrhea, urinary incontinence, weight decrease

Box 17-7 | *Communication Techniques for Persons With Alzheimer's Disease*

1. Always approach from the front—no surprise appearances.
2. Speak in a normal tone of voice, and greet the person as you would anyone else.
3. Face the person as you talk.
4. Minimize hand movements.
5. Avoid a setting with a high level of sensory stimulation, such as a big room with many people, a high traffic area, or a noisy place.
6. Maintain eye contact, and smile. A frown will convey negative feelings.
7. Use simple familiar words and short, simple sentences.
8. Ask yes-or-no questions.
9. Allow plenty of time for a response.
10. Repeat important information.
11. Be respectful of personal space, and observe the client's reaction as you move closer. Maintain a distance of 1 to 1½ feet initially.
12. If a person is a pacer, walk with him or her, in step, while you talk.
13. Use distraction if a situation looks like it may get out of hand, such as if the person is about to hit someone or is trying to leave the home or facility.
14. Use a low-pitched, slow speaking voice, which older adults hear best.
15. Ask only one question at a time. More than one question increases confusion.
16. Repeat key words if the person does not understand the first time.
17. Nod and smile only if what the person said is understood.

Modified from ElderCareOnline at www.ec-online.net.

wandering. Individuals remain ambulatory throughout the middle stage, but they are at a much greater risk for falls and accidents as a result of their confusion.

Wandering is a serious and common problem with AD persons. "The Alzheimer's Association estimates that 60% of people with that disease will wander and become lost in the community at some point" (Rowe, 2003). Because of this, the Safe Return Program (1-800-272-3900; www.alz.org) was established by the Alzheimer's Association to assist in the safe return of people with dementia who become lost.

Problems with aggression, wandering, and shouting accompany the middle to late stages of AD. These behaviors are seen as offensive and frightening by most caregivers. To understand these behaviors, nurse researchers developed the need-driven dementia-compromised behavior model. The model views offensive behaviors as communications of unmet needs. Behaviors result from the interaction of one's background factors (characteristics that shape lasting behavior patterns) with changeable environmental triggers called proximal factors. Table 17-3 explains the factors of the need-driven dementia-compromised behavior model. By viewing disruptive behaviors as expressions of needs, caregivers are able to respond in ways that meet those needs, thus decreasing inappropriate behaviors. Other therapies that have been helpful for clients with AD are listed in Table 17-4.

Box 17-8 *Orienting Environmental Cues*

- Keep environment simple and "user friendly."
- Keep the environment safe: ramps for stairs, grab bars in bathroom, no throw rugs, etc.
- Put large signs that identify each room on the doors.
- Label each drawer with its contents. Use large letters and simple words. Tape the list to the drawer.
- Have clocks and calendars with large letters and numbers in several rooms.
- Color-code hot and cold faucets red and blue, respectively. Adjust water heater to 120° Fahrenheit.
- Install a brightly colored toilet seat (it is easier to see).
- Keep rooms brightly lit with no glare.
- Use night-lights in hallways, bedrooms, and bathrooms.
- Cover doors with curtains or posters to discourage wandering.

SAMPLE CLIENT CARE PLAN 17-1

Self-Care Deficit

ASSESSMENT *History.* Tess is a 70-year-old retired accountant who is being admitted with a diagnosis of Alzheimer's disease. She had been cared for in her daughter's home until she began to wander. Now the family fears for her safety.
Current Findings. Functional assessment reveals an ambulatory woman who is unable to follow directions. She is oriented to person only and has self-care deficits in bathing, dressing, eating, and toileting.

Multidisciplinary Diagnosis	*Planning/Goals*
Self-care deficit related to cognitive impairment	Tess will dress correctly daily. Tess will consume 50% or more of each meal by September 15.

Therapeutic Interventions

Intervention	Rationale	Team Member
1. Lay out clothes in order of dressing, underclothes first to sweater last.	Provides routine, easier to dress appropriately.	Nsg
2. Assist as needed, and praise all efforts.	Positive feedback increases the likelihood that the desired behaviors will be repeated.	All
3. Determine her favorite foods.	She will eat the foods she likes.	Diet, Nsg
4. Evaluate speech and swallowing.	Determines level of impairment.	ST
5. Assist Tess with eating.	Ensures nutrition is received.	Nsg
6. Document intake, output, and amount of food consumed.	Monitors fluid and nutritional status.	Diet, Nsg

Evaluation

By the seventh day on the unit, Tess was dressing herself appropriately with cues from caregivers. She currently consumes more than 70% of her meals when she is fed.

? CRITICAL THINKING QUESTIONS

1. How does providing a daily routine benefit Tess?

2. What can be done to provide support for Tess' daughter?

A complete client care plan includes several other diagnoses and interventions.
Nsg, Nursing staff; *Diet,* dietitian; *ST,* speech therapist.

By the time clients enter the third stage of AD, they are usually unable to walk, totally incontinent, and incapable of self-care. Memory is completely lost. Speech becomes limited to one or two words and is soon lost altogether. Clients become unable to swallow or eat, which leads to a high risk for malnutrition, pneumonia, and bedsores. Placement in a long-term care facility becomes necessary because full-time care and monitoring are now required. Eventually, the individual slips into a coma and dies.

CAREGIVER SUPPORT

"Caring for an elderly person with dementia radically changes the life of the primary caregiver" (Sclan and Kanowski, 2001). Caring for a loved one with AD is probably the most difficult of all caregiving experiences. It has often been said that AD is worse on the caregivers who must stand by and watch the person they love fade into a vague, unconscious existence.

The majority of people with AD are cared for in the home by family, friends, and home care agencies. Tremendous physical and emotional burdens accompany the home care of a loved one with AD. Caregivers must learn to find a balance between personal needs and providing care for their loved ones. Various sources of support help family members through this difficult journey.

Informal support groups consist of family members, friends, people at work, social groups, and faith communities. Members of these groups knew the individual with AD before the illness. Often, they are a great source of respite, strength, socialization, and support for the primary caregivers.

Formal support groups are offered by various home care agencies, elder care centers, and hospices. The local Alzheimer's Association supports family members and provides information about dementia. It offers both emotional and educational support groups. Stress management groups are helpful in recognizing stress and developing successful coping strategies. Many long-term care facilities now offer **respite** care where the loved one with AD is safely cared for while caregivers receive a much needed break. Never forget that those who care for the cognitively impaired need your attentions as much as your client does. The support from family, friends, and resource people makes a difference in the quality of life for those caring for loved ones with AD.

Caregiver Education

Studies have found that when caregivers are educated, stress levels in the home decrease. Caregiver training prepares family members to provide care for their loved one. Topics such as environmental safety, personal care, coping with difficult behaviors, and care provider stress are addressed, and sources of support are explored.

AD and other dementias are serious problems, but with continued research and good care we may someday be able to lessen the sad effects of these devastating conditions.

Table 17-3 *Need-Driven Dementia-Compromised Behavior Model**

BACKGROUND FACTORS	PROXIMAL FACTORS†
Shape long-standing behavior pattern	Induce a need state and bring out dementia-related (disruptive) behaviors
Health state: Gender, race, ethnicity, marital status, occupation, religion	**Physical need state:** Hunger, thirst, elimination, pain, education, discomfort, sleep disturbance
Psychosocial variables: Personality, behavioral responses to stress	**Physical environment:** Light level, sound level, heat/cold
Dementia-compromised functions: Circadian (body) rhythm, motor ability, memory, language	**Social environment:** Staff mix, staff stability, environment, presence of others

From Kolanowski AM: An overview of the need-driven dementia-compromised behavior model, *J Gerontol Nurs* 25:7, 1999.
*Behaviors (aggression, wandering, shouting, etc.) are the result of the factors given.
†Caregivers intervene by identifying the proximal factors and helping clients meet their needs, thus decreasing unwanted behaviors.

Table 17-4 *Therapeutic Interventions for Alzheimer's Disease*

WHAT IS IT?	HOW DOES IT WORK?
Validation therapy	Caregiver buys into client's illusions and plays along (validates it) until opportunity to refocus behaviors is present, based on the premise that the client's illusion cannot be changed, but it can be directed
Music therapy	Use of familiar tunes to induce relaxation, alter moods, improve social interactions, and change maladaptive behaviors
Life review	A systematic reflection on one's personal history in which one learns to evaluate, integrate, and accept life as it has been lived; increases quality of life and helps prevent despair and depression
Comfort touch	Skin-to-skin touch with the purpose of bringing comfort; results in improved well-being, self-esteem, and socialization
Doll therapy	Use of dolls and stuffed animals to provide tactile stimulation and comfort
Audio presence intervention	Playing of tape-recorded memories by family members to help decrease agitation

Key Points

- AD and other dementias are behavioral or mental health problems caused by a medical condition.
- The most significant losses in aging are slower response times and short-term memory.
- The causes of confusion are damage, delirium, dementia, depression, and deprivation.
- Many medications and drugs cause confusion, especially in the elderly because metabolism is slower, drugs are eliminated more slowly, and they can reach toxic levels quickly.
- The signs and symptoms of delirium include disorganized thinking, a decreased attention span, lowered or fluctuating level of consciousness, disturbances in the sleep-wake cycle, disorientation, and changes in psychomotor activity.
- The treatment of delirium depends on its cause. The first priority is to treat the source. The second focus of care is supportive.
- Dementia is a loss of multiple abilities, including short- and long-term memory, language, and the ability to understand. Persons with dementia are unable to process, retrieve, and use information. All have progressive problems with memory, judgment, and abstract thinking.
- AD is characterized by memory loss, difficulty performing familiar tasks, problems with language, poor judgment, problems with abstract thinking, misplacing things, disorientation to time and place, loss of initiative, changes in mood or behavior, and changes in personality.

- Dementia can be primary, as with AD, or it may occur as a result of disease, such as HIV (secondary).
- AD is characterized by memory loss, difficulty performing familiar tasks, problems with language, poor judgment, problems with abstract thinking, misplacing things, disorientation to time and place, loss of initiative, changes in mood or behavior, and changes in personality.
- AD is accompanied by losses in every area of functioning.
- The progression of AD is divided into three stages—early, middle, and late.
- The need-driven dementia-compromised behavior model views disruptive behaviors as communications of unmet needs. Behaviors result from the interaction of one's background factors with proximal factors. Clients' needs are defined and met, thus decreasing the disruptive behavior.
- Informal support groups consist of family members, friends, and people who knew the individual with AD before the illness. Formal support groups are offered by various home care agencies, elder care centers, hospices, and the Alzheimer's Association.

---

evolve Be sure to visit the companion Evolve site at http://evolve.elsevier.com/Morrison-Valfre/ for additional online resources.

18 Managing Anxiety

evolve http://evolve.elsevier.com/Morrison-Valfre/

Objectives

Upon completion of this chapter, the student will be able to:

1. Describe the continuum of responses to anxiety.
2. Identify three types of coping mechanisms used to decrease anxiety.
3. Explain how anxiety is experienced in each stage of the life cycle.
4. Compare the difference between normal anxiety and an anxiety disorder.
5. Discuss the difference between phobic and obsessive-compulsive behaviors.
6. Examine three features of posttraumatic stress disorder.
7. List two therapeutic interventions for the client with rape-trauma syndrome.
8. Explain the importance of monitoring medication use for clients with high levels of anxiety.
9. Examine three methods for recognizing and preventing anxiety.

Key Terms

addictive behaviors (p. 199)
agoraphobia (Ă-or-ə-FO-bē-ə) (p. 197)
anxiety (p. 191)
anxiety disorder (p. 197)
anxiety state (p. 191)
anxiety trait (p. 191)
avoidance behaviors (p. 196)
compulsion (p. 198)
coping mechanisms (p. 192)
defense mechanisms (p. 193)
flashbacks (p. 199)
obsession (p. 198)
panic attack (p. 197)
phobia (FŌ-bē-ə) (p. 198)
signal anxiety (p. 191)
traumatic stress reaction (p. 199)

Anxiety is a feeling of uneasiness, uncertainty, and helplessness. It is a state of tension sometimes associated with feelings of dread or doom. Anxiety is the **normal emotional response** to a real or imagined threat or stressor.

Anxiety serves several purposes. It is a warning of impending danger. Mild anxiety can increase learning by helping with concentration and focus. Anxiety can also provide motivation. However, uncontrolled anxiety often leads to ineffective and maladaptive behaviors. Anxiety is a normal part of survival and growth. How individuals use and control anxiety is one of the measures of mental health and illness.

CONTINUUM OF ANXIETY RESPONSES

Reactions to anxiety occur along a continuum of behavioral responses (Stuart and Laraia, 2005) (Figure 18-1). Adaptive responses to anxiety result in positive outcomes. New learning and greater self-esteem result from coping successfully with anxiety. Positively focused anxiety helps us to adapt, learn, and grow from our experiences. However, maladaptive responses to anxiety are ineffective attempts to cope. They do nothing to resolve the problem or eliminate uneasy feelings.

Responses to anxiety occur on four levels, ranging from mild to panic (Table 18-1). During periods of anxiety, physical, intellectual, emotional, and behavioral responses help us cope. In periods of severe anxiety, the autonomic nervous system stimulates the fight-or-flight response, which triggers many physical changes. Use Table 18-1 as a basis for assessing the anxiety levels of clients. Decreasing anxiety is an important intervention in every health care situation.

TYPES OF ANXIETY

Anxiety occurs as the result of a perceived threat to one's self. The threat itself may be real or occur in response to what we think is happening. The actual object of anxiety often cannot be identified, but the feelings associated with the experience are all too real.

For the sake of discussion, anxiety is classified by types. Signal anxiety is a learned response to an anticipated event. The usually calm student who becomes nauseated during examinations illustrates signal anxiety. An anxiety state occurs when an individual's coping abilities become overwhelmed and emotional control is lost. Many emergencies, accidents, and traumas are associated with anxiety states. Last is an anxiety trait, which is a learned component of the personality. Persons with anxiety traits react with anxiety in relatively low stress situations. The adolescent who always gives reasons for his or her behavior, even when not requested, illustrates an example of an anxiety trait.

TYPES OF ANXIETY RESPONSES

"People usually experience anxiety about events they cannot control or predict or about events that seem threatening or dangerous" (*Microsoft Encarta Online Encyclopedia*, 2007). We all experience anxiety. New situations, unfamiliar environments, or tasks for which we are not prepared are often associated with anxiety.

The physical symptoms of anxiety include muscle tension, fidgeting, headaches, and problems with sleep. Higher levels of anxiety trigger the fight-or-flight reaction and result in nausea, dizziness, sweating, increased heart rate, and elevated blood pressure.

Most individuals deal with anxiety by using a number of behaviors or coping mechanisms to help

decrease discomfort. All coping methods reduce anxiety, but if used to extreme, serious mental and physical health problems can result.

COPING METHODS

Coping mechanisms in the **physical** realm include efforts to directly face and handle the problem. The woman who fights the thief who is attempting to snatch her purse, for example, is directly dealing with the source of her anxiety. Many individuals exercise to reduce anxiety. Physical exercises, such as running or other aerobics, can reduce the effects of the fight-or-flight response by lowering blood pressure and neurochemical levels. Stretching and yoga exercises release muscle tension and encourage relaxation.

Intellectual coping mechanisms are aimed at making the threat less meaningful by changing one's perception. If we do not define the event as threatening, anxiety is not produced. A good example is the individual who sees everyone in his audience smiling when he is about to give a speech. The threat (audience disapproval) is reduced by the perception of smiling faces. Another coping mechanism in the intellectual realm is meditation, which helps clear and refocus one's mental energies.

Spiritual coping methods include faith, prayer, and ritual. Attending religious services or communing

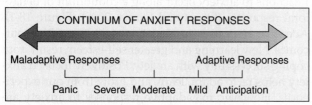

FIGURE **18-1** Continuum of anxiety responses.

Table 18-1 | *Levels of Anxiety*

ANXIETY LEVEL	PHYSIOLOGICAL	COGNITIVE/PERCEPTUAL	EMOTIONAL/BEHAVIORAL
Mild	Vital signs normal. Minimal muscle tension. Pupils normal, constricted.	Perceptual field is broad. Awareness of multiple environmental and internal stimuli. Thoughts may be random, but controlled.	Feelings of relative comfort and safety. Relaxed, calm appearance and voice. Performance is automatic; habitual behaviors occur.
Moderate	Vital signs normal or slightly elevated. Tension experienced may be uncomfortable or pleasurable (labeled as "tense" or "excited").	Alert; perception narrowed, focused. Optimum state for problem solving and learning. Attentive.	Feelings of readiness and challenge, energized. Engage in competitive activity and learn new skills. Voice, facial expression interested or concerned.
Severe	Fight-or-flight response. Autonomic nervous system excessively stimulated (vital signs increased, diaphoresis increased, urinary urgency and frequency, diarrhea, dry mouth, appetite decreased, pupils dilated). Muscles rigid, tense. Senses affected; hearing decreased, pain sensation decreased.	Perceptual field greatly narrowed. Problem solving difficult. Selective attention (focus on one detail). Selective inattention (block out threatening stimuli). Distortion of time (things seem faster or slower than actual). Dissociative tendencies; vigilambulism (automatic behavior).	Feels threatened; startles with new stimuli; feels on "overload." Activity may increase or decrease (may pace, run away, wring hands, moan, shake, stutter, become very disorganized or withdrawn, freeze in position/unable to move). May seem and feel depressed. Demonstrates denial; may complain of aches or pains; may be agitated or irritable. Need for space increased. Eyes may dart around room, or gaze may be fixed. May close eyes to shut out environment.
Panic	Above symptoms escalate until sympathetic nervous system release occurs. Person may become pale, blood pressure decreases, hypotension. Muscle coordination poor. Pain, hearing sensations minimal.	Perception totally scattered or closed. Unable to take in stimuli. Problem solving and logical thinking highly improbable. Perception of unreality about self, environment, or event. Dissociation may occur.	Feels helpless with total loss of control. May be angry, terrified; may become combative or totally withdrawn, cry, run. Completely disorganized. Behavior is usually extremely active or inactive.

From Fortinash KM, Holoday Worret PA: *Psychiatric nursing care plans*, ed 5, St. Louis, 2007, Mosby.

with nature can reduce anxiety. Many cultural rituals also help individuals cope.

Emotional responses include crying, communicating or sharing one's anxious feelings, and using ego defense mechanisms.

DEFENSE MECHANISMS

The psychological strategies that help to lessen anxious feelings are called (ego) defense mechanisms. These psychological self-preserving behaviors reduce or avoid negative states such as conflict, frustration, anxiety, and stress. They are used when one feels threatened. Employing defense mechanisms helps to avoid negative emotional states, but usually individuals are not consciously aware of their use. No matter which mechanism is used, the goal is to reduce uncomfortable negative emotions. Table 18-2 lists several commonly used ego defense mechanisms.

CRISIS

When one's ability to cope with anxiety is overwhelmed, a crisis results. Defense mechanisms are no longer useful. No efforts to cope with the situation lessen one's anxiety. During a crisis, new coping behaviors must be developed to successfully resolve the source problem. Review Chapter 8 for a more thorough discussion of crisis and its therapeutic interventions.

Ineffective Coping

Anxiety is a normal part of everyday life. It occurs in all cultures (see Cultural Considerations 18-1).

Anxiety is a protective state that motivates us to pursue goals and respond to threats. However, too little or too much anxiety can lead to ineffective coping behaviors and cause more problems. Too little anxiety can result in a lack of attention or focus in important

Table 18-2 | *Common Defense Mechanisms*

MECHANISM	DEFINITION	EXAMPLE
Compensation	Attempt to overcome feelings of inferiority or make up for deficiency	A girl who thinks she cannot sing studies to become an expert pianist.
Conversion	Channeling of unbearable anxieties into body signs and symptoms	A boy who injured an animal by kicking it develops a painful limp.
Denial	Refusal to acknowledge conflict and thus escapes reality of situation	A child covered with chocolate refuses to admit eating candy.
Displacement	Redirecting of energies to another person or object	A husband shouts at his wife, the wife then berates her child, who then scolds the dog.
Dissociation	Separation of emotions from situation; isolation of painful anxieties	A soldier casually describes the battle in which he lost his legs.
Fantasy	Distortion of unacceptable wishes, behaviors	A teenager doing poorly in school daydreams about owning a private jet airplane.
Identification	Taking on of personal characteristics of admired person to conceal own feelings of inadequacy	Adolescents dress and behave like the members of a popular singing group.
Intellectualization	Focusing of attention on technical or logical aspects of threatening situation	A wife describes the details of nurses' unsuccessful attempts to prevent the death of her husband.
Isolation	Separation of feelings from content to cope unemotionally with topics that would normally be overwhelming	A soldier humorously describes how he was seriously wounded in combat.
Projection	Putting of one's own unacceptable thoughts, wishes, emotions onto others	A woman is afraid to leave her house because she knows people will ridicule her.
Rationalization	Use of a "good" (but not real) reason to explain behavior to make unacceptable motivation more acceptable	A student justifies failing an examination by saying that there was too much material to cover.
Reaction formation	Prevention of expression of threatening material by engaging in behaviors that are directly opposite to repressed material	A young man with homosexual feelings, which he finds to be threatening, engages in excessive heterosexual activities.
Regression	Coping with present conflict, stress by returning to earlier, more secure stage of life	A 4-year-old boy whose parents are going through a divorce starts to suck his thumb and wet his pants.
Restitution	Giving back to resolve guilt feelings	A man argues with his wife and then buys her roses.
Sublimation	Unconscious channeling of unacceptable behaviors into constructive, more socially approved areas	A hostile young man who enjoys fighting becomes a football player.
Substitution	Disguising of motivations by replacing inappropriate behavior with one that is more acceptable	A man who is attracted to pornography campaigns to ban adult book stores in his community.
Suppression	Removal of conflict by removing anxiety from consciousness	A woman with a family history of breast cancer "forgets" her appointment for a mammogram.
Symbolization	Use of an unrelated object to represent hidden idea	A girl who feels insignificant draws a picture of her family in which she is the smallest character.
Undoing	Inappropriate behavior that is followed by acts to take away or reverse action and decrease guilt and anxiety	A man physically abuses his wife and then cleans her wounds and nurses her back to health.

Cultural Considerations 18-1

Anxiety appears to occur in most, if not every, culture. Expressions of anxiety, however, differ greatly:

Japanese people tend to somatize or handle anxiety by becoming physically ill.

Mothers in the Dominican Republic cope with the anxiety of the "evil eye" by wearing red and saving the infant's umbilical cord.

Greek men consider body hair a sign of manhood. Shaving their hair in preparation for a surgical procedure can result in great anxiety.

Case Study 18-1

Cathy's appointment with her physician was for 10 AM. By the time she had waited for more than 2 hours, Cathy was feeling frustrated. After a 2½-hour wait, she was downright anxious. Just as she began to leave, her name was called and she was ushered into a rather impersonal examination room where she changed into the paper gown and waited, shivering, for her physician.

After what seemed another hour, the door finally opened. Her physician, a woman of many words, began the interaction with "My gads, what a day! One thing goes wrong in the morning, and I spend the rest of the day chasing myself to catch up."

Noting her physician's tension and rapid speech, Cathy responded, "You certainly look tired. Sounds like you have been working too hard." Her physician countered with, "That's not the half of it," and then proceeded to share each of her day's frustrations.

- Who was the therapeutic one in this situation?
- How did the physician's behavior affect therapeutic interactions with this client?
- How do you think the interaction affected Cathy's anxiety?

situations. Too much anxiety can overwhelm and immobilize an individual and result in an inability to accomplish important tasks. When ego defense mechanisms become the primary means of dealing with anxiety, they replace problem solving and other positive ways of coping. The use of ineffective coping behaviors can lead to too much anxiety and result in an anxiety disorder.

SELF-AWARENESS AND ANXIETY

A basic characteristic of anxiety is that it is contagious. Like a cold or influenza virus, anxiety is easily transmitted to others. Clients have an uncanny ability to focus on the anxiety levels of their health care providers. Sometimes the client becomes the therapeutic agent for an anxious caregiver.

The therapeutic relationship is built on trust. Inherent in that trust is the care provider's responsibility to listen and communicate effectively. High levels of anxiety can impair our ability to interact therapeutically with the client. For this reason, it is important for caregivers to recognize and cope effectively with their own anxieties. Remember, we may not choose our anxieties, but we do choose how we deal with them. Case Study 18-1 provides an example of how a health care provider's anxiety can affect the therapeutic relationship.

THEORIES RELATING TO ANXIETY

A number of theories have been developed since Sigmund Freud first listed anxiety as a defense mechanism. Today the causes of anxiety are still uncertain, but research indicates that a combination of biological, psychosocial, and environmental factors is involved. A few of the more well-known theories of anxiety are discussed here.

BIOLOGICAL MODELS

The biological group of theories attempts to find a biological or physical basis for anxiety. The work of Charles Darwin first posed the possibility of a link between emotions and the ability to adapt. Later, Hans Selye demonstrated a connection between the perception of stress and physical changes in the body with his fight-or-flight response. During the 1990s, called "the decade of the brain," many advances in the understanding of emotions and mental illness were made. Today we are beginning to gain an understanding of the role emotions play in health and illness as researchers unveil new information.

One of the most popular current theories of anxiety relates to the role of neurochemicals. Research into the role of these body chemicals, called neurotransmitters, has resulted in evidence that emotions may be linked to changes in brain development and biochemistry (Hyman, 1998). Anxiety is thought to result from the dysfunction of two or more neurotransmitters. Some studies have demonstrated inappropriately activated norepinephrine and imbalances between this and other neurotransmitters. Further research is being done to investigate specific medications designed to alter neurotransmitter activity. Other ongoing studies are investigating the role of the autonomic nervous system in the development of anxiety. Many medical disorders, hormonal imbalances, problems with substance use, and even fatigue are related to anxiety.

PSYCHODYNAMIC MODEL

According to Freud, anxiety results from a conflict between two opposing forces within the personality—the ego and the id. Neurotic or maladaptive behaviors are the result of attempts to defend oneself against anxiety, just as adaptive behaviors do. Psychotherapists today have broadened the psychoanalytical theory to define anxiety as the result of a conflict between two opposing forces within an individual.

INTERPERSONAL MODEL

With the interpersonal model, anxiety is explained in terms of interactions with others. Anxiety develops when early childhood interactions with significant others result in negative outcomes, such as disapproval. Over time, an individual's responses to anxiety form the basis for low self-esteem and poor self-concept.

Interpersonal theorists work with a broad definition of anxiety. Harry Stack Sullivan believed that children acquire the values of their parents because they are dependent on others for approval or disapproval. In adulthood, individuals cope with anxiety based on their perceptions and on how they were taught to cope with conflict as children. Using this interpersonal model, one can see the importance of early assessment and intervention for children who are anxious.

BEHAVIORAL MODEL

The behavioral theories consider anxiety a learned response. Children who experienced anxiety in one situation link those feelings to more general situations. Anxiety results when individuals encounter a signal that reminds them of earlier anxious times. Thus individuals learn to react with anxiety by linking anxious experiences.

OTHER MODELS

Other theories explain anxiety as the result of a loss of life's meaning (**existential** theory). Environmental models tie anxiety with uncontrollable events or situations. Fires, floods, and other natural disasters, along with assaults and human-induced traumas, all serve as stressors for the individual.

Many health care providers have chosen to view anxiety from a **holistic** mode. Anxiety is viewed as having an impact on every realm of human functioning. Physical reactions, such as the fight-or-flight reaction, result from anxiety. Strong emotional responses occur when one is anxious. Social areas of functioning can become impaired because of anxiety, and even one's spirituality comes into question during times of great or prolonged anxiety. By considering each area of functioning, care providers are better able to plan and implement effective therapeutic interventions for relieving anxiety.

ANXIETY THROUGHOUT THE LIFE CYCLE

Anxiety is a universal experience. It begins early in life, as soon as one becomes capable of realizing that something could go wrong. Responses to anxiety grow and evolve with the individual. Behavioral reactions to anxiety change as effective (anxiety-reducing) actions are added to current coping mechanisms. Responses or behaviors that are ineffective or serve no purpose are discarded. An understanding of how individuals at various developmental stages perceive and cope with anxiety helps care providers plan and implement individualized care for all clients.

ANXIETY IN CHILDHOOD

Children learn to cope with anxiety by watching and imitating others. Most children are happy, active individuals with few anxieties. However, if their needs for nurturing are not met, high levels of anxiety can result. Children's needs for love and belonging are so great that later-life emotional problems are often related to unmet needs in childhood. "Although children are not strangers to stress, some children appear to be more vulnerable than others" (Hockenberry and others, 2007). Recognizing signs of childhood stress and intervening early are important. They prevent anxiety from becoming overwhelming and help teach children how to cope successfully.

Anxiety is experienced in relation to a child's **developmental level**. Infants feel a sense of discomfort if their needs are not immediately met. Toddlers become anxious when they perceive something larger or more ferocious than themselves that is capable of harming them. Their anxiety relates to power and lasts until the balance of power can be restored. Anxiety in preschool children revolves around the experience of separating from the security of parents. As children learn that separations are not permanent, anxieties lessen and coping abilities improve. School-age children learn to cope with the anxieties of becoming members of a group outside the family.

The development of certain habits early in childhood appears to help children relieve anxiety. Thumb sucking, nail biting, hair pulling, and rhythmic body movements are examples of behaviors that seem to soothe and lessen anxiety for young children. Excessive anxiety appears to develop when children resist their feelings of anxiety and focus them elsewhere. Problems associated with anxiety in childhood include compulsions, phobias, separation anxiety disorder, overanxious disorder, and avoidant disorders.

Separation anxiety disorder is diagnosed when children are unable to be without their parents for any length of time. By about 6 months of age, infants are able to recognize their mother's absence from the room and protest. They soon become very aware of their mother's activities. They learn to identify behaviors that indicate their mother is leaving the area. By 11 months, most children begin to protest before their mother leaves. During the next 4 years, children learn to tolerate varying degrees of separation from parents. By school age, most children separate from parents easily and their focus changes to coping with school life.

Children with separation anxiety disorder, however, experience severe anxiety that can develop into panic when separated from significant others. Physical complaints such as headaches, nausea, or vomiting are common when children anticipate separation. Nightmares occur frequently. Associated fears of death, animals, monsters, and harmful situations are seen in children with separation anxiety disorder.

Overanxious disorder appears during childhood with unrealistic levels of anxiety lasting longer than 6 months—a long time in the life of a child. These children worry about everything from past events to future expectations. Overanxious disorder often occurs in children whose parents focus on overachievement and downplay their children's actual accomplishments.

Children can also experience severe anxiety during times of great change in the family. Reactions to divorce, death, or separation often lead to situational anxiety or avoidance behaviors in which the child refuses to cope with the anxiety-producing situation by ignoring it.

Sadly, children are not immune to the effects of unresolved anxiety. Occurrences of posttraumatic stress disorder, depression, and suicide are on the rise in children. Children with behavioral problems often have underlying anxieties. For children to grow and mature into effective, adaptable individuals, we must recognize and treat the signs of anxiety early. The old proverb "A stitch in time saves nine" is worth remembering when working with children.

ANXIETY IN ADOLESCENCE

Coping skills learned in childhood continue to be refined throughout adolescence. If teens have successfully handled anxieties in childhood, the distresses of becoming adults offer opportunities for personal growth and maturation. Adolescents who ineffectively cope with anxiety often express themselves inappropriately. Running away from home; becoming angry, defiant, aggressive, or manipulative; experimenting with drugs; and engaging in high-risk behaviors often occur. They frequently use denial to cope and resist attempts to explore the anxiety-producing perceptions that lead to understanding. When anxieties are extreme, adolescents may engage in self-mutilating behaviors or develop the behaviors of anorexia nervosa or bulimia (see Chapter 23).

Many initial symptoms of schizophrenia and other psychoses begin in adolescence. Signs of maladaptive behaviors, such as flights from reality, ritualistic behaviors, or withdrawal from others, may actually be symptoms of serious mental health problems.

Unfortunately, adolescents are a forgotten population when it comes to mental health care. Many children and adolescents with serious emotional or behavioral disorders receive little or no mental health treatment. Health care providers who work with adolescents must assess adolescents' anxiety levels and offer early intervention and education before anxiety becomes the fuel for more serious mental health problems.

ANXIETY IN ADULTHOOD

By young adulthood, coping behaviors are well established. Adults commonly encounter situations that provoke anxiety as they move through their worlds of work, family, and community. Some adults appear to lead a "charmed life," with few stresses and anxieties. Others seem to continually struggle, only to rebound from one misfortune after another. Like their younger counterparts, adults handle anxiety using earlier, established coping mechanisms.

Adults must cope with many anxiety-producing situations. Developmental tasks, such as establishing a career and family, present numerous stressors. The loss of income, spouse, or physical ability can lead to severe anxiety. Uncontrollable situations, such as fires, floods, earthquakes, or wars, often result in long-lasting anxiety. Unless resolved, it can evolve into posttraumatic stress syndrome. When adult anxieties are not successfully managed, a number of mental health problems may result. Generalized or situational anxiety disorders are diagnosed when individuals become overwhelmed and nonfunctional because of their anxieties. Other maladaptive responses include panic disorders, phobias, behavioral addictions, obsessions, and compulsive activities.

ANXIETY IN OLDER ADULTHOOD

Older adults tend to express anxieties in less overt ways than younger people do. Elders often deny their anxiety. They may **somatize** (express physically) their feelings. Social desirability factors, such as looking good to others and projecting an image of self-reliance, commonly influence their expressions of anxiety.

Although few actual statistics are available, anxiety appears to be a common problem for many older adults. Elders face a combination of anxiety-producing life hazards. They must cope with an uncertain future as well as the problems of the present. Issues about loss of health, self-determination, and control can cause much anxiety in elderly individuals.

Many of today's older adults have experienced difficult times when work and food were scarce. Socially, they were taught that it is inappropriate to share one's fears and anxieties. Because older adults are less likely to share feelings directly, it becomes more difficult to recognize the signs of anxiety in elderly clients.

Behaviors indicating the presence of anxiety include apathy; changes in eating, sleeping, and ability to concentrate; impatience; and fatigue. To promote an atmosphere that allows for expression of what is being experienced, state your observations of behaviors that indicate anxiety. One of the most effective methods for assessing anxiety in older adults is to simply ask the client to explain his or her anxious feelings. Elderly people usually appreciate the interest of concerned caregivers.

ANXIETY DISORDERS

If anxiety is a normal human response, when does its expression become a disorder? An anxiety disorder exists when anxiety is expressed in ineffective or maladaptive ways and one's coping mechanisms (behaviors) do not successfully relieve the distress. People cope with anxiety using every area of functioning. In the **physical** realm, one deals directly with the source. **Intellectual** efforts analyze the situation, problem solve, or change the meaning of the problem. Many individuals call on their **spiritual** resources in an effort to cope with anxiety-producing problems. When efforts in these areas fail, ego defense mechanisms attempt to reduce the emotional distress.

The diagnosis of an anxiety disorder is based on a description of the behaviors that express distress. The *Diagnostic and Statistical Manual of Mental Disorders* (DSM-IV-TR) classifies anxiety disorders by type: generalized, panic, phobic, obsessive-compulsive, behavioral, and posttraumatic. Because these disorders are encountered in every culture, society, and health care setting, it is important to understand their nature.

GENERALIZED ANXIETY DISORDER

Anxiety disorders usually occur in adolescence or early adulthood. A **generalized anxiety disorder** is diagnosed when an individual's anxiety is broad, long-lasting, and excessive. It is primarily a disturbance in the emotional area of functioning. Eventually it affects every other aspect of one's world. People with generalized anxiety disorder are worried and anxious more often than not. They tend to **fret** about numerous things and find it difficult to control their worries. They are so anxious they often cannot concentrate on a task long enough to complete it. Emotional responses are far out of proportion to the actual situation. Physical signs and symptoms usually accompany the anxiety. They can range from muscle tension to full fight-or-flight responses. Generalized anxiety disorder occurs frequently in persons with irritable bowel syndrome, headaches, sleep disturbances, and substance abuse.

Generalized anxiety in children is diagnosed as **overanxious disorder of childhood.** These children tend to worry about their school performance and social interactions, whereas adults with generalized anxiety concentrate on worrying about everyday events.

PANIC DISORDERS

Panic disorders offer a challenge to health care providers because their signs and symptoms are difficult to distinguish from actual physical dysfunctions. A panic attack is a brief period of intense fear or discomfort. It is always accompanied by various physical and emotional reactions (Box 18-1). The duration of the actual attack is short (1 to 15 minutes), with a peak in anxiety after about 10 minutes.

Box 18-1 *Panic Attack Criteria*

A panic attack is a period of intense fear or discomfort in which at least four of the following symptoms develop abruptly and reach a peak within 10 minutes:
1. Palpitations, pounding heart, or accelerated heart rate
2. Sweating
3. Trembling or shaking
4. Feelings of shortness of breath, smothering
5. Feeling of choking
6. Chest pain or discomfort
7. Nausea or abdominal distress
8. Feeling dizzy, unsteady, light-headed, or faint
9. Derealization (feelings of unreality) or depersonalization (being detached from oneself)
10. Fear of losing control or going crazy
11. Fear of dying
12. Paresthesias (numbness, tingling sensations)
13. Chills or hot flushes

From Stuart GW: *Handbook of psychiatric nursing*, ed. 6, St. Louis, 2005, Mosby.

Panic disorders are more common than once thought. Research has shown that many clients seen in primary care settings suffer from panic disorders. These disorders are often misdiagnosed or inadequately treated. Panic disorders are more common in women (70%), people who are separated or divorced, and people between ages 24 and 44 years (American Psychiatric Association, 2000). Typically, an individual with a panic attack presents with physical complaints that may indicate a life-threatening situation.

There are two kinds of panic disorders: those associated with agoraphobia and those that are not. Agoraphobia is anxiety about possible situations in which a panic attack may occur. People with agoraphobia avoid people, places, or events from which escape would be difficult or embarrassing. Fear accompanies a sense of helplessness and embarrassment with the thought of a panic attack occurring. Typically, agoraphobia is associated with public situations, such as being in a crowd, standing in line, or traveling on a bus or plane. Standing on a bridge or being afraid to leave the house alone is also associated with agoraphobia. The presence of chronic stressors complicates the picture for treatment and improvement.

Treatment for panic disorders has three goals: educate clients about the nature of the disorder, block the panic attacks pharmacologically, and assist clients in developing more adaptive ways of coping with their anxieties. Cognitive therapy helps individuals identify their emotions and behaviors. Psychotherapy allows them to explore social or personal difficulties. Education and emotional support are important therapeutic measures for clients who experience panic disorders. Many have found meditation, biofeedback, aromatherapy, and other stress-reducing techniques helpful.

PHOBIC DISORDERS

A **phobia** is an internal fear reaction. Phobias involve specific situations or objects. They can stem from a fear of people, animals, objects, situations, or occurrences. For example, a **social phobia** is an unrealistic and persistent fear of any situation in which other people could be judging. Individuals with social phobias are constantly worried about looking foolish. They fear their hands will tremble if they try to write, their voice will quaver if they attempt to talk, or they will vomit if they start to eat. Some are especially anxious in the presence of authority figures or persons with high social contacts. Even eye contact (or the lack of it) from others can be misunderstood as scrutiny and rejection. When the anxieties associated with the social phobia are intense, a full-blown panic attack often results. Persons with severe social phobias often avoid contact with anyone outside their immediate family. Life for many socially phobic individuals can be a lonely and isolated existence.

Phobias differ from common fears. First, phobias are obsessive in nature. Individuals with phobias tend to dwell on their object of fear almost to the point of fascination. Thinking may take the form of fantasies about the fear, such as the person with thanatophobia (fear of dying) rehearsing his or her funeral.

People with phobias handle their anxieties differently. "A phobia typically produces so high a level of anxiety that it is immobilizing, preventing the person from acting in a way that could prove effective in alleviating the anxiety" (Craighead and Nemeroff, 2002). The anxiety or fear that is normally protective immobilizes the individual with a phobia.

The characteristics of phobias vary with the culture. In some cultures, fears of hexes, spells, magical spirits, and unseen forces result in phobic reactions. Health professionals should remember cultural backgrounds when assessing clients for phobic responses to anxiety (see Think About 18-1).

OBSESSIVE-COMPULSIVE DISORDER

An **obsession** is a distressing persistent **thought.** A **compulsion** is a distressing recurring **behavior.** An obsession must be persistent, recurring, inappropriate, and distressing. Compulsions are not just habits. They are specific behaviors that must be performed to reduce anxiety. All of us have repeated worries and routines that we recognize as not entirely sensible. However, persons with **obsessive-compulsive disorder** (OCD) are consumed by self-destructive, anxiety-reducing thoughts and actions. For behaviors to be called obsessions and compulsions, they must meet the criteria listed in Box 18-2.

Obsessive-compulsive disorders were thought to be relatively rare, but recent studies have demonstrated that OCD occurs in many more individuals than previously thought. Symptoms of OCD can occur as early as

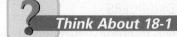
Think About 18-1

The client believes that his abdominal abscess is caused by a hex placed on him by his neighbor because of an ongoing dispute over the placement of the shared fence. Last week, a particularly angry interaction took place. His neighbor shouted curses and threatened to have a hex placed on him. Less than 24 hours later, the client began to experience abdominal pain, which he endured for 3 days before seeking treatment.

At this time, you are preparing the client for surgery to drain the abscess. Noting his anxious expression, you ask what is bothering him. He replies by telling you that the surgery will not cure his condition until the hex is removed, and the only way to do that is to appease his neighbor.
- How would you react to your client's anxiety associated with the hex?
- Which therapeutic interventions would you choose if you were this client's care provider?

Box 18-2 | **Obsessions and Compulsions Criteria**

OBSESSIONS
1. Recurrent and persistent thoughts, impulses, or images that are experienced as intrusive or inappropriate and cause marked anxiety or distress. The thoughts, impulses, or images are not simply excessive worries about real-life problems.
2. The person attempts to ignore, suppress, or neutralize such thoughts.
3. The person recognizes that the thoughts, impulses, or images are a product of his or her own mind.

COMPULSIONS
1. Repetitive behaviors (e.g., hand washing, ordering, checking) or mental acts (e.g., praying, counting, repeating words silently) that the person feels driven to perform in response to an obsession or according to rules that must be applied rigidly.
2. The behaviors or mental acts are aimed at reducing distress or preventing some dreaded event or situation; however, these behaviors or mental acts either are not connected in a realistic way with what they are designed to neutralize or they are clearly excessive.

From Stuart GW: *Handbook of psychiatric nursing,* ed 6, St. Louis, 2005, Mosby

3 years of age, but usually they begin in adolescence. Men and women seem to be equally affected, although symptoms frequently appear an average of 5 years earlier in men. A high rate of OCD occurs in persons with other mental health problems, especially depression and schizophrenia.

The most common obsessions relate to cleanliness, dirt, and germs; aggressive and sexual impulses; health concerns; safety concerns; and order and symmetry. Obsessions can take the form of thoughts, doubts, fears, images, or impulses. People with OCD use the ego defense mechanisms of repression to cope with distressing obsessions. They focus anxieties into compulsive actions **(displacement)** and engage in undoing behaviors to relieve stress. They know, intellectually, that their attempts to relieve anxiety are maladaptive, but they feel emotionally compelled to yield to their distressing obsessions. Many people with OCD are unable to maintain social relationships because their compulsions are too time consuming or inappropriate.

OCD is seen in families. Many studies are exploring possible genetic and hormonal causes. Treatment for OCD consists of a combination of drug and behavioral therapy. A number of antidepressants and selective serotonin reuptake inhibitor (SSRI) antidepressant medications have been used successfully to treat OCD.

BEHAVIORAL ADDICTIONS

Obsessive-compulsive activities may also take the form of certain addictive behaviors, such as gambling, shopping, working, or engaging in excessive sexual activity. Compulsive gambling or wagering is a problem for many people as more and more states legalize gambling. Estimates put the number of compulsive gamblers in the United States at more than 10 million people and that number is increasing rapidly. If left unchecked, obsessive-compulsive activities can destroy personal, professional, and financial relationships. Compulsive sexual activity has the added risk factors of contracting and spreading sexually transmitted diseases.

TRAUMATIC STRESS REACTION

A traumatic stress reaction is a series of behavioral and emotional responses following an overwhelmingly stressful event. People at high risk for being exposed to traumatic stress are persons with current mental health problems, victims or observers of violence, victims of sexual assault (especially as a child), victims of spouse abuse, and homeless persons. Traumatic stress reactions must be considered in anyone who has been sexually assaulted. Reactions to traumas, specifically rape-trauma syndrome, follow a predictable clinical course: fear and anguish, recovery and repair, and adaptation.

Following a traumatic event, "the initial response generally consists of an outcry of anguish or fear. Then the patient tries to recover from the traumatic event and repair the immediate damage" (Forster and King, 1994). During the repair and recovery stage, most individuals make reasonably adaptive responses, but some will react ineffectively and develop chronic stress reactions or posttraumatic stress disorder. The adaptation phase is heralded by a return to real-world situations and appropriate coping behaviors. Providing psychological stability, emotional support, and advocacy are the most important therapeutic interventions for clients with traumatic stress reactions.

POSTTRAUMATIC STRESS DISORDER

Individuals with posttraumatic stress disorder (PTSD) have been exposed to a traumatic experience that was outside the realm of normal life experiences at some time in their lives. Intense fear, horror, or helplessness was experienced. Posttraumatic stress disorder is the reliving of the traumatic events or situations. Symptoms of PTSD include flashbacks, which are vivid recollections of the event where the individual relives the frightening experience. Flashbacks can last from a few seconds to longer than one-half hour. During a flashback, the experience is vividly real and life threatening to the individual. Health care providers must remember this fact when coping with a client who is experiencing a flashback. Interventions must ensure everyone's safety and reorient the client to his or her present surroundings.

Anxiety, depression, and nightmares can complicate the picture. Individuals may reduce their involvement with others as their responsiveness to life numbs. Frequently, people with severe PTSD isolate themselves from society by living in sparsely populated rural areas. Children with PTSD express themselves through disorganized or agitated behaviors. Long-term interventions include pharmacological and psychological therapy and emotional support.

THERAPEUTIC INTERVENTIONS

The most effective way to cope with anxiety is to **prevent** it. Learn to recognize the signs and symptoms of anxiety in yourself and others. Include an anxiety-level assessment for every client. Be especially alert to the signs of anxiety in children. Teaching children to cope appropriately with their anxieties can prevent or minimize a number of mental health problems later in life.

Therapeutic interventions for individuals with maladaptive responses to anxiety involve a combination of mental health therapies and medications. Psychotherapy helps clients to discover the basis for their anxiety. Two behavioral therapies that are successful in treating phobias are systematic desensitization and flooding.

With **systematic desensitization,** clients learn to cope with one anxiety-provoking stimulus at a time until the stressor is no longer associated with anxiety. This step-by-step method gradually removes the anxiety from the distress-causing event and allows clients to develop more effective ways of perceiving their anxiety.

Flooding is just the opposite. This method for treating phobias rapidly and repeatedly exposes clients to the feared object or situation until anxiety levels diminish. Other treatments, such as cognitive-behavioral therapy, are designed to help clients learn how their

Box 18-3 *NANDA-I Nursing Diagnoses Related to Anxiety Responses*

Anxiety*
Breathing pattern, ineffective
Communication, impaired verbal
Coping, ineffective
Diarrhea
Energy field, disturbed
Fear*
Health maintenance, ineffective
Incontinence, stress urinary
Injury, risk for
Insomnia
Post-trauma syndrome
Powerlessness
Risk-prone health behavior
Sensory perception, disturbed (specify)
Social interaction, impaired
Social isolation
Thought processes, disturbed
Urinary elimination, impaired

From NANDA International: *NANDA-I nursing diagnoses: definitions and classification 2007-2008,* Philadelphia, 2007, NANDA International.
NANDA-I, NANDA International.
*Primary nursing diagnosis for anxiety.

illogical thinking leads to maladaptive behaviors. Meditation and other complementary therapies are proving to be effective.

Anxiety is also treated with various medications, including benzodiazepines, antidepressants, antihistamines, propranolol, and the anxiolytic drug called buspirone (BuSpar). Because each type of drug is associated with possibly severe side effects, nurses must monitor their clients' responses to drug therapy (see Drug Alert 18-1). The side effects of commonly used antianxiety agents, benzodiazepines, and suggested therapeutic interventions are listed in Table 18-3.

After a complete nursing history and thorough physical examination, the most appropriate problem statements and nursing diagnoses (Box 18-3) are selected (Bulechek and Bulechek, 2008). Information is then

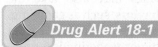

Drug Alert 18-1

CAUTION: Benzodiazepines and other anxiety-reducing medications can be dangerous when taken in combination with alcohol. Clients must be instructed about the possibility of sedation, decreased mental activity, and decreased coordination when alcohol is consumed while taking these drugs.

Table 18-3 *Side Effects of Benzodiazepines and Nursing Care*

SIDE EFFECTS*	NURSING (THERAPEUTIC) INTERVENTIONS
CENTRAL NERVOUS SYSTEM Dizziness, drowsiness, sedation, headache, tremors, depression, insomnia, hallucinations	Ensure safety, prevent falls, assist with ambulation, use side rails. Reassure that symptoms are common when first beginning the medication. Assess mental status routinely.
GASTROINTESTINAL Dry mouth, anorexia, nausea, vomiting, constipation, diarrhea	Give with food or milk. Ensure frequent oral care. Offer hard candy, gum, sips of water frequently.
CARDIOVASCULAR Electrocardiogram changes, *orthostatic hypotension, tachycardia*	Monitor intake and output if anorexia, vomiting, diarrhea. Assess blood pressure, pulse (lying and standing); if systolic pressure drops ≥20 mm Hg, hold drug, notify physician. Monitor complete blood count and other laboratory studies during long-term therapy.
EYES, EARS, NOSE, THROAT *Blurred vision,* ringing in ears	Provide reassurance. Ensure safety.
INTEGUMENT (SKIN) Itching, rash, dermatitis	Encourage use of tepid baths without soap. Assess rash, and report to physician.
EMOTIONAL Feelings of detachment, irritability, increased hostility	Encourage social interactions. Assess for loss of control over emotions and aggression.
LONG-TERM EFFECTS Increased drug tolerance, physical and psychological dependency, rebound anxiety and insomnia	Drug dose is tapered slowly after 4 mo of treatment. Help client identify difference between symptoms of drug withdrawal and original feelings of anxiety.

*The most common side effects are in italics.

brought to the health care team, and overall client goals are established and therapeutic interventions chosen.

One of the first priorities of care is to protect the client from injury to self and others. Establishing a trusting therapeutic relationship helps clients to explore their distresses and learn to link their behaviors to the sources of their anxiety. Problem-solving techniques assist clients in developing more effective coping mechanisms. Relaxation techniques, such as medita-tion, and stress-reducing exercises help clients counter their anxieties. Sample Client Care Plan 18-1 provides an example of a care plan for anxiety responses.

Health care providers are in an excellent position to help clients cope effectively with the effects of stress and anxiety. Handling small, everyday distresses successfully is the key to preventing complicated mental health problems that arise as maladaptive expressions of anxiety.

SAMPLE CLIENT CARE PLAN 18-1

Anxiety

ASSESSMENT *History.* Joe is a 44-year-old man who lost his wife, job, and car within the past 3 months. Last night, after Joe and his buddies "had a few drinks," Joe became suspicious and accused his friends of trying to steal "what little I have left. I just know something awful is going to happen." Today Joe is seeking treatment for his upset stomach and inability to sleep.

Current Findings. An untidy man who appears older than his stated age. There is an odor of alcohol. Vital signs are increased, with a pulse rate of 116 beats/min. He complains of shortness of breath, upset stomach, frequent urination, and lack of sleep. When questioned about the recent changes in his lifestyle, he replies, "It's no big deal. I'll get by."

Multidisciplinary Diagnosis	*Planning/Goals*
Anxiety related to loss of wife and job	Joe will identify the causes of his anxiety and make two attempts to decrease the level of anxiety he is experiencing by October 10.

Therapeutic Interventions

Intervention	Rationale	Team Member
1. Establish trust with Joe.	Trust helps client to explore new ways of coping.	All
2. Contract with him to refrain from hurting himself and others for the duration of therapy.	To ensure safety of Joe and others during expressions of anxiety.	Nsg
3. Use active listening to encourage Joe to link his anxiety with recent experiences.	Allows time to assess Joe's perspective; helps Joe to connect his emotions with his feelings of anxiety.	All
4. Assess Joe's statements of self-worth, and reinforce personal strengths that he has identified.	Helps determine Joe's perception of himself; energy flows where it is focused.	All
5. Help Joe identify areas of his life over which he has control.	Learning to direct one's energies decreases anxiety, promotes relaxation, and increases sense of control.	All
6. Give positive feedback for attempts to reduce anxiety.	One small success builds on another when recognized.	All
7. Encourage Joe to continue already established relationships.	Established relationships can be a source of comfort and support.	All
8. Help identify areas of strength and limitations in social interactions.	Positive reinforcement encourages appropriate actions; the first step in changing behaviors is identifying them.	Soc Svc, Nsg
9. Encourage Joe to undergo job skill and employment testing.	A source of income helps satisfy basic needs.	Soc Svc, OT
10. Monitor for therapeutic response, side effects of BuSpar.	Drug has several side effects that can be disturbing for client.	Nsg

Evaluation

Joe attended four counseling sessions before he recognized that he was anxious. By the seventh session, he was able to reduce his anxiety about 15% of the time.

❓ CRITICAL THINKING QUESTIONS

1. What is the purpose of helping Joe link his feelings of anxiety to recent events?

2. How does identifying strengths help decrease anxiety?

A complete client care plan includes several other diagnoses and interventions.
Nsg, Nursing staff; *Soc Svc,* social services; *OT,* occupational therapist.

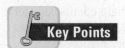
Key Points

- Anxiety is a diffuse feeling of uneasiness, uncertainty, and helplessness; it is a normal emotional response to a threat or stressor.
- Adaptive responses to anxiety result in positive outcomes, new learning, and greater self-esteem.
- Maladaptive responses to anxiety are ineffective attempts to cope that do nothing to eliminate feelings of anxiety.
- To decrease stress, people use physical, intellectual, spiritual, and emotional coping mechanisms.
- An understanding of how individuals at various developmental stages perceive and cope with anxiety is important for health care providers.
- The specific causes of anxiety are still uncertain, but research indicates that a combination of physical, psychosocial, and environmental factors is involved.
- An anxiety disorder exists when one's coping mechanisms or behaviors do not relieve anxiety's distress.
- A generalized anxiety disorder is diagnosed when anxiety is broad, long-lasting, and excessive.
- A panic attack is a brief period of intense fear or discomfort accompanied by physical and emotional reactions.

- A phobia is an unnatural fear of people, animals, objects, situations, or occurrences.
- An obsession is a distressing, recurring, persistent thought.
- A compulsion is a distressing recurring behavior.
- Posttraumatic stress disorder (PTSD) is the reliving of previously experienced traumatic events or situations.
- One of the first priorities of care is to protect the client from possible injury to self and others.
- Medications for treating anxiety include the benzodiazepines, antihistamines, propranolol, buspirone, and antidepressants.
- Establishing a trusting therapeutic relationship is a therapeutic intervention that helps clients to explore their distresses and learn to connect behaviors with the sources of their anxiety.
- Problem-solving techniques assist clients in developing new, more effective coping mechanisms.
- Relaxation techniques help clients counter the anxieties currently being experienced.

evolve Be sure to visit the companion Evolve site at http://evolve.elsevier.com/Morrison-Valfre/ for additional online resources.

evolve http://evolve.elsevier.com/Morrison-Valfre/

Objectives

Upon completion of this chapter, the student will be able to:

1. Explain the difference between health and illness.
2. Outline the five stages of illness.
3. Identify how denial is used as a protective mechanism during illness.
4. Explain why hospitalization is considered a situational crisis.
5. Describe the three stages of the hospitalization experience.
6. Compare hospitalization for psychiatric problems with hospitalization for physical problems.
7. Discuss how emotional support of significant others affects the outcome of a client's illness.
8. Identify three nondrug methods for managing pain.
9. Examine the importance of discharge planning for hospitalized persons.

Key Terms

body image (p. 205)
denial (p. 206)
discharge planning (p. 212)
health (p. 203)
hospitalization (p. 206)
illness (p. 203)
pain management (p. 211)
sick role (p. 204)
situational crisis (p. 206)

Do you remember the first time you visited a hospital? Perhaps you were a visitor or maybe a patient. Can you recall how you felt? First, the hospital appeared to be huge. Even small hospitals are confusing, with mazes of hallways and mysterious little rooms everywhere. The odors were different—extra clean, antiseptic smells, like no other odors. The workers there were all dressed in ceremonial garb and paraded through the hallway mazes with businesslike efficiency. Then there was the equipment—the machines and strange items that do one thing or another. It seemed that every piece came with a bell, whistle, or other annoying tone to periodically remind us of its presence. Generally, a health care facility can be a scary, intimidating place, not one in which most people choose to spend time.

For those of us in the health care professions, however, the hospital (or nursing home or clinic) is a known environment, filled with the familiar. We often forget that the thought of "going to the hospital" brings immediate anxiety to the hearts of many. For these people, hospitalization can be an overwhelming and threatening experience (see Case Study 19-1). This chapter explores the mental health aspects of illness and the situational crisis of hospitalization. It describes the process of illness and its psychosocial adaptations, and it offers several therapeutic interventions for decreasing or eliminating the anxieties that accompany the illness and hospitalization experiences. Most important, it reminds us of the discomforts shared by the individuals who must cope with and adapt to the inpatient environment—a world we health care providers take for granted.

THE NATURE OF ILLNESS

Health is a dynamic state of physical, mental, and social well-being, as well as the absence of disease or abnormal conditions (Potter and Perry, 2009). Our state of health constantly changes as we respond and adapt to the challenges of life. This constant change process is called homeostasis, and it serves us well throughout our lives. When individuals become unable to adapt or regain the balance of homeostasis, they become ill and must mobilize critical energies to return to a state of health.

Illness is a state of imbalance. It is an "abnormal process in which aspects of the social, physical, emotional, or intellectual condition and function of a person are diminished or impaired, compared with that person's previous condition" (Anderson, Anderson, and Glanze, 2006). When you are ill or sick, you feel poorly. The body is not working correctly, energy is sapped, and spirits are low. Activities performed yesterday without a thought now loom as obstacles. Getting dressed for work becomes such a challenge that you seriously wonder how you will make it through the day. You need some rest, but your will is reminding you of your commitments and obligations. Does this sound familiar?

Case Study 19-1

Bob is an 82-year-old retired printer, living in a small retirement village with his wife, who has diabetes. He has enjoyed excellent health throughout his life. Other than periodic visits to his physician, he has had no contact with the medical community.

One evening, Bob noticed that he was bleeding when he urinated. After referral to a specialist, he was scheduled for a simple operative procedure to remove the extra tissue that was blocking the flow of urine and causing the bleeding. Bob and his wife were instructed to arrive at the hospital early on the following morning.

On admission, the nurse, noting Bob's age, assumed that he had some experience in a hospital—after all, he was more than 80 years old. Bob was quickly admitted and prepared for surgery.

The surgical procedure was completed without problems. Bob was taken to the recovery room in good condition with a Foley catheter to straight drainage and an intravenous line in his right forearm. The first hour following the procedure was uneventful; however, the minute Bob regained consciousness, he insisted on going home. Nurses reassured him that he would be discharged as soon as the physician saw him. He nodded and then dozed off. Seeing him sleeping, they turned their attention to other clients.

Bob suddenly hopped off the gurney and detached himself from the intravenous line and Foley catheter. He was last seen walking out the door to his car in his hospital gown and bleeding from the urethra. As a result of this mishap, Bob was chased down, "captured" against his will, and hospitalized for 3 days to control the bleeding from the traumatic catheter removal. You can imagine what a challenging time that was for Bob and his wife, not to mention his health care providers.

Regretfully, not one health care provider assessed this man's previous experiences relating to hospitalization or medical treatment. Bob was under the false assumption that once the task was completed, he was free to return home.
- What actions could have prevented this situation from occurring?
- How could the lessons from this study be applied to your practice?

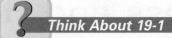

Think About 19-1

Remember the last time you were feeling ill but you went to work or school anyway.
- How well did you perform that day?
- How sharp was your mental acuity?
- How did you cope with the physical, intellectual, and emotional demands of the day?

Illness is the body's way of communicating its need for attention. It will adjust to the demands placed on it until it is no longer capable of compensating (see Think About 19-1). Illness also has strong psychosocial aspects. The example of the person with hallucinations who collapses from malnutrition because his visions told him he should not accept food from others reminds us of the complexity of the mind-body interaction.

STAGES OF THE ILLNESS EXPERIENCE

The subjective experiences associated with illness and disability are very personal. Some individuals consider being ill a minor annoyance, whereas others analyze their sickness for hidden evidence of certain doom. The illness experience is roughly divided into five stages. Each stage is associated with certain perceptions, decisions, and behaviors (Table 19-1).

Because nurses and other health care providers support clients throughout their institutional stays, it is important to be familiar with the emotional and behavioral reactions during each phase of the illness experience, be it physical or mental in origin.

Stage 1: Symptoms

The illness experience begins when a person becomes aware that something is not right. It may be a physical or emotional discomfort, but something is perceived as wrong. During this stage, one becomes aware of an undesirable change. He or she analyzes and evaluates the change and makes a decision that the change indicates an illness. Actions are then taken to remedy the situation based on the decision and the accompanying emotional response.

Many factors, such as the nature of the symptoms, the knowledge of the individual, and the availability of treatment resources, enter into determining if an illness exists. Emotional responses often govern behavior during this stage. If symptoms are mild, one may self-medicate with various over-the-counter drugs, visit a local cultural folk healer, pray or meditate, or ignore the situation. For more serious symptoms, the individual may seek medical care or continue to deny a problem exists. When an individual recognizes the presence of a health problem, he or she begins to move into the second stage.

Stage 2: The Sick Role

Once a person acknowledges the presence of an illness, he or she seeks to confirm it by talking with other people. Family members, fellow workers, and friends are consulted for their opinions. The social group supports the presence of an illness, and the individual either assumes the **sick role** (actions and behaviors of a person who is ill) or continues to deny the illness.

Assuming the sick role serves several purposes. First, the person is excused from everyday duties and responsibilities. Other people "take up the slack" by assuming the ill person's duties. Second, permission is given for the individual to rest and conserve energy for healing. Third, the social responsibilities of interacting with others are relieved during the illness. In

Table 19-1 *Stages of the Illness Experience*

STAGE	DECISION	BEHAVIOR
Symptom experience	Aware that something is wrong	Symptom control, folk medicine, self-medicates
Assumes sick role	Gives up normal roles	Seeks support for sick role
Medical care contact	Seeks professional advice	Seeks sick role approval from an authority, negotiates treatments and procedures
Dependent patient role	Accepts health care treatment	Receives treatment, follows regimen
Recovery and rehabilitation	Gives up sick role	Resumes normal roles and responsibilities

short, permission is given for the individual to focus on restoring health.

Stage 3: Medical Care

If symptoms of the illness persist and home remedies fail, the person usually becomes motivated to seek medical intervention. The authoritative advice of a health professional confirms the presence of an illness, provides treatment, and informs the individual about the causes, course, and future implications of the illness. At this time, the individual can either accept the diagnosis and follow the plan of treatment or continue to deny the problem. Many people consult several different health care professionals (shop around) in an attempt to receive a diagnosis more to their liking or until they finally accept the professionals' opinions.

Stage 4: Dependency

In the dependency stage, the ill individual accepts the attentions of other people. A dependent role is assumed in which one must rely on the kindness and energies of others. "Care, sympathy, and protection from the demands and stresses of life" (Potter and Perry, 2005) are provided by family, friends, or health care providers. The individual is relieved of obligation, allowed to be passive and dependent, but expected to get well. The sick person may feel ambivalent: grateful for the help but resentful of the limitations imposed by the illness. People in this stage have a particular need to be informed and emotionally supported.

Stage 5: Recovery and Rehabilitation

Movement into the recovery and rehabilitation stage can occur suddenly (e.g., a response to drug therapy or the breaking of a fever) or more slowly (e.g., recovery from a stroke or mental disorder). If recovery is rapid and complete, the individual gradually gives up the sick role and resumes his or her normal obligations and duties. For those whose recoveries are prolonged, long-term care is usually necessary. Whenever possible, arrangements are made for people to recover in their homes. When this is not an option the individual is usually transferred to another institution for further rehabilitation or care.

Not all people pass through every stage of the illness experience, and progression through the stages occurs at a very individual rate. However, caregivers who understand the emotional aspects of the illness experience are better able to plan and implement effective client care.

IMPACTS OF ILLNESS

Illness is not an isolated event. It affects the activities of the individual as well as those who come in contact with the sick person. When illness occurs, it challenges the resources and changes the activities of all those involved. Illness has an impact on the individual. Short-term acute illnesses, such as the flu or a cold, have little effect on behavior, but a serious health problem (physical or mental) can lead to major emotional and behavioral changes. Individuals may react to illness with anxiety, anger, denial, shock, or withdrawal (Box 19-1).

An illness involving a change in physical appearance will have a strong impact on the individual's **body image** (one's concept of his or her body). Threats to body image occur with surgery, extensive diagnostic procedures, and acute and chronic illness. One's self-concept also becomes threatened if the illness progresses beyond the expected time. Tension and conflict with other family members can further erode the ill person's confidence, and a depressed mood may begin to take hold.

Psychosocially, illness has an impact on the family. Changes in routine add more pressure to an already threatened family. Because the obligations and responsibilities of the ill individual cannot be met, family members often take on heavier workloads during times of illness. If the illness is prolonged, family members may experience situational stress, leading to an imbalance in family stability (Edelman and Mandle, 2002) until new roles and habits are established.

Illness has many faces. Remember, when assessing the physical signs and symptoms of illness, we are touching only the tip of the iceberg. Underneath lie the emotions, reactions, and behaviors that arrive with the package called "illness."

Illness Behaviors

During each stage of the illness experience, people are faced with several emotional choices. Some emotions serve to protect us from further stresses or mobilize resources to be devoted to healing. Emotions can be destructive, however, if they block efforts toward

■

Box 19-1 *Behavioral and Emotional Changes Associated With Illness*

Anxiety: Stress, feelings of apprehension, uncertainty about the illness. Responses to anxiety vary with the individual and the stage of the illness.

Anger: A response to feeling mistreated, injured, or opposed; may be directed inward or outward, may be irrational (has no basis in fact), and may affect the person's social functioning.

Denial: Refusal to acknowledge painful facts. Short-term denial helps mobilize resources, but long-standing denial results in maladaptive behaviors.

Shock: An overwhelming emotional state; individual is unable to process the information within the environment; may trigger both effective and maladaptive behaviors. (Refer to the stages of crisis discussed in Chapter 5.)

Withdrawal: The removal of self from others; individual refuses to interact; is often a sign of depression. Family members and/or the ill person may withdraw from each other.

Data from Potter PA, Perry AG: *Basic nursing: essentials for practice*, ed 6, St. Louis, 2005, Mosby.

---

resolving health problems. For example, the emotion of denial can be useful or paralyzing.

Denial is a psychological defense mechanism (see Chapter 18) used to ward off the painful feelings associated with problems. Denial can be helpful when it allows the time to collect and reorganize thoughts and plans, but it can be deadly when it clouds judgments and prevents individuals from taking the needed steps to restore themselves to health. Clients in denial require patience and understanding. They are struggling with the emotional aspects of illness and attempting to restore themselves to a more comfortable state of functioning.

Fortunately most people experience illness, recover to previous levels of functioning, and move on with their lives. They have taken part, actively or passively, in returning themselves to a state of homeostasis. Becoming ill and experiencing disability is not a comfortable experience. Health care providers, especially nurses, should remember that illness is the most important priority for the individual who is experiencing it.

THE HOSPITALIZATION EXPERIENCE

The great majority of illnesses are treated successfully in the home. However, some individuals are placed in an inpatient setting for treatment. Hospitalization is the placing of an ill or injured person into an inpatient health care facility that provides continuous nursing care and an organized medical staff.

People have vastly different experiences relating to stays in a hospital. Attitudes are also affected by what one hears. The relative who drags out minor historical facts about the hospital experiences of every family

member and the horror stories from tabloid newspapers adds to one's concerns about receiving care in a hospital.

People who are hospitalized experience several emotional threats to their well-being and progress through different stages throughout their hospital stays. During each stage, certain anxieties and emotional issues surface and challenge the client's coping abilities. Care providers should be aware of these issues and include them in the client's plan of care. Persons who are hospitalized are faced with physical, emotional, and environmental problems all at the same time. For most of us, being hospitalized is seen as a crisis, an event with which we are unable to cope.

SITUATIONAL CRISIS

People are generally hospitalized in one of two ways: either the admission is planned in advance or an emergency requires special health care resources. In the case of the planned admission, one has time to experience the anxieties and work with the complications that will occur as a result of the individual's absence. Although emotional reactions may be intense and the event may be viewed as a crisis, persons who elect to be hospitalized have the luxury of time to prepare themselves and their loved ones, both physically and emotionally. For those individuals brought to the hospital through the emergency department, no time is allowed for preparation. Their lives have suddenly been disrupted. If the health problems require complicated or long-term treatment, major adjustments in lifestyles must be made quickly.

Review the principles of crisis intervention discussed in Chapter 8, and apply them to the crisis of being hospitalized. Remember, a situational crisis is one that relates to external or environmental problems. In the case of the client who has been coping with an illness or dysfunction before admission, the precrisis behaviors consist of efforts to deal with the health problem. For the individual whose admission was an emergency, the precrisis behaviors were a healthy person's usual activities of daily living with no thought given to illness or injury.

The actual crisis in both cases, however, is about being removed from one's familiar home environment to be cared for by strangers in an impersonal, uncomfortable setting. All hospitalized clients have one thing in common—the feeling of being out of control and dependent on the mercy, knowledge, and expertise of unknown care providers. If caregivers are sensitive to the fact that their clients are experiencing a crisis, therapeutic interventions will meet with greater success.

Stages of Hospitalization

The process of becoming a patient is peppered with problems. The dilemma becomes more anxiety provoking as the admission process transforms a person from an individual into a patient or client. The name band around the wrist provides a means of identity that removes the requirement of a vocal inquiry because now caregivers can identify one by an armband. The demand for paperwork diminishes a person into an account number and saps what little energy is present. Next, an institutional gown helps the sick person to exchange his role as a functioning adult for that of a patient (Figure 19-1). The individual goes to bed and is surrounded by caregivers. In this vulnerable position, a person is expected to submit passively to the scrutiny of body and behavior. All this is expected to be done gracefully and cooperatively, denying the fear, anger, and humiliation that are actually being experienced. The sick individual has made an agreement, a deal of sorts, whereby privacy is offered in exchange for treatments and interventions that will return him or her to wellness. The focus of treatment may be on the physical body, but care providers must stay aware of the psychosocial aspects of clients' health problems and hospitalization experiences.

Individuals who are experiencing hospitalization progress through three stages. The first stage is the sense of being **overwhelmed.** The intensity of being separated from loved ones and left alone in an unfamiliar environment leaves many individuals exhausted. Energies needed to cope with the illness were diverted to surviving the admission process, separating from loved ones, and tolerating various diagnostic procedures. As a result, many clients withdraw into themselves and interact only when necessary. They must focus their attention inward in an effort to replace the energies that have been drained by the experiences of illness, crisis, and hospitalization.

During the second stage, **stabilization,** the hospitalized person gradually gains the strength to reestablish some personal identity. Individuals can become self-centered in this phase. The intellectual understanding that one is not the only person requiring care exists, but the emotional needs for reassurance and personal interest frequently must be asserted.

Adaptation marks the third stage. In this stage, the individual has regained enough of a personal identity to adapt. He or she often becomes interested in and willing to learn about health problems, coping techniques, or preventive measures. Energies are replenished, the body feels better, and emotional responses are stable. Reorganization has taken place, and most people are again able to function effectively. For those persons who are transferred to another institution, the crisis begins again.

Common Reactions to Hospitalization

The rule of thumb for clients' reactions is "every person will react in his or her way." The manner in which individuals respond to the stresses of being hospitalized is determined by how they react to

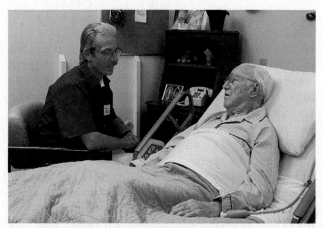

FIGURE **19-1** Becoming a patient.

other threats or crises. The executive who controls a company commonly reacts by attempting to gain control over his or her hospital environment. The woman dominated by her spouse makes few decisions without his opinion, and the helpless individual often becomes more so in the hospital. Please remember that even though some of your clients' behaviors may be distasteful, they are coping to the best of their abilities.

Hospitalization may also hold symbolic meaning. For some persons, hospitalization confirms the fear that this is no ordinary illness, that there may be something seriously amiss. For others, especially elderly people, the hospital is the place where one goes to die. It is also seen as a place of respite where one is removed from the stresses of daily living. Attitudes and meanings concerning inpatient treatment for mental health problems differ from those relating to institutional stays for physical problems.

PSYCHIATRIC HOSPITALIZATION

The experience of entering a psychiatric treatment facility differs from hospitalization for physical reasons in several ways. The individual and family must cope with the stigma of mental illness. Friends may be reluctant to discuss the illness or feel awkward about offering their support. Employers may question the individual's fitness for the job, and insurance companies may deny payment for treatment.

The ill person has received a diagnostic label that will follow him or her for years. Admission may be seen as a confirmation that one is truly crazy. There are also numerous stories about life in psychiatric hospitals.

If clients are alert and aware, they may fear other clients' behaviors. Odd or inappropriate behaviors can create anxiety and feelings of needing to protect oneself. Frequent contact and support from the health care staff during the admission and adjustment period help clients cope with the anxieties of psychiatric hospitalization.

THERAPEUTIC INTERVENTIONS

Nurses and other caregivers play a vital role in the care of sick persons within the hospital setting. Clients remember the people who provided their care. The caregiver who went that extra mile for a personal favor, the therapist who made certain a client's pet was fed, and the nurse who sat at the bedside when a client was too anxious to sleep are remembered clearly. Unfortunately, the opposite is also true. Clients frequently remember the short temper, the cutting words, and the negative nonverbal messages faster than acts of kindness and concern. Psychosocial attention is just as important as good physical care. All health care providers need to be willing to meet both the physical and nonphysical needs of all clients. Box 19-2 lists nursing diagnoses (problem statements) that apply to the experience of illness and hospitalization.

PSYCHOSOCIAL CARE

Good physical care is always the first place to start in meeting the emotional needs of ill persons. Therapeutic care communicates a willingness to focus attention on the client, offers opportunities for interaction, and allows nurses to assess the client's adaptation to the changes resulting from treatment. Good psychosocial care begins with an assessment of the client's coping status (Ferszt, 1995). Perform a crisis assessment using criteria listed in Table 19-2. This allows you to identify problems **before** a crisis develops and plan preventive interventions.

Box 19-2 | *NANDA-I–Approved Nursing Diagnoses*

Activity intolerance	Diarrhea
Activity intolerance, risk for	Disuse syndrome, risk for
Airway clearance, ineffective	Diversional activity, deficient
Allergy response, latex	Energy field, disturbed
Allergy response, risk for latex	Environmental interpretation syndrome, impaired
Anxiety	Failure to thrive, adult
Anxiety, death	Falls, risk for
Aspiration, risk for	Family processes: alcoholism, dysfunctional
Attachment, risk for impaired parent/child	Family processes, interrupted
Autonomic dysreflexia	Family processes, readiness for enhanced
Autonomic dysreflexia, risk for	Fatigue
Behavior, risk-prone health	Fear
Body image, disturbed	Fluid balance, readiness for enhanced
Body temperature, risk for imbalanced	Fluid volume, deficient
Bowel incontinence	Fluid volume, excess
Breastfeeding, effective	Fluid volume, risk for deficient
Breastfeeding, ineffective	Fluid volume, risk for imbalanced
Breastfeeding, interrupted	Gas exchange, impaired
Breathing pattern, ineffective	Grieving
Cardiac output, decreased	Grieving, complicated
Caregiver role strain	Growth, risk for disproportionate
Caregiver role strain, risk for	Growth and development, delayed
Communication, impaired verbal	Health maintenance, ineffective
Communication, readiness for enhanced	Health-seeking behaviors
Conflict, decisional	Home maintenance, impaired
Conflict, parental role	Hopelessness
Confusion, acute	Hyperthermia
Confusion, chronic	Hypothermia
Constipation	Identity, disturbed personal
Constipation, perceived	Incontinence, functional urinary
Constipation, risk for	Incontinence, reflex urinary
Coping, compromised family	Incontinence, stress urinary
Coping, defensive	Incontinence, total urinary
Coping, disabled family	Incontinence, urge urinary
Coping, ineffective	Incontinence, risk for urge urinary
Coping, ineffective community	Infant behavior, disorganized
Coping, readiness for enhanced	Infant behavior, readiness for enhanced organized
Coping, readiness for enhanced community	Infant behavior, risk for disorganized
Coping, readiness for enhanced family	Infant feeding pattern, ineffective
Denial, ineffective	Infection, risk for
Dentition, impaired	Injury, risk for
Development, risk for delayed	Injury, risk for perioperative-positioning

Box 19-2   *NANDA-I–Approved Nursing Diagnoses—cont'd*

Insomnia	Self-esteem, situational low
Intracranial adaptive capacity, decreased	Self-esteem, risk for situational low
Knowledge, deficient	Self-mutilation
Knowledge, readiness for enhanced	Self-mutilation, risk for
Loneliness, risk for	Sensory perception, disturbed
Memory, impaired	Sexual dysfunction
Mobility, impaired bed	Sexuality pattern, ineffective
Mobility, impaired physical	Skin integrity, impaired
Mobility, impaired wheelchair	Skin integrity, risk for impaired
Nausea	Sleep, readiness for enhanced
Neglect, unilateral	Sleep deprivation
Noncompliance	Social interaction, impaired
Nutrition, imbalanced: less than body requirements	Social isolation
Nutrition, imbalanced: more than body requirements	Sorrow, chronic
Nutrition, imbalanced: risk for more than body requirements	Spiritual distress
	Spiritual distress, risk for
Nutrition, readiness for enhanced	Spiritual well-being, readiness for enhanced
Oral mucous membrane, impaired	Sudden infant death syndrome, risk for
Pain, acute	Suffocation, risk for
Pain, chronic	Suicide, risk for
Parenting, impaired	Surgical recovery, delayed
Parenting, readiness for enhanced	Swallowing, impaired
Parenting, risk for impaired	Therapeutic regimen management, effective
Peripheral neurovascular dysfunction, risk for	Therapeutic regimen management, ineffective
Poisoning, risk for	Therapeutic regimen management, ineffective community
Post-trauma syndrome	Therapeutic regimen management, ineffective family
Post-trauma syndrome, risk for	Therapeutic regimen management, readiness for enhanced
Powerlessness	
Powerlessness, risk for	Thermoregulation, ineffective
Protection, ineffective	Thought processes, disturbed
Rape-trauma syndrome	Tissue integrity, impaired
Rape-trauma syndrome, compound reaction	Tissue perfusion, ineffective
Rape-trauma syndrome, silent reaction	Transfer ability, impaired
Relocation stress syndrome	Trauma, risk for
Relocation stress syndrome, risk for	Urinary elimination, impaired
Role performance, ineffective	Urinary elimination, readiness for enhanced
Self-care deficit, bathing/hygiene	Urinary retention
Self-care deficit, dressing/grooming	Ventilation, impaired spontaneous
Self-care deficit, feeding	Ventilatory weaning response, dysfunctional
Self-care deficit, toileting	Violence, risk for other-directed
Self-concept, readiness for enhanced	Violence, risk for self-directed
Self-esteem, chronic low	

Data from NANDA International: *NANDA-I nursing diagnoses: definitions and classification 2007-2008,* Philadelphia, 2007, NANDA International.
NANDA-I, NANDA International.

Table 19-2   *Crisis Assessment*

ASSESSMENT STEPS	DESCRIPTION
Assess client's history of loss.	What types of losses (physical, psychological, social, or spiritual) has client experienced in past?
	Who or what has helped client through crises in past?
	Older and younger persons have more difficulty coping with crisis.
Assess what illness means to client.	What is client's understanding of current situation?
	What has client been told about condition, treatment, chances for recovery?
	How have client and family been affected?
Assess for other risk factors.	Assess client's level of support from supportive significant others and friends.
	How easily does client adapt to new situations?
	Assess for other crises. Other problems can exist in addition to the crisis.
	Older adults and children have more trouble cooperating and following therapeutic plans.

Modified from Ferszt GG: Performing a crisis assessment, *Nursing* 25:88, 1995.

Next, get to know your clients as individuals and real persons. Use active listening skills to encourage clients to discuss their anxieties and concerns. Clarify clients' perceptions of the problems and their roles in treatment (Campbell and Anderson, 1999). **Listen** more than you talk. Most clients need to share their emotions about the illness experience. No matter what your personal opinions are, do not pass judgment on your clients' emotions and behaviors. Creating an accepting environment gives clients permission to share themselves and helps to build trust in the therapeutic relationship.

Assist clients in coping with the fight-or-flight response brought about by the illness or hospitalization. According to the theorist Lazarus, stress is defined by the individual's cognitive evaluation of the situation and the importance or significance he or she attaches to it. Some individuals interpret the hospitalization experience as comforting and healing, whereas others may feel it is the first step toward dying. Teach and encourage clients to practice muscle relaxation techniques, imagery, and conscious sedation techniques to help ease their stresses. If the client practices a certain spiritual belief, notify the appropriate priest, minister, or spiritual practitioner. Also, be alert for any cultural practices that bring emotional support and comfort (see Cultural Considerations 19-1). The therapeutic (nursing) process applied to the hospitalized client is illustrated in Box 19-3.

Support clients throughout each stage of the illness experience. Be alert to the behaviors associated with each stage of illness and hospitalization. Assist clients with the emotional discomforts of illness, whether physical or psychological. Sample Client Care Plan 19-1 addresses some of these factors.

Supporting Significant Others

An individual's family is an important group in one's life. The traditional family consisted of a mother, father, siblings, and relatives. Newer family forms, such as the single-parent family, the same-gender couple family, and the blended family, are replacing it. The children of previous relationships are now often "blended" into new family groups. Clients' families can have a significant impact on the outcome of their illnesses.

In many societies, the man is a symbol of strength and stability. When men from these societies are ill or hospitalized, their roles as providers change and they become receivers. Because they are unable to fulfill their roles, they feel inadequate and humiliated. The role changes leave family members bewildered and uncertain. If the condition is serious or chronic, loved ones are also faced with the issues of long-term care placement or death. In addition, each family member is trying to cope with all the internal emotional problems associated with the illness of a loved one.

Care providers should be alert to how the family's interactions affect their client. Family members should

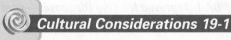

Cultural Considerations 19-1

Appalachian families have a general distrust of health care providers and organizations. Sickness is seen as "the will of God," and there is a fear of "being cut on." The family is of great importance, and members depend greatly on each other. Care for ill members is provided by the family, and hospitalization is considered the step before dying. If a person from Appalachia is hospitalized, expect the extended family to accompany the patient.

Box 19-3 | ***Therapeutic (Nursing) Process for Hospitalized Clients***

ASSESSMENT
1. Perform a complete physical and psychosocial assessment, including previous hospitalizations. Have client describe each hospitalization and his or her reactions to and opinions of the experience.
2. Ask client to describe any particular concerns or fears about being hospitalized.
3. Ask if there is a special routine or ritual that is important to the client.

PLANNING
1. Based on the data obtained in the interview, develop a plan to decrease the client's concerns and anxieties related to hospitalization.
2. Involve client and significant others in the planning process.

NURSING DIAGNOSES
See Box 19-2 for a list of possible diagnoses.

INTERVENTIONS
1. Convey respect and politeness when interacting with clients.
2. Maintain a pleasant environment. Pay attention to noise levels, lighting, staff interactions.
3. Encourage client to cooperate and participate in his or her care.
4. Use therapeutic communications, and offer emotional support. Listen to what the client is saying.

EVALUATION
1. Evaluate the client's responses to the therapeutic interventions. Does the client demonstrate a decrease in his or her level of anxiety? Have the client's concerns been addressed?
2. Ask the client to evaluate his or her hospital experience.

---

be included and consulted for details about the client's care. All family members should be kept informed about the client's progress.

Also, remember that family members are people in crisis themselves. Gentle interventions provide some much-needed emotional support. When family members are satisfied that their loved one is receiving good care, the decrease in anxiety can help promote clients' recoveries.

SAMPLE CLIENT CARE PLAN 19-1

Hospitalization

ASSESSMENT *History.* Mac is a 72-year-old man who has enjoyed excellent health until approximately 6 weeks ago when he noticed a lump in the right abdominal area. Because of the possibility of extensive surgery, the physician would prefer to perform the biopsy at the hospital. Mac is being admitted the evening before surgery for preparation. *Current Findings.* A nervous, pale man, appearing his stated age. Appearance, speech, and motor activity are all within normal limits. Mac states he is "a little concerned" about the surgery. Although alert, oriented, and cooperative, he has difficulty following instructions.

Multidisciplinary Diagnosis	*Planning/Goals*
Anxiety related to situational crisis of illness, hospitalization, and outcome of surgery	Mac will verbalize his concerns over his outcome and management of care by August 28. Mac will understand and cooperate with his care by August 22.

Therapeutic Interventions

Intervention	Rationale	Team Member
1. Address client by his preferred name.	Demonstrates respect and ensures that dignity will be maintained.	All
2. Obtain history of previous hospitalizations.	Helps plan care based on individual needs and experiences.	Nsg
3. Actively listen to and accept Mac's feelings of anxiety and the threat it poses to his self-esteem.	Conveys respect, self-worth; assures him that his concerns will be addressed.	All
4. Explain each procedure, and gain cooperation before beginning.	Helps decrease anxiety and fear of the unknown.	All
5. Assist Mac to identify and build on past successful coping mechanisms	When added to newly learned ones, past successful coping mechanisms. Equip Mac with more effective skills.	All
6. Help Mac identify new ways to cope with his anxiety.	Helps him manage anxiety.	Psy
7. Inform Mac frequently of his status and progress made during hospitalization.	Knowledge of one's condition decreases anxieties associated with the lack of control during hospitalization.	All

Evaluation

By the morning of surgery, Mac was able to discuss his concerns with the nurse. Recovery from anesthesia was uneventful.

? CRITICAL THINKING QUESTIONS

1. How would the fact that Mac had never been hospitalized affect his anxiety?

2. How would the fact that Mac had never been hospitalized affect your planning of his care?

A complete client care plan includes several other diagnoses and interventions.
Nsg, Nursing staff; *Psy,* psychologist.

Pain Management

An important component of any illness, hospitalization, or surgery relates to the concept of pain—that unpleasant sensation of nerve endings being unkindly stimulated. Pain is associated with many illnesses and hospital stays. It is a subjective experience and can be felt only by the individual experiencing it. People view pain individually based on their own experiences, attitudes, and anxieties.

To manage clients' pain effectively, nurses must discover their clients' expectations of pain, what they think may happen to them, and how much they expect it will hurt. Many clients believe that, if they complain, the physicians and nurses will be distracted from their real job—helping them to heal. Taking the time to learn about the clients' viewpoints will help you plan and implement more effective pain relief measures.

An essential step in helping clients control their pain (**pain management**) is mutual goal setting. Using a pain scale of 0 to 10, the client is asked to pick a target, a "pain score." The objective is to keep pain at or below the pain score level throughout the illness or hospital stay. This concrete goal helps both nurses and clients set realistic, attainable goals for pain management. For diagnostic procedures associated with pain, conscious sedation may be ordered (Messinger and others, 1999).

Assess your client's pain frequently. Try natural remedies to decrease the discomforts before resorting to pain medications. Massage, visualization, distraction, and therapeutic touch have all been found helpful in relieving pain. Pain has an emotional component attached to it. If nurses and other care providers can decrease the anxiety associated with pain, the chances of a speedy recovery are much greater, because energy that was once used to control pain can now be focused on healing.

DISCHARGE PLANNING

To help clients cope with the hurdles of illness or dysfunction, early identification of and intervention for their problems following hospitalization are essential. This process is called discharge planning. After the initial admission assessment, possible home care needs are identified. Then referrals are made to appropriate resources. For example, home care nursing is arranged for the client who must recover from a fracture at home, or the social worker is notified of a client's need for psychiatric day care or housing. For clients who are living with others, discharge planning helps discover educational needs relating to the care of the recovering individual.

Illness affects the entire family group. New anxieties about the individual returning home must be addressed before release from the hospital. During the client's hospitalization, make an effort to discuss home care requirements with the family. Note and correct any misleading or inaccurate information. Take time with family members to teach health care practices related to client care. Most loved ones are more than willing to learn about good home care practices.

For people living alone, especially older adults, discharge planning is vital if individuals are to return to their homes after leaving the health care institution. Basic needs are a high priority for persons living alone. When those needs are met, anxieties are diminished, and people can get on with the business of living. Discharge planning is an important component of every client's care plan and a valuable tool for assessing and meeting clients' after-hospitalization needs.

Illness and hospitalization are stressful. Although thousands of people are treated in hospitals yearly, every admission is a crisis. Do not become so comfortable in your work environment that you cannot appreciate your clients and their situations.

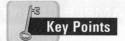

Key Points

- Health is a dynamic state of physical, mental, and social well-being.
- Illness is an abnormal process in which aspects of the social, physical, emotional, or intellectual condition and function of a person are diminished or impaired.
- The illness experience is roughly divided into five stages, with each stage associated with certain perceptions, decisions, and behaviors.
- During each stage of the illness experience, people are faced with several emotional choices and with reactions frequently involving feelings of denial, anger, frustration, shame, and helplessness.
- Denial is a psychological defense mechanism used to ward off the painful feelings associated with hospitalization.
- The situational crisis of inpatient treatment is about being removed from one's familiar home environment to be cared for by strangers in an impersonal, uncomfortable building.
- The stages of the hospitalization experience are being overwhelmed, stabilization, and adaptation.
- It is important for clients to be emotionally supported through the psychiatric hospitalization experience because of the associated stigma and anxiety.
- Family interactions affect clients. Family members should be included and consulted for details about the client's care. They should be kept informed about the client's progress.
- Health care providers must remember that psychosocial attention is just as important as good physical care.
- Pain has an emotional component. Decreasing the anxiety associated with pain through the use of massage, visualization, distraction, and therapeutic touch increases chances of a speedy recovery because the energy used to control the pain can be focused on healing.
- Discharge planning is the early identification of and intervention for possible problems following hospitalization.
- Psychosocial care for hospitalized clients focuses on supporting clients and their families throughout the illness experience.

evolve Be sure to visit the companion Evolve site at http://evolve.elsevier.com/Morrison-Valfre/ for additional online resources.

20 Loss and Grief

Objectives

Upon completion of this chapter, the student will be able to:

1. Describe two characteristics of loss.
2. Illustrate four behaviors associated with loss.
3. Describe the stages of the grieving process.
4. Explain the differences among anticipatory, healthy, and unresolved grief.
5. Compare the reactions of being diagnosed with a potentially fatal illness with those of having a terminal diagnosis.
6. Describe how cultural factors can influence attitudes about death, grief, and mourning.
7. Outline each stage of the dying process.
8. Explain the meaning of a "good death."
9. Describe the support given by nurses who provide hospice care for terminally ill persons.

Key Terms

anticipatory grief (p. 216)
bereavement (bĭ-RĒV-mĕnt) (p. 215)
bereavement-related depression (p. 216)
complicated grief (p. 216)
dying process (p. 219)
external losses (p. 213)
grief (p. 215)
grieving process (p. 215)
hospice (p. 220)
internal losses (p. 213)
loss (p. 213)
mourning (MŎR-nĭng) (p. 215)
terminal illness (TĔR-mĭ-nəl) (p. 218)

Life is a series of situations, experiences, challenges, joys, and losses—a dynamic process that requires continual adaptation and adjustment. Life is filled with gains and losses on every level of functioning. Although change is interwoven throughout each life, reactions to change and the accompanying losses vary according to our sociocultural perceptions. We all tend to react to our world as we were taught. Culture influences attitudes about proper living, relationships with others, and what is considered important in life. It also has a strong impact on a society's attitudes and practices relating to loss, the expression of a loss, and dying individuals.

This chapter explores reactions to loss. It offers several suggestions for assisting clients and their loved ones through the emotions of loss, and it encourages you to consider a "client-centered peaceful death" as an appropriate therapeutic goal.

THE NATURE OF LOSS

The word **loss** has several meanings. It is a form of the verb *to lose,* which means to bring about the destruction of; to become unable to find, to misplace; a failure to keep, win, or gain; or to have taken from one by accident, separation, or death. Add to this the attached emotional perceptions, and one can see how loss becomes a very individual and personal experience.

Losses are an unavoidable part of life. Everyone must cope with them. Emotional reactions and their resultant behaviors are learned from childhood observations and experiences. How individuals cope with problems, successes, and losses is influenced by the success or failure of past experiences and current attitudes. People react and behave during times of loss in highly individual ways. Responses to loss can range from quiet withdrawal to angry rampages, depending on how the loss is perceived, valued, and supported by others.

Losses can be classified as external or internal (self) losses. **External losses** include those losses outside the individual. They relate to objects, possessions, the environment, loved ones, and support. **Internal losses** are more personal and include the losses that involve some part of oneself. An understanding of the characteristics of loss is important if caregivers are to provide the psychosocial interventions that are so important in helping clients (and themselves) cope effectively with the emotional times during loss.

CHARACTERISTICS OF LOSS

In the health care professions, loss is defined as a "state in which something valued that was formerly present is changed or gone. It can no longer be seen, felt, heard, known, or experienced." This broad statement requires some analysis.

First, loss is an actual or potential state. A loss can be real—an actual threat or a situation based in reality.

For example, the family whose home burns in flames is experiencing an actual loss. Potential losses are defined by the individual experiencing them. The industrial worker who is facing a layoff is coping with the possibility of losing his means of providing for his family. A college student who loses her confidence is faced with a less overt, but still important, potential loss. Losses can also be imagined—perceived as a loss. The case of a newlywed who loses her breast to cancer and imagines that her husband will reject her (even though that is not actually the case) illustrates an imagined loss that resulted from an actual loss.

How a loss is defined depends on the value, importance, and significance of the item to the individual. Often the significance of a loss will be different for the client and the care provider. For example, the young mother who has just experienced her fourth miscarriage may define her loss differently from the nurse who has never been pregnant. Remember to assess the **meaning** of loss for each client.

The last portion of the definition, "can no longer be seen, felt, heard, known, or experienced," explains the state of loss. When the valued person, object, or concept is gone, something is changed. This change leads to certain emotional reactions and responses we call grief.

Losses may also be **temporary** or **permanent, expected** or **unexpected.** They may occur suddenly or gradually. Illness, for example, results in the temporary loss of roles and obligations, but the loss of a limb is definitely a permanent loss. Expected losses arrive with many situations. To illustrate, a chronically ill 70-year-old does not expect to compete in the Senior Olympics because he knows he has gradually lost physical abilities. The individual diagnosed with a terminal illness is coping with an expected loss. Unexpected losses are just that. They are the unknown occurrences that arrive suddenly and without warning. The automobile accident, the diagnosis of human immunodeficiency virus (HIV), or the suicide of a cherished friend each illustrates unexpected losses.

Losses can also be **maturational,** in which an individual must give up something to gain a higher level of development. The 18-year-old who is moving into her own apartment loses the comfort and security of family to establish herself as an independent adult. The loss here is ideally offset by the gains in self-development and maturity.

Situational losses occur in response to external events. In a situational loss, the individual has no control over the event leading to the loss. The death of a loved one, a natural disaster, and the divorce of family members are typical situational losses.

BEHAVIORS ASSOCIATED WITH LOSS

Each person reacts to loss based on his or her level of development, past experiences, and current support systems. To help clients cope with their losses, it is important to understand how people at various developmental stages react to loss.

Children's understanding of and reactions to loss change as they mature. Newborns and infants feel the loss of their caregivers but show little emotional reaction to the loss as long as their basic needs are being met. Toddlers are concerned with themselves. Although they may repeat phrases such as "Daddy is gone," they have no grasp of the real meaning of loss. Because of their sense of time, preschoolers cannot understand a permanent loss such as death. Preschoolers use magical thinking (they believe that their thoughts can control events) to explain their losses. This can result in a child carrying the burdens of shame, doubt, and guilt when his or her thinking is associated with the loss. To illustrate, Jerry, a 3-year-old, believes that if he were not such a bad boy, his mother would not have gone away. Younger children may react to the same loss more intensely than older children or adults because they have fewer coping mechanisms.

School-age children have some idea about cause and effect, but they still associate bad thoughts or misdeeds with losses. At this age, children experience great feelings of grief over the loss of a body part or function. They may feel overwhelming responsibility and guilt about an event, but they respond well to simple, logical explanations. Children around 6 or 7 years old often apply a broad definition to loss, especially death, by giving responsibility for the loss to the devil, God, or the bogeyman. By 9 or 10 years of age, most children have an adult concept of loss and death. They realize that some losses are permanent, whereas others are only temporary. Their attitudes, reactions, and responses to their losses are now firmly established.

Adolescents react to loss with adult thinking and childlike emotions. Although they can understand the concepts of loss and death, they are the age-group least likely to accept the situation. Adolescents grieve acutely over the loss of a body part or function and fear rejection from their peers. Death is particularly difficult to accept at this age because the developmental task of adolescence is to define who one is and to establish an identity. Threats of loss at this age may make a person stand out from the peer group, so many adolescents ignore or minimize the loss or deny their own mortality.

Adults facing loss are able to perceive events more abstractly than younger individuals. They can tell the difference between temporary and permanent losses. Most are able to accept their losses and grow from the experiences. As they continue to encounter and cope with various losses, most adults develop a "hardiness," a sense of self-confidence and understanding about life and death. This strength helps stave off the depression so common in older adults who have experienced significant losses. Hardy people are able to problem solve. They are in control of their emotions, their lives, and their reactions to loss. By the time most individuals have reached old age, their emotional hardiness has carried them through many of life's losses.

THE NATURE OF GRIEF AND MOURNING

Although the terms grief, mourning, and bereavement are used interchangeably, each has a separate meaning. Grief is the set of **emotional reactions** that accompany a loss. Mourning is the **process** of working through or resolving one's grief, and bereavement is the **behavioral state** of thoughts, feelings, and activities that follow a loss. The period of grief and mourning after a loss can be intense and painful. It may last for a short period or remain as a deep emotional scar. Feelings of loss, grief, and mourning are deeply personal, and each of us has his or her own way of coping with these emotions. There is no right or wrong way to grieve.

THE GRIEVING PROCESS

To work through the emotional responses to loss, one must experience the grieving process—a method for resolving losses and healing or recovering. Grieving, mourning, and bereavement are normal, healthy responses to loss. Working through the grieving process allows people to "piece themselves back together," to reintegrate their lives, to find meaning in new relationships, and to reestablish a positive picture of themselves. It is a healing process that encourages individuals to continue on, even after the loss. The care provider's role during the grieving process is to provide emotional support and an atmosphere that helps clients accomplish the painful work of grieving (Meiner and Lueckenotte, 2006).

The grieving process was first studied by Sigmund Freud in the early 1900s. Since then, many theories have been developed to explain the work of grieving. Although various theories consider different aspects of grieving, all include stages that we experience while resolving our grief (Figure 20-1).

STAGES OF THE GRIEVING PROCESS

The first step in the process of grieving (denial) begins with a feeling of shock. One wants to reject the loss, to say "no," to refuse to give up the cherished object or person. Individuals may not even acknowledge that a loss has occurred. They behave as if nothing has happened or pretend that the loved object or person is still present. Denial at this stage provides an emotional buffer that allows people time to mobilize resources for the work ahead.

As the realization that the loss can no longer be ignored sets in, denial turns to yearning. During this stage, the reality of the loss begins to be realized and the griever becomes overwhelmed. Crying, self-blame, and anger are common, and some may even strike out at self or others. The griever "falls apart"—becomes disorganized, depressed, and unable to complete daily living activities. He or she may try to postpone coping with the loss by ignoring it. The person in this stage may feel that life is not worth living and consider or attempt suicide (Box 20-1). This is an extremely difficult time for people. They need the emotional support and caring of friends and family to remind them of all that still remains, even after loss and suffering.

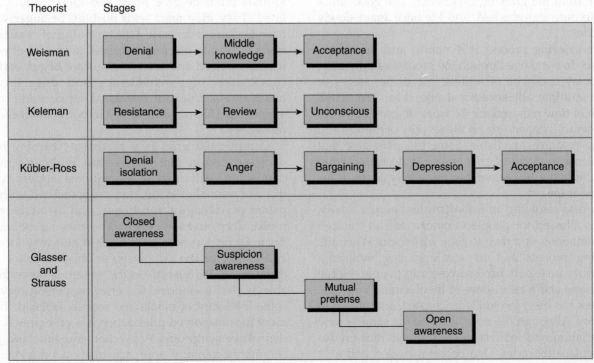

FIGURE **20-1** Theories—Stages of dying and grief.

Box 20-1 *Suicide Alert*

Individuals experiencing acute emotions of grief and loss often feel that life is not worth continuing. Any medications, over-the-counter drugs, or other chemicals in the environment have the potential of being used for a suicide attempt. Grieving persons have been known to ingest medications prescribed for the deceased with the purpose of committing suicide during the grieving process.

Sometimes grief is so intense that they will resort to slitting their wrists or using a weapon on themselves. Health care providers should be alert to the signs and symptoms of possible suicidal actions. See Chapter 27 for a more thorough discussion of suicide.

As the impact of the loss is experienced in daily living, the third stage, **depression and identification,** settles over the grieving individual. The work of mourning begins as the full impact of the loss is realized. Feelings of guilt and remorse are frequent as attempts are made to cope with the painful void left by the loss. The grieving individual may withdraw from social interactions, engage in unhealthy behaviors, or experience overwhelming loneliness. As time passes, however, most people become willing to share their memories and rely on the emotional support of others.

Acceptance and recovery begin when grieving individuals begin to focus their energies toward the living. The loss is a reality, but life continues, so they begin to reinvest their feelings in others and nurture their remaining relationships. Steps are taken to reorganize their lives by filling the void created by the loss. Eventually, a new self-awareness and inner strength evolve from the grieving experience. The good times start to outweigh the bad, and life once again slowly stabilizes.

The grieving process is dynamic, and most individuals do not move through the process step-by-step. They may backslide or regress into earlier stages or make multiple adjustments at one time. The actual length of time required for the work of grieving varies considerably, depending on the severity of the loss and coping resources available. Some theorists state that the intense reactions of grief gradually decrease within 6 to 12 months, but active mourning may continue for 5 years or longer.

Because resolving an important loss occurs slowly, time is allowed for people to mourn, to sort through their emotions, and then to cope with them. When the grieving process and its accompanying mourning behaviors are experienced successfully, people emerge with hope and a new sense of involvement with life. The loss has been recognized, accepted, and placed in memory. Although life may never be the same, a new appreciation and interest in current activities gradually replace the grief. One becomes healed and able to continue.

An individual who becomes aware of an impending loss, such as the loss of a body part or the diagnosis of a terminal condition, may experience **anticipatory grief**—the process of grieving before the actual event occurs. During divorce proceedings, for example, many persons grieve for the part of life that has been lost and what they know will be lost in the future. Anticipatory grieving allows individuals time to prepare for the loss.

Unresolved Grief

Mental health problems can result when the grieving process is prolonged or impairs functioning over time. Unresolved grief, also termed dysfunctional grief or complicated bereavement, describes unhealthy or ineffective grief reactions. People who experience unresolved grief are unable to shift their attention from their loss to the realities of everyday life. They become so preoccupied with the loss that they are unable to function effectively. There are two types of unresolved grief: bereavement-related depression and complicated grief. Both are associated with distress about the loss, changes in eating or sleeping patterns, and changes in activity levels.

With **bereavement-related depression**, the grieving person feels the loss so intensely that feelings of despair and worthlessness overwhelm everything in life. Every day is a gray fog with no light as one looks toward the future. Life becomes a burden, and each new day is faced with remorse. This attitude overshadows all else. The grieving individual experiences changes in eating, sleeping, and activity levels; angry or hostile moods; and an inability to concentrate or complete work tasks. To complicate matters, individuals often become more and more socially isolated. They may react with hostility or anger when friends express concern. This type of grief commonly leads to suicide but responds well to treatment when it is recognized and interventions are begun early. A combination of psychotherapy and drug therapy has been effective, but emotional support and social support are factors of primary importance in clients' recoveries.

Complicated grief is a persistent yearning for a deceased person that often occurs without signs of depression. Although the symptoms appear to be those of normal grieving, they are associated with impaired psychological functioning and disturbances of mood, sleep, and self-esteem. The grieving individual becomes preoccupied with the loss and may idealize and search for the lost person or object or relive past experiences. Because life in the present is not as desirable as past memories, the grieving person may become intolerant of others and socially isolated. Treatment for unresolved grief depends on the presence of depressive symptoms. A psychotherapeutic and psychopharmacological approach treats depression. The grief is helped by emotional support and someone to

Your client displays all the signs and symptoms of complicated grief. It is recommended that she attend a support group for widows, but she refuses. With gentle questioning, she confides that she has no money for transportation to the meetings and she will not ask for help.
• What therapeutic interventions would help this client meet the goal of regularly attending the support group meetings?

Cultural Considerations 20-1

In Sri Lanka, a small island off the southeastern tip of India, quality is strongly preferable to quantity of life. Most of Sri Lanka's citizens are Buddhist (69%) and believe in reincarnation (the rebirth of a soul in a different body). They believe the suffering of this life will be relieved in the next incarnation so there is no need for heroic lifesaving measures.

Dying persons in this culture are prepared for death by helping them remember past good deeds of their lives and achieve a comfortable mental state. Because the body is no longer required after death, cremation is the preferred burial custom.

listen. Support groups and opportunities for social interactions add to the effectiveness of treatment in most cases (see Think About 20-1).

The therapeutic interventions for both types of unresolved grief involve listening, providing emotional support, and referral to appropriate resources. Nurses and direct caregivers are often the first to identify the signs and symptoms of unresolved grieving because of the focus on clients' activities of daily living. Therapeutic listening helps in understanding the needs of the grieving individual. It also offers an opportunity to provide emotional support and comfort. Sometimes when grieving individuals are encouraged to verbalize their feelings, the real healing begins. Health care providers are instrumental in referring their clients to the therapists, support groups, and educational opportunities that may help them work through the grieving process.

Caregivers' Grief

Caregivers experience the same grief as others when faced with loss. Many nurses work with dying clients, some on a daily basis. Relationships are formed between caregivers and clients that develop into understanding and rapport. The focus is on the client, and the caregiver acts therapeutically, but the bond between individuals grows with the relationship. When that relationship is lost, even if it was an expected loss, caregivers grieve, and that is a necessary process for health.

However, the care provider's role in offering support and comfort to grieving loved ones can become complicated if one's personal feelings of grief overshadow one's effectiveness. Caregivers should share in the grief experience, but they need to remember that the primary goal is to provide support for the remaining loved ones. Many health care facilities offer support groups for nurses and other caregivers who work with dying clients in an effort to assist them with their own grief experiences. Learn to appreciate the experiences of dying and grieving clients. Understand the steps of the grieving process. Discover how you cope with losses. Finally, do not forget to find a way to renew your energies. When we know and accept our own attitudes and feelings about loss and grieving, we are better able to provide the therapeutic interventions so needed by others.

THE DYING PROCESS

Dying is the last stage of growth and development. Like birth, it is an intensely personal process. Unlike birth, however, an individual is often aware and consciously takes part in the process. Death means different things to each of us. For some, it is a welcome relief from suffering. For others, it is the ultimate fear. The process of dying remains unchanged, but attitudes, beliefs, and behaviors surrounding death are as variable as the individuals who practice them (see Cultural Considerations 20-1).

Death may occur suddenly or gradually. It may be expected or arrive as a total surprise. One may be fortunate enough to die in familiar surroundings, attended by loved ones and friends, or one may be forced to face the fate of dying alone and unloved. During earlier days in American history, most families cared for their elders and ill members at home. Children witnessed the births of their siblings and the deaths of their grandparents. It was all accepted as part of living. Today children know little about dying because older adults no longer live in the family home. More than two thirds of all deaths now occur in health care facilities, hospitals, and nursing homes (Ebersole and Hess, 2005).

AGE DIFFERENCES AND DYING

The impact of death is only as strong as one's understanding of it. Before the age of 8 years, most children do not understand the permanency of death, but they do experience a sense of doom and danger associated with dying. By 12 years of age, children are aware that death is irreversible, but they do not relate to their own deaths. Adolescents and young adults do not relate to death unless forced. As people grow older, they begin to lose family and friends and must begin to face their own mortality.

A special word about the dying child is needed here. Children are remarkably observant and have an intuitive ability to understand the seriousness of their illness and its outcomes. However, their immediate concerns focus on how the illness affects their activities of daily living and limits their abilities. Children are also very aware of the family's reactions and hesitate to discuss issues they think may be upsetting to the family. Whenever possible, parents should be encouraged to communicate with the dying child. Open discussions of the illness and its outcome help children cope with the feelings of isolation, anxiety, and guilt over causing distress in the family. Sharing feelings and insecurities helps to bond family members together and to give them strength from each other. Children who are able to share their emotions have fewer behavioral problems, less depression, and higher self-esteem than those who suppress their feelings (Calandra, 1993). They adapt to the difficulties of their disease and its treatment better than those who must cope with the isolation of dying emotionally alone. Siblings of the dying child also need extra attention during this time because feelings of jealousy, anger, and guilt are often present.

TERMINAL ILLNESS

A **terminal illness** is a condition in which the outcome is death. The diagnosis of a terminal illness is perhaps one of the most difficult challenges an individual must face in his or her lifetime. In today's world, the diagnosis of HIV/acquired immunodeficiency syndrome (AIDS) is especially devastating for young adults. The course of the disease is long, with periods of physical improvement and hope alternating with illness and suffering. Grieving occurs throughout the course of the illness.

How a person responds to and prepares for death depends on two factors: the meaning of death and the coping mechanisms used throughout life to deal with problems. If the individual is comfortable and satisfied with life, death is accepted without fear; but if the person lived struggling and fighting, the experience of dying will be much the same. People tend to cope with dying in the same ways in which they coped with living.

The diagnosis of a fatal illness or condition is received with disbelief and shock—true crisis. This is a time of great uncertainty because client and family are struggling to cope with the illness, its effects, and its final outcome. Crisis interventions can be very effective at this stage.

As the condition progresses, denial and hope allow the client and family to slowly adjust to the reality of the situation. Hope is future oriented and helps individuals endure the suffering of the present because it offers the possibility that soon things will be better. Denial offers a way of coping with each little loss until the reality of the situation is finally accepted. During this time, the individual is encouraged to continue with daily activities until he or she is no longer able. In time, both the family and individual either accept the outcome and prepare for death or continue to deny the reality of the situation until it is no longer possible.

Receiving the diagnosis of a potentially fatal illness can bring forth a variety of reactions. Individuals who are young and feel healthy may refuse to accept that a problem exists. For others, the diagnosis of a potentially terminal condition acts as a wake-up call and a motivator to make major lifestyle changes. Case Study 20-1 illustrates such a situation.

People often make the major changes necessary to prevent the condition from becoming fatal. Others value their present ways of living too much or feel that the work is not worth the extra time gained. The decisions about one's remaining time belong to and should be made by the individual. Caregivers should accept and support clients' decisions about terminal illness. The goals of care are then structured to provide the best possible interventions within the realities of each situation.

Case Study 20-1

Brittany was just 35 years old when she received the diagnosis of severe coronary artery disease. She became short of breath one day while doing household chores and decided that she must be hanging on to the cold she had gotten from her 8-year-old a few weeks before. She decided to schedule an appointment with her family physician.

Dr. Dunn had worked with Brittany's family for many years. He knew about her smoking, eating, and exercise habits. He had encouraged her to consider weight loss and had referred her to a smoking cessation program several times in the past few years, but to no avail. After a thorough physical examination and an electrocardiogram, Dr. Dunn scheduled Brittany for a cardiac catheterization at the local hospital the following day. Brittany left the office in shock, stunned by the realization that she may actually not live long enough to see her children grow into adults. She knew inside her heart that this was the warning call to take her life and health more seriously. She only hoped that she had the strength to make the changes she knew would be required if she wanted to live longer.

The results of Brittany's cardiac catheterization showed that three of her coronary arteries were seriously blocked and the blood supply to her heart was inadequate. Her physician recommended surgery but firmly stated that this was only a temporary measure. Without major lifestyle changes, the problem would reappear. At this point Brittany had to make some life-and-death decisions. As she saw it, she had two options: to continue with her easygoing, comfortable lifestyle and run the risk of dropping over with a heart attack at an early age or to change her diet, stop her unhealthy habits, begin to exercise, and learn to defuse her stress.

• What therapeutic interventions would help Brittany make a sound decision?

CULTURAL FACTORS, DYING, AND MOURNING

Although death is a personal experience, it occurs within a cultural and social context. Cultural practices regarding dying, grief, and mourning have a strong influence on behaviors. To illustrate, many modern North Americans see death as the final loss in life. East Indian Hindus, however, believe that all creatures are in a process of spiritual evolution that extends through the boundaries of time and space. They view death as a passage from one existence to another (Giger and Davidhizar, 2008).

Culture also dictates many funeral, burial, and mourning practices. The length of time for mourning and public displays of grief is culturally determined. Special clothing is commonly worn during the grieving process to symbolize loss. To illustrate, traditional Chinese wear white as a sign of mourning, whereas black is the required color for mourning in North America and Russia.

The beliefs, rituals, and practices of one's culture may be very important to one individual and barely matter to another member of that same culture. Nurses must be careful to assess and understand the meaning of each client's cultural, religious, and social practices (Geissler, 2003). Many variations exist in every group of people, no matter which culture. Do not assume how a client feels about his or her cultural beliefs and practices. Find out what is important and, if at all possible, incorporate it into the client's plan of care. Never take a person's cultural background for granted.

STAGES OF DYING

Unless death arrives suddenly, both individuals and loved ones progress through several psychological stages. These stages or phases, called the **dying process**, allow people to cope with the overwhelming emotional reactions associated with dying and losing loved ones. Several theories about the process of dying have been developed, but the most well known theory is Elisabeth Kübler-Ross' five stages of dying: denial, anger, bargaining, depression, and acceptance (Kübler-Ross, 1969). Later theorists simplified Kübler-Ross' five stages into three basic phases of resistance, working, and acceptance.

During the resistance stage, the individual fights the issue through denial, avoidance, anger, and bargaining. The working, or review, stage broadens consciousness as one's life is reviewed. The resistance disappears, and the individual begins to deal with unfinished business. He or she reclaims a part of the self and becomes more in tune to the self of the present rather than of the past.

In the last stage, called acceptance, the individual is comfortable and acknowledges death. He or she can discuss death with peace and calm. Increasingly greater amounts of time are spent focusing inward, moving one's energies away from reality. Some individuals have near-death experiences that they describe as a passage into another realm of consciousness or a "vivid personal journey...when they were on the brink of death" (Hayes and others, 1998). Eventually, the dying person fades from this life, leaving only the body behind.

A broader perspective of the dying process is offered by Glaser and Strauss (1965). Their models of awareness of dying can be applied to family, friends, and those who care for the dying individual. They describe the closed awareness model as one in which medical personnel and family know that the condition is fatal but still "keep the secret" or withhold the information from the client. Once the dying individual becomes suspicious of the truth, a battle for control of information ensues. This closed awareness model was commonly practiced by health care providers in the past. Frequently, clients were not told of the seriousness of their illness because it was believed that the news was too upsetting. Most terminally ill persons know that they are dying. Many still experience death locked into a denial supported by care providers and loved ones.

The mutual pretense model is a "let's pretend" kind of awareness. Both caregivers and the dying individual are aware of the impending death, but nobody talks about it. Although no one really expects the client to recover, it is easier to pretend that things will get better. Unfortunately, the true feelings of everyone remain hidden, unspoken, and unresolved.

In the open awareness model, the approaching death is openly acknowledged and accepted. The client is resigned to dying and accepts each day as it can be lived. Family members, health care providers, and the dying have permission to discuss their fears, concerns, and experiences. The open awareness method of coping allows mutual support and comfort to be given and received. It also encourages loved ones to grieve with, rather than for, the dying individual.

THERAPEUTIC INTERVENTIONS

One of the most rewarding areas in health care is assisting an individual to experience a "good" death, one in which the dying and the living participate fully and completely. With a good death, individuals control their own destiny. Clients decide when to stop aggressive treatments, refuse the one last surgical procedure, or end the discomfort of a painful therapy. Peace, serenity, and acceptance replace denial, fighting, and anger. Individuals value and cherish each day but look forward to the day when their suffering will end. They are not afraid of death—rather, it is the last step of the growth process, which draws a productive and fruitful life to a close.

Nurses and other health care providers bring their own attitudes, values, beliefs, and biases to the care of the dying. The way caregivers perceive "the act of dying, as painful, upsetting, indifferent, or a blessing, influences the treatment the dying patient will receive in the last days, whether in the hospital or nursing home" (Ebersole and Hess, 2005). Explore your own attitudes about death; the quality of your clients' care depends on it.

Never limit your clients by placing labels on them. It is easy for nurses to focus on the dying person's biological or physical needs. It is nonthreatening to help relieve the physical symptoms associated with dying, but it is another thing to become involved in a meaningful therapeutic relationship that supports the dying individual. Box 20-2 lists nursing diagnoses (problem statements) that relate to dying clients.

HOSPICE CARE

In the past, most dying individuals were cared for in the home by family and friends. As society gradually became more mobile, families separated from relatives when they moved to different locations. Dying at home was no longer an alternative for many people, so they were sent to hospitals and long-term care facilities. Health care providers assisted their clients through the dying process, providing comfort where they could, but realizing that there must be better ways to meet life's final challenge.

Finally, during the 1960s, a model for humane care of the dying was developed and tested at Saint Christopher's Hospice in London, England. Since then the number of hospices has grown tremendously. In the United States today, more than one-half million clients are receiving hospice care. The term hospice symbolizes a philosophy of care for people with terminal illnesses or conditions and their loved ones. The National Hospice Organization (NHO), an organization dedicated to promoting the principles and standards of high-quality hospice care, has developed guidelines for hospice care in the United States. Other countries have similar organizations.

The goal of hospice care is to make the remainder of an individual's life as meaningful and comfortable as humanly possible. Hospice care differs from institutional care in several ways. The focus of care reorients from curative to palliative (providing comfort). Hospice services are available 24 hours per day in institutional or home settings.

Hospice care helps the family retain control for the dying individual, and it allows individuals to experience death with the dignity they deserve. Hospice care helps redefine family relationships because care of the dying individual requires great energies of loved ones and friends. Many nurses and other care providers are choosing to specialize in hospice care today because it is such a rewarding area of practice.

MEETING THE NEEDS OF DYING CLIENTS

Dying clients have special needs during their final days (Figure 20-2). One of the most urgent needs is to be free from pain and discomfort. This is usually accomplished by around-the-clock administration of pain-relieving medications. Addiction is not an issue in caring for the terminally ill population.

Box 20-2 *NANDA-I Nursing Diagnoses Related to Dying*

Anxiety
Behavior, risk-prone health
Caregiver role strain
Coping, ineffective
Decisional conflict
Denial, ineffective
Grieving
Grieving, complicated
Hopelessness
Insomnia
Knowledge, deficient
Nutrition, imbalanced: more or less than body
   requirements
Powerlessness
Self-esteem disturbance
Social interaction, impaired
Social isolation
Spiritual distress
Violence, risk for self-directed

Data from NANDA International: *NANDA-I nursing diagnoses: definitions and classification 2007-2008*, Philadelphia, 2007, NANDA International.
NANDA-I, NANDA International.

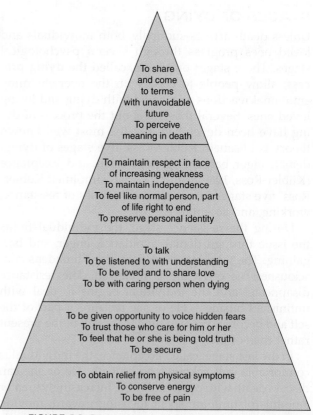

FIGURE **20-2** Hierarchy of a dying person's needs.

Freedom from loneliness is not always so easily accomplished. Many dying individuals have already suffered numerous losses, both physical and emotional. The strange surroundings of an institution and unfamiliar caregivers can add to a person's sense of isolation and loneliness. Dying clients need to know that someone who really cares for their welfare is there to help. Health care providers should assess for loneliness in clients and offer personal attention.

Individuals with terminal illnesses also need to preserve their self-esteem. The pride of a lifetime of work and struggle can be easily shattered by the thoughtless words or actions of a caregiver. Respect is always an important factor in caring for clients, especially older adults. One of the most important principles to remember when working with terminally ill clients is that a dying person lives with the same needs as the rest of us. Life and its needs for love, friendship, and self-esteem continue even when an individual is in the process of dying.

As death approaches, many physical and emotional changes begin to take place (Tables 20-1 and 20-2). This

Table 20-1 | *Signs and Symptoms Associated With Dying*

SYMPTOMS	RATIONALE	INTERVENTIONS
Coolness, color and temperature change in hands, arms, feet, and legs	Peripheral circulation diminishes to facilitate increased circulation to vital organs	Place socks on feet. Cover with light cotton blanket.
Increased sleeping	Conservation of energy	Spend time with the client; hold client's hand; speak normally to the client even though there may be a lack of verbal response or consciousness.
Disorientation, confusion of time, place, or person	Metabolic changes	Identify self by name before speaking to client; speak softly, clearly, and truthfully.
Incontinence of urine and feces	Increased muscle relaxation and decreased consciousness	Maintain vigilance, and change bedding as appropriate.
Congestion	Poor circulation of body fluids, immobilization, and inability to expectorate secretions causing gurgling, rattles, bubbling	Elevate the head, and gently turn the head to the side to drain secretions.
Restlessness	Metabolic changes and a decrease in oxygen to the brain	Calm the client by speech and action. Reduce light; gently rub back, stroke arms, or read aloud; play soothing music. DO NOT USE RESTRAINTS.
Decreased intake of food and liquids	Body conservation of energy for function	Do not force client to eat or drink. Give ice chips, soft drinks, juice, and popsicles as appropriate. Apply petroleum jelly to dry lips. If client is a mouth breather, apply protective jelly more frequently as needed.
Decreased urine output	Decreased fluid intake and decreased circulation to kidney	None
Altered breathing pattern	Metabolic and oxygen changes to respiratory centers	Elevate the head of bed; hold hand, speak gently.

Table 20-2 | *Emotional and Spiritual Symptoms of Approaching Death*

SYMPTOMS	RATIONALE	INTERVENTIONS
Withdrawal	Prepares the client for release and detachment and letting go of relationships and surroundings	Continue communicating in a normal manner using a normal voice tone. Identify self by name: hold hand, say what you want person to hear from you.
Visionlike experiences (dead friends or family, religious vision)	Preparation for transition	Do not contradict or argue regarding whether this is or is not a real experience. If the client is frightened, reassure that he or she is not crazy but that these aberrations do occur.
Restlessness	Tension, fear, unfinished business	Listen to client express fears, sadness, and anger associated with dying. Give permission to go.
Decreased socialization	As energy diminishes, the client withdraws and begins to make the transition	Express support; give permission to die.
Unusual communication: out-of-character statements, gestures, requests	Signals readiness to let go	Say what needs to be said to the dying client; kiss, hug, or cry with him or her.

Modified from McCracken AL, Gerdsen L: Sharing the legacy: hospice care principles for terminally ill elders, *J Gerontol Nurs* 17:4-8, 1991.

is a time to provide comfort and solace and meet the physical needs of care, but most important, it is a time to support those who must say good-bye and those who are left behind.

LOSS, GRIEF, AND MENTAL HEALTH

Loss is a part of living. The behaviors associated with grief and mourning assist us with healing after suffering a loss. For many people, death represents the ultimate loss. How effectively individuals cope with their losses has a large effect on their mental and emotional health. Sample Client Care Plan 20-1 offers an example of a care plan for an individual who is coping with grief.

Many behaviors associated with the grieving process could be diagnosed as mental health disorders except for the fact that they are short lived. Mental health problems arise only when a person is stuck or immobilized during a stage of the grief reaction. Clinically, the *Diagnostic and*

Statistical Manual of Mental Disorders (DSM-IV-TR) diagnoses of bereavement and bereavement-related depression apply only to those grieving individuals who are significantly impaired in their abilities to accomplish the activities of daily living for longer than 2 months (American Psychiatric Association, 2000).

For persons who currently have a mental health disorder, the stresses of loss and grief can overwhelm delicate coping mechanisms and lead to further problems. For example, the 23-year-old with schizophrenia who has lived with her family all her life will have great difficulties in grieving for the loss of her mother. Caregivers must remember that people with existing mental health problems require much emotional support during periods of loss or grieving.

How each human being copes with loss is unique and individual. Coping mechanisms may be effective and result in growth and healing. They may also be

---

SAMPLE CLIENT CARE PLAN 20-1

Grieving

ASSESSMENT *History.* Jerry, 14 years old, lost his leg in an automobile accident 8 weeks ago. His attitude toward the loss of his leg was casual at first, but soon he became angry and withdrawn. Complaints of chronic fatigue, poor appetite, and an inability to concentrate have prompted his mother to seek health care.
Current Findings. An alert adolescent boy who complains that he is unable to sleep. Speech is slow with delayed responses. Left leg is amputated above the knee. Uses crutches for mobility.

Multidisciplinary Diagnosis	*Planning/Goals*
Complicated grieving related to loss of body part and physiological functioning	Jerry will attend each counseling session. Jerry will identify his feelings of loss and anger by February 21.

Therapeutic Interventions

Intervention	**Rationale**	**Team Member**
1. Establish trust and open communication.	Adolescents must trust in the relationship before they commit themselves.	All
2. Assure Jerry that his feelings are important, and give permission to discuss them.	Shows interest and respect; helps maintain self-worth and dignity.	All
3. Assist Jerry in acknowledging his feelings associated with losing his leg	Helps Jerry to connect his anger with the loss and begin the work of grieving.	All
4. Help Jerry and family understand that anger is a normal response to loss.	Assures him that his emotions are a normal part of the grieving response.	All
5. Assist Jerry in finding appropriate outlets for his anger rather than projecting it onto others.	Provides structure, gives a sense of control, helps him focus on more effective ways of emotional expression.	Psy, Soc Svc
6. Encourage Jerry to make plans for the future and set goals.	Goals help change the focus from the past to the future.	Psy, Nsg

Evaluation

Jerry missed the first two appointments but has kept every appointment for the past month. Jerry is able to identify three reasons why he feels angry and frustrated. Jerry was unwilling to make any plans for the future at time of evaluation.

❓ **CRITICAL THINKING** QUESTIONS

1. How would you help Jerry cope with his anger?

2. What interventions may help Jerry look toward the future?

A complete client care plan includes several other diagnoses and interventions.
Psy, Psychologist; *Soc Svc,* social services; *Nsg,* nursing staff.

inadequate or dysfunctional, resulting in distress, depression, or other mental health problems. Nurses need to assess their clients' abilities and resources to cope with their losses. By encouraging effective coping skills and providing physical and emotional support, health care providers become able to help their clients (and themselves) successfully work through life's losses and grief.

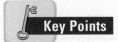

Key Points

- A loss can be actual, potential, or imagined; temporary or permanent; maturational or situational; expected or unexpected. Losses may occur suddenly or gradually.
- The significance of the loss is determined by the person experiencing it.
- Each person reacts to loss based on his or her level of development, past experiences, and current support systems.
- Grief is the set of emotional reactions accompanying loss.
- The steps of the grieving process are shock, disbelief, and denial; anger, bargaining, and reviewing; depression; and acceptance.
- Mourning is the process of working through or resolving one's grief.
- Bereavement is the emotional and behavioral state of thoughts, feelings, and activities that follow a loss.
- Anticipatory grief is the process of grieving before the actual event occurs.
- Two types of dysfunctional (unresolved) grief are known as bereavement-related depression and complicated grief.

- The care provider's role in offering support and comfort to grieving loved ones can become complicated if one's personal grief overshadows his or her effectiveness.
- To cope with your own feelings of grief, learn to appreciate the experiences of dying and grieving clients. Understand the steps of the grieving process. Discover how you cope with losses. Find a way to renew your energies.
- Dying is the last stage in the development of an individual.
- How an individual responds to and prepares for death depends on what death means and the coping mechanisms used throughout life.
- Terminally ill children who are able to share their feelings have fewer problems and adapt better than those who must cope with emotional isolation.
- One of the most rewarding experiences in health care is assisting an individual in experiencing a client-centered, peaceful death, one in which the dying and the living participate fully and completely.
- The term *hospice* has come to mean a philosophy of care for people with terminal illnesses or conditions and their loved ones.
- Dying clients have special needs during their final days, including freedom from pain and discomfort, freedom from loneliness, and preservation of self-esteem.
- One of the most important principles to remember is that a dying person lives with the same needs as the rest of us.

---

evolve   Be sure to visit the companion Evolve site at http://evolve.elsevier.com/Morrison-Valfre/ for additional online resources.

Objectives

Upon completion of this chapter, the student will be able to:

1. Describe the continuum of emotional responses.
2. Compare four theories relating to emotions and their disorders.
3. Explain how emotions affect individuals throughout the life cycle.
4. Compare the differences between a depressive episode and a depressive disorder.
5. List the diagnostic criteria for bipolar disorders.
6. Explain seasonal affective disorder.
7. Discuss behaviors associated with postpartum depression.
8. Identify three drug classes used for the treatment of depression and other mood disorders.
9. Apply four nursing (therapeutic) interventions for clients with mood disorders.

Key Terms

affect (p. 227)
bipolar disorders (p. 229)
cyclothymic (sī-klō-THĪ-mĭk) **disorder** (p. 229)
depression (p. 227)
dysthymia (dĭs-THĪ-mē-ə) (p. 227)
emotion (p. 224)
hypomania (hī-pō-MĀ-nē-ə) (p. 229)
mania (MĀ-nē-ə) (p. 227)
manic depression (p. 229)
mood disorder (p. 227)
postpartum depression (p. 230)
religiosity (rĭ-LĬJ-ē-ĂHS-ĭt-ē) (p. 235)
seasonal affective disorder (p. 230)
situational depression (p. 225)

The emotional realm affects all other areas of human functioning. Emotions can lead to physical changes, new intellectual perspectives, and altered social roles. An emotion is a feeling—a nonintellectual response. Emotions are **reactions** to various stimuli based on individual points of view. Think About 21-1 presents an example of how perceptions affect emotional reactions.

CONTINUUM OF EMOTIONAL RESPONSES

The spectrum of human emotion ranges from elation to despair. Emotional responses can be growth promoting and adaptive, or they can lead to ineffective behaviors that could soon become maladaptive. Figure 21-1 illustrates the continuum of emotional responses. As individuals repeatedly react to behaviors, interactions, society, and the environment, they establish patterns of emotional responses that become moods. Over time, moods evolve into an overall view or outlook on life. From this outlook, people interpret and react to the world about them. Some of the reactions are emotional, and the cycle continues.

THEORIES RELATING TO EMOTIONS AND THEIR DISORDERS

A **mood** is described as a "prolonged emotional state that influences one's whole personality and life functioning" (Rollant, 1998). Mood disorders were once considered simple, correctable imbalances in behavior. Today, evidence suggests that a combination of physical, psychological, and environmental factors is involved in the development of mood disorders. Many theories about the cause of mood disorders have been presented throughout the years, but none fully explains the complexities of these conditions.

BIOLOGICAL EVIDENCE

Much has been learned about the physical nature of mood disorders. The causes are complex. When sad moods deepen and persist, the individual is unable to restore emotional equilibrium (balance) because of unusual stress or poor internal regulation. Box 21-1 lists the possible causes of mood disorders.

Defects in the immune system have been implicated in depression. Genetics may be a factor in mood disorders because high rates of depression and bipolar illness are seen in individuals who have relatives with mood disorders.

Studies of the effects of neurochemical messengers (neurotransmitters) and hormones on behavior have revealed that behaviors and body chemistries are interrelated. The monoamines norepinephrine and serotonin

Think About 21-1

James and Justin, two neighborhood teens, are working on building a model airplane in Justin's backyard. A piece of the model breaks, and they begin to argue about each other's clumsiness. The emotions grow, and soon scuffling, swearing, and fighting ensue. The commotion brings both fathers to the scene. Justin's father shakes his fist and shouts, "That's a boy! Punch him good. No son of mine is going to let someone get the best of him!" James' father, also seeing the scene, reacts with, "Boys! Stop fighting! There are better ways to solve your problems than beating each other up."
- How did each father's perception of the situation differ?
- What do you think caused the difference in their reactions?
- What do you think James and Justin learned from observing each father's response?

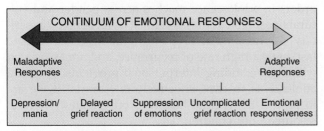

FIGURE 21-1 Continuum of emotional responses.

are major neurotransmitters that excite or inhibit the brain circuits involved in mood regulation. Monoamines are longer-acting neurotransmitters that actually modify the sensitivity of the neurons. When an imbalance in this complex system occurs, depression can result.

One of the ways the pituitary gland controls the secretions of hormones in the body is by balancing thyroid and adrenal hormones. This balance is often poorly regulated in those with mood disorders. Serotonin, estrogen, and progesterone imbalances may help explain the fact that women are more than twice as likely to develop depression (Scott, 1998).

Investigators have also found that the biological rhythms of depressed persons differ from those of nondepressed persons. Depression is also related to physical illness. Many individuals who are being treated for a physical condition show signs of depression. As research efforts continue, new information about the biology of mood disorders will be uncovered.

OTHER THEORIES

Psychoanalytical theories see mood disorders as anger turned inward. **Behaviorists** view depression as a group of learned responses, whereas **social theorists** consider depression the result of faulty social interactions. A holistic viewpoint is usually used by health care providers because it considers all areas (realms) of human functioning and provides a framework from which to work with the whole person.

Box 21-1 *Possible Causes of Mood Disorders*

- Genetic susceptibility
- Biochemical imbalances (neurotransmitters, hormones)
- Environmental and other stressors
- Childhood and adult experiences
- Social circumstances

Many social factors have an influence on the development of mood disorders. Family relationships are important. Adults who were not nurtured as children are at higher risk for depression. Losses, role changes, and physical illnesses have an impact on the development of emotional problems. Poor social support, such as few friends and no significant others, heightens the loneliness of individuals, and repeated reactions to stress and crises wear down one's emotional resistance. Although the exact cause of depression and other mood disorders remains unclear, we do know that early recognition and treatment greatly improve the lives of people with severe and prolonged emotional problems.

EMOTIONS THROUGHOUT THE LIFE CYCLE

Because emotional responses are a realm of human functioning, they grow and develop as the individual does. When we are young, emotions are often experienced but seldom controlled. Emotional control is slowly gained as individuals test and learn about the appropriateness of their emotionally expressive behaviors. By adulthood, most societies expect people to control their emotions and express them in appropriate ways. (Review Box 15-2 for the characteristics of successful adults.)

EMOTIONS IN CHILDHOOD

When infants' basic needs are met, they feel a sense of contentment. Any delay in meeting those needs, however, is often announced by verbal expressions of frustration or even anger. Toddlers struggle to cope with many newly experienced emotions, such as fear, helplessness, and anxiety. Many of these feelings are acted out because young children are often unable to express themselves verbally. School-age children learn to identify, express, and control their emotions. The emotional intensity of adolescence offers new challenges for learning emotional control.

Most depressive responses in children are tied to a specific event or situation. This type of depression is called acute depression or **situational depression** because it can be traced to a recognizable cause. The depression is relieved once the stressors are removed or decreased. Situational depression occurs in all age-groups.

Children who are depressed have a distinct way of thinking. Depression involves feelings of hopelessness, low self-esteem, and a tendency to take the blame for every negative event (Hockenberry and others, 2007). They often respond with irritability, tearfulness, and sadness. Schoolwork and friendships suffer as increasing amounts of time are spent alone, especially watching television. Some children become clinging and dependent. Others engage in aggressive or disruptive behaviors. Many show changes in eating and sleeping behaviors. Fortunately, most acute episodes of childhood depression fade with family and social support.

During childhood, individuals begin to establish their self-esteem, coping mechanisms, and problem-solving abilities. If they have been successful in developing these skills, they are well prepared to handle the emotional distresses of later life. If self-esteem fails to grow or coping mechanisms and problem-solving abilities fail to develop, a mood disorder or other mental health problem may arise. The incidence of depression in childhood is increasing, and health care providers should include an assessment of mood for all young clients.

EMOTIONS IN ADOLESCENCE

During the teen years, individuals struggle to identify, gain control over, and express emotions. The moods of adolescents commonly swing from feeling vulnerable and dependent to knowing that they are the smartest one in the family. Most adolescents establish their personal and social identities without significant psychological problems or emotional disorders. However, a growing number of teens are showing evidence of depression.

Depression in adolescence is usually related to four factors: self-esteem, loneliness, family strengths, and parent-teen communications. Age and gender are lesser factors, but women with depression outnumber men by two to one. Many individuals tend to react with a sense of helplessness and feelings of depression when self-esteem is low. They perceive the world as bleak and themselves as small and insignificant. Feelings of a poor self-image feed other negative emotions, and a cycle of depression and low self-esteem is established. Grades drop as interest in school activities fades.

Loneliness is an aspect of depression in all age-groups, but especially in adolescence. People need other people. As loneliness increases, so does depression. The emotionally isolated teen may be surrounded by others yet still feel like an outcast.

Family relationships also have an influence on adolescent depression. Studies of mothers of depressed adolescents revealed that higher standards of achievement were expected, but the children were seldom rewarded. Often adolescents rebel against what they feel are impossible standards by withdrawing into depression.

Parent-adolescent communication patterns also have an impact on the teen's ability or willingness to

---

Box 21-2 *Adults at Risk for Depression*

- Women
- People between the ages of 35 and 44 years
- Whites and Hispanics
- Individuals with fewer than 12 years of school
- People who live in major urban areas
- People with physical illnesses
- Recently widowed older adults
- People who live in the western region of the United States

Data from Keltner NL, Schwecke LH, Bostrom CE: *Psychiatric nursing*, ed 5, St. Louis, 2007, Mosby.

---

discuss problems. Teens who can discuss their concerns with understanding parents have lower rates of depression.

The occurrence of depression and other mood disorders in adolescence reaches across gender and cultural lines. Teen depression must be recognized as serious. Depressions arising during adolescence tend to last, have a high rate of recurrence, and are associated with long-standing interpersonal problems. Teaching adolescents to cope effectively is essential if we are to protect the mental health of our greatest "natural resource," our children.

EMOTIONS IN ADULTHOOD

During adulthood, society expects people to practice emotional control. Unfortunately, many adults have difficulties with emotional control, and mood disorders are among the most common serious mental health problems today (Box 21-2).

Adults must cope with a wide range of situations, events, developmental tasks, and responsibilities, as well as the emotional reactions that accompany each. Family interactions have a strong influence on adults. Many are also challenged with the problems of physical illness or dysfunction. Sometimes the practice of certain behaviors, such as drug use, dieting, or refusal to seek help for distressing symptoms, can result in the development of a mood disorder. Unfortunately, the public (and clients themselves) stigmatize people with mood disorders. Mood disorders are seen as being caused by a lack of willpower or a character flaw. Thus adults with depression or bipolar disorder must endure the additional burden of being stereotyped as "mentally ill." Being sensitive to this issue assists health care providers in providing support for adults with emotional difficulties.

EMOTIONS IN OLDER ADULTHOOD

Depression is very common in elderly people. Major depression affects as many as 40% of older Americans. The highest rates are found in elderly women, medically ill persons, and individuals who receive long-term care.

Depression is not a normal consequence of aging. Most older adults live full, active, and rewarding lives.

When depression or another mood disturbance occurs suddenly in an older adult, it is most likely linked to a physical cause. Depression can be treated, but a failure to recognize its symptoms prevents many elders from receiving therapy.

Older adults often express their feelings of depression in more subtle ways than younger persons do. Most do not complain or volunteer to share their feelings. Signals of depression in the elderly population include changes in daily routine, eating, sleeping, or activity patterns; decreased concentration, communications, and motivation; feelings of envy, failure, indecision, guilt, and hopelessness; loss of interest, self-confidence, and self-esteem; and worry or talk about death. Active listening, gentle questioning, and alert assessments help nurses detect signs of depression.

CHARACTERISTICS OF MOOD DISORDERS

Affect is the outward expression of one's emotions. Affects can be described as blunted (restricted), flat, inappropriate, and labile (rapidly changing). A **mood disorder** is defined as a disturbance in the emotional dimension of human functioning. Mood disorders have also been called **affective disorders.** Problems with emotions occur when one is extremely happy or sad. We all experience emotional extremes; but when feelings interfere with effective living, they become maladaptive.

Problems with emotions range from mania to depression. **Mania** refers to an emotional state in which a person has an elevated, expansive, and irritable mood accompanied by a loss of identity, increased activity, and grandiose thoughts and actions. **Depression,** the opposite of mania, is characterized by feelings of sadness, disappointment, and despair. It is an illness that affects more than 10% of the adult population. More than 20 million people in the United States will suffer from a depressive illness each year (National Institute of Mental Health [NIJMH], 2004). Depression occurs in all races, ethnic groups, age-groups, and socioeconomic levels. It affects twice as many women as men. It is easy to see that emotional problems are a large part of the distresses experienced by people.

MOOD DISORDERS

According to the *Diagnostic and Statistical Manual of Mental Disorders* (DSM-IV-TR), mood disorders are divided into two basic categories: depression and mania (Figure 21-2). Depression is further classified into depressive episodes and depressive disorders, based on time and recurring behavior patterns. Mania is seen in bipolar disorders, which are divided into bipolar I, bipolar II, and cyclothymic disorders.

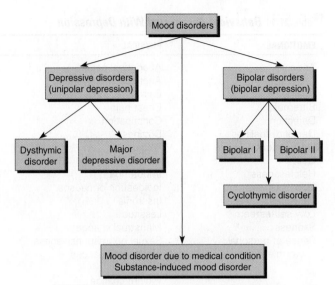

FIGURE **21-2** Classification of mood disorders.

Depression is a "whole body" illness that involves emotional, physical, intellectual, social, and spiritual problems. It can be transitory (lasting only a few days), or it can plague an individual for many years. It is one of the most common and treatable mental disorders (Isaacs, 1998).

Table 21-1 lists many of the behaviors associated with depression. Study it carefully. A client's nonverbal messages may be the only clues to the presence of this disabling mood disorder.

Depression can occur on several levels. Mild depression is short-lived and usually triggered by life events or situations outside the individual. For example, mild depression is common after suffering an important loss. With mild depression, individuals frequently complain of feeling lost, let down, or disappointed. Drug or alcohol use may increase during this time. Mild depression is usually self-limiting and subsides as interest in life returns to normal.

In contrast, moderate depression (**dysthymia**) persists over time. Feelings of depression begin to seriously interfere with activities of living because individuals lack the energy to make it through the day. Physically, they are fatigued (anergia) and drag themselves around. Eating and sleeping difficulties and changes in sexual functioning and menstrual cycles begin to surface (Perry, 1999). Emotionally, these individuals are also drained of energy. They feel despondent, dejected, gloomy, and unable to find joy in life (anhedonia). Feelings of helplessness, low self-esteem, ineffectiveness, and worthlessness reinforce their negative outlooks. Judgment and decision making are clouded by gloom. With moderate depression, intellectual efforts are focused on proving how really bad they are. Slowed thoughts and impaired concentration add to the picture of ineptness. Problem-solving skills fail, hopelessness sets in, and escape from emotional turmoil seems impossible. Persons with moderate levels of depression

Table 21-1 *Behaviors Associated With Depression*

EMOTIONAL	PHYSICAL	INTELLECTUAL	BEHAVIORAL
Anger	Abdominal pain	Ambivalence	Aggressiveness
Anxiety	Anorexia or overeating	Confusion	Agitation
Apathy	Backache	Inability to concentrate	Alcoholism
Bitterness	Chest pain	Indecisiveness	Altered activity level
Dejection	Constipation	Loss of interest and motivation	Drug addiction
Denial of feelings	Dizziness	Pessimism	Intolerance
Despondency	Fatigue	Self-blame	Irritability
Guilt	Headache	Self-depreciation	Lack of spontaneity
Helplessness	Impotence	Self-destructive thoughts	Overdependency
Hopelessness	Indigestion or nausea	Uncertainty	Poor personal hygiene
Loneliness	Insomnia		Psychomotor retardation
Low self-esteem	Lassitude		Social isolation
Sadness	Menstrual changes		Tearfulness
Sense of personal	Sexual nonresponsiveness		Underachievement
worthlessness	Sleep disturbances		Withdrawal
	Vomiting		
	Weight change		

Modified from Stuart GW, Laraia MT: *Principles and practice of psychiatric nursing*, ed 8, St. Louis, 2005, Mosby.

are at higher risk for suicide as their depression increases.

MAJOR DEPRESSIVE EPISODE

When depression is severe and lasts more than 2 weeks, it is called a major depressive episode. Severe depression encompasses one's whole being—every realm of human functioning. "The zest for life has vanished. It left without notice. Hours, days drag into weeks, months, even years. The simplest tasks loom over us like impossible demands. Energy is gone. Hope and joy are only meaningless words. Truly, darkness rules" (National Depressive and Manic-Depressive Association, 2007).

Behaviors associated with severe depression range from paralysis to agitation. Feelings of worthlessness, guilt, and despair are expressed in every thought, every movement, and every activity. Physical appearance declines. Eating and sleeping become distasteful chores. Poor concentration and an inability to follow through on tasks lead to feelings of powerlessness and helplessness. Suicidal thoughts are entertained. Frequently, suicide is seen as the only way to cope with the misery. Individuals suffering a major depressive episode drag through each day, unable to function, caring about nothing, and interested only in their suffering. As truly distressed human beings, they are caught in a downward emotional cycle.

Major depressive episodes can occur in response to situations, events, and developmental tasks. They are frequently seen in combination with other mental health problems.

MAJOR DEPRESSIVE DISORDER

When major depressive episodes routinely repeat themselves (for more than 2 years), a **depressive disorder** is diagnosed. Persons with major depressive

disorders have a high mortality rate. "Up to 15% of individuals with severe major depressive disorder die by suicide. Statistical evidence also suggests that there is a fourfold increase in death rates in individuals with major depressive disorder who are over age 55 years" (American Psychiatric Association, 2000). Major depressive disorder occurs twice as often in adolescent girls and adult women as in men. Symptoms may begin at any age, but the average age of symptom onset is in the early 20s. The course of the disorder is variable. Some individuals experience depressive episodes separated by many years, whereas others suffer more frequent episodes as they grow older. Families with one depressed member are at an increased risk for other members developing the disorder. Some families appear to be genetically vulnerable to depression.

Severe, prolonged depression results in many physical changes and increases one's risk for illness. Studies have demonstrated an association between depression and low immune system functions. Researchers who observe depressed individuals over time have found that depressed persons face more physical and mental impairments than individuals with chronic illnesses. Major depressive disorders are truly debilitating.

DYSTHYMIC DISORDER

A dysthymic disorder is daily moderate depression that lasts for more than 2 years. People with dysthymic disorder are chronically sad and self-critical. They see themselves as incapable and uninteresting. They experience many symptoms of moderate depression, such as low energy levels, poor decision-making skills, and eating or sleeping difficulties. Because the feelings of depression have lasted so long, they become a part of everyday experiences. Individuals with dysthymia have learned to see the world from a negative point of view and will often tell you that they have always

Table 21-2 | *Levels of Manic Behavior*

LEVEL OF MANIA	DESCRIPTION OF BEHAVIORS
Hypomania	Outgoing, happy-go-lucky, free of worry; catchy euphoria (observers feel euphoric), confident, uninhibited; unconcerned about feelings of others; increased motor activity, sexual drives, distractibility, sense of importance; decreased ability to concentrate; moves quickly from one topic to another (flight of ideas); becomes easily irritated
Mania	"High," expansive, unstable affect; angers quickly; pressured speech, flight of ideas, delusions of persecution and grandiosity; dresses inappropriately (layers of clothing, bizarre outfits, excessive makeup and jewelry); inappropriate behaviors (meddles in others' affairs, spends money recklessly, engages in risky activities); sexually driven; little food or sleep but still hyperactive
Delirium	Period of extreme excitement, anger, elation; has grandiose or religious delusions; becomes disoriented, incoherent, agitated; may injure self or others; poor hygiene, disheveled, physically drained; death from exhaustion may occur if mania goes untreated

been this way. During periods of intense stress, these persons may experience major depressive episodes in addition to their existing dysthymia.

Dysthymic disorders can begin in childhood or as late as early adulthood. Because they develop slowly, dysthymic disorders are often difficult to recognize and diagnose. Persons with dysthymia can often carry out their daily living activities, but they are seldom able to enjoy them.

BIPOLAR DISORDERS

The hallmark of a **bipolar disorder** is sudden and dramatic shifts in emotional extremes. Persons with bipolar disorders live in a world that seesaws between the emotional extremes of mania and depression. Thoughts, moods, and behaviors swing from normal to grandiose to depressed. A return to normal functioning follows (the "in-between time"), and then the cycle begins again. Time intervals between manic episodes vary. Individuals who cycle rapidly have a poorer prognosis.

Mania is defined as "an abnormally and persistently elevated, expansive, or irritable mood" (American Psychiatric Association, 2001). During periods of mania, behaviors build in intensity as the individual moves through three stages (Table 21-2). **Hypomania**, an exaggerated sense of cheerfulness, begins the cycle. Soon cheerfulness progresses to the unstable "high" of mania. If allowed to continue, delirium and death from exhaustion may result.

During the manic phase, behaviors become more and more impaired. If not treated, the manic phase of bipolar illness can last as long as 3 months. Eventually the depressive phase begins again. Hospitalization is often required to break the cycle of mania and to protect the person from the negative consequences of poor judgments and actions. An episode of mania is presented in Case Study 21-1.

Bipolar disorders (also called **manic depression**) exist in two forms. Bipolar I disorder is characterized by episodes of depression alternating with episodes of mania. It is the more severe and incapacitating form of bipolar illness. Delusions are common during periods of mania. Hallucinations can occur.

 Case Study 21-1

Kevin felt extraordinarily good—full of confidence and vigor. He even convinced himself that this would be his lucky day. By the time he started dressing, he had already decided to "skip" work. He was going to the casino because he could do no wrong today. Too impatient to eat or finish dressing, he bolted from the house and jogged the 4 miles to the casino.

By noon, Kevin had lost his pocket money and had consumed four scotch and sodas. He became angry with the cashier when she refused to cash a check without identification. "She should certainly know who I am. Why should I need identification? Everyone in town knows who I am! How dare they demand to see my identification!" Kevin shouted as he paced agitatedly.

After being forcibly removed from the casino, Kevin began a tour of every business in town. He demanded to see the owners and then offered them a contract to share a portion of his winnings if they financed his gambling now. By the time he visited the fourth establishment, the police were waiting.

Kevin made his offer to both police officers and was promptly admitted to the local hospital for mental health care. After 3 days of hospitalization, Kevin traded his extraordinarily good feelings for depressive ones.

• What clues (signs or symptoms) in Kevin's behavior indicate that he was in the manic phase of bipolar illness?

Individuals with bipolar II disorder experience major episodes of depression alternating with periods of hypomania. Bipolar II disorder often results in 1 to 2 weeks of severe lethargy, withdrawal, and melancholy. This is followed by several days of elevated or irritable mood, constant activity, and risky decision making. Although the depths of depression and mania may not be as severe as with bipolar I disorder, the effects are just as devastating.

CYCLOTHYMIC DISORDER

The extreme emotional swings of bipolar disorders are less intense in persons with cyclothymic problems. As the name implies, a **cyclothymic disorder** is a pattern that involves repeated mood swings alternating between hypomania and depressive symptoms. With cyclothymia, there are no periods of "normal" functioning. No day is free of symptoms because individuals bounce from "too high" to "too low." Many persons with cyclothymic problems eventually progress to full-blown (clinically definable) bipolar disorders.

OTHER PROBLEMS WITH AFFECT

Many other emotional problems exist in society today. Seasonal affective disorder (also known as winter depression) occurs in many people from October to April. Levels of mild and moderate depression are experienced during long winter days. Symptoms begin to lift with the coming of spring. Daily exposure to full-spectrum light **(phototherapy)** lessens the symptoms of sadness and social withdrawal in persons with seasonal affective disorder.

Phototherapy or light therapy has also been found to be useful in treating women with late luteal phase dysphoric disorder—the depression associated with the onset of menses. Every month, these women experience the melancholy and sadness of depression. In these cases the cause, however, lies within the rhythms of their hormone cycles.

A connection between hormonal balance and emotions is implicated in postpartum depression. Tearfulness, irritability, hypochondria, sleeplessness, impairment of concentration, and headache in the days and weeks following childbirth are characteristic (Perry, 1999). Mild postpartum depression often clears within days, but symptoms lasting longer than 2 weeks should be investigated. Women at higher risk for postpartum depression include those who have experienced complicated pregnancies or difficult deliveries. Women who are not emotionally prepared for motherhood are also at greater risk.

A substance-induced mood disorder is defined as a persistent emotional disturbance that can be directly traced to the physiological effects of a chemical. Many illegal chemicals (street drugs), such as amphetamines, cocaine, marijuana, and heroin, as well as alcohol, bring about changes in mood. In addition, many therapeutic medications are related to the development of mood disorders. Drug Alert 21-1 lists several common medications that have depressive effects.

MEDICAL PROBLEMS AND MOOD DISORDERS

Depression is a common condition among hospitalized persons. Most physically ill people are depressed to some degree. Because the whole person is involved, a physical illness always has emotional consequences. Many physical problems and medical conditions are associated with mood disorders. It is common for people to feel depressed when ill or feeling poorly. Depression is a response to chronic illness or lingering disability as

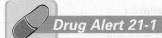
Drug Alert 21-1

Medications That May Be Linked to Depression

Analgesics (for treating pain)
Antibiotics (for treating infections)
Anticonvulsants (for treating seizures)
Antihypertensives (for treating high blood pressure)
Antiinflammatory agents (for treating swelling and inflammation)
Antineoplastic agents (for treating cancer)
Antiparkinsonian agents (for treating Parkinson's disease)
Antituberculosis agents (for treating tuberculosis [TB])
Cardiovascular agents (for treating heart problems)
Central nervous system agents (for treating obesity, eating disorders, sleeping disorders, and various mental health problems)

people anticipate their losses and lifestyle changes. Because it is often encountered within health care settings, an important responsibility of each health care provider is to assess for signs and symptoms of mood disorders in every client, from the youngest to the oldest.

THERAPEUTIC INTERVENTIONS

Mood disorders present many treatment challenges. Perhaps the greatest challenge is that fewer than one half of the people with mood disorders receive help. Feelings of hopelessness and the stigma of having a mental illness prevent many people from seeking treatment. Others are misdiagnosed or treated for a medical illness because their symptoms are mainly physical. Men are less likely to receive treatment because they often hide their emotions behind alcohol, drugs, or aggression. Depression responds well to treatment, especially if begun early. Serious disturbances of severe depression and bipolar disorders, however, may involve years of therapy.

TREATMENT AND THERAPY

The therapeutic plan for clients with mood disorders is divided into three phases. The **acute treatment phase** lasts 6 to 12 weeks. The goal during this phase is to reduce symptoms and inappropriate behaviors. Inpatient hospitalization may be required when clients are too impaired to continue with the activities of daily living or too suicidal to be left alone.

The goal of the **continuation phase** is to prevent relapses into distressing emotional states. This period usually lasts 4 to 9 months and is done on an outpatient basis. Medications and psychotherapy are continued. Clients are educated about the nature of their conditions and their medications and encouraged to try new coping behaviors.

Table 21-3 | *Phases of Treatment for Depression*

PHASE	TIME PERIOD	GOAL OF TREATMENT
Acute treatment	6-12 wk	To reduce symptoms and inappropriate behaviors
Continuation	4-9 mo	To prevent relapses into distressing emotional states
Maintenance	Indefinite	To prevent recurrences

The **maintenance treatment phase** concentrates on preventing recurrences in clients with prior episodes of depression or mania. Maintenance psychotherapy and medications help prevent new episodes or recurrences (Table 21-3).

Current standard treatments for mood disorders include psychotherapy, pharmacological therapy, and electroconvulsive therapy. During each phase of treatment, nurses and other health care providers play important roles because they are the ones who help teach, encourage, and guide clients toward living effectively with their disorders.

Psychotherapies

Various psychotherapies are effective in treating mild and moderate depression. Cognitive-behavioral therapy is used to help clients identify and correct self-defeating thoughts and actions that keep self-esteem low. Interpersonal therapy assists clients with relationships and interactions, and psychodynamic therapy encourages the growth of personal insight. Support groups and organizations are also very helpful for clients and families coping with mood disorders.

Electroconvulsive Therapy

Electroconvulsive therapy (ECT) is the introduction of a controlled grand mal seizure by passing an electrical current through the brain. ECT appears to work by raising the levels of the neurotransmitter norepinephrine, which are low in many people with depression. ECT is used only after attempts to stabilize the depression with various medications have failed.

Each ECT treatment requires about 15 minutes, but the actual shock lasts for only a few seconds. Generally, 6 to 12 treatments are administered over a course of several weeks, and most individuals receive ECT two or three times per week.

ECT is not prescribed for clients with a recent myocardial infarction (MI) (heart attack), heart disease, high or low blood pressure, stroke, or congestive heart failure. The treatment slows heart rate and lowers blood pressure. This is followed by a reflex rise in heart rate and blood pressure. It is contraindicated in people with increased intracranial pressure and tumors of the nervous system. Each client is evaluated for ECT on an individual basis, and the benefits must outweigh the risks before treatment is prescribed.

ECT may be administered on an outpatient or inpatient basis. The preparation of the client includes physical and emotional care, as well as education about the expected side effects of ECT. Consent forms are signed, and the client is reminded that confusion and memory loss are common after treatment. Outpatient clients must be accompanied by someone to care for them following treatment.

Clients must eat nothing by mouth for at least 8 hours before treatment. Baseline vital signs are obtained. The client is then attached to cardiac, blood pressure, and oxygen monitors. Short-acting muscle relaxants, sedatives, and an anesthetic agent are administered intravenously.

Electroencephalogram (EEG) monitors and electrodes are positioned at certain points on the head by the physician. An airway is established, and an electrical shock, resulting in a controlled seizure of about 30 to 60 seconds, is delivered. Often the only evidence of a seizure is a flexing of the client's big toes. Brain waves are monitored throughout the procedure, and the client sleeps for about 1 hour following the treatment.

Common side effects of ECT include headache, confusion on awakening from the treatment, and short-term amnesia, but the client's mood improves rapidly. Many individuals can be managed on an outpatient basis with good postprocedure nursing management and appropriate client teaching. The responsibilities of the nurse when working with clients undergoing ECT include initiating intravenous therapy, administering ordered medications, and monitoring the client's responses before, during, and after treatment.

DRUG THERAPIES

Medications are a mainstay in the treatment of mood disorders. However, their use must be carefully assessed, monitored, and evaluated because of side effects and drug misuse. The most commonly used drugs for treating mood disorders are antidepressants and mood-stabilizing drugs known as antimanics. All work to increase neurotransmitter levels in the body, which leads to improvement of depression.

Antidepressants

Based on their chemical composition, antidepressants are divided into the following groups: tricyclics, nontricyclics, monoamine oxidase inhibitors (MAOIs), selective serotonin reuptake inhibitors (SSRIs), and atypical antidepressants. Each alters a part of the brain's neurochemical balance.

Many antidepressants require 2 to 4 weeks before their effects are noted and the client's well-being improves. For this reason, some clients believe that antidepressants are ineffective. They require education and reminders that these drugs require time to take effect and encouragement to continue taking their medications.

Tricyclic antidepressants were once the first choice for the treatment of depression The SSRIs are now more often prescribed because of their low incidence of side effects. Last choice for use is the MAOIs because of their severe and potentially fatal side effects. New antidepressants that are chemically unrelated to the other classes have been introduced into the market. Nurses who administer these chemicals are responsible for maintaining current knowledge about their uses and effects.

Tricyclic antidepressants can produce severe central nervous system (CNS) depression when they interact with barbiturates, certain anticonvulsants, drugs, and alcohol. SSRIs act specifically to prevent the uptake of the neurochemical serotonin. They have fewer side effects than the tricyclics. Headache, nausea, nervousness, and insomnia are the most common side effects.

When MAOI antidepressants are combined with certain substances and foods containing the enzyme tyramine, the nervous system can become overexcited. This can lead to severely elevated blood pressure levels and hypertensive crisis. Refer back to Chapter 7 for a review of antidepressants, diet restrictions, and education for clients receiving MAOIs. Profound CNS depression or severe anticholinergic effects can occur.

Elderly male clients receiving antidepressants should be observed for urinary retention, which can develop quickly. Side effects, such as blurred vision and dry mouth, can cause problems with compliance because individuals stop taking their medications as a result of these bothersome effects. Atypical and other antidepressants achieve the same effect using different mechanisms of action. Box 21-3 lists various antidepressant and mood-stabilizing drugs.

Basically antidepressants exert their unwelcome side effects on both the central and peripheral nervous systems. Therapeutic interventions are often needed to help clients adjust to their medications. Table 21-4 lists common side effects and related nursing care.

Because antidepressants may alter liver and kidney functions, hepatic and renal studies should be obtained monthly. Nurses should review all laboratory results for each client. Often blood levels of certain drugs are measured to determine the amount of drug still in the system. Toxic antidepressant levels can result if clients are not carefully monitored. Headaches, palpitations, changes in levels of consciousness, and stiffness in the neck should be reported to the physician immediately because they are signs of serious side effects.

Antimanics

Lithium is a naturally occurring salt that helps to control the exaggerated thoughts and behaviors associated with mania. Because lithium does not bind to body proteins (as do many other drugs), it does not need to be metabolized by the liver. Lithium is distributed

---

| Box 21-3 | *Antidepressants and Mood-Stabilizing Drugs* |

TRICYCLIC ANTIDEPRESSANTS

amitriptyline (Elavil)	clomipramine (Anafranil)
doxepin (Adepin, Sinequan)	imipramine (Tofranil)
trimipramine (Surmontil)	desipramine (Norpramin)
nortriptyline (Pamelor)	protriptyline (Vivactil)

MONOAMINE OXIDASE INHIBITORS (MAOIs)

isocarboxazid (Marplan)	phenelzine (Nardil)
tranylcypromine (Parnate)	

SELECTIVE SEROTONIN REUPTAKE INHIBITORS (SSRIs)

fluoxetine (Prozac)	fluvoxamine (Luvox)
paroxetine (Paxil)	sertraline (Zoloft)

OTHER ANTIDEPRESSANTS

amoxapine (Asendin)	bupropion (Wellbutrin)
trazodone (Desyrel)	venlafaxine (Effexor)

MOOD-STABILIZING DRUGS

lithium (Lithobid, Lithonate)	divalproex (Depakote)
carbamazepine (Tegretol)	olanzapine (Zyprexa)
clonazepam (Klonopin)	

From Stuart GW, Laraia MT: *Principles and practice of psychiatric nursing,* ed 8, St. Louis, 2005, Mosby.

---

throughout the body fluids, where it competes with sodium. It is excreted by the kidneys more rapidly than sodium. Therefore an important interaction between the level of lithium in the blood and common table salt exists.

When clients who are taking lithium ingest large amounts of salt, lithium levels usually drop because of rapid kidney excretion of lithium. The opposite is also true. When clients decrease their salt intake or lose salt through sweating, diarrhea, or altered kidney function, lithium levels in the blood are likely to increase. Because the range between therapeutic response and toxic effects is very narrow, clients must be instructed to avoid changing their diet or activity habits abruptly.

The narrow therapeutic index of lithium requires close observation of client responses. If blood levels of the drug are too low, manic behavior returns; if levels are too high, an uncomfortable and possibly life-threatening toxicity may result.

Most side effects of lithium are directly related to dosage and blood serum levels (Table 21-5). Polyuria (large urinary output) and polydipsia (increased thirst) are frequently seen in people beginning lithium therapy. Unwanted gastrointestinal tract reactions include a metallic taste, dry mouth, thirst, nausea, diarrhea, a bloated feeling, and weight gain. Sleepiness, light-headedness, drowsiness, and a mild hand tremor are common during the first weeks of therapy.

Because the signs and symptoms of lithium toxicity are the same as the side effects during the first weeks of therapy, all caregivers should be aware of clients' responses to their lithium therapy. Most side effects disappear or decrease to a tolerable level by the sixth

Table 21-4 | Side Effects of Antidepressants and Nursing Care

SIDE EFFECTS	NURSING CARE
TRICYCLIC ANTIDEPRESSANTS	
Fatigue, sedation, slow psychomotor reactions, poor concentration, tremors, ataxia	Give at bedtime; increase dose slowly; teach caution when using machinery; write instructions; document behaviors.
Suicidal gestures	Institute suicide precautions; drug increases energy for suicide.
Anticholinergic effects: dry mouth, decreased tearing, blurred vision (common)	Encourage frequent oral care, water, gum; use artificial tears; ensure that vision clears in 2 wk; report eye pain immediately.
Constipation, urinary hesitancy or retention, excessive sweating	Monitor food and fluid intake; promote high-fiber diet (more than 30 mg/day); encourage water intake of at least 2500 ml/day; teach importance of adequate fluids, clothing, and sensible exercise; avoid hot showers, baths, dehydration; monitor urinary output, especially in older men.
NONTRICYCLIC ANTIDEPRESSANTS	
Dizziness, drowsiness, anxiety, confusion, tremors, weakness, dry mouth, nausea, diarrhea, increased appetite, paralytic ileus, urinary retention	Ensure safety; monitor mental status, moods, affect, level of consciousness, increased symptoms; weigh weekly; monitor for weight gain; encourage fluids to 2500 ml/day; monitor intake and output.
Orthostatic hypotension, tachycardia, palpitations	Teach client to rise slowly; monitor and report vital signs.
MONOAMINE OXIDASE INHIBITORS (MAOIs)	
Increased CNS stimulation	Reassure client; monitor for psychosis, seizures, hypoactivity.
Postural hypotension	Teach client to rise slowly; assure client that symptoms will decrease.
Muscle twitching	Vitamin B$_6$ (300 mg/day) is helpful.
Fluid retention, urinary hesitancy	Monitor intake and output; administer thiazide diuretics as ordered.
Insomnia	Give last dose as early as possible; encourage relaxation in evening.
Food-drug interaction with tyramine (common amino acid)	Avoid tyramine-rich foods; avoid drugs with epinephrine or stimulants.
SELECTIVE SEROTONIN REUPTAKE INHIBITORS (SSRIs)	
Dry mouth	Encourage fluids, good oral care.
Nausea, diarrhea	Give drug with meals; maintain bland diet; encourage good hydration; administer lower dose.
Drowsiness, dizziness, nervousness	Give at bedtime; keep active during day; institute safety precautions; instruct client to avoid machinery.
Sweating	Maintain good hygiene; wear cotton clothing; encourage fluids.
Headaches	Teach relaxation techniques; administer mild analgesic for headache.
Insomnia	Give medications early; encourage good sleep habits and relaxation.
NONSELECTIVE REUPTAKE INHIBITORS (VENLAFAXINE)	
Increased blood pressure	Monitor vital signs; report to physician if blood pressure stays high; may reduce dose.
Weakness, sweating, sleepiness, dry mouth, nausea, vomiting, constipation, anorexia, blurred vision, anxiety, tremors	Refer to nursing care for other drug classes of antidepressants.

CNS, Central nervous system.

Table 21-5 | Side Effects of Lithium and Nursing Care

SIDE EFFECTS	NURSING CARE
Abdominal discomfort, nausea, soft stools, diarrhea	Give lithium with food or milk; reassure that signs and symptoms are temporary and should subside.
Edema, especially feet	Reassure that signs and symptoms are temporary; check with physician about salt restriction.
Hair loss, hypothyroidism	Obtain thyroid function tests; reassure that condition is temporary; if continues, notify physician, who may discontinue drug.
Muscle weakness, fatigue	Provide reassurance; give more frequent divided doses per physician order.
Polyuria (can progress to diabetes insipidus)	Provide reassurance; increased output is expected; monitor intake and output; report if output greater than 3000 ml/24 hr.
Thirst	Encourage client to quench thirst but maintain stable fluid intake.
Tremors	Provide reassurance; eliminate caffeine; give slow-release form per physician order.
Weight gain	Provide reassurance that weight gain is common; moderately restrict calories; advise client against restricting fluids or salt.

week of treatment. If they continue, be alert for the possibility of early lithium toxicity.

Blood tests for thyroid and kidney function, in addition to lithium levels, are routinely performed. Therapeutic blood levels of lithium range from 0.6 to 1.2 mEq/L. Toxic reactions occur when lithium levels in the blood are greater than 1.5 mEq/L. Lithium toxicity can be life threatening, and no specific antidote exists. Because of this, one of the nurse's most important responsibilities is to frequently assess each client's response during treatment and monitor for signs and symptoms of toxicity. See Table 21-6 and review Chapter 7 for more information about client care and education. Study the procedure for a prelithium workup. Be alert to the special educational needs of clients who require lithium.

Once the client is no longer manic, the need for lithium drops dramatically. Toxicity may set in rapidly unless the dose is reduced. Clients must be carefully monitored during the first weeks of lithium therapy. If little response is noted by the sixth week of treatment, the physician usually considers other mood-stabilizing drug therapies such as those listed in Box 21-3.

NURSING (THERAPEUTIC) PROCESS

Therapeutic care for clients with disturbances in mood includes the whole person. Clients are first assessed for level of depression or mania. Next, a thorough history and physical examination help to establish the database. Nursing diagnoses and therapeutic interventions are then chosen based on the client's most distressing problems (Box 21-4).

A holistic approach for clients with emotional problems is very effective. Therapeutic interventions for the **physical** realm focus on helping clients with personal hygiene, maintaining adequate nutrition, and encouraging physical activity. If clients are suicidal, special precautions and observations are implemented.

In the **emotional** realm, care revolves around the therapeutic relationship. Acceptance and support are powerful tools in this area. Once trust is established, clients need encouragement and emotional support to cope with their problems.

Extreme emotional responses alter one's ability to think logically long enough to complete a task. In the **intellectual** realm of care, care providers should remember that these clients need extra patience. Use gentle, nonjudgmental guidance when they are attempting to follow through on tasks. Give instructions slowly and clearly. Repeat them as needed, and do not become impatient. Remember, it is difficult to cope when one cannot think straight.

Socially, most individuals with mood disorders are lonely and afraid of associating with others. Once medications have begun to stabilize the client's moods, gentle encouragement to begin interacting with others is often needed.

Mood disorders involve the **spiritual** realm too. Many individuals with depression often question their spiritual

---

Box 21-4 *NANDA-I Nursing Diagnoses Related to Emotional Responses*

Anxiety	Powerlessness*
Communication, impaired verbal	Self-care deficit, bathing/hygiene, dressing/grooming, feeding, toileting
Coping, community	
Coping, ineffective individual	
Grieving	Self-esteem disturbance, low, situational/chronic
Grieving, complicated*	Sexual dysfunction
Hopelessness*	Social isolation
Injury, risk for	Spiritual distress*
Insomnia	Thought processes, disturbed
Loneliness, risk for	
Nutrition, imbalanced, more/less than body requirements	Violence, risk for self-directed

Data from NANDA International: *NANDA-I nursing diagnoses: definitions and classification, 2007-2008,* Philadelphia, 2007, NANDA International. *NANDA-I,* NANDA International. *Primary nursing diagnoses for disturbances in mood.

Table 21-6 *Signs and Symptoms of Lithium Toxicity*

LEVEL OF TOXICITY	SIGNS AND SYMPTOMS
MILD TOXICITY Blood serum fluid levels 1.5 mEq/L	Apathy, sluggishness, drowsiness, and lethargy; diminished concentration; mild incoordination, muscle weakness, muscle twitches, coarse hand tremors
MODERATE TOXICITY Blood serum levels 1.5 to 2.5 mEq/L	Nausea, vomiting, severe diarrhea; slurred speech, blurred vision, ringing in the ears; apathy, drowsiness, lethargy, moderate sluggishness; muscle weakness, irregular tremors, ataxia, frank muscle twitching, increased tonicity
SEVERE TOXICITY Blood serum levels above 2.5 mEq/L	Nystagmus; irregular muscle tremors, fasciculations (twitches of single-muscle groups), hyperactive deep tendon reflexes; oliguria, decreased urine output, severe changes in level of consciousness, hallucinations; grand mal seizures, coma, death

beliefs. Manic clients commonly have delusions of **religiosity**, believing they have powers to communicate with God or become a spirit. Therapeutic listening is a helpful intervention, but do not hesitate to contact a cleric if the client so requests. Sample Client Care Plan 21-1 offers a plan for clients with a mood disorder. Remember, each actual plan will be unique according to the needs of the individual client.

Emotions, both positive and negative, add texture and meaning to the tapestry of our lives. We may not yet understand the exact connections between mind and body. We do know, however, that our emotions are determined in large part by the way we think, the way we perceive the world, and our "self-talk." So powerful is this optimistic or pessimistic view that it determines not only our emotions, but also the very

---

SAMPLE CLIENT CARE PLAN 21-1
Major Depressive Episode

ASSESSMENT *History.* Leanne is a 22-year-old woman with a diagnosis of major depressive episode following the loss of her infant son. Her childhood was uneventful except for a domineering father. She reports no abuse during childhood but admits to being intimidated by her father's loud voice and gruff manner.

During her first year in college, she met and married Mark, a senior majoring in marketing. The first 10 months of the marriage went well, until Leanne discovered she was pregnant. The news of her pregnancy infuriated Mark, who insisted that she "do something." Leanne insisted on keeping the baby but was plagued by the guilt of adding an extra burden to Mark's load throughout the pregnancy. On May 10, she delivered a son.

Leanne's postpartum course was difficult. She was trying to care for her son, attend school, and appease her husband who had become somewhat more interested in the baby. One morning she noticed that her son was too quiet. Attempts to revive him were unsuccessful, and the diagnosis of sudden infant death syndrome was made on autopsy. Three weeks later, Mark filed for divorce, stating that Leanne was not a "good mother."

Current Findings. A disheveled-appearing young woman with uncombed hair and wrinkled clothes. Speech is soft, almost inaudible. Does not maintain eye contact. Eyes red and swollen. Offers no information but when questioned admits to "being a complete failure" and "not worth the space I'm taking up." She describes her history as "filled with failures."

Multidisciplinary Diagnosis	*Planning/Goals*
Hopelessness related to loss of significant others as evidenced by an inability to perform activities of daily living.	Leanne will use two effective coping methods to counteract her feelings of hopelessness by November 29. Leanne will express three hopeful thoughts by December 15.

Therapeutic Interventions

Intervention	Rationale	Team Member
1. Assess risk for suicidal behaviors.	Suicide rates are high in depressed persons.	Nsg, All
2. Establish a no–self-harm contract with Leanne.	Demonstrates caring and helps prevent suicidal gestures.	Psy, Nsg
3. Assist with activities of daily living as needed.	Supports Leanne until she is able to care for herself.	Nsg
4. Monitor fluid and food intake.	Depressed persons often do not eat or drink.	Nsg, Diet
5. Use active listening to encourage her to identify and express feelings.	Gives her an opportunity to explore and vent her emotions realistically.	All
6. Assess progress through the grief reaction and offer appropriate support.	Unresolved grief can cause depression; Leanne may not have grieved for the loss of her child yet.	Psy, Nsg
7. Help her to focus on the positive aspects and support systems in her life.	When energies are positively focused, success is encouraged.	All

Evaluation

After 5 days on the unit, Leanne assumed self-care activities and appeared well groomed throughout the remainder of her stay. By December 1, Leanne was able to discuss her feelings with two staff members. On December 14, Leanne joined a support group for mothers who have lost children.

? CRITICAL THINKING QUESTIONS

1. What care provider behaviors can demonstrate to Leanne that she is not worthless?

2. How does the goal of "expressing hopeful thoughts" help Leanne cope with her current depression?

A complete client care plan includes several other diagnoses and interventions.
Nsg, Nursing staff; *Psy,* psychologist; *Diet,* dietitian.

condition of our physical and mental health. Stay healthy by thinking positively. You and your clients will both benefit.

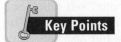

Key Points

- An emotion is a nonintellectual response in the affective realm of human functioning.
- A mood disorder is a disturbance in the emotional dimension of human functioning.
- Emotional responses grow and develop with the individual.
- Current evidence suggests that a combination of physical, psychological, and environmental factors is involved in the development of mood disorders.
- Depression is a "whole body" illness that involves emotional, physical, intellectual, social, and spiritual problems.
- Depression can be experienced as mild, moderate, or severe.
- When depression is severe and lasts more than 2 weeks, it is called a major depressive episode.
- When major depressive episodes routinely repeat themselves (for more than 2 years), a depressive disorder is diagnosed.
- A dysthymic disorder is daily moderate depression that lasts longer than 2 years.

- The hallmark of bipolar disorders is sudden and dramatic shifts in emotional extremes.
- Bipolar I disorder is characterized by episodes of depression alternating with episodes of mania.
- With bipolar II disorder, individuals experience major episodes of depression alternating with periods of hypomania.
- Other problems with depression include seasonal affective disorder, postpartum depression, and depression associated with menses, medical conditions, or substance use.
- The therapeutic plan for clients with mood disorders is arranged into three phases: acute treatment phase, continuation phase, and maintenance phase.
- Various psychotherapies are effective in treating mild and moderate depression.
- The most commonly used drug classes for treating mood disorders are antidepressants and mood-stabilizing drugs.
- Electroconvulsive therapy is used to relieve depression by inducing a controlled grand mal seizure by passing an electrical current through the brain.
- Therapeutic care for clients with disturbances in mood relates to each realm of functioning.

evolve Be sure to visit the companion Evolve site at http://evolve.elsevier.com/Morrison-Valfre/ for additional online resources.

22 Physical Problems, Psychological Sources

Objectives

Upon completion of this chapter, the student will be able to:

1. Explain the purpose of the physiological stress response.
2. Illustrate how stress can affect immune system functions.
3. Describe five physical responses related to the physiological stress response.
4. Examine three theories that explain the role of emotions in the development of illnesses.
5. Compare three culturally related somatization disorders.
6. Explain the differences between conversion disorders and somatization disorders.
7. Describe the most essential feature of hypochondriasis.
8. Compare the differences between hypochondriasis and malingering.
9. Plan three therapeutic goals when caring for clients with psychophysiological disorders.

Key Terms

body dysmorphic (dĭs-MŎR-fĭk) **disorder** (p. 244)
conversion disorder (p. 242)
factitious disorder (p. 241)
hypochondriasis (HĪ-pō-kŏn-DRĪ-ə-sĭs) (p. 243)
la belle indifference (lă BĔL ĭn-DĬF-ĕr-ĕnts) (p. 243)
malingering (p. 245)
physiological (FĬZ-ē-ō-LŎJ-ĭ-kəl) **stress response** (p. 238)
primary gain (p. 240)
psychophysical (SĪ-kō-FĬZ-ĭ-kəl) **disorders** (p. 239)
psychosomatic (SĪ-kō-sō-MĂT-ĭk) **illnesses** (p. 239)
secondary gains (p. 240)
somatization (SŌ-mə-tĭ-ZĀ-shən) (p. 240)
somatoform (sō-MĂT-ō-fŏrm) **disorder** (p. 240)

For centuries, humankind has questioned the interactions of mind and body and the roles emotions play in health. In ancient China, around the year 2000 BC, the emperor Huang Ti recorded his keen observations of the physical illnesses arising from emotional causes in his book titled *Classic of Internal Medicine*. Hippocrates instructed people to care for the spirit as well as the body. Throughout the Middle Ages, magical and symbolic thinking kept body and mind inseparably

linked. People whose behavior or physical appearance differed were condemned as witches and workers of the devil.

Toward the end of the nineteenth century, scientific advances were made in biology, chemistry, and microbiology that shifted the focus of research to the cause and treatment of physical disease. By the time Freud's theories were introduced, the study of human beings had evolved into two distinct divisions: the biological (physical) and all other aspects of functioning (psychological). Complex human beings were now officially categorized into convenient sections for study, discussion, research, and treatment.

Today, however, researchers and practitioners alike are remembering that no such divisions between the mind and body exist. Human beings are dynamic, complicated physical organisms that are affected by many nonphysical events. Each of us is a unique individual—a combination of genetics, culture, and experience. Each of us has psychological aspects to our being and our own way of coping with the stresses of life.

This chapter explores the connection between the physical and psychological aspects of people. It is an important chapter because clients with psychologically based physical problems are encountered in every practice setting. Health care providers who understand the role emotions play in the development of health problems are better able to assess client needs and plan more effective care.

ROLE OF EMOTIONS IN HEALTH

Health is a concept embodying the whole person. It is a state of well-being in which the psychological realm is in balance with the physical realm. It is a state of homeostasis. All animals, including humans, must live with and adapt to stress. The antelope on the African savanna must deal with the stress of becoming some carnivore's lunch every day of its life. To do this, the antelope is equipped with a delicate internal mechanism of neurochemicals, all wired to the appropriate organs. When the animal is stressed, a response is activated and the antelope can run faster, jump higher, and endure the chase longer. In short, animals have evolved a stress response mechanism that protects them during times of threat or illness. It is called the **fight-or-flight response,** and it is an essential part of every animal's survival mechanisms.

ANXIETY AND STRESS

Human beings are also equipped with a physiological stress response mechanism. This biochemical fight-or-flight system is a biological survival tool designed to provide the energy for fighting opponents or running to save one's skin. The physical stress response served early humans effectively. However, as people became civilized and adopted rules for behavior, fighting and running were replaced by more socially acceptable (but biochemically stifling) behaviors. Today the stressors of modern life are many, but outlets for the stress response are few.

In his book *Stress of Life,* Hans Selye "proposed that all humans show the same general bodily response to stress" (Craighead and Nemeroff, 2002). Selye studied the biochemical reactions of the stress response and their effects on various body systems; he called these reactions the **general adaptation syndrome.** Today it is known that stress activates primitive regions in the brain that also control eating, aggression, and immune responses. These responses to the stresses of modern life are biochemically identical to the responses that early humans experienced when fighting to stay alive. The problem today is that the fight-or-flight response occurs in non–life-threatening situations, stimulating the body for actions that never occur. The stress response mechanism can even work overtime when individuals are routinely exposed to stressors.

When an individual perceives stress, tension, or anxiety, the body initiates a cascade of biochemicals. The body's central command post, the hypothalamus, communicates to the pituitary gland, which in turn notifies the adrenal glands. The adrenal glands manufacture and release the body's four major stress hormones—dopamine, epinephrine, norepinephrine, and cortisol. Body functions are so responsive to these chemicals that even small changes in their levels can have a significant impact on one's state of health. Responses to stress exist along a continuum ranging from high-level adaptive responses to life-threatening disorders (Figure 22-1).

Scientific investigation is beginning to show that the immune system is affected by stress levels. Several studies have demonstrated that significant immune function and blood pressure changes occur in people who displayed hostile or negative behaviors during periods of conflict. One study revealed that married couples who frequently argued had less effective immune systems. Other studies have demonstrated the importance of a positive attitude in physical healing.

The psychological side of an individual has a strong impact on the ability to identify and successfully cope

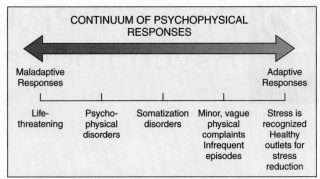

FIGURE **22-1** Continuum of psychophysical responses.

with stress. People who are able to recognize and defuse their stressors early seldom experience the physical effects of stress. Others struggle with stressors and the body's response to them. Some individuals focus their stress into body activities and functions, thus developing physical problems that arise from psychological sources. These problems are called **somatoform, psychosomatic,** or **psychophysical** disorders.

CHILDHOOD SOURCES

How an individual perceives and responds to stress is established in childhood (Figure 22-2). The link between mind and body is made early in infancy. Infants require the routine attentions of a consistent caregiver—someone who feeds, cuddles, and protects them. As children learn to cope with stresses, the brain becomes patterned. Biochemical reactions to stress alter the physical patterns of the brain and sensitize children to future stressors. This patterning sets up automatic chemical responses to stress. With each exposure to stress, the body responds with its biochemical program, even though the individual may not consciously feel stressed. Children who have experienced an unstable home environment, for example, may react to stress with exaggerated hormonal mechanisms as adults.

People experience stress related to their levels of development. In infancy, mechanisms for coping with stress are limited. The only means of expression is through the body, so infants create physical signs and symptoms to help cope with their stresses. Problems such as colic, atopic dermatitis, allergic reactions (Figure 22-3), and obesity may all arise from the effects of stress. Older children can express their stresses by developing allergic skin reactions, asthma, gastrointestinal tract complaints, or joint aches and pains.

Families who emotionally support and encourage their children to effectively cope with their stresses have few physical complaints. Families filled with conflict and uncertainty often live with numerous physical problems, as well as psychological distresses. Most psychosomatic problems and somatoform disorders (physical problems with emotional sources) start in childhood and become established during adolescence.

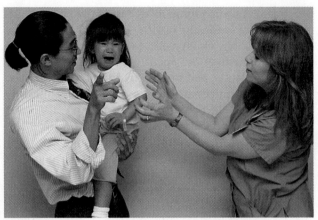

FIGURE **22-2** The stress response is established early in childhood.

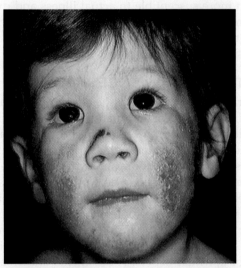

FIGURE **22-3** Infantile atopic dermatitis, which can be a manifestation of stress.

By adulthood, individuals can be significantly impaired in their daily living activities because of their reactions to stress.

COMMON PSYCHOPHYSICAL PROBLEMS

The physical signs and symptoms of emotional distress are very real to the individual who is experiencing them. The discomfort of an upset stomach is the same, whether caused by too much pizza or a disturbing piece of news. The effects of emotionally caused illnesses are the same as those arising from physical sources.

When the body is under continual or repeated stress, it responds by overactivating its stress response mechanism, which can result in many physical signs and symptoms of an illness, disease, or disability. (Refer to the stress adaptation theory in Chapter 5.) In the past, these symptoms were often referred to as psychosomatic illnesses, meaning emotionally (psycho) related physical (somatic) disorders. Unfortunately, this term has come to mean an imaginary illness in popular

---

Box 22-1 *Physical Conditions Affected by Psychobiological Factors*

CARDIOVASCULAR	SKIN
Migraine headaches	Neurodermatitis
Tension headaches	Eczema
Hypertension (high blood pressure)	Psoriasis
	Pruritus (itching)
Angina (chest pain)	
	GENITOURINARY
MUSCULOSKELETAL	Impotence
Rheumatoid arthritis	Frigidity
Low back pain	Premenstrual syndrome
RESPIRATORY	**ENDOCRINE SYSTEM**
Hyperventilation	Hyperthyroidism
Asthma	Diabetes
GASTROINTESTINAL	
Anorexia nervosa	
Obesity	
Peptic ulcer	
Irritable bowel syndrome	
Colitis	

From Stuart GW: *Handbook of psychiatric nursing*, ed 6, St. Louis, 2005, Mosby.

vocabulary. The more recent term, **psychophysical disorders**, was coined to refer to stress-related physical problems. The physiological stress response affects many body systems (Box 22-1).

One of the systems that experiences much of the stress response is the gastrointestinal tract. Common stress-related problems include indigestion, vomiting, constipation, and diarrhea. Ulcerative colitis and gastric, peptic, and duodenal ulcers can also occur when the gastrointestinal tract is the focus of one's stress. The respiratory system can develop asthma, and the cardiac system can raise blood pressure when subjected to prolonged stress. Many mental health conditions, such as anxiety, are expressions of stress.

THEORIES OF PSYCHOPHYSICAL DISORDERS

Although we know that emotions play an important role in the development or prevention of illness, just how this connection works is uncertain. Several theories attempt to explain this relationship.

The **stress response theory** states that individuals are biochemically patterned to react to stress. During times of stress, the autonomic nervous system prepares the body for fight or flight. Because the threat is not external, no physical outlet for the biochemical response is usually possible. Consequently, nothing is done to relieve the conflict, and soon a cycle of biochemical stimulus-response is established. This pattern eventually results in physical disturbances within the body.

Carl Jung's theory focuses on the **symbolism attached to a symptom** or illness. For example, the young executive who needs to vent his rage but feels that displays of anger are inappropriate may develop ulcerative colitis or high blood pressure as a way of coping with his anger.

Erich Fromm's theory states that certain **personality types** are prone to develop certain illnesses. The hard-working, independent, overly ambitious executive is at high risk for the development of cardiac problems because of his aggressive personality. The quiet, uncomplaining, overburdened clerk may suffer from ulcers, joint problems, or skin rashes.

Last is the theory of **organic weakness,** which states that every individual has one body system that is more sensitive than other systems. When a person has underlying emotional problems that affect functioning, he or she may develop a physical illness as a means of coping with the unconscious problem.

Although these theories may appear unrelated, all of them have several concepts in common. First, unconscious emotional conflict that increases anxiety is the basis for many psychophysical problems. Second, the development of physical symptoms is the result of attempts to lower anxieties associated with conflict. Third, the illness is real to the person, regardless of whether organic changes exist or not. In some cases, physical changes can be life threatening, so never treat a client's complaints casually. Finally, frequently the onset of the illness or problem is related to a stressful event.

The physical signs and symptoms of an illness often relieve an individual's anxieties by masking inner emotional turmoil. This anxiety-reducing benefit is called primary gain because the symptoms reduce anxiety. There are other benefits, called secondary gains, to assuming the sick role. These include being relieved of responsibilities, receiving the special attentions of others, and having dependency needs met. Most of the time, these gains tend to reinforce the pattern of psychophysical symptoms and encourage illness behaviors to continue.

SOMATOFORM DISORDERS

Somatization is a term for feeling physical symptoms in the absence of disease or out of proportion to an ailment. It is a common stress-reducing mechanism. Its use may or may not result in pathological functioning. Persons with a somatoform disorder demonstrate no objective causes or physical dysfunctions for their signs and symptoms. A somatoform disorder is a condition in which a person's symptoms suggest the presence of a medical illness (Miller, 2003). The diagnosis of a somatoform disorder is made by first excluding any possible physical dysfunctions, the presence of drugs or other toxic substances, or other mental health problems that may be related to the symptoms. Finally, if no diagnosable medical condition accounts for the client's physical condition, the diagnosis is usually one of the somatoform disorders.

Somatization is common in the United States. Almost 80% of basically healthy people have somatic symptoms in any given week. Many health care dollars (about one in five) are spent treating non–physically based complaints, and nearly half of the patients seen in physicians' offices are the "worried well" (Holloway and Zerbe, 2000). Somatization costs more than just money. Often individuals with somatoform disorders will subject themselves to painful or dangerous diagnostic procedures and treatments. Cardiac pain, for example, must be investigated in order to determine whether its origin is emotional or physical.

The signs and symptoms of illness may be the client's way of coping with emotional distress. Emotional stress depletes the body's energies and results in decreased immune functions, which can make the person more susceptible to actual illness and disease. Remember, people with somatoform disorders also fall ill to the same maladies as everyone else, so do not dismiss any client's complaints as trivial.

CULTURAL INFLUENCES

Cultural differences are associated with certain illnesses, both physical and mental. Many somatization disorders are culturally related, and their treatment depends on understanding the problem within the client's cultural context or framework (Table 22-1).

Health care providers who work with clients from different cultures must be aware of the meaning or importance that the problem holds for the person (Giger and Davidhizar, 2008) (see Cultural Considerations 22-1). Many somatic illnesses are based in cultural or spiritual beliefs. Assessments and treatment plans must not threaten or challenge these beliefs if therapeutic interventions are to be effective. Culturally appropriate nursing interventions are based on knowledge of and respect for another's way of living (Geissler, 2003). The effective health care provider does not hesitate to learn as much as possible about other cultures.

CRITERIA FOR DIAGNOSIS

Expressing emotions through the body (somatization) is a common coping mechanism that fulfills needs and relieves anxiety. Because every physical sign or symptom may have a biological cause, each complaint must be investigated thoroughly before it is labeled as emotionally based. Therefore the first criterion for diagnosis is that **no organic medical condition** to explain the symptoms can be found.

The second criterion is that **the disorder significantly disrupts or impairs one's level of functioning.** Because of the somatoform problem, the person is unable to engage in activities of daily living, perform work, or engage in social activities. This adds significant distress to an already emotionally charged situation.

The third criterion for diagnosis is that **the client is unaware of or unable to express his or her emotional**

Table **22-1** | *Culturally Related Somatic Disorders*

CULTURAL GROUP	DESCRIPTION
Japanese	**Gaman** means to internally suppress emotions, especially anger.
	Emotional distresses are expressed through physical signs or symptoms.
	Illness is a socially acceptable way of receiving care.
	Body functions are of concern, especially blood pressure.
	Headaches are related to depression.
Southeast Asians	Mental distress is not discussed but expressed via various physical ailments.
	Koro is fear of penis shrinking into abdomen, which results in death.
Hispanics	**Mal ojo** (the evil eye) is associated with fever, headaches, diarrhea, restlessness, irritability, and weight loss.
East Indians (India)	**Dhat** syndrome consists of male reproductive signs and symptoms caused by fear and concern about losing semen.
Koreans	The body is the property of the ancestors.
	Mental and emotional illnesses are expressed as physical (somatic) complaints.

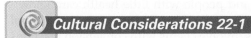

Cultural Considerations 22-1

Assessment of a client's culture* should focus on the following:
- Biological variations
- Communications
- Cultural uniqueness
- Environmental control
- Social orientation
- Space
- Time

*See Figure 4-1 for a complete cultural assessment.

distress. Acknowledging emotional distress is often considered a weakness, especially for men. Experiencing physical problems, however, enables individuals to accept the attention and the sympathy that anxiety or emotional expression would not elicit. Somatization is a way for many emotional problems to make themselves known.

The *Diagnostic and Statistical Manual of Mental Disorders* (DSM-IV-TR) lists six types of somatoform disorders: somatization disorder, undifferentiated somatoform disorder, conversion disorder, pain disorder, hypochondriasis, and body dysmorphic disorder. Most eating and sleeping disorders arise from emotional sources (see Chapter 23). Individuals with factitious disorder intentionally produce signs and symptoms of illness or disability in order to assume the sick role. Because most of these clients are seen in general medical settings, such as clinics and physicians' offices, it is important for all caregivers to be familiar with somatoform disorders.

SOMATIZATION DISORDER

Somatization disorder has been historically referred to as **Briquet's syndrome,** or **hysteria.** As a polysymptomatic disorder, the condition is associated with many signs and symptoms. It begins before 30 years of age, sometimes as early as adolescence or childhood, and can persist for many years. Somatization disorder occurs more frequently in women and appears to have a family pattern. It is seen in 10% to 20% of the daughters of women diagnosed with the disorder. The male relatives of these women show an increased risk for antisocial personality disorders and substance-abuse problems (American Psychiatric Association, 2000). Both genetic and environmental factors contribute to the risk for developing a somatization disorder.

Individuals with somatization disorder often possess a long history of vague complaints. Their complaints are usually described in colorful and exaggerated terms but offer few facts. Although the descriptions of their illnesses may be vivid, they actually give a poor history of their medical problems. In addition, individuals with somatization disorder seek treatment from several physicians at the same time. This dangerous practice can lead to hazardous events for these clients if the combined drugs and therapies are not compatible (see Drug Alert 22-1).

The most common client complaints are a combination of gastrointestinal tract and sexual problems, with pain and false neurological symptoms. Case Study 22-1 illustrates a typical case. For a diagnosis of somatization disorder to be made, the client must meet the criteria listed in Box 22-2.

Signs of anxiety and depression are very common in people with somatization disorders. They may also behave in impulsive, antisocial, or suicidal manners. Frequently, their lives are associated with chaos, marital discord, and social problems with lifestyles as complicated as their medical histories.

Three features may help health care providers to differentiate a somatization disorder from a medical problem (Kirmayer, Robbins, and Paris, 1994). First, the **involvement of multiple organ systems** suggests somatization disorder. Second, the disorder is characterized by an **early onset** and **chronic condition** in which no physical changes occur over time. Third, the **absence of any significant laboratory values** indicates that the underlying problems may be emotionally based. It is important to remember that the onset of multiple complaints in an older person is almost always caused by a medical condition, not somatization. Also, having a somatization disorder does not protect individuals from developing a physical problem.

Clients with somatization disorder are difficult to diagnose and even more challenging to effectively

Drug Alert 22-1

Nurses need to ask all clients if they are currently seeing any other health care providers, natural healers, or other practitioners.

Multiple drug use is common. Obtain a full drug history from each client, including the use of over-the-counter drugs, home remedies, and herbs.

Case Study 22-1

Sarah was a single 31-year-old woman who came to the clinic with complaints of diarrhea, nausea, pain, and weight loss over a period of 5 years. During the health history, Sarah revealed that she was the only one of five children still living at home with her mother. Sarah described her younger years as always being "sickly," but she could not identify any specific health problems.

Her father, whom Sarah described as "silent and cold," died when she was 15 years old. She remembers feeling little loss at her father's death. Sarah's relationship with her mother became very important following the death of her father. Sarah and her mother did everything together, even to the point of sharing the same bed. On graduation from high school, Sarah worked in a candy shop for a few years but found the work too demanding and quit. She has not been employed for more than 7 years.

It seems that just before the symptoms of her illness began, Sarah's aunt became widowed and decided to move in with Sarah and her mother. Aunt Sally arrived with much of her furniture, including a pair of twin beds. Soon thereafter, the mother sold the large double bed and substituted the twin beds, forcing Sarah to sleep alone. Although she did not protest, Sarah felt angry and deserted. A few weeks later, she developed abdominal pain, diarrhea, and nausea.
- How do you think the onset of Sarah's symptoms relates to her family situation?
- Consider which therapeutic (nursing) interventions would be most effective with Sarah.

treat. "Conflict between patients' experience of illness and physicians' diagnostic categories, and fear of blaming the patient, complicate naming and characterizing the illness" (Epstein, Quill, and McWhinney, 1999). These individuals are not consciously aware of the conflicts related to their difficulties. Long-term therapy is usually indicated when clients are willing to recognize and work with the emotional conflicts that are the basis of their physical problems.

CONVERSION DISORDER

The term *conversion* is derived from Freud's theory of conversion hysteria, which stated that a psychosexual conflict is focused or converted into a physical disturbance. Today, this relatively uncommon condition,

---

Box 22-2 | *Criteria for Diagnosis of Somatization Disorder*

1. A history of pain related to at least four different sites (e.g., headache, backache, or joint, extremity, chest, or abdominal pain) or functions (e.g., menstrual, sexual, or urinary dysfunctions).
2. A history of at least two gastrointestinal tract symptoms (other than pain), such as nausea, abdominal bloating, vomiting, diarrhea, and food intolerance.
3. A history of one sexual or reproductive problem other than pain. For women, these include irregular or difficult menses, heavy menstrual bleeding, or vomiting throughout pregnancy. For men there may be erectile or ejaculatory problems. Both men and women are often sexually indifferent.
4. A history of at least one symptom that suggests a neurological disorder, such as impaired coordination, localized weakness, and double vision.

---

called a **conversion disorder**, is considered to be a somatoform disorder in which the individual presents problems related to the sensory or motor functions (Table 22-2).

Conversion disorders appear more commonly in persons of lower socioeconomic status, those living in rural areas, and people with little health care knowledge. Approximately 1% to 3% of referrals to mental health clinics involve clients with conversion reactions (Kirmayer and others, 1994). When clients with conversion disorders are assessed, it is important to consider their social and cultural backgrounds.

Men and women differ in relation to conversion disorder. As many as 10 women for every 1 man are diagnosed with conversion disorders. In men, conversion disorders are often associated with military service, industrial accidents, and antisocial personalities. The onset of problems is usually during late childhood through early adulthood, but almost always after 10 and before 35 years of age. There have been reports, however, of conversion reactions in persons in their 90s. Children usually present with gait problems or seizures. In older individuals, the signs and symptoms usually appear as sensory or motor disturbances. Symptoms often appear suddenly, but they can also begin slowly and increase over time and typically last only a short time. In hospitalized clients, symptoms often disappear within 2 weeks. However, recurring episodes are common, and as many as 25% of clients have a return of symptoms within 1 year.

Conversion disorders are thought to be the result of an emotional (psychic) conflict. Situational factors, such as environmental stressors or interpersonal conflicts, can frequently trigger the appearance of conversion reactions. For a conversion disorder to be diagnosed, the client must meet four criteria (Box 22-3).

Conversion signs and symptoms tend to be more in keeping with the individual's ideas of what the

Table 22-2 *DSM-IV-TR Diagnoses for Somatoform Disorders*

DSM-IV-TR DIAGNOSES	ESSENTIAL FEATURES
Somatization disorder	A history of many physical complaints beginning before the age of 30 yr, occurring over a period of several years, and resulting in treatment being sought or significant impairment in social or occupational functioning. The patient must display at least four pain symptoms, two gastrointestinal symptoms, one sexual symptom, and one symptom suggesting a neurological disorder.
Conversion disorder	One or more symptoms or deficits affecting voluntary motor or sensory function suggesting a neurological or general medical condition. Psychological factors are judged to be associated with the symptom or deficit because the initiation or exacerbation of the symptom or deficit is preceded by conflicts or other stressors. The symptom or deficit cannot be fully explained by a neurological or general medical condition and is not a culturally sanctioned behavior or experience.
Hypochondriasis	Preoccupation with fears of having, or ideas that one has, a serious disease based on the person's misinterpretation of body symptoms. The preoccupation persists despite appropriate medical evaluation and reassurance and has existed for at least 6 mo. It causes clinically significant distress or impairment in functioning.

Modified from American Psychiatric Association: *Diagnostic and statistical manual of mental disorders*, ed 4, text revision, Washington, DC, 2000, The Association.

problems should be. For example, a "paralyzed" arm that is raised over the head by the caregiver remains suspended for a moment, and then falls to the side rather than on its owner's head or an extremity that is "paralyzed" moves automatically when the client is not paying attention to the arm. Individuals with conversion "seizures" vary in their seizure activity and few, if any, changes are noted on an electroencephalogram (EEG). In short, the course of the signs and symptoms are not in keeping with physically based disease processes but rather the client's ideas.

An interesting feature of conversion disorders is la belle indifference, which is a lack of concern or indifference about the signs or symptoms. Some individuals with conversion disorders appear totally indifferent to their symptoms, whereas others present their complaints in dramatic or hysterical manners. Symptoms are more apparent during times of extreme psychological stress, such as the loss of a loved one or change in fortune. People with conversion disorders are often very suggestible, and their symptoms can be modified or intensified by the reactions of others in their environments. Laboratory and other diagnostic examinations show no specific abnormalities. In fact, it is the absence of diagnostic findings that helps to establish the diagnosis.

Treatment goals focus on eliminating the possibility of any physical causes and then assisting clients in identifying the conflicts responsible for their signs and symptoms. Individuals and their families are frequently referred for psychotherapy, wherein antidepressants and antianxiety agents are often prescribed. Behavior modification techniques are successful in some cases.

HYPOCHONDRIASIS

Hypochondriasis is a somatoform disorder in which one has an intense fear of or preoccupation with having a serious disease or medical condition based in a

Box 22-3 *Criteria for Diagnosis of a Conversion Disorder*

1. At least one of the signs or symptoms involves the voluntary motor or sensory system and suggests the presence of a neurological problem.
2. The signs and symptoms are brought on or worsened by the presence of a conflict or other stressor.
3. The signs and symptoms are not intentionally produced.
4. The signs and symptoms cause significant distress and impairment in daily functions.
5. After extensive investigation, the signs and symptoms cannot be explained by a pathological condition or the effects of a substance and are not culturally appropriate behaviors.

misinterpretation of body signs and symptoms. Hypochondriasis is a persistent fear that something is physically wrong, even when all diagnostic test results are negative and reassurances have been given by various physicians. Although the individual can acknowledge the possibility that the symptoms are being exaggerated or blown out of proportion, he or she continues to hold onto the belief that something is physically wrong.

Symptoms commonly relate to minor abnormalities (a sore on the skin, a cough), body functions (heartbeat, sweating), or vague physical sensations, such as "tired blood" or "aching veins." The meaning, source, and nature of the symptoms cause great concern to the client despite repeated negative test results and reassurances from health care providers. These people commonly "doctor shop," seeing several physicians at the same time. Often their relationships with health care providers become strained because clients with hypochondriasis feel they never receive the proper medical care and usually resist referral to mental health care settings.

Hypochondriasis can begin at any age, but the symptoms most commonly occur in early adulthood. It is more frequent in persons who were exposed to a serious illness or life-threatening condition in childhood. The course of the disorder follows a seesaw pattern and tends to become chronic. In some cases, the disorder is first diagnosed following a severe stressor, such as the death of a loved one. Although exact statistics are not available, it is estimated that from 4% to 9% of the clients seen in a general medical practice are suffering from hypochondriasis.

People with hypochondriasis often have strained interpersonal relationships. Because they are so focused on themselves, many expect special consideration and treatment. Family and social lives can become quite disturbed because they center around clients' pictures of their health. Individuals may be able to remain employed if the appearance of symptoms is limited to nonwork time. Hypochondriacs frequently miss work. In the most severe cases, people become complete invalids. To be clinically diagnosed with hypochondriasis, the client must meet five criteria (Box 22-4).

Anxiety, depression, and compulsive personality traits are often present along with hypochondriasis. These clients are frequently demanding and a challenge to treat because they can be critical and suspicious of all offered health care. Patience, therapeutic communication skills, and alert observations are needed when caring for individuals with hypochondriasis.

Because of the chronic nature of the disorder and the fact that these clients are "doctor shoppers," hypochondriasis is difficult to treat. Many times clients show poor insight or little concern about the source of their preoccupations. Psychotherapy and emotional support assist some clients in identifying the sources of their problems. Antianxiety and antidepressive medications may be prescribed. Because of the chronic and interfering nature of the disorder, long-term therapy and support are indicated.

OTHER SOMATOFORM DISORDERS

Table 22-2 presents a summary of the essential features of the three most common somatoform disorders. Two less common but important somatoform disorders

---

Box 22-4 *Criteria for Diagnosis of Hypochondriasis*

1. A preoccupation with fears of having a serious disease based on a misunderstanding of body messages.
2. The preoccupation is not delusional (clients can admit that they have an unreasonable concern).
3. The preoccupation persists despite negative diagnostic testing results.
4. The preoccupation causes significant distress or impairment in the client's activities of daily living.
5. The preoccupation has been present for at least 6 months.

---

relate to the perceptions of pain and disfigurement. **Somatoform pain disorder** may be diagnosed when pain or discomfort is the major focus of distress and no other cause of the pain can be identified. Many times these individuals benefit from attending pain clinics.

Body dysmorphic disorder is characterized by a preoccupation with a physical difference or defect in one's body. The most common site of concern is the face or head. Clients may be concerned about their ears, noses, thinning hair, drooping chin, crooked teeth, or numerous other imperfections. They describe their distress as tormenting, devastating, or intensely painful. Because of their concern and embarrassment over their perceived defect, these individuals often describe themselves as "ugly" or "unacceptable" and often avoid work, social, or public gatherings. Their distress can lead to repeated hospitalizations for treatment of the perceived defect as well as suicide attempts.

FACTITIOUS DISORDERS AND MALINGERING

Factitious disorders and malingering differ from somatoform disorders in that signs and symptoms are **intentionally** produced. People who are malingering or engaging in factitious behaviors are purposefully and willfully producing the signs or symptoms of illness for some form of gain. Both psychological and physical signs and symptoms can be expressed. Clients are rarely diagnosed with factitious disorder because they tend to move from physician to physician and undergo various operative procedures in different facilities. Some spend the major focus of their lives seeking admission or staying in health care facilities.

Factitious disorder by proxy, also called Munchausen's syndrome by proxy, is the deliberate production of signs and symptoms in another person. Situations most often involve a caregiver (mother, babysitter) who induces signs of illness in a child and then presents the child for medical care. The type and severity of signs and symptoms vary with the medical knowledge of the offender. Diagnosis is difficult because offenders commonly remove their victims as soon as the disorder is suspected.

Clinical Presentations

The difference between a factitious disorder and malingering lies with the **intent** of the individual. The most important feature of a factitious disorder is that symptoms are purposefully produced to assume the sick role. Presenting complaints include psychological signs and symptoms, self-inflicted illnesses or injuries, and exaggerated symptoms of actual physical problems. Examples include complaining of acute abdominal pain, producing abscesses by injecting saliva under the skin, ingesting medications to produce dramatic side effects, or pretending to have a seizure with no actual history of epilepsy. The motivation for their behaviors is to assume the sick role.

The medical history of individuals with factitious disorders may be dramatic and colorful, but clients are vague and inconsistent when questioned. Often they lie entertainingly about any aspect of their condition. Some may have extensive knowledge of hospital routines, diagnostic testing, and medical terminology. When the cause of the original symptoms is ruled out, individuals often develop new complaints and eagerly undergo invasive procedures. If they are confronted with evidence of their behaviors, they strongly deny it and discharge themselves from the institution or change health care providers.

On the other hand, the malingering individual produces symptoms to meet a recognizable goal. The student who fakes a stomachache to be excused from school for the day is a common example of malingering. Producing symptoms to avoid military service, the police, jury duty, or social obligations are examples. Not infrequently, clients will produce symptoms with the goal of receiving compensation, food, or shelter for the night. However, once the motive becomes apparent to others, the symptoms usually disappear because they no longer serve a purpose.

IMPLICATIONS FOR CARE PROVIDERS

Caring for clients with somatoform disorders is both challenging and rewarding. The first goal of care (in every case) is to rule out the presence of any physical disease or dysfunction. As physicians order and interpret diagnostic tests, nurses and other caregivers observe and assess clients and their activities. Data are gathered and analyzed, physical dysfunctions are ruled out, and health care team and nursing diagnoses are established (Box 22-5).

The development of trust is an important goal in the treatment of clients with somatoform disorders. Clients' sufferings are very real to them, and health care providers must be aware of how their behaviors and attitudes affect the clients for whom they care.

All care providers should attempt to understand the purposes served by clients' symptoms and work to encourage a trusting relationship. Encourage the expression of feelings and emotional states rather than physical complaints. Also, teach the importance of good nutritional, exercise, and sleep habits using the client's anxiety level as a guide for teaching. Meet physical needs when necessary, but encourage independence. Help clients fill their social needs, and encourage them to explore more adaptive ways of handling their stresses. Box 22-6 summarizes key interventions for clients with

somatoform disorders. Sample Client Care Plan 22-1 illustrates a client plan of care. Finally, acknowledge clients as individuals and responsible adults who are capable of changing and developing more effective coping mechanisms.

Box 22-5 *NANDA-I Nursing Diagnoses Related to Psychophysical Responses*

Anxiety
Behavior, risk-prone health*
Body image, disturbed
Constipation
Coping, ineffective
Denial, ineffective
Diarrhea
Diversional activity, deficient
Family processes, interrupted
Fear
Gas exchange, impaired
Health maintenance, ineffective
Hopelessness
Insomnia
Nutrition, imbalanced: less than body requirements
Pain, chronic*
Mobility, impaired physical
Powerlessness
Self-care deficit
Self-esteem, chronic low
Self-esteem, situational low
Skin integrity, impaired
Social interaction, impaired
Social isolation
Spiritual distress

Data from NANDA International: *NANDA-I nursing diagnoses: definitions and classification 2007-2008*, Philadelphia, 2007, NANDA International. *NANDA-I*, NANDA International.
*Primary nursing diagnoses for maladaptive psychophysiological responses.

Box 22-6 *Key Interventions for Clients With Psychophysical Problems*

Convey an attitude of acceptance and understanding.
Meet all physical needs of the client during acute feelings of illness.
Minimize secondary gains once the acute phase of the illness is resolved.
Use the client's level of anxiety as a gauge to determine the amount and type of health teaching.
Acknowledge the client as a responsible adult while indirectly addressing dependency needs.
Encourage the client to talk about his or her feelings.
Assist the client and family in enlarging their social network.

From Taylor CM: *Essentials of psychiatric nursing*, ed 14, St. Louis, 1994, Mosby.

SAMPLE CLIENT CARE PLAN 22-1

Psychophysical Responses

ASSESSMENT *History.* Jasmine is a 20-year-old college student. Last year, during final examination week, she developed frequent bouts of nausea followed by vomiting. Once final examinations were over, her symptoms subsided until about 3 days ago.

Current Findings. A tense, young woman, sitting stiffly in the chair and wringing her hands. On questioning, Jasmine reveals that she has "never had problems with her stomach." She believes that her nausea and vomiting are related to the "institutional food" she eats while on campus. She is here at the clinic to "get some of those nausea pills." Final examinations for her four classes are scheduled for next week. Jasmine states that school stresses "really have nothing to do with my stomach problems. It's the food that's the real problem here."

Multidisciplinary Diagnosis	*Planning/Goals*
Risk-prone health behavior related to anxiety about school examinations	Jasmine will express her feelings verbally rather than through nausea and vomiting by July 2.

Therapeutic Interventions

Intervention	Rationale	Team Member
1. Assist Jasmine in identifying stressful situations by reviewing the events surrounding the development of nausea and vomiting	Identifying events relating to internal conflicts helps reduce the anxiety that results in nausea and vomiting.	Psy, Nsg
2. Help her see thoughts, feelings, and behaviors.	Helps Jasmine to gain control over her expressions of emotions.	All
3. Explore more effective ways of coping with her anxieties.	Preserves dignity and self-respect; encourages effective coping behaviors.	Psy, All
4. Help her choose two new coping mechanisms for dealing with the stress of examinations.	Equips Jasmine with multiple ways to manage her anxieties and demonstrates the use of more effective behaviors.	Psy, Nsg
5. Actively encourage Jasmine to test the new coping mechanisms and provide feedback.	Change requires time, emotional support, and positive reinforcement from others.	All
6. Encourage physical activity and relaxation exercises.	Wellness requires a balance between physical and psychosocial needs.	Nsg
7. Assess eating and sleeping habits, and encourage her to follow a routine schedule.	A healthy, well–cared-for body functions more effectively during stress.	Nsg

Evaluation

During final examination week, Jasmine had two episodes of nausea but no vomiting. By the next final examination period, Jasmine had replaced nausea and vomiting with a 1-mile walk and 10 minutes of relaxation exercise during each examination day.

❓ CRITICAL THINKING QUESTIONS

1. How did Jasmine's coping behaviors affect her activities of daily living?

2. How would you assist her in developing more effective coping mechanisms?

A complete client care plan includes several other diagnoses and interventions.
Psy, Psychologist; *Nsg,* nursing staff.

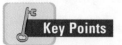
Key Points

- No real divisions between mind and body exist.
- The physical signs and symptoms of psychic (emotional) distress are very real to the individual who is suffering from them at the time.
- When the body is under stress, it activates its stress response mechanism, which protects the individual by preparing the body to fight or flee.
- When an individual perceives stress, the body initiates a cascade of biochemicals and releases the body's four major stress hormones—dopamine, epinephrine, norepinephrine, and cortisol.

- Common stress-related problems include indigestion, vomiting, constipation, diarrhea, asthma, high blood pressure, and mental health conditions.
- Theories about stress include the stress response, symbolism, personality, and organic weakness theories.
- Many somatization disorders are culturally related and include Japanese, *gaman;* Southeast Asian, *koro;* Hispanic, *mal ojo;* and East Indian, *dhat.*
- Somatization is the term for feeling physical symptoms in the absence of disease or out of proportion to a given ailment.
- A somatoform disorder is diagnosed when no diagnosable organic medical condition can be found, the

disorder significantly impairs one's level of functioning, and the client is unaware of or unable to express his or her emotional distress.

- Clients with a conversion disorder present with problems related to sensory or motor functions.
- Hypochondriasis is an intense fear of or preoccupation with having a serious disease or medical condition based on a misinterpretation of body signs or symptoms.
- The most important feature of factitious disorder is that symptoms are purposefully produced so that the individual can assume the sick role.

- The malingering individual produces symptoms to meet a recognizable external goal.
- The goals of care for every client with a somatoform disorder are to rule out the presence of any physical disease or dysfunction and to develop trust in the therapeutic relationship.

evolve   Be sure to visit the companion Evolve site at http://evolve.elsevier.com/Morrison-Valfre/ for additional online resources.

23 Eating and Sleeping Disorders

Objectives

Upon completion of this chapter, the student will be able to:

1. List three criteria for the diagnosis of an eating disorder.
2. Compare anorexia nervosa and bulimia.
3. Forecast the prognosis (outcome) for a client with an untreated eating disorder.
4. Explain why obesity can be considered an eating disorder.
5. Examine the main therapeutic goal for treating clients with eating disorders.
6. Develop four therapeutic interventions for clients with eating disorders.
7. Describe three functions of sleep.
8. Discuss the signs and symptoms of a client experiencing insomnia.
9. Plan four therapeutic (nursing) interventions to assist clients with sleeping problems.

Key Terms

anorexia (ĂN-ō-RĔK-sē-ə) **nervosa** (p. 249)
binge eating (p. 251)
body image (p. 248)
bulimia (bū-LĔM-ē-ə) (p. 250)
cataplexy (KĂT-ə-plĕk-sē) (p. 258)
compulsive overeating (p. 253)
dyssomnias (dĭs-SŎM-nē-əs) (p. 257)
eating disorder (p. 249)
insomnia (p. 257)
narcolepsy (p. 257)
obesity (p. 252)
parasomnias (PĂR-ə-SŎM-nē-əs) (p. 258)
pica (PĪ-kă) (p. 254)
polysomnogram (PŎL-ē-SŎM-nō-grăm) (p. 257)
purging (p. 251)
rumination (ROO-mĭ-NĀ-shən) **disorder** (p. 254)
sleep disorder (p. 254)

Every person has a body image—the collection of perceptions, thoughts, feelings, and behaviors that relate to one's body size and appearance. Body image is an important part of self-concept. **Positive body images** lead to behaviors that express confidence and self-assurance. **Negative body images** can lead to problems such as shyness and social isolation. Anxiety, depression, anorexia nervosa, bulimia, obesity, and other mental health problems are all interwoven with body image.

In the privacy of our thoughts, we all carry on conversations with ourselves. Our internal dialogue that focuses on the body and appearance is our "private body talk." It is the content of this private talk that helps determine how we feel about our bodies.

Body image is also historically defined. Throughout European history, a large, fleshy body was a sign of wealth and prosperity. Only the wealthy could afford rich foods and extra pounds of body fat. Poor people were thin because they never got enough to eat. The same ideals followed our ancestors to the Americas. The wealthy remained well fed and overweight, while the remainder of the population worked hard and carried little extra fat.

By the early 1900s, things began to change. Economic situations became more secure, and people ate better. The style and attitude evolved from "fat's where it's at" to "thin is in," and the day of the dieter began. Since the early part of the last century, the emphasis on body appearance has centered on one's weight as a definition of beauty.

Most modern societies place a high value on the thin body. Little tolerance is shown for individuals whose bodies are outside the range of "normal." Today, anorexia nervosa is much more common in societies in which there is an abundance of food and a focus on being thin as a measure of attractiveness. A fear of obesity leads many persons to engage in unhealthy or destructive lifestyles.

It seems that few people in modern societies are content with how their bodies look. Almost one third of Americans are dissatisfied with their weight. People who see themselves as too thin try to gain weight. People whose body images portray them as too fat try to lose weight.

Children learn early about which body images are desirable. It is not unusual to see boys imitating some muscular popular hero or young girls dieting so that they may look like the latest underfed model. Because late childhood and early adolescence are times for defining oneself, body image plays an important role (Hockenberry and others, 2007). The desire for the perfect body can push young individuals toward many unsound physical and emotional habits.

This chapter focuses on the eating and sleeping problems considered mental health disorders. As

Table **23-1**	*Theories About Eating Disorders*

THEORY	DESCRIPTION
Psychological	
Behavioral	Eating disorders are attempts to reduce anxiety; discomfort with body image creates more anxiety, feelings of guilt and disgust, and loss of self-protecting boundaries.
Cognitive	Eating disorders are the result of deficits in attention, concentration, and vigilance related to underlying anxiety and depression.
Developmental	Individual fails to develop an appropriate sense of self and body; has problems with autonomy and self-identity; disorder is often brought about by a significant loss or crisis.
Sociocultural	Eating disorders are a response to a daily social emphasis on a stereotypical ideal of thinness; social stereotypes serve as stressors that drive women and girls to harmful dieting behaviors; anorexia nervosa is a way of mastering some control over the pressure on women to be successful in all areas of life.
Neurobiological	The causes for eating disorders involve complex relationships among the body's neurotransmitters; there is evidence of altered serotonin function; many of the same neuroendocrine findings are found in persons with depressive and bipolar disorders; cortisol levels are altered in depression and eating disorders; anorexia nervosa decreases levels of luteinizing hormone and follicle-stimulating hormone, which results in menstrual irregularities.

Modified from Irwin EG: A focused overview of anorexia nervosa and bulimia, *Arch Psychiatric Nurs* 7:342, 1993.

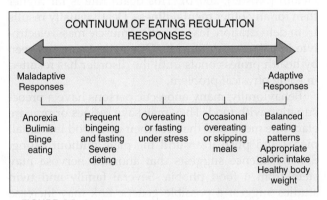

FIGURE **23-1** Continuum of eating regulation responses.

with everything in life, an occasional skipped meal or overindulgence is not a problem (Figure 23-1), but when behaviors associated with eating or sleeping interfere with an individual's quality of daily life, they become mental health disorders.

EATING DISORDERS

An **eating disorder** is an ongoing disturbance in behaviors associated with the ingestion of food. The most common eating disorders are anorexia nervosa and bulimia. Although obesity is not officially classified as an eating disorder, it presents problems for many individuals. According to the *Statistical Abstract of the United States: 2007* (U.S. Census Bureau, 2006), almost 30% of all adults believe their actual weight is more than their desirable weight.

For adolescents, the statistics relating to weight loss behaviors are alarming. Attempts to lose weight are very common among adolescents and adults. Girls as young as 8 years old are dieting, and the number of teens with serious eating disorders is increasing. Adolescents exercise, skip meals, take diet pills, and vomit

to control their weight. The desire for thinness leads many young people into unhealthy behaviors. These can eventually lead to severe mental health problems and life-threatening situations. Eating disorders are one result of the quest for the perfect body.

Although the cause remains unknown, several theories and much research have attempted to explain the nature of eating disorders (Table 23-1).

ANOREXIA NERVOSA

One of the most serious eating disorders is **anorexia nervosa**, a condition in which an individual does not maintain a normal body weight because of an intense fear of becoming fat. Actually, the term *anorexia* (which in Greek means "want of appetite") is inaccurate because there is seldom an actual appetite loss associated with the disorder. The refusal to gain weight is a part of a strategy to solve a deep psychological problem and maintain some form of control. Because of the secrecy and social stigma associated with them, the exact number of persons with eating disorders is unknown.

Anorexia nervosa was first described more than 100 years ago as a mania to be thin. Since then the number of people with this once-rare disorder has steadily grown to about 1 in 250 persons. Today approximately 90% to 95% of people with anorexia nervosa are female, but men are not immune to the disorder. In fact, anorexia nervosa is a serious disorder that affects more than 1 million males yearly (Crosscope-Happel and others, 2000). Anorexia nervosa is seldom seen before puberty and rarely appears after 40 years of age. The average age of onset is about 17 years, but anorectic behaviors may be seen in 12-year-olds. People who are concerned with their appearances for professional reasons, such as models, athletes, or flight attendants, are at a higher risk for developing anorexia nervosa. Early signs and symptoms of anorexia nervosa occur in children with depressive symptoms and obsessive behaviors. Children from dysfunctional or abusive families

Cultural Considerations 23-1

The incidence of anorexia nervosa is rising in Hong Kong. As a result of "increasing Westernization of Hong Kong society, anorexia is taking on a Western pattern" (Lai, 2000). Other countries that are adapting to Western influences are also seeing a rise in the incidence of eating disorders.

Box 23-1 *Criteria for Diagnosis of Anorexia Nervosa*

1. A refusal to maintain body weight that is more than 15% below normal.
2. Even though the individual is underweight, an intense fear of becoming fat exists.
3. A distorted (inaccurate) significance placed on body weight and shape (person "feels fat" and perceives self as fat despite being underweight).
4. An absence of at least three menstrual cycles in a female who has previously menstruated.

---

are at a greater risk for developing the disorder. Anorexia primarily occurs in industrialized, Western societies, but it is seen with increasing frequency in other cultures (see Cultural Considerations 23-1).

Certain **personality factors** appear to be associated with anorexia nervosa. The classic description of a person with anorexia nervosa is a tense, alert, hyperactive, rigid young woman who thinks, talks, and walks rapidly. She is very ambitious and drives herself to perfection. She is sensitive, insecure, and serious with a conscience that works overtime. Her neatness, self-will, and stubbornness make her difficult to treat. A lack of warmth and friendliness allows her to make few friends. As she struggles to gain a self-respecting identity, she engages in "a relentless and successful pursuit of thinness that results in psychological and physiological disturbances" (Walsh, 1998).

The main issue is one of control, and the anorectic individual becomes constricted, conforming, and obsessed with the need to control body weight. Some teenagers have a fear of growing up and sexually maturing. Anorexia nervosa allows them to prevent the onset of adulthood by delaying menses and the development of secondary sexual characteristics.

Clinical Presentation

Weight concerns put adolescents at a high risk for developing anorexia nervosa. Dieting, body dissatisfaction, current body weight below body weight ideals, and unusual eating patterns do not necessarily indicate an eating disorder. However, when the quest for thinness results in the refusal to maintain a normal body weight, anorexia is the result. To be diagnosed with anorexia nervosa, the individual must meet the four criteria listed in Box 23-1.

People with anorexia nervosa have a self-esteem that depends highly on body size and shape. They often go to great measures to monitor their bodies, such as weighing three or four times each day, measuring body parts, and frequently looking in the mirror to check for areas of fat. The ability to lose weight is considered a sign of control and extraordinary self-discipline. Conversely, even the smallest gain in weight is seen as a threat and a failure of self-control. Some individuals may actually acknowledge their extreme thinness, but they typically deny the seriousness of their condition. Figure 23-2 shows a typical anorectic woman before and after treatment.

Anorexia nervosa is a **life-threatening disorder.** One study demonstrated that the mortality rate for anorexia due to complications of starvation, cardiac arrest, or suicide, is substantial, approximately 5% per decade of follow-up (National Institute of Mental Health [NIMH], 2007b). This death rate is far higher than for any other mental illness. Death usually results from dehydration, loss of critical muscle mass, electrolyte imbalances, or suicide. Often clients are not seen by health professionals until the disorder has resulted in some physical problem.

Behaviorally, many anorectic persons have a preoccupation with food. They may save recipes or prepare elaborate meals and then cut their own food into small pieces and push it around the plate without eating. Some evidence suggests that anorexia nervosa may stem from a food phobia. Several family and twin studies suggest a possible genetic link may increase the risk of developing anorexia (NIMH, 2007b). Obsessive behavior with food often extends into other obsessive-compulsive activities, such as a preoccupation with studying, exercising, or cleaning. Often individuals have poor sexual adjustment, with delayed sexual development or little interest in sex.

An inability to effectively cope or solve problems commonly exists. The history frequently is positive for anxiety, depression, or substance abuse. People with anorexia nervosa need intervention, but they often deny the seriousness of their problems until extensive physical damage has taken place. Nurses in every setting must be alert for the clues of anorexia nervosa because early intervention will often save a life that otherwise may literally waste away.

BULIMIA

Bulimia is a disorder of binge eating and the use of inappropriate methods to prevent weight gain. Although anorexia nervosa may be a more dramatic problem, bulimia occurs more commonly. The estimated incidence of bulimia varies with the population, method, and criteria used for study. Estimates of the incidence of bulimia in college-age women are as high as 19%.

Bulimia is most often found in young, white, middle-class and upper-class women. Men account for

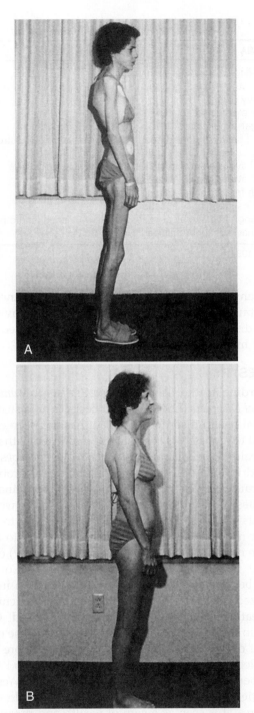

FIGURE **23-2** Anorectic woman before **(A)** and after **(B)** treatment.

Binge eating is defined as consuming (within a certain time) an amount of food that is definitely larger than most individuals would eat in similar circumstances. During a binge, an individual often consumes large amounts of certain foods, usually carbohydrates. It is not unusual for the binger to eat as many as 5000 calories in donuts, cakes, or other sweets. The binge lasts about 1 to 2 hours and then is followed by feelings of guilt and attempts to rid the body of the food just consumed.

Two subtypes of bulimia are classified according to the presence or absence of purging behaviors. **Purging** is an attempt to rid the gastrointestinal tract and body of unwanted food. The most common purging behaviors are vomiting and the use of diuretics and laxatives. Less commonly, some people use syrup of ipecac or enemas to purge.

The individual with "nonpurging" bulimia does not purge after a binge but uses other inappropriate methods to prevent weight gain, such as fasting between binges and exercising excessively.

The personality traits of persons with bulimia differ from those with anorexia nervosa. The average individual with bulimia is a woman who is slightly older and more outgoing than her anorectic counterpart. She is socially and sexually active. She actually experiences hunger and feels distressed about her abnormal eating behaviors. Often her body weight is normal or even slightly above average. Other mental health problems, such as substance abuse, self-mutilation, or hysteria, may be present at the same time. Refer to Table 23-2 for a comparison of the key features of anorexia nervosa and bulimia.

When it comes to body image, people with bulimia typically view themselves as fat or thin. Being in the middle, or average, is not considered. Commonly, a woman with bulimia fears that she must follow a diet for the rest of her life if she gives up binge eating.

Perfectionism is important with bulimia and contributes to maintaining bulimic behaviors. Bulimic women frequently have unrealistic expectations about themselves and how their lives should go. They become frustrated by their own inabilities to reach unrealistic goals. If they experience failure, they conclude that they were unable to reach the goal because they were weak, not trying hard enough, inadequate, or unlovable or had some other negative failing. In short, these are the "I should have ..." types who are never satisfied with their own efforts. Even when successful, they seldom can enjoy their accomplishments because they tell themselves that they should have done it better, sooner, or more efficiently. The desire to become the perfect person commonly leads to feelings of failure and uselessness. When life is based on the all-or-nothing principle, anything short of perfect is considered a failure. Unfortunately, this means most of their time is spent in feeling that they are truly "nothing." Perfection, in reality, is not attainable.

about one of nine cases. There is an increased frequency of anxiety, depression, and drug abuse among individuals with bulimia. "Adolescents with chronic depressive symptoms may be at elevated risk for the development of bulimia" (Zaider, Johnson, and Cockell, 2002). About one third to one half also meet the diagnostic criteria for a personality disorder. Because it is difficult to detect, many individuals with bulimia go untreated. Like anorexia nervosa, bulimia appears to be more of a problem in modern industrialized countries.

Table 23-2 *Key Features of Anorexia and Bulimia*

ANOREXIA NERVOSA	BULIMIA
Rare use of vomiting, diuretics, laxatives	Vomiting or diuretics, laxative abuse
More severe weight loss	Less weight loss
Slightly younger	Slightly older
More introverted	More extroverted, social
Hunger denied	Hunger experienced
Eating behavior may be considered normal and source of esteem	Eating behavior considered foreign and a source of distress
Sexually inactive	More sexually active
May be obsessive or compulsive	May have hysterical or borderline, as well as obsessive, behaviors
Death from starvation or suicide	Death from hypokalemia or suicide
Amenorrhea	Menses irregular or absent
Fewer behavioral abnormalities	Stealing, drug and alcohol abuse, self-mutilation, and other behavioral abnormalities

Modified from Physicians of the Geisinger Health System: *Help for anorexia nervosa*, 1997.

Clinical Presentation

The most essential feature of bulimia is recurring episodes of binge eating. Individuals are usually ashamed of their binges and often eat in secret. Episodes of binge eating may or may not be planned in advance. During the bingeing episodes, the individual feels out of control and often attacks eating in a frenzied state.

Bingeing is followed by recurring inappropriate behaviors to prevent weight gain. The most popular method of purging is to induce vomiting (80% to 90%), which relieves the physical discomfort of a full stomach and the emotional fear of gaining weight. "In some cases vomiting becomes a goal in itself, and the person will binge in order to vomit or will vomit after eating a small amount of food" (American Psychiatric Association, 2000). Other methods of purging include the misuse of laxatives, diuretics, enemas, and syrup of ipecac. Some people use a combination of methods to purge, engage in strenuous exercise at inappropriate times, or follow semistarvation diets after a bingeing episode.

In order for a diagnosis to be established, the eating binges must occur at least twice per week for at least 3 months (Box 23-2). Patterns of binge eating range from several episodes each day to a regular and persistent pattern. Often episodes are triggered by a stressful event or experience.

Individuals place excessive emphasis on body shape and weight in determining their self-esteem. They are dissatisfied with their imperfect bodies, have a fear of gaining weight, and often restrict their caloric intake or choose low-calorie foods between binge-eating episodes.

When purging behaviors are frequent, fluid and electrolyte abnormalities can result. The few persons who use syrup of ipecac are at risk for developing serious cardiac and skeletal muscle wasting. Although death from bulimia is rare, the underlying psychiatric problems are often more severe than those seen with anorectic persons.

Many times, the signs and symptoms of anorexia and bulimia occur together in the same individual. Both disorders are complex and often interrelated with other mental health problems.

OBESITY

According to the *Diagnostic and Statistical Manual of Mental Disorders* (DSM-IV-TR), obesity is not listed as a mental health disorder because it has not been established that obesity is consistently associated with mental health or behavioral problems. However, obesity is linked to many physical and psychological problems that cause distress for most overweight individuals.

Obesity is defined as an excess of body weight. Clients are classified as mildly obese (20% to 40% above normal weight), moderately obese (41% to 100% above normal weight), and severely (morbidly) obese (more than 100% above normal weight). Concern with being overweight is common in modern industrialized societies in which the luxuries of chronic overeating and underexercising are practiced. Children in the United States are growing fatter. The number of overweight children age 6 to 11 has more than doubled in the past 20 years. For teens age 12 to 19 that number has tripled (Shields, 2007). In non-Western societies, obesity is a relatively rare condition. In some cultures, it is seen as a sign of wealth and prosperity (see Cultural Considerations 23-2).

Obesity is the result of too many calories consumed or not enough calories burned (Figure 23-3). Like the person with bulimia or alcoholism, many overweight individuals lose control over their eating. Although the eating patterns of obese individuals do not pose an immediate threat, being chronically overweight can eventually result in severe physical and emotional problems. Throughout the industrialized world today, much time and money are spent in the pursuit of losing weight.

There are several causes of obesity. In addition to overeating, other factors have been discovered that may help explain obesity. Complicated neurochemical mechanisms that help to control appetite and eating

Box 23-2 *Criteria for Diagnosis of Bulimia*

1. Recurring episodes of binge eating
2. Bingeing followed by recurring inappropriate behaviors to prevent weight gain
3. Eating binges at least twice per week for at least 3 months
4. Excessive emphasis placed on body shape and weight in determining self-esteem

Cultural Considerations 23-2

The island nation of Nauru lies in the western Pacific Ocean south of the equator. Most Nauruans lead an inactive life-style because the island's phosphate mines are worked by immigrant miners. Almost all food and water are imported from Australia.

Eating processed foods is considered a sign of wealth. Obesity is considered attractive, and overweight women are sought as wives. Nauru has the highest rate of diabetes in the world.

behaviors are being studied. Heredity also appears to play a role in the development of obesity. The children of obese parents tend to be overweight themselves. Obese persons have larger fat cells in their bodies. Finally, a lack of sufficient exercise also contributes greatly to obesity.

Faulty eating behaviors appear to begin in childhood. Many overweight persons once relied on food to numb the discomforts of growing up. Throughout childhood, eating helped to relieve the emotional distresses of life. This pattern of lessening emotional pain by eating is called compulsive overeating. In time, food becomes like a drug, with a "fix" that temporarily lessens the psychological discomforts of an ever-growing desire for more food.

As the individual continues to find comfort in food, he or she grows physically more obese and less attractive to others. (Remember our cultural stigmas against obesity.) This behavior serves only to increase feelings of worthlessness, and the person again eats to relieve the pain. A vicious circle soon becomes established where the individual replaces social relationships with the comforts of food. Compulsive overeating can become a lonely way of life.

Clinical Presentation

The first signs of obesity are seen early in life. An estimate may be made by comparing one's height and weight with a standardized chart. Children who are 20% over normal for their height and weight should undergo further evaluation. The evaluation should include a "height and weight history of the child, parents, and siblings, as well as eating habits, appetite, and hunger patterns, and physical activity" (Hockenberry and others, 2007).

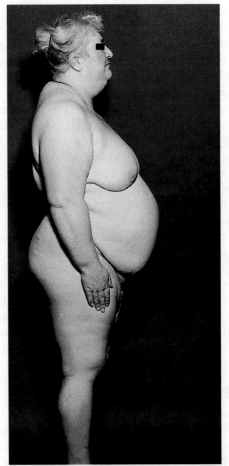

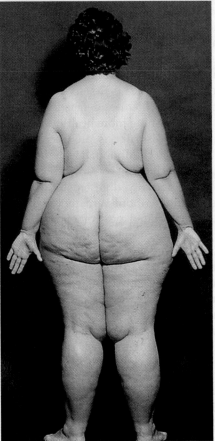

FIGURE **23-3** Obesity.

As overweight children grow and mature, they begin to sense society's disapproval of their obesity. Youngsters may begin to diet and exercise or react by continuing to find comfort in food. Dieting and other weight-loss methods soon become a way of life for many overweight young people.

During adolescence, weight becomes an important part of a newly forming body image. Teens may rebel against parental nagging to lose weight or become unwilling to control their caloric intake. They may resort to unhealthy methods, such as prolonged fasting or purging, to gain some control over their weight. Often, they will ignore their obesity and eat as though a problem does not exist.

The cycle of "I'm not attractive, so I'll eat because it makes me feel better" becomes an ingrained way of coping in childhood. Many overweight individuals become even more obese as they grow older. Eventually, the many chronic health problems associated with obesity begin to appear. These problems increase anxiety and further encourage the individual to seek the comfort that food has so frequently brought in the past. The cycle continues, and problems grow.

OTHER EATING DISORDERS

Two less common eating disorders are pica and rumination. Pica is the persistent eating of nonfood items that lasts for more than 1 month. Substances such as clay, laundry starch, insects, leaves, or pebbles are chosen for ingestion. The person with pica still eats and enjoys food. He or she just has an overwhelming need to eat the nonfood item. Many times the cause of pica can be traced to a vitamin, mineral, or calorie deficiency. Case Study 23-1 presents an interesting case history of pica. Treatment for pica is first to rule out the presence of any physical problem or deficiency. Then clients are assisted in establishing more healthful eating habits.

Rumination disorder is an uncommon problem most often seen in childhood. It is defined as the regurgitation and rechewing of food. According to the DSM-IV-TR, "partially digested food is brought up into the mouth without apparent nausea, retching, disgust, or associated gastrointestinal disorder. The food is then either ejected from the mouth or, more frequently, chewed and reswallowed."

When rumination disorder affects infants, death from malnutrition can result. In older children and adults, malnutrition is less of a problem. This disorder can occur continuously or appear at intervals. Psychosocial problems, such as lack of attention, neglect, or a stressful environment, may be risk factors. Other feeding disorders of early childhood are discussed in Chapter 13.

GUIDELINES FOR INTERVENTION

The main therapeutic goal for all eating disorders is to establish behaviors that promote health for the individual. Although it sounds simple, this is a lofty goal.

 Case Study 23-1

Loren was assigned to rounds with the mobile clinic nurse, whose responsibility was to provide prenatal services for a group of poor women from a rural farming region. As he rode through the countryside, he was surprised to see how many pregnant women and children were working in the fields. He asked the clinic nurse how long field workers were expected to work during their pregnancies. He was surprised to find that they were in the fields until the onset of labor. "How do they get enough to eat when they are working in the fields?" he wondered.

The mobile clinic nurse, sensing Loren's curiosity, assigned him to obtain dietary histories from as many of the farm workers as he could. By the time Loren had completed four histories, he was amazed. Not only were the workers' daily diets poor, but also many of the pregnant clients made it a habit to carry laundry starch into the fields with them. During the day, as they became hungry, they would eat a handful of laundry starch and drink a few sips of water.

When Loren finally mustered enough courage to ask one of the women why she ate laundry starch, she told him that it "takes the edge off my hunger and lets me work a little longer. Some of the ladies even eat clay, if it's a good kind."

It seemed that eating the laundry starch provided these women with a substitute for more expensive calories. The need to eat clay may have indicated the presence of a mineral deficiency.

• How do you think the infants will be affected by their mothers' dietary habits?

People with eating disorders have learned to cope with their stresses by focusing on food in one way or another. Those with anorexia nervosa attempt to cope by controlling, and the highest form of control is the ability to rule over one's body size. Individuals with bulimia learn to numb emotional pain by eating large amounts of food, and then they suffer through overwhelming guilt. Many persons who experience the discomforts of obesity have developed compulsive overeating habits to fill their needs for love and belonging.

Treatments and Therapies

Treatment for eating disorders requires medical and mental health interventions. There are three immediate (short-term) treatment goals. The highest priority is to **stabilize existing medical problems.** The second goal is to **reestablish normal nutrition** and eating patterns. Last is to help the client **resolve the psychological/emotional issues** that underlie his or her disordered eating behaviors.

Medical care centers on nutritional management. Individuals with severe weight loss may require total parenteral nutrition (TPN). With TPN, all necessary nutrients are administered through an intravenous line placed in a large blood vessel. For less severely malnourished clients, intravenous therapy or tube feedings may be ordered. However, the main focus is to encourage the client to voluntarily consume food.

Clients are weighed daily, and supplemental vitamins are usually prescribed. Each client is closely observed for secret anorectic or bulimic behaviors. The long-term goals (for both underweight and overweight clients) focus on teaching clients about good nutrition and assisting them in developing appropriate eating habits.

The goals of mental health care focus on helping clients improve their self-esteem and develop more effective coping skills. Once clients are physically stable, they are encouraged to adopt proper eating habits. Behavior modification techniques may help to reinforce healthful eating behaviors. Signs of depression are diagnosed and treated. Often family therapy is helpful. Individual or group therapy helps clients to focus on the psychological conflicts that underlie their inappropriate eating behaviors. Drug therapy can be quite effective, but only if it is combined with some form of psychotherapy (see Drug Alert 23-1). Amphetamines have been successfully used to treat obesity. However, their potential for addiction is high, and they are not frequently prescribed. Antidepressants or lithium has been used with success in the treatment of bulimia.

Nurses and other health care providers play an important role in caring for individuals with altered eating patterns in both the hospital and community settings. The main goal is to assist clients in identifying and coping with the problems that led to inappropriate eating behaviors. Possible nursing diagnoses relating to eating disorders are listed in Box 23-3.

To accomplish the goals of care, rapport and trust with clients must first be established. Then clients are assisted in identifying how food is used to provide comfort and reduce anxiety. During the working phase of the therapeutic relationship, clients are helped to replace distorted body image ideas with thoughts and behaviors that build self-esteem. Problem-solving skills are taught, and clients are encouraged to identify the social support systems that promote healthful practices. Refer to Sample Client Care Plan 23-1 for clients with eating disorders.

Every individual with an eating disorder needs the understanding and compassion of health care providers. Hopefully, health care providers can help make the struggles of clients with eating disorders a little less difficult by nurturing and supporting more effective coping behaviors.

SLEEP DISORDERS

Sleeping patterns and routines change as we grow older. The 16 hours of nightly sleep required by infants dwindle to less than 8 hours by adulthood. The afternoon naps of childhood are soon replaced by the all-day demands of school and work. The ritual of the

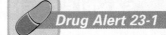
Drug Alert 23-1

Administering antidepressants to clients with anorexia nervosa before they regain weight may be hazardous if the individual has a history of cardiac problems or presently has a low serum potassium level. For this reason, the physician may order a trial dose of the antidepressant.

Be sure to check the laboratory results of clients with eating disorders. Withhold the medication and notify the physician if the potassium level drops below normal limits.

Box 23-3 *NANDA-I Nursing Diagnoses Related to Eating Disorders*

Activity intolerance
Behavior, risk-prone health
Body image, disturbed*
Coping, ineffective*
Denial, ineffective
Failure to thrive, adult
Fluid volume, risk for deficient
Health maintenance, ineffective
Identity, disturbed personal
Noncompliance
Nutrition, imbalanced: less than body requirements *
Self-esteem, chronic low*
Sexuality pattern, ineffective
Social isolation
Thought processes, disturbed
Violence, risk for self-directed

Data from NANDA International: *NANDA-I nursing diagnoses: definitions and classification 2007-2008,* Philadelphia, 2007, NANDA International. *NANDA-I,* NANDA International.
*Primary nursing diagnoses for eating disorders.

bedtime hour disappears altogether. By the time many persons reach adulthood, their sleeping habits may have changed dramatically. Most young adults have few difficulties with sleeping. However, sleep disorders begin to occur more frequently as adults grow older. By older adulthood, it is unusual to have a full night of uninterrupted sleep.

Although no one knows exactly why we must sleep every night, researchers have found that sleep serves several purposes. During sleep, body functions and metabolic rate slow and the workload on the heart decreases. Muscles relax, and the body conserves energy during sleep. One theory states that sleep is important for the renewal and repair of body cells and tissues. Sleep also "appears to be a critical cycle of brain activity important for learning, memory, and behavioral adaptation" (Potter and Perry, 2009).

Dreaming is also important for health. Dreaming helps us gain insights, solve problems, work through emotional reactions, and prepare for the future. Many cultures place great meaning in dreams and use them to cope with the problems of everyday reality (see Think About 23-1).

SAMPLE CLIENT CARE PLAN 23-1

Eating Disorder

ASSESSMENT *History.* Erica is a 15-year-old who is 20 lb under her usual body weight. She has always been a "chubby child" who had no problems eating until the beginning of this school year. Three months ago Erica told her mother to stop fixing "all those fattening foods" and began refusing most of her meals.

Current Findings. A thin, tired-appearing adolescent girl who appears older than her stated age. Face is hollow, eyes are sunken, and skin is dry. Hair is fine and brittle. Skin is covered with lanugo (fine hair). Vital signs are low for age and size. When questioned, Erica states that she "feels fine" and does not "know what all the fuss is about." "Just because I choose to lose a few pounds everybody gets upset. Sounds like this is their problem more than mine. I'm really still way too fat."

Multidisciplinary Diagnosis	*Planning/Goals*
Impaired nutrition: less than body requirements related to distorted self-image	Erica will voluntarily consume 2000 calories/day by July 4. Erica will gain 1 lb of body weight per week.

Therapeutic Interventions

Intervention	Rationale	Team Member
1. Establish trust and gain Erica's cooperation.	Erica must first agree to work with the staff if other interventions are to achieve therapeutic results.	All
2. Perform a complete nutritional assessment.	Establishes a baseline from which to judge progress.	Diet, Nsg
3. Help Erica identify the consequences of her eating behaviors.	Helps her acknowledge the problem and its effects on her life.	Psy, Nsg
4. Monitor physical status daily for signs of malnutrition.	To prevent further physical problems and decline.	Nsg, MD
5. Explore other ways to achieve control over the parts of Erica's life that are causing distress.	When control is achieved in one area, it tends to spread to other areas; control builds self-image and confidence.	All
6. Involve family members in therapy if possible.	Erica may benefit from supportive family members; offers an opportunity to assess family interactions.	Psy, Nsg

Evaluation

During the first week, Erica consumed an average of 1000 calories per day with much encouragement. By July 3, Erica was voluntarily consuming about 1800 calories per day. Weight gain averaged ½ pound per week.

? CRITICAL THINKING QUESTIONS

- How do you think Erica's attitude influences her treatment?

- Why do you think control is an important issue for Erica?

A complete client care plan includes several other diagnoses and interventions.
Diet, Dietitian; *Nsg*, nursing staff; *Psy*, psychologist; *MD*, physician.

Think About 23-1

It has been said that dreams are the result of reflection or suggestion.
- What do you think is meant by this statement?
- Do you believe that dreams have meanings? Why or why not?

Sleep occurs in cycles of about 24 hours, depending on each individual's personal body rhythms. There are two phases to sleep: nonrapid eye movement (NREM) sleep and rapid eye movement (REM) sleep. NREM sleep is divided into four stages.

The average adult's sleep pattern begins with a presleep period, lasting about 10 to 30 minutes. During this time, a gradual drowsiness develops until the

individual "drops off to sleep" or enters stage 1 of NREM sleep. As the sleeper moves through each stage of NREM, the quality of sleep becomes deeper. During stage 4, the sleeper is most difficult to arouse. After reaching stage 4, the sleep pattern reverses itself and the sleeper moves back through stage 3 into stage 2, where REM sleep takes place. Figure 23-4 illustrates the normal adult sleep cycle and its stages. If the sleeper is interrupted or awakened at any time during the cycle, he or she must return to stage 1 and begin the process again. If the disturbances occur frequently enough, the individual will experience the signs and symptoms of sleep deprivation. Everyone has an occasional poor night's sleep. For people with sleeping disorders, however, this experience becomes an unwelcome and unwanted way of life.

A sleep disorder is a condition or problem that repeatedly disrupts an individual's pattern of sleep.

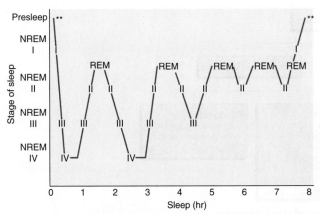

FIGURE 23-4 Normal adult sleep cycle.

Problems with sleep are very common in modern societies where the pace of life is fast and demanding. Sleep disorders occur more frequently in elderly individuals, but all age-groups are affected.

The diagnosis of a sleep disorder is based on a thorough history, physical examination, and the results of several tests. A polysomnogram monitors the client's electrophysical responses during sleep. It includes measurements such as brain wave activity (electroencephalogram), muscle movement (electromyogram), and extraocular eye movements (electrooculogram). Many medical centers have specially designed sleep laboratories where clients can be monitored for the quantity, quality, and characteristics of their sleep.

The two basic types of sleep disorders are primary sleep disorders and those related to other conditions, called secondary sleep disorders (Figure 23-5). Primary sleep disorders are thought to be related to abnormal functioning of the sleep-wake or timing mechanisms of the body. The two subdivisions of primary sleep disorders are called the dyssomnias and the parasomnias.

DYSSOMNIAS

Dyssomnias are characterized "by abnormalities in the amount, quality, or timing of sleep" (American Psychiatric Association, 2000). Dyssomnias include problems such as insomnia, hypersomnia, narcolepsy, and breathing-related and circadian rhythm sleep disorders. Insomnia occurs most frequently.

Insomnia is a disorder of falling asleep or maintaining a sound sleep. It is often associated with increased physical and mental alertness at night and sleepiness during the day. The individual who cannot regularly fall asleep often becomes preoccupied and distressed. This contributes to more anxiety about sleep and sets up a vicious cycle in which the harder one "tries" the more difficult it becomes to fall asleep. Often, people are worried, anxious, or concerned about something when they prepare for sleep.

As nights of interrupted sleep continue, one becomes negatively conditioned toward sleep and begins to expect a poor night's sleep. Eventually, chronic insomnia develops and persists long after the problem that caused the initial sleep loss is solved. Chronic insomnia often leads to decreased well-being during waking hours. It is accompanied by a lack of energy or motivation; decreased attention span and poor concentration; and a general worsening of moods and emotional reactions.

Insomnia is relatively rare in childhood and adolescence. Approximately 30% to 40% of adults have problems with insomnia, and the incidence increases with age. It occurs more often in women and usually begins in young adulthood or middle age with an initial period of poor sleep that progressively worsens over a period of months. Some people experience periodic episodes of insomnia. Others develop a chronic ineffective sleep pattern that may last for years. Many have a history of being "light sleepers" who are easily disturbed by environmental noises or other distractions.

Primary hypersomnia is an excessive sleepiness that usually begins between 15 and 30 years of age, slowly progresses over a period of weeks or months, and then becomes chronic and stable. Hypersomnia is characterized by prolonged sleep episodes or daytime sleeping that occurs daily for at least 1 month. Excessive sleepiness severe enough to cause significant impairment of daily living activities and excessive sleepiness that is not caused by any other physical or mental health disorder are also characteristic of hypersomnia.

In persons with hypersomnia, nighttime sleep may last from 8 to 12 hours, but it is often followed by difficulty awakening in the morning and excessive sleepiness during normal waking hours. During the day, these people may take long naps that last for more than 1 hour. After awakening, individuals do not feel refreshed or alert.

Hypersomnia can lead to significant distress in functioning. The long sleep and difficult morning awakenings make it nearly impossible to meet morning business or social obligations. Low levels of alertness result in decreased concentration, poor efficiency, and few memories of the day's events. Unplanned episodes of sleep can lead to embarrassing and even dangerous situations, such as falling asleep while driving. Daytime sleepiness can result in automatic behavior where tasks are carried out with little or no memory of having done them. Sadly, people with excessive sleepiness are often thought of as lazy or indifferent.

Narcolepsy is an uncommon condition in which an individual has repeated attacks of sleep. Symptoms usually become apparent during adolescence, but a careful history often reveals a pattern of sleepiness dating back to preschool years. The onset of the disorder often follows a change in the person's sleep-wake schedule or a very stressful event.

The periods of sleepiness in narcolepsy are described as irresistible. Individuals fall asleep for about 10 to 20 minutes in any situation, whether it is appropriate to sleep or not. Episodes occur from two to six

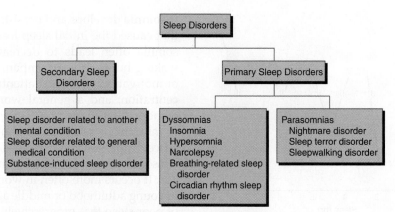

FIGURE **23-5** Classification of sleep disorders.

times per day. Some people with narcolepsy can "fight off" their sleep attacks, whereas others plan naps throughout the day to manage the condition.

Two other distressing features of narcolepsy are cataplexy and inappropriate rapid eye movement. Cataplexy is a sudden episode of muscle weakness and loss of muscle tone that lasts for seconds to minutes. These episodes are often brought about by an intense emotion. **Inappropriate rapid eye movement** occurs during the transition between sleep and wakefulness during which dreamlike hallucinations or paralysis of voluntary muscles occurs.

Breathing-related sleep disorders are more common than once thought. They are defined as sleep disruptions caused by abnormal ventilation during sleep. The most common form is called **obstructive sleep apnea syndrome.** During sleep, a partially obstructed upper airway causes periods of apnea that repeatedly awaken the individual. Sleeping patterns are characterized by periods of loud snoring, followed by periods of apnea lasting as long as 90 seconds. The apneic event ends when the individual gasps, moans, mumbles, or shakes with loud, air-gulping snores. Although the person may not fully awaken during these events, sleep is disrupted enough to result in excessive sleepiness during the day. People who are extremely overweight are at risk for this disorder. The term **pickwickian syndrome** was coined to describe this disorder, based on an obese character in a Charles Dickens novel.

Another dyssomnia is circadian rhythm sleep disorder, a persistent pattern of sleep disruption that results from a mismatch between personal body rhythms and environmental demands. This disorder is most often seen in persons who do shift work or must travel frequently.

Disruptions in sleep can also be caused by physical factors, **restless legs syndrome,** or nocturnal myoclonus. Restless legs syndrome is described as disagreeable sensations, such as pricking, tingling, itching, or crawling, that occur while falling asleep or during sleep. The sensations are relieved by moving the legs or walking and return when the legs are still. Nocturnal myoclonus

is also called idiopathic periodic limb movements. These repeated, brief jerks occur mostly in the legs at the beginning of sleep and decrease during stage 4 NREM sleep. Because the movements take place every 20 to 60 seconds, they disturb normal sleep patterns.

PARASOMNIAS

Sleep disorders characterized by abnormal behavioral or physical events during sleep are called **parasomnias.** It is believed that parasomnia sleep disorders are caused by the inappropriate activation of certain brain centers that govern physical and emotional functions (Hobson and Silvestri, 1999). New research points to a disruption in the body's master clock, located within the brain's hypothalamus (NIMH, 2007a). People with parasomnias most often complain of unusual behaviors during sleep instead of daytime sleepiness. The most common parasomnias are nightmare disorder, sleep terror disorder, and sleepwalking disorder.

The most important feature of **nightmare disorder** is repeated frightening dreams that lead to abrupt awakenings. The individual is fully alert on awakening and significantly distressed from the experience. Awakenings may be accompanied by fight-or-flight responses, such as sweating, rapid respirations, and rapid heartbeat. Often a sense of anxiety lingers after the individual is awake and he or she finds it difficult to return to sleep. The nightmares produce images that are often remembered in detail after awakening.

Sleep terror disorder is repeated nightmares and abrupt awakenings accompanied by a panicky cry or scream and intense fear. During the episode the person cannot be comforted or awakened without difficulty. Usually the individual does not awaken but returns to sleep. There is no memory of the event on awakening. Sleep terrors usually occur only once per night during stages 3 and 4 of NREM sleep. They are often accompanied by the physical signs of intense stress, such as increased heart rate, respirations, and muscle tone.

Sleepwalking disorder is characterized by episodes of complex motor movement during sleep. Individuals who sleepwalk rise from their beds and begin to walk around. They often have a blank stare and are not responsive to communication or efforts to awaken them. If awakened during or after an episode, they remember little about the event and may have a brief period of confusion until they become oriented. Sleepwalking is first seen between the ages of 4 and 8 years. It peaks by about 12 years of age and usually disappears by adolescence. First-time episodes of sleepwalking rarely occur in adults.

OTHER SLEEP DISORDERS

An unusual sleep disorder is gaining attention. **Nocturnal sleep-related eating disorder (NSRED)** is binge eating during sleep. It is "characterized by the rapid and uncontrolled ingestion of food during partial or full awakening from sleep, with variable recall of the episode" (Montgomery, Haynes, and Gardner, 2002). During the sleep-eating episode, the individual quickly consumes a bizarre selection of high-calorie foods and nonfood items, such as cleaning products, animal food, or cigarettes. Diagnosis is difficult because of the client's inability to remember or embarrassment.

Other sleep disorders can be traced to specific causes. These include sleep disorders related to a general medical condition, a mental health condition, or the use of chemical substances. Sleep disorders can result from many physical problems. The presence of a neurological, cardiovascular, or respiratory disorder or an infection has a significant effect on sleep. Pain from musculoskeletal disease and anxiety related to coughing or difficult breathing can lead to prolonged periods of inadequate sleep.

Many mental health disorders are associated with sleep-related problems. Insomnia or hypersomnia is often seen in clients with major depressive, mood, anxiety, adjustment, somatoform, panic, and personality disorders. During flare-ups of schizophrenia, people have significant periods of insomnia.

Sleeping problems can occur during substance use (intoxication) or periods of withdrawal from the substance. Many prescription medications are associated with sleep disorders, including drugs that treat hypertension, cardiac problems, inflammatory processes, neurological conditions, and respiratory diseases. Chemicals such as alcohol, cocaine, and various street drugs affect sleep. Even the medications prescribed to induce sleep (hypnotics and sedatives) produce unwanted effects on the sleep cycle. Nurses and other caregivers must be aware of how various medications and chemicals affect each client's sleep.

GUIDELINES FOR INTERVENTION

The first step in the treatment of sleep disorders is to teach prevention. Because many people do not regularly receive a good night's sleep, the need for good sleep hygiene habits is great. One of the best treatments for insomnia is to establish and maintain a regular sleeping routine by preparing both body and mind for the night's

---

| Box 23-4 | *Sleep Hygiene Strategies* |

Set a regular bedtime and wake-up time, 7 days per week.

Exercise daily; however, vigorous exercise too close to bedtime may make falling asleep difficult.

Schedule time to wind down and relax before bed.

Avoid worrying when trying to fall asleep.

Guard against nighttime interruptions. Earplugs may help with a noisy partner. Heavy window shades help to screen out light. Create a comfortable bed.

Maintain a cool temperature in the room. A warm bath or warm drink before bed often helps.

Excessive hunger or fullness may interfere with sleep. Avoid large meals before bed. If hungry, a light carbohydrate snack may be helpful.

Avoid caffeinated drinks, excessive fluid intake, stimulating drugs, and excessive alcohol in the evening and before bedtime.

Excessive daytime napping may make it difficult for some people to fall asleep at night.

Do not eat, read, work, or watch television in bed. The bed should be used only for sleep and sex.

Maintain a reasonable weight. Excessive weight may result in daytime fatigue and sleep apnea.

Get out of bed and engage in other activities if unable to fall asleep.

From Stuart GW: *Handbook of psychiatric nursing*, ed 6, St. Louis, 2005, Mosby.

---

upcoming rest. Health care providers are in ideal positions to educate clients about the importance of receiving enough quality sleep. Box 23-4 offers several suggestions for developing effective sleep practices.

The main goal of care is to assist the client in obtaining a restful night's sleep. Short-term goals focus on helping clients establish a regular and healthy sleep pattern. Nursing diagnoses for sleep disorders include insomnia, high risk for injury, fatigue, disturbed thought processes, ineffective coping, ineffective breathing pattern, and deficient knowledge related to sleep hygiene practices.

Therapeutic interventions are aimed at promoting comfort, controlling physical disturbances, and maintaining a quiet, restful environment. Hypnotics (sleeping pills) may be administered as ordered, but only after all other methods of inducing sleep have failed. Special care must be taken when administering hypnotics or sedatives to older persons because they react strongly to these classes of medications.

Research has demonstrated that morning bright light therapy improves the sleeping patterns of older adults with dementia by helping reestablish natural biological rhythms (Mishima and others, 1994). Other studies have revealed that the body has a naturally occurring sleep hormone, called **melatonin,** which helps to control our biological clocks. These findings may prove to be promising developments in the treatment of sleep disorders.

Become aware of the importance of keeping the client's environment dark during sleep and brightly lit during daylight hours. Read about the new developments in the treatment of sleeping disorders, and apply them to yourself and your clients. We are learning more every day about the mysteries of sleep.

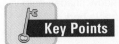

Key Points

- Body image is the collection of perceptions, thoughts, feelings, and behaviors that relate to body size and appearance.
- An eating disorder is an ongoing disturbance in behaviors associated with the ingestion of food.
- The criteria for a diagnosis of an eating disorder are as follows: the problem interferes with a person's quality of daily life; the person does not maintain a normal body weight; there is a distorted significance placed on body weight and shape; and the person engages in inappropriate episodes of eating.
- One of the most serious eating disorders is anorexia nervosa, a condition in which an individual refuses to maintain a normal body weight because of an intense fear of becoming fat.
- Bulimia is a disorder of binge eating and the use of inappropriate methods to prevent weight gain.
- Untreated eating disorders have a high mortality rate.
- Obesity is defined as an excess of body weight. Although not officially classified as an eating disorder, it presents problems for a great number of people.

- The main therapeutic goals for treating all eating disorders are to establish eating behaviors that promote health and to assist clients in identifying and coping with the problems that led to their inappropriate eating behaviors.
- During sleep, body functions and metabolic rate slow. Muscles relax, and the body conserves energy. Renewal and repair of body cells and tissues occur. Sleep also appears to be a critical cycle of brain activity important for learning, memory, and behavioral adaptation.
- Dreaming allows us to gain insights, solve problems, work through emotional reactions, and prepare for the future.
- A sleeping disorder is a condition or problem that repeatedly disrupts an individual's pattern of sleep.
- Dyssomnias are characterized by abnormalities in the amount, quality, or timing of sleep.
- Symptoms of insomnia include a preoccupation with the inability to sleep. This sets up a vicious cycle in which persons become negatively conditioned toward sleep. Chronic insomnia leads to decreased feelings of well-being and a lack of energy or motivation; decreased attention span, energy, and concentration; or worsening of moods and emotional reactions.
- Sleep disorders characterized by abnormal behavioral or physical events during sleep are called parasomnias.
- Sleep disorders can also result from medical, psychological, or drug-induced conditions.
- Therapeutic interventions to promote sleep are to promote comfort, control physical disturbances, and maintain a quiet, restful environment.

---

evolve Be sure to visit the companion Evolve site at http://evolve.elsevier.com/Morrison-Valfre/ for additional online resources.

Objectives

Upon completion of this chapter, the student will be able to:

1. Examine the meaning of the term *self-concept*.
2. Describe the continuum of self-concept responses.
3. Compare the development of self-concept throughout the life cycle.
4. Classify the main characteristics of dissociative disorders.
5. Describe four types of dissociative disorders.
6. Explain the outstanding feature of a dissociative identity (multiple personality) disorder.
7. State the main goal of treatment for clients with dissociative disorders.
8. Plan three nursing diagnoses for clients with dissociative disorders.
9. Develop a care plan for a client who has been diagnosed with a dissociative disorder.

Key Terms

amnesia (ăm-NĒ-zhə) (p. 265)
depersonalization (p. 264)
dissociation (dĭ-SŌ-sē-Ā-shən) (p. 263)
dissociative (dĭ-SŌ-sē-ə-tĭv) **disorder** (p. 264)
dissociative identity disorder (DID) (p. 266)
fugue (fyūg) (p. 264)
identity diffusion (p. 263)
personal identity (p. 261)
self-concept (p. 261)
self-esteem (p. 261)
self-ideal (p. 261)
trance (p. 266)

Human beings differ from animals in a significant way: they have a concept of **self.** As children grow, they learn to identify and define themselves as individuals. They develop a picture (a point of view) of who they are. Then they use that picture as a framework for perceiving, experiencing, and evaluating the world. This point of view becomes one's self-concept.

Self-concept is defined as all the attitudes, notions, beliefs, and convictions that make up a person's self- knowledge. "It includes the individual's perceptions of personal characteristics and abilities, interactions with other people and the environment, values,

associated experiences and objects, and goals and ideals" (Stuart and Laraia, 2005).

The development of self-concept is influenced by many factors. The **culture** into which an individual is born and the **society** in which one lives have a strong impact on self-concept. The attitudes and beliefs of parents, siblings, and other **significant people** influence how an individual defines himself or herself. The **experiences** of life also shape and influence one's picture of the self.

Self-concept is the frame of reference through which people view the world. It is the sum of several components, including **body image** (the attitudes and feelings one has for his or her body), **self-esteem** (an individual's judgment of his or her own worth), **self-ideal** (personal standards of how one should behave), **personal identity** (composite of behavioral traits and characteristics by which one is recognized as an individual), and **role performances** (socially expected behavioral patterns). All these parts of an individual fuse and blend over time into the unique characteristics called self-concept.

CONTINUUM OF SELF-CONCEPT RESPONSES

People behave in a manner based in large part on their self-concepts. The range of behavioral responses relating to self-concept can be seen as occurring on a continuum. At the adaptive end, a healthy self-concept leads one toward self-actualization. Low self-concept results in maladaptive behavioral responses as individuals struggle to define who they are (Figure 24-1).

THE HEALTHY PERSONALITY

Persons with healthy personalities are able to effectively perceive and function within their worlds (Fortinash and Holoday-Worret, 2008). They have achieved a sense of peace and harmony within themselves that allows them to successfully cope with life's anxieties, traumas, and crises. A realistic self-ideal and a clear personal identity help to provide a sense of purpose and direction in life. High self-esteem and confidence levels provide the strength to handle anxieties and learn from life's highs and lows. Socially, they are satisfied with the roles they play in society.

261

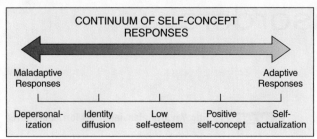

FIGURE **24-1** Continuum of self-concept responses.

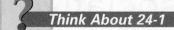

They have the ability to intimately relate to others and to share themselves without fear. In short, individuals with healthy personalities are able to struggle with life's problems while feeling good about living (see Think About 24-1).

SELF-CONCEPT THROUGHOUT THE LIFE CYCLE

Self-concept develops over time, shaped by the influences within one's environment. The theorist Erik Erikson, in describing his eight stages of human development, stated that a psychosocial crisis or core task must be resolved for further personality development. As each task is completed, one's self-concept is affected. Mastery of core tasks builds self-confidence, worth, and esteem (Hockenberry and others, 2007). If, however, one is unable to cope with a core task, ineffective or maladaptive behaviors result. This process, according to Erikson, continues throughout life.

SELF-CONCEPT IN CHILDHOOD

Infants do not view themselves as separate from the rest of the world. Only after a period of time do they begin to distinguish themselves as different from their mothers. Infants learn to **trust** others when their needs are consistently met. After a series of social experiences, they develop stable relationships and learn to feel good about themselves. Rejection by significant others at this time has a strong negative effect on an individual's self-concept.

Toddlers' tasks are to explore the limits of their abilities, and these tasks include the nature of their impact on others. Toddlers become independent by exploring their environments and testing their capabilities. They develop autonomy and a sense of self through experimenting with a variety of behaviors. Actions that get results are effective, even if inappropriate, and they are added to the general knowledge of the child. Behaviors that are not rewarded or do not get results are discarded. In this way, children learn about "right and wrong" and then use this information as a framework for their self-ideal. When parental reactions are routine and consistent, children develop a stable sense of who they are and a stable self-concept. When the reactions of significant others change or differ, children become confused and have

trouble establishing a positive identity and healthy self-concept.

School-age children become aware of different perspectives on life. They learn about social norms, peer pressures, and moral issues. Skill building and broadening social relationships keep them occupied with self-evaluations. Self-concept continues to develop as school-age children assess their skills and interactions with others and form mental pictures of themselves. If the picture is positive, the move into adolescence is graceful; but if self-concept is low or threatened, adolescence is filled with anxiety and turmoil.

SELF-CONCEPT IN ADOLESCENCE

By the early teen years, the comfortable self-concept of childhood is challenged. As adolescents mature, they begin to develop a more complex picture of themselves. Self-concept becomes more individual and based on one's special characteristics rather than on similarities shared by others. Thinking becomes more abstract, and much self-reflection is needed to digest all the physical, emotional, and social changes that are taking place.

During adolescence, self-concept is influenced by many things. Relationships with family and peers play an important role in helping to define teens' confidence levels. The development of a sexual identity and the adjustment to a new adult body image must be included in the new concept of self. The struggle is to define oneself by combining previous roles and new emotions into a reasonably consistent and pleasing sense of self. Without the love, nurturing, and guidance of concerned adults, many teens do not finish the task of developing a comfortable self-concept. They become ill prepared to assume the many responsibilities of adult life because the struggle to find themselves continues.

SELF-CONCEPT IN ADULTHOOD

Adults with strong, positive self-concepts can freely explore their environments because they have a background of success and effectiveness. Positive experiences further enhance self-concept, and the cycle of learning, succeeding, and growth repeats itself.

If the concept of oneself is low or negative, individuals develop views of themselves as inadequate or unable. They become easily threatened, which in turn increases anxiety levels. High anxiety forces them to become preoccupied with defending themselves. Soon this cycle becomes a way of life. Individuals find themselves caught in the trap of looking only at the negative or "down" side of life. The cycle of few successes and negative reinforcement becomes established, which reinforces a poor self-concept. Most adults, however, function somewhere between these two extremes.

SELF-CONCEPT IN OLDER ADULTHOOD

Self-concept is established in childhood, developed in adolescence, strengthened in adulthood, and refined in older adulthood. In later life, many occurrences and situations can threaten a positive self-concept. **Ageism,** the stereotyping of older persons as feeble, dependent, and nonproductive, contributes to older adults' self-concepts. Threats to the stability of one's lifestyle, such as changes in occupation, social standing, or environment, often lead to changes in self-concept. Health care providers can enhance older clients' feelings of self-worth through active listening and demonstrations of concern.

DISSOCIATIVE DISORDERS

Dissociation is an attempt to cope with deep-seated emotional anxiety or distress. Low self-esteem is a problem for many persons. It involves feelings of being weak, inadequate, and helpless. Usually, low self-esteem is expressed through various levels of anxiety. Low self-esteem is a common component of many mental health problems. Feelings of self-rejection and dislike are expressed through various behaviors (Box 24-1).

Identity diffusion is the failure to bring various childhood identifications into an effective adult personality. Individuals with identity diffusion are not sure who they really are because they have been unable to build a "picture" of themselves. They drift through life, like a boat without a rudder, unable to set a course or steer around obstacles.

Although these people feel emptiness and anxiety, they often exploit others. Feelings of empathy are often lacking. This leads to problems with intimacy and a lack of caring. Because the self-ideal is confused, moral codes or standards of behavior are often missing (Keltner, Schwecke, and Bostrom, 2007). Frequently, they are so desperate to define themselves that they attempt to bind their self-concepts to another. This type of identity diffusion is called **personality fusing.** When behaviors interfere with an individual's ability to function, a mental health problem exists. The mental health problems that relate to anxiety and self-concept are called the dissociative disorders.

CHARACTERISTICS

Dissociation is an "interruption of a person's fundamental mental aspects of waking consciousness" (National Alliance for the Mentally Ill, 2003). It is a complex

---

Box 24-1 *Behaviors Associated With Low Self-Esteem*

CRITICISM OF SELF AND OTHERS
"Doomed to failure" outlook; negative thinking
Sees normal life stresses as impossible barriers

DECREASED PRODUCTIVITY
Does not complete tasks; works below level of actual abilities
Postpones decisions

DENIES SELF PLEASURE
Feels need to be punished, so refuses pleasure
Rejects personal strengths and assets

DESTRUCTIVE TOWARD SELF AND OTHERS
May displace self-hate onto others
Becomes accident prone or engages in dangerous activities
Suicide is ultimate act of self-rejection

DISTURBED INTERPERSONAL RELATIONSHIPS
Exploits others
May be demeaning, cruel, withdrawn, or isolated

EXAGGERATED SENSE OF SELF-IMPORTANCE
Makes up for low self-esteem with grandiose thinking; may boast, brag, or describe special abilities
Sets unrealistic goals; has unrealistic dreams

FEELINGS OF GUILT, INADEQUACY, AND WORRY
Uses destructive activities to punish self
Rejects self through nightmares, obsessions, phobias, or reliving of distressing memories
Is irritable and easily angered

NEGATIVE OUTLOOK ABOUT ONE'S BODY, ABILITIES, AND LIFE
Has polarized view of life; everything is either right or wrong, good or bad
Rejects aspects of self that have potential for growth and refuses to consider real strengths and assets
Has physical complaints and problems

WITHDRAWAL
Becomes socially isolated
May withdraw from reality when anxiety of self-rejection reaches severe levels
May have delusions, hallucinations, dissociation, jealousy, suspicion, paranoia

Modified from Stuart GW, Laraia MT: *Principles and practice of psychiatric nursing,* ed 8, St. Louis, 2005, Mosby.

---

neuropsychological process that ranges from normal, everyday experiences to those that disrupt daily living. Dissociation is a common, natural experience. Examples of normal dissociations are daydreaming or becoming so absorbed in an activity that one loses a sense of time and surroundings. Dissociation is also used as a coping mechanism to protect us from trauma. The victim of a mugging or severe accident is often unable to remember events surrounding the incident. Individuals who were abused in childhood may have only a few small, unrelated memories.

Children dissociate more easily than adults do. Faced with overwhelming abuse or trauma, children often psychologically flee their distresses by blocking emotionally damaging information from awareness. Dissociation, when used as a defense in childhood, can later grow into a dissociative disorder.

A dissociative disorder is a disturbance in the normally interacting functions of consciousness: identity, memory, and perception. The most anxiety-producing aspects of the self are walled off or split from the remainder of the personality in an attempt to cope with severe anxiety or emotional trauma.

Although dissociative disorders were once considered rare, new evidence reveals that they are becoming more common in the United States, especially in those who were neglected or abused in childhood. Dissociative disorders are diagnosed more frequently in women.

In countries such as Japan, England, and France, the incidence of diagnosed dissociative disorders is low. In other cultures, dissociative trances are a part of religious or spiritual practices. Devout people enter into altered states or trances in which they interact with spirits or beings. Care providers who work with clients from different cultural backgrounds must be alert to the customs and practices of the culture. Several interesting culturally defined mental health disorders involving dissociative states are described in Table 24-1.

When the disturbance of a dissociative disorder occurs primarily with memory or consciousness, amnesia or fugue (inability to remember important personal events or travels) results. If the disturbance is with one's identity, parts of the self assume separate personalities, and a dissociative identity (multiple personality) disorder is diagnosed. Posttraumatic stress disorder, although considered an anxiety disorder, is actually a recall of past traumatic events alternating with detachment or dissociation. Traumatic experiences are the basis of all dissociative disorders. Behaviors are the result of repeated splitting of traumatic memories. Just as the body walls off the infection of an abscess, the mind walls off the extreme distresses of trauma and anxiety. Four types of dissociative disorders are classified by the *Diagnostic and Statistical Manual of Mental Disorders* (DSM-IV-TR). They are depersonalization disorder, amnesia, fugue, and identity disorder.

DEPERSONALIZATION DISORDER

During an episode of depersonalization, one feels detached or unconnected to the self. The individual may feel like a robot, working on automatic. There may be a sensation of being an outside observer and of not being involved. Depersonalization is a response to severe anxiety associated with a blocking of awareness and a fading of reality. One is unable to tell the difference between internal and external stimuli because the self-concept becomes disorganized. The body takes on an unreal quality, and the world becomes a dream.

Depersonalization serves as a defense mechanism. However, it does nothing to relieve the cause of the distress, so it soon becomes a maladaptive behavior. In cases in which depersonalization becomes a mental health problem, individuals attempt to "escape" distress and anxiety by losing their identities. Table 24-2 lists the physical, emotional, intellectual, and behavioral characteristics of this behavioral pattern.

Depersonalization is commonly associated with other mental disorders, including acute stress disorder,

Table 24-1 *Cultural Aspects: Culturally Defined Mental Health Disorders With Dissociative States*

DISORDER	CULTURE(S)	DESCRIPTION
Amok	Malaysia, Laos, Philippines, Polynesia, Puerto Rico, Navajo	Period of brooding followed by outbursts of aggressive, violent behavior; found only in males
Ataque de nervios	Latinos	Uncontrollable shouting, crying, fainting, and suicidal gestures following stressful event
Falling out	Southern United States, Caribbean groups	Sudden collapse; eyes are open, but individual is unable to see; hears and understands but feels powerless to move
Latah	Japan *(imu)*, Philippines *(mali-mali)*, Thailand	Excessive reactions to sudden fright; trancelike behavior with command obedience, echolalia
Pibloktoq	Arctic and subarctic Eskimos	Extreme excitement and irrational behavior followed by seizures and coma lasting up to 12 hr
Qi-gong psychotic reaction	Chinese	Acute episode of psychotic behaviors following folk practice of *Qi Gong*, the exercise of vital energy
Shin-byung	Korean	Anxiety and somatic complaints that progress to dissociation and possession by ancestral spirits
Spell	African-American, European, Americans from southern United States	Trance in which communication with deceased relatives or spirits takes place
Zar	Egypt, Ethiopia, Iran, Sudan	Spirit possession that interferes with daily activities; may develop long-term relationship with spirit and withdraw from reality

Modified from American Psychiatric Association: *Diagnostic and statistical manual of mental disorders*, ed 4, text revision, Washington, DC, 2000, The Association.

panic disorder, obsessive-compulsive disorder, and schizophrenia. These mental health problems can suddenly develop after a life-threatening event or develop slowly following years of distress.

DISSOCIATIVE AMNESIA

Amnesia is a loss of memory. Dissociative amnesia is characterized by an inability to remember personal information that cannot be explained by ordinary forgetfulness. It is an attempt to avoid extreme stress by blocking memories from consciousness. Individuals with dissociative amnesia usually have gaps in their ability to recall certain events during their childhood. Most of these memory lapses relate to extremely stressful events. For example, a rape victim often has no memory of the attack but still experiences the emotional numbness and depression associated with the trauma. Sights, sounds, odors, and images can trigger emotional distresses long after the event has occurred. Actual memories are too painful to consider, so they stay submerged—walled off but still capable of inflicting pain.

These clients require high levels of emotional support. Client safety becomes a primary therapeutic goal because suicide attempts are common. Although memory may be gone, the emotional distress still remains. Clients' connections with other human beings are sometimes the only link on the road back to mental health.

DISSOCIATIVE FUGUE

One of the most interesting dissociative disorders is the rare, but dramatic, amnesic fugue. The word *fugue* means an escape from reality. The main characteristic of dissociative fugue is sudden, unexpected travel with an inability to recall the past. A fugue occurs in response to an overwhelmingly stressful or traumatic event. It is an extreme expression of the fight-or-flight mechanism, engaged to protect the individual.

Persons with dissociative fugue may travel from a few miles away from home to another continent. Individuals behave quite normally during periods of travel but are confused about their personal identities, which is what frequently brings them to the attention of authorities. Some individuals assume entirely new identities, complete with a new occupation and new significant others. Case Study 24-1 describes an interesting case of fugue.

During an actual fugue, few personality changes are noticeable. Individuals may be more friendly and outgoing, but their behaviors remain appropriate. After the return to the prefugue state, individuals may experience aggressive impulses, conflict, depression, guilt, and suicidal wishes. There may be loss of memory of

Case Study 24-1

Amy was only 3 years old when she was first abused by her father. By 4 years old, she was hiding whenever she heard his footsteps coming down the hall. By 6 years old, Amy slipped out the window to escape. On those occasions when he could not be avoided, Amy played a game in her mind in which she would fly away to a land where everyone was kind and carried no evil. She would wish and dream and hope during those times, ignoring the pain and distress of being repeatedly molested.

By the time Amy was 13 years old, she had run away from home. Luckily, she found a youth shelter early in her wanderings where staff members were understanding and had a genuine interest in seeing Amy survive her adolescence. She stayed at the shelter for about 7 months, learning the skills needed for adulthood. Soon Amy became very efficient in coordinating and supervising the daily household events.

Because of her newly learned organizational abilities, Amy was offered a job as a teacher's assistant at the local grade school. There she remained for many years. By the time she was 30 years old, Amy had buried the memories of her abuse and forgotten the pain of her childhood. She was married and looking forward to a bright future.

Amy's father became seriously ill the following year. He was alone and in need of care. After no communications with Amy in 20 years, he wrote to ask if he could come and live with Amy and her family.

The letter arrived, and Amy stared, horrified, at the return address. Six months later, she remembers nothing more: not the trip to San Francisco, not the bus ride to Colorado, not even her new fiancé. Today she can hardly remember who she really is.

- What happened after Amy read the return address on the letter?
- If Amy were admitted to your unit, what psychosocial interventions would you include in the care plan?

Table 24-2	**Behaviors Associated With Depersonalization**	
AREAS OF FUNCTIONING	**DESCRIPTION**	
Affective (emotional)	Feels identity is lost	
	Lacks sense of inner togetherness	
	Unable to feel pleasure or pride	
	Feelings of detachment, fear, insecurity, shame, unreality	
Behavioral (social)	Affect blunted; emotionally unresponsive and passive; not lively or spontaneous	
	Communications odd or difficult to follow	
	Loss of drive, decision-making abilities, impulse control	
	Social isolation and withdrawal	
Cognitive (intellectual)	Confusion; distorted thinking and memory	
	Impaired judgment; disoriented to time	
Perceptual (physical)	Dreamlike experiences of world	
	Difficulty telling self from others	
	Disturbed body image and sexuality	
	May experience auditory and visual hallucinations	

Modified from Stuart GW, Laraia MT: *Principles and practice of psychiatric nursing,* ed 8, St. Louis, 2005, Mosby.

the events that occurred during the time of the fugue. Recovery is usually rapid, but some amnesia may remain. Psychosocial care and emotional support are important elements in recovery.

DISSOCIATIVE TRANCE DISORDER

A trance is defined as a state resembling sleep in which consciousness remains but voluntary movement is lost. In many cultures, trances are expressions of spiritual or religious beliefs. Cultural trances are entered into voluntarily and cause no distress or harm to the individuals. Channelers, psychics, spirit guides, shamans, and the like rarely suffer from mental impairments. Cultural influences also have an impact on the type of trance, the associated sensory disturbances, and the behaviors exhibited during the trance. **Culturally normative trances** involve signs, symptoms, and behaviors that are expected by other members of the culture. During these trances, individuals do not lose their identities.

Possession trances involve the appearance of one or more distinct identities that direct the individual to perform sometimes complex behaviors and activities, such as culturally appropriate conversations, gestures, or facial expressions. Amnesia following either type of trance state is not uncommon, but it occurs more frequently with possession trances.

A **dissociative trance disorder** exists when trances cause "clinically significant distress or functional impairment" (American Psychiatric Association, 2000). Dissociative trance disorders are listed in the DSM-IV-TR in the category of "diagnoses in need of further study." However, the fact remains that if trances cause a great deal of anxiety and distress in an individual, he or she can likely benefit from psychotherapeutic interventions.

DISSOCIATIVE IDENTITY DISORDER

When stress or trauma is repeated and severe, the personality attempts to protect itself. Abused children use dissociation to escape and defend themselves from the anxiety, trauma, and helplessness of reality. Major studies have confirmed that dissociative identity disorders are the result of severe physical, sexual, or emotional abuse.

A dissociative identity disorder (DID) is defined as the presence of two or more identities or personalities that repeatedly take control of the individual's behavior. DID develops as a defense against prolonged and inescapable trauma. The diagnosis of DID, which was formerly called "multiple personality disorder," occurs more often in the United States than other countries. Some mental health professionals think that this is a result of better diagnostic tools, whereas others think that DID is overdiagnosed or view it as a culturally related syndrome.

The essential features of DID are associated with the presence of other personalities in one individual.

Individuals with DID often have a personal history full of time losses, unexplained possessions or changes in relationships, out-of-body experiences, and the awareness of other parts of the self. A history of abuse or trauma is not always identified because emotions are deeply buried.

When different personalities do emerge, each has its own way of thinking about and relating to the world. Each personality is unique and often represents the individual at different developmental stages. The identities may be helpful, controlling, seductive, or destructive, but each serves a specific protective purpose. They may differ in age, gender, knowledge, state of health, speech, and behaviors. The primary personality (called the **host**) may or may not be aware of the presence of the other personalities (called **alters**). Usually the transition from one personality to the other is sudden and related to stress. Sometimes the identities cooperate with each other, but more often they attempt to take control and refuse to share knowledge with the others. Hostility or open conflict can result among the more powerful personalities.

Individuals with dissociative problems, especially DID, often have symptoms of posttraumatic stress syndrome (nightmares, flashbacks, extreme startle responses). Other mental or physical health problems are frequently present, especially with some of the identities found in DID. The main goal of treatment is to help the client integrate or combine the personalities into one functional individual, capable of coping with life's stresses in a healthy manner.

THERAPEUTIC INTERVENTIONS

Treatment for dissociative disorders involves long-term therapy in an outpatient setting. Hospitalization is required in only three situations:
1. When anger, aggression, or violence is directed toward self or others and presents a danger
2. When individuals are unable to function because of memory loss, rapid switching between identities, flashbacks, or overwhelming emotions
3. When medications need to be evaluated or adjusted

The stages of treatment for dissociative disorders relate to assessment, stabilization, and reworking past traumas. The most effective results are seen when clients are able to work with stable, established multidisciplinary treatment teams.

TREATMENTS AND THERAPIES

Therapy for clients with dissociative disorders begins with assessment and stabilization. Because the work of coping with deeply seated trauma is difficult and emotionally demanding, an environment in which clients can safely examine their conflicts must first be established. A careful assessment includes the client's history, symptoms, support systems, medical status, relationships, and problems, and the presence of substance abuse and sleeping or eating disorders. Family history should include both the family of origin and the current family situation. Videotaping the alters often results in more diagnostic information.

During the stabilization phase, the diagnosis is established as the client gradually reveals the complexities of his or her nature. After each treatment team member assesses the client, a plan for stabilization is jointly developed. Therapies are carefully chosen and may include individual psychotherapy, group therapy, family therapy, psychoeducation, and various expressive therapies, such as art, poetry, and dance. Contracts to ensure safety during therapy are established. During this time, clients and care providers develop trust in each other and build client support networks. Although this part of treatment may last for more than 1 year, it is an essential step for the work to come.

The next phase of treatment involves revisiting and reworking past traumas. Once the client develops an awareness of other personalities and their purposes, the painful material is slowly and gently analyzed. Each identity is treated equally with respect and is encouraged to communicate with the others. Feelings of shame, guilt, anger, and grief are encountered as each traumatic event is relived. With time, patience, and hard work, the client eventually begins to integrate or combine the personalities into a unique individual who is able to effectively cope with life's stressors. This is the main treatment goal for clients with dissociative disorders.

Pharmacological Therapy

No specific medication exists at this time to treat amnesia, fugues, or other dissociative behaviors. Treatment is often based on symptoms. If high anxiety is apparent, antianxiety agents may be prescribed. When depression is intense, an antidepressant may be ordered. If hallucinations or delusions are commonly present, an antipsychotic medication may be administered. All medications are prescribed for only short periods to encourage the use of inner coping skills.

Nursing (Therapeutic) Process

As with all other mental health clients, assessments are routinely performed. Clients with dissociative disorders can present different pictures to various staff members to manipulate and divide their care providers. They may offer one side of themselves during one minute, and then, in the next moment, a personality that wants to pick a fight emerges. Assessments should describe the client's behaviors, communications, anxiety, depression, social functioning, and the presence of amnesia (Shives, 2008). A much clearer picture is given with descriptions than with psychiatric "buzz words" or jargon.

Nursing diagnoses for clients with dissociative disorders are related to self-concept responses and depend on the identified problems of each client. The expected outcome for each diagnosis is a client who is able to obtain his or her maximum level of effective functioning and self-actualization. Primary or main nursing diagnoses include disturbed personal identity, disturbed body image, low self-esteem, and ineffective role performance. Refer to Box 24-2 for examples.

After clients have established trust with the staff, interventions are directed at helping them examine their situations and related feelings within an environment of safety and support. This process assists the growth of personal insight, which is the first step toward making behavioral changes. A problem-solving approach helps clients to gradually expand self-awareness, explore and evaluate the self, and eventually plan for actions that result in behavior changes. Clients are emotionally supported and encouraged to actively take part in therapy.

Some clients with dissociative disorders engage in self-destructive behaviors. They may cut, bite, or repeatedly hit themselves or pull out their hair. Self-destructive behavior is of great concern, and several interventions have been devised to assist clients in achieving control over these behaviors.

First, clients must be routinely assessed for self-destructive thoughts. The easiest way to find out if such thoughts are occurring is to ask the client. Contracts and agreements between client and staff help staff and client to develop trust in the therapeutic relationship and

---

Box 24-2 *NANDA-I Nursing Diagnoses Related to Dissociative Disorders*

Anxiety
Behavior, risk-prone health*
Body image, disturbed
Coping, ineffective
Denial, ineffective
Environmental interpretation syndrome, impaired
Family processes, interrupted
Fear
Hopelessness
Memory, impaired*
Personal identity, disturbed*
Powerlessness
Role performance, ineffective
Self-esteem, low, chronic
Self-mutilation, risk for
Social interaction, impaired
Social isolation*
Violence, risk for self-directed

Data from NANDA International: *NANDA-I nursing diagnoses: definitions and classification 2007-2008*, Philadelphia, 2007, NANDA International. *NANDA-I*, NANDA International.
*Primary nursing diagnoses for dissociative disorders.

■

environment. During the admission process, ways of dealing with destructive behaviors should be discussed with the client. If necessary, one-to-one support is provided until the client can achieve self-control.

If the client is willing, a daily journal of thoughts and feelings is kept. This practice has been found to be a helpful self-control activity. Care providers should be limited to a few personnel to provide a stable therapeutic environment (see Sample Client Care Plan 24-1).

The care and treatment of individuals with dissociative problems are complex, time consuming, and

challenging. Individuals diagnosed with dissociative disorders are suffering from one of the worst human fears—not knowing oneself and being out of control of oneself. Although behaviors may be odd, unusual, or dramatic, each serves a purpose and communicates something about the person. Health care providers are challenged with the twin tasks of accepting and understanding the messages sent by dissociated individuals. Treatment of clients with backgrounds of trauma is often frustrating. At the same time, it can be an extremely rewarding experience.

SAMPLE CLIENT CARE PLAN 24-1

Maladaptive Self-Concept

ASSESSMENT *History.* Christine is a 35-year-old wife and mother of three children, 15, 10, and 7 years old. Although she experienced severe sexual and physical abuse as a child, she has managed to complete college, marry, and raise her family. She is being admitted to the clinic's mental health services for "several episodes of losing myself" that she has experienced in the past 5 months.

Current Findings. A well-groomed woman who is distressed because she was unable to remember to pick up her daughter's dress at the cleaners yesterday. Because of this, her daughter refused to attend the school dance and threatened to run away. Lately Christine has felt like an "outside observer of my own life," "like a robot on automatic." During these episodes she is aware of reality but feels as though everything is mechanical. She feels that she may be "going insane" because the "spells" are becoming more and more frequent since her daughter has begun dating.

Multidisciplinary Diagnosis	*Planning/Goals*
Disturbed personal identity related to increased anxiety and past history of abuse	Christine will decrease the number of depersonalization episodes to fewer than one per week by May 20. Christine will be able to recognize her anxiety and take steps to decrease it before it progresses to a depersonalization episode.

Therapeutic Interventions

Intervention	Rationale	Team Member
1. Establish therapeutic relationship; confirm her identity; support adaptive behaviors, identify strengths.	Provides a way of offering emotional support; builds trust; supports current adaptive behaviors.	All
2. Assist Christine in describing thoughts and feelings.	Identification is the first step toward focused change.	All
3. Identify stresses that bring about her "spells."	Known stressors can be handled more effectively.	Psy, Nsg
4. Help to clarify faulty beliefs about self.	Builds confidence; helps focus energies in positive direction.	All
5. Encourage Christine to make a plan for decreasing her anxiety during times her daughter is on a date; role-play mother-daughter roles.	Recalling and using successful strategies help to decrease anxiety levels, thus preventing depersonalization episodes.	Psy, Nsg
6. Reinforce strengths, assets, and problem-solving abilities; encourage Christine to focus on her "positives."	Helps to improve coping abilities and ease the pain of feeling powerless.	All

Evaluation

Christine was able to decrease her episodes of depersonalization to less than one per week by May 29.

? CRITICAL THINKING QUESTIONS

1. In what ways will long-term therapy benefit Christine?

2. How would care providers go about helping Christine identify stressors in her daily life?

A complete client care plan includes several other diagnoses and interventions.
Psy, Psychologist; *Nsg,* nursing staff.

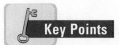
Key Points

- Self-concept is defined as all the attitudes, notions, beliefs, and convictions that make up an individual's self-knowledge. It develops over time, shaped by one's developmental level and environmental influences.
- The continuum of self-concept responses ranges from a low self-concept, which results in maladaptive behavioral responses, to a healthy self-concept, which leads one toward self-actualization.
- Self-concept develops over time and is shaped by the influences within one's environment.
- Infants learn to trust others when their needs are consistently met.
- Toddlers develop autonomy by exploring their environments and testing their capabilities.
- School-age children assess their skills and interactions with others and form mental pictures of themselves.
- The adolescent's struggle is to define oneself by combining previous roles and new emotions into a consistent sense of self.
- Adults with strong, positive self-concepts can freely explore their environments. Those with low self-concepts view themselves as inadequate or unable.
- Many occurrences and situations can threaten a positive self-concept of older adults.

- Low self-esteem is a common component of many mental health problems.
- Identity diffusion is the failure to bring various childhood identifications into an effective adult personality.
- Dissociation is an interruption of a person's fundamental aspects of waking consciousness.
- Dissociative amnesia is characterized by an inability to remember personal information that cannot be explained by ordinary forgetfulness.
- The main characteristic of a dissociative fugue is sudden, unexpected travel, with an inability to recall the past.
- A trance is a state resembling sleep in which consciousness remains but voluntary movement is lost.
- A dissociative identity disorder (DID) is defined as the presence of two or more identities or personalities that repeatedly take control of the individual's behavior.
- Treatment for dissociative disorders involves long-term psychodynamic/cognitive therapy.
- There are no specific psychotherapeutic drugs for the treatment of dissociative disorders.
- Therapeutic interventions for clients with dissociative disorders focus on safety, trust, communication, and problem solving.

evolve   Be sure to visit the companion Evolve site at http://evolve.elsevier.com/Morrison-Valfre/ for additional online resources.

25 Anger and Aggression

evolve http://evolve.elsevier.com/Morrison-Valfre/

Objectives

Upon completion of this chapter, the student will be able to:

1. Explain the differences among anger, aggression, and assertiveness.
2. Describe how anger is expressed by children, adolescents, young adults, and older adults.
3. Examine the impact of anger and aggression on society.
4. Compare three theories that attempt to explain the causes of aggression.
5. Describe each of the five stages of the assault cycle.
6. Explain the main characteristics for three mental health disorders that relate to anger or aggression.
7. Outline the process for assessing clients who are angry or aggressive.
8. Develop four therapeutic interventions for clients who are experiencing anger or acting aggressively.
9. Consider seven techniques for recognizing and coping with your own anger.

Key Terms

acting out (p. 271)
aggression (ə-GRĔSH-ən) (p. 270)
anger (p. 270)
assault (p. 271)
assertiveness (p. 271)
battery (p. 271)
impulse control (p. 271)
intermittent explosive (Ĭn-tĕr-MĬT-ĕnt ĕk-SPLŌ-sĭv)
   disorder (p. 275)
passive aggression (p. 271)
violence (p. 271)

Anger is a normal emotional response to a perceived threat, frustration, or distressing event. It commonly occurs in reaction to feeling threatened or losing control. Anger is felt, experienced, suffered, and expressed in many ways. In a crisis situation, anger is often one of the first coping behaviors employed.

Anger can be directed outward through aggressive or violent behaviors, or it may be expressed through passive-aggressive behaviors. Anger can also be focused onto oneself. Some individuals turn their anger inward and become suicidal or depressed. Some live bouncing between aggression and helplessness, whereas others channel their anger into physical complaints and

problems. Figure 25-1 illustrates the continuum of anger responses.

Anxiety and loss of control are associated with anger. Anger can include feelings of hopelessness, powerlessness, and regret. It can arise intentionally as one "stews" about an event or situation, or it can result from unplanned circumstances. People tend to label anger as justified or unjustified according to their personal values. Anger can be rational and planned, or it can arrive in a blind fury of irrational rage.

Anger serves several purposes. It can be used as a **coping mechanism** to meet needs. According to Maslow's hierarchy (ladder) of human needs, when basic needs are threatened a person may react with anger. The client who feels powerless at the news of his prolonged recovery may react by insulting others, or the child who flies into temper tantrums may be attempting to meet basic needs.

People can be **motivated** or encouraged to act by anger. Consider the college student who, as a child, felt the anxiety and helplessness of watching her mother being abused. Now she studies to become a lawyer and champion of abused people. In this case, the use of anger motivated positive actions.

Table 25-1 lists many expressions of anger. Many of the listed emotions and actions are appropriate expressions of anger. However, when anger provides the motivation for inappropriate behaviors or violence, it becomes defined as a problem.

Aggression is a forceful attitude or action that is expressed physically, symbolically, or verbally. Passive aggression involves indirect expressions of anger through subtle, evasive, or manipulative behaviors. Acting out is the use of inappropriate, detrimental, or destructive behaviors to express current or past emotions.

Aggressive behaviors often are the result of angry feelings that are converted into action and expressed. Socially approved aggression is a basic element of many sports, such as football, hockey, and soccer (Stuart and Laraia, 2005). Aggressive behavior is socially approved for certain groups, such as news people hot on the trail of some developing story. However, aggressive behaviors become inappropriate when they affect other people or their possessions. Several terms describe the characteristics of anger (Box 25-1). The legal concepts of assault and battery were established to define inappropriate aggression and to protect people from those who act on their emotions in ways that are threatening to others.

Finally, the term **assertiveness** defines the quality for which we strive. Assertiveness is the ability to directly express one's feelings or needs in a way that respects the rights of other people yet retains one's dignity.

ANGER AND AGGRESSION IN SOCIETY

Anger and its expressions have a strong impact on a society. The histories of many cultures are peppered with accounts of uprisings and wars. Children were often sacrificed to the gods to keep them from becoming angry. Cultural expressions of anger differ, and care providers need the ability to recognize the signs of anger in the cultural groups with whom they work (see Cultural Considerations 25-1).

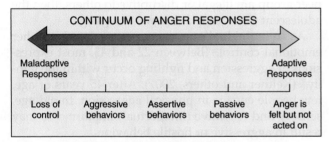

FIGURE **25-1** Continuum of anger responses.

GENDER AGGRESSION

"Violence against wives has been tolerated since the beginning of history" (Landers, Jacobs, and Siegel, 1995). Ancient and well-accepted beliefs that men were superior led to values that supported the abuse of women. Beatings and floggings of women were accepted practices throughout ancient Greek and Roman societies. By the fourteenth century, it was legal in France for a man to beat his wife as long as he did not maim or kill her. In 1427, a nobleman encouraged his fellow Italians to treat their wives with as much concern and consideration as they did their livestock and fowl.

Box 25-1 *Terms Relating to Anger*

Expressions of anger depend on **impulse control**, the ability to express one's emotions in appropriate or effective ways.

Acting out is the use of inappropriate or destructive behaviors to express emotions.

Passive aggression involves indirect expressions of anger through subtle, evasive, or manipulative behaviors.

Violence is behavior that threatens or harms other people or their property. A violent act is actions of force that result in abuse or harm.

Assault is a legal term that describes any behavior that presents an immediate threat to another person.

Battery is the unlawful use of force on a person without his or her consent.

Table 25-1 *Expressions of Anger*

TURNED OUTWARD		TURNED INWARD	
OVERT ANGER	**PASSIVE AGGRESSION**	**SUBJECTIVE**	**OBJECTIVE**
Verbalization of anger	Impatience	Feeling upset	Crying
Irritation	Sulking	Tension	Self-destructive behavior
Pacing with agitation	Frustration	Unhappiness	Self-mutilation
Swearing	Tense facial expressions	Feeling hurt	Substance abuse
Hostility	Pessimism	Disappointment	Suicide
Contempt	Resentment	Guilt	
Clenched fists	Jealousy	Feelings of inferiority	
Insulting remarks	Bitterness	Low self-esteem	
Intimidation	Complaining	Sense of failure	
Bragging about violent acts	Deceptive sweetness	Humiliation	
Provoking behaviors	Unreasonableness	Somatic symptoms	
Sadistic acts	Intolerance	Feeling harassed	
Maliciousness	Resistance	Envy	
Verbal abuse	Stubbornness	Feeling violated	
Temper tantrums	Intentional forgetting	Feeling alienated	
Violation of others' rights	Noncompliance	Feeling demoralized	
Screaming	Procrastination	Feeling depressed	
Deviance	Antagonism	Resignation	
Rage	Belittling remarks	Powerlessness	
Argumentativeness	Sarcasm	Helplessness	
Overt defiance	Fault finding	Hopelessness	
Threats: words or weapons	Manipulation	Desperation	
Damage to property	Power struggles	Apathy	
Assault	Unfair teasing		
Rape	Sabotage of others		
Homicide	Domination		

From Keltner NL, Schwecke LH, Bostrom CE: *Psychiatric nursing*, ed 5, St. Louis, 2007, Mosby.

In nineteenth-century America, the high incidence of violence against women and children became unacceptable. By 1871, states began to enact statutes that denied the husband's right to physically abuse his wife. Today in the United States, wives can legally sue their husbands for abusing them. However, the problems of violence against women and children continue to occur throughout the world far too often.

Gender aggression and abuse are still practiced everywhere. Many aggressive acts against women are centered around the concepts of virginity and fidelity. Young women in parts of Africa and the Middle East are forced to undergo circumcision and other mutilating genital surgeries. Women of all ages can suffer from the effects of gender violence (Table 25-2).

AGGRESSION THROUGHOUT THE LIFE CYCLE

Expressions of anger begin in infancy and end with death. Infants express unmet needs through diffuse rage reactions with "loud, uncontrollable crying and screaming, profuse perspiration, difficulty in breathing (sometimes turning blue), and flailing of arms and legs" (Keltner, Schwecke, and Bostrom, 2007).

Toddlers engage in temper tantrums (Figure 25-2) where they learn to focus their aggression on the person or thing they believe is responsible for their anger (Potter and Perry, 2009). Toddlers observe the behaviors of others in their environment and pattern their own actions after them. If toddlers observe shouting, fighting, or other forms of aggression, they understand that aggressive behaviors are acceptable.

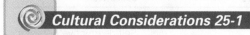

Cultural Considerations 25-1

Koreans express anger and other distresses by becoming physically ill.
Asian individuals may smile when angry.
Filipino people may react to anger by becoming passive aggressive.

In some families, a show of aggression is encouraged in children as a way of teaching them to "stand up for their rights." Television is another source of aggression. Many studies have shown that violence on television has a direct effect on the children who watch the programs (Hockenberry and others, 2007).

During preschool years, children often direct their anger toward others, especially peers or younger children. Children in the early school-age years assault or hit each other frequently. By preadolescence most children stop hitting and learn to channel their aggression into physical activities, such as competitive sports or physical conditioning. Slander, gossip, and practical jokes provide other outlets for aggressive feelings during the school years. However, bullying is becoming an increasing problem in schools today.

By adolescence, fighting is organized, controlled, and purposeful. The peer group becomes the greatest source of influence on the teen. If the activities of the peer group are illegal or disruptive to others, then the adolescent peer group is known as a **gang.**

As an individual's age increases, so does his or her emotional control. "Between 22 and 45, most expressions of aggression and fighting occur within the family" (Keltner and others, 2007). After 45 years of age, few people engage in physical aggression. In old age, sensory and cognitive (intellectual) impairments may result in aggressive or hostile behaviors.

SCOPE OF THE PROBLEM TODAY

Today aggression and violence are worldwide concerns. Wife beating is still common in many countries. In Papua New Guinea almost 67% of wives suffer from abuse. In the United States, 4,266,000 violent crimes were reported in 1999. Homicide (murder) is the tenth leading cause of death for all citizens. Injuries are the second leading cause of death for American Indians. For black males and 5- to 15-year-old children, murder was the third leading cause of death (U.S. Census Bureau, 2001).

Statistics are impressive, but they cannot tell the stories of how aggression and violence have changed

Table 25-2 *Gender Violence Throughout the Life Cycle*

PHASE	TYPE OF VIOLENCE PRESENT
Prebirth	Sex-selective abortion (China, India, Republic of Korea); battering during pregnancy (emotional and physical effects on woman; effects on birth outcome); forced pregnancy (e.g., mass rape in war)
Infancy	Female infanticide; emotional and physical abuse; differential access to food and medical care for female infants
Girlhood	Child marriage; genital mutilation; sexual abuse by family members and strangers; differential access to food and medical care; child prostitution
Adolescence	Dating and courtship violence (acid throwing in Bangladesh, date rape in the United States); economically coerced sex (African secondary school girls with "sugar daddies" to afford school fees); sexual abuse in the workplace; rape; sexual harassment; forced prostitution; trafficking in women
Reproductive age	Abuse of women by male partners; marital rape; dowry abuse and murders; partner homicide; psychological abuse; sexual abuse in the pworkplace; sexual harassment; rape; abuse of women with disabilities
Elderly	Abuse of widows; elder abuse (in the United States, the only country where data are available, elder abuse affects mostly women)

the lives of so many individuals. It is our task, as health care providers and human beings, to help others focus their aggression into more effective (and less violent) ways of coping with today's complex world.

THEORIES OF ANGER AND AGGRESSION

Theories about human aggression and violence attempt to explain why certain persons behave the way they do. Many theories about the nature of aggression have been devised, but most fall into one of three basic models: biological, psychosocial, and sociocultural theories.

BIOLOGICAL THEORIES

Models that see the cause of aggression and violence as physical or chemical differences are called biological or individual theories. Currently research is focusing on the areas of the brain that influence emotional control and aggressive behaviors. The roles of certain neurotransmitters are being investigated as possible factors in the development of violence. Biological theories explain aggressive behavior as a psychopathology—a disorder in the biological or physical makeup of a person.

Charles Darwin favored his animal model, which stated that aggression strengthened human beings

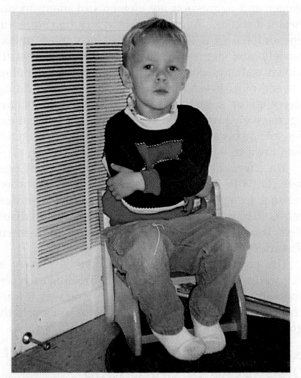

FIGURE **25-2** Preschoolers generally direct their aggression toward peers. Time-outs are a disciplinary measure used to remove the child from an activity and allow him or her to calm down and consider what was wrong in his or her actions.

through natural selection. Sigmund Freud believed that the greater the death wish, the greater the need for aggressive behavior. Other biological theories explain aggression as an innate (instinctual) drive. One thing, however, is certain: physical problems that cause aggressive behaviors do exist.

PSYCHOSOCIAL THEORIES

The models based on psychosocial theories focus on an individual's interactions with the social environments. Violence arises from interpersonal frustrations. Psychosocial theories of aggression state that aggressive behaviors are learned responses.

SOCIOCULTURAL THEORIES

With the sociocultural theories, aggression is explained from a social and cultural group viewpoint. Cultural theories state that aggressive or violent acts are a product of cultural values, beliefs, norms, and rituals. Many cultures have rules that endorse the use of violence.

The **functional model** states that aggression and violence fill certain functions in a society, serving as catalysts or motivators for action. Aggressive behaviors are often used to achieve fame, fortune, and power. Athletes, for example, must be aggressive if they are to excel.

Conflict theories assume that aggression is a natural part of all human interactions. They state that individuals, groups, and societies seek to further their own causes. This results in disagreements, conflicts, and aggressive actions. Because conflict is a natural part of human associations, conflict theories believe that aggression will never be eliminated. It can only be controlled.

The premise of the **resource theory** is that aggression is a fundamental part of society. Therefore the person who has the most resources can muster the greatest force or power. With this model, aggression is the result of having many resources and the power that goes with them.

The last theory of aggression is the **general systems model.** Here the feedback loop is used to demonstrate how aggression and violence perpetuate (feed on) themselves. Violence is viewed as a product of a system that must be stabilized and managed.

Many factors contribute to the use of aggressive behaviors. Attitudes about work, education, the media, and religion all influence the development of anger, hostility, and aggression. Population problems, such as overcrowding, can promote aggressive behaviors. Available community resources, or the lack of them, also play important roles in the occurrence of violent or criminal acts. Many attempts have been made to explain the nature of aggression and violence. No matter what the cause, however, society must learn to recognize and cope with the aggressive behaviors of some of its members.

THE CYCLE OF ASSAULT

Assaults are aggressive behaviors that violate others' person or properties. Behaviors that are considered assaultive include causing physical pain; certain criminal acts, such as rape, murder, suicide, robbery, theft, assault, and battery; passive-aggressive actions; and many forms of emotional abuse.

Studies have demonstrated that assault and violence occur in a predictable pattern of emotional responses. Each response pattern is called a stage. There are five stages in the assault cycle: trigger, escalation, crisis, recovery, and depression. Figure 25-3 illustrates the cycle of assault. This section describes each stage.

TRIGGER STAGE

During the trigger stage, a stress-producing event occurs. Stress responses, such as anger, fear, or anxiety, then occur. Coping mechanisms—behaviors to deal with the situation—are chosen in an attempt to achieve control. Individuals may withdraw, become irritable, start complaining. For most people these coping behaviors are appropriate reactions to stress. For persons who are assaultive, however, the choice of coping behaviors becomes automatic and focused outward. Their abilities to problem solve or choose effective options decrease as aggressive responses increase. **Crisis interventions** are very successful if begun early in this stage.

ESCALATION STAGE

The escalation stage is the building stage during which each behavioral response moves a step closer to total loss of control. Attempts to use aggressive behaviors to gain control become repeatedly ineffective. This results in increasing frustration and greater anger. Intense emotions further flame the fires of aggression. Behaviors include rapid pacing, fist pounding, and complaining loudly. The person may swear, scream, and become irrational. Intervention is crucial at this stage if violence is to be prevented.

CRISIS STAGE

During the crisis stage, the potential for danger is increased. This is a period of emotional or physical blowout when actual assaultive behaviors occur. The ability to reason is lost, and many individuals act out, physically harm other people and animals, or destroy property. Others become verbally abusive or scream

and shout. People in this stage are unable to listen to reason, follow directions, or engage in mental exercises. They are so controlled by their anger that they cannot respond to most outside stimuli. The best interventions at this stage are to protect the individual and others in the environment from physical harm. External control by caregivers is needed.

RECOVERY STAGE

The recovery stage is the cooling-down period that follows an emotional explosion. The individual slowly calms and returns to normal behavioral responses and actions. Interventions during this stage include assessing for injuries or trauma and providing a safe, quiet environment in which the person can recover.

DEPRESSION STAGE

The last stage of the assault cycle involves a period of guilt and attempts to reconcile (make up) with others. Aggressors are aware of the assault and genuinely feel bad about it. They may cry, apologize frequently, or provide loving care for the victim. They may spend large amounts of money on gifts or other offerings seeking forgiveness. With the passage of time, the assaultive event is slowly placed in the past. Life returns to normal; that is, until the next trigger is cocked, and the cycle repeats itself over and over again.

ANGER-CONTROL DISORDERS

Anger and aggression are elements of many mental health disorders. Aggressive behaviors are commonly encountered in clients with substance abuse, mood, anxiety, and depressive disorders. The potential for violence always exists in individuals with schizophrenia and other psychotic disorders. Clients with eating, sleeping, or somatoform disorders seldom behave aggressively toward others, but they are at a great risk for suicide because they focus their anger and aggression inward.

The *Diagnostic and Statistical Manual of Mental Disorders* (DSM-IV-TR) lists three categories of disorders relating to aggressive behaviors. **Conduct disorders** most often occur in childhood. **Impulse-control disorders** usually develop later in life, and **adjustment disorders** can occur at any time.

The potential for aggressive actions is present in every client, regardless of diagnosis. Treating each person with respect and concern goes a long way toward removing that potential. It also helps establish the groundwork for effective therapeutic interventions.

AGGRESSIVE BEHAVIORAL DISORDERS OF CHILDHOOD

Being a child is like being a stranger in a foreign land, unable to speak the language and unaware of the proper behaviors. To function as healthy adults, children need

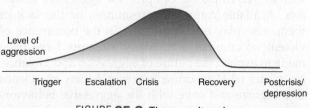

Level of aggression

Trigger　Escalation　Crisis　Recovery　Postcrisis/depression

FIGURE **25-3** The assault cycle.

limits and rules that are lovingly, repeatedly, and consistently applied throughout their childhoods. They need to learn the customs, which behaviors are "right" or appropriate and which behaviors are "wrong." They require the energies of adults to help guide them through the foreign lands of childhood and adolescence. Without this attention and guidance, children learn to cope in the best ways they can, even if these ways lead to ineffective or destructive behavioral disorders. Two diagnoses that relate to childhood and adolescent aggression are conduct disorder and oppositional defiant disorder.

Conduct disorder is characterized by a pattern of behavior "in which the basic rights of others or major age-appropriate societal norms or rules are violated" (American Psychiatric Association, 2000). Behaviors associated with this disorder fall into four main groups: **aggressive conduct, nonaggressive conduct, deceitfulness,** and **serious rules violations.** Individuals with conduct disorder naturally relate aggressively to others even when the situation is nonthreatening. They have no empathy for others and lack appropriate guilt feelings. The inability to tolerate frustration leads to temper outbursts and reckless behaviors. Inappropriate behavior patterns occur in homes, school, and communities.

Conduct disorders are usually diagnosed in late childhood or early adolescence. Most people "outgrow" the problem by adulthood and are able to live effectively. However, a significant number go on to develop social and legal problems. Often they are diagnosed with **antisocial personality disorders** as adults.

Oppositional defiant disorder is a pattern of negative, aggressive behaviors that focuses on authority figures in the child's life. Children with this problem are constantly involved in power struggles, always fighting for control and attention. Their behaviors are stubborn, uncooperative, resistant, and hostile. The signs and symptoms of oppositional defiant disorder are often seen by 8 years of age, and, without effective intervention, the behaviors often escalate or grow into conduct disorders. (See Chapter 13 for a discussion of conduct disorders in children.)

IMPULSE-CONTROL DISORDERS

The essential feature of an impulse-control disorder is "the failure to resist an impulse, drive, or temptation to perform an act that is harmful to the person or to others" (American Psychiatric Association, 2000).

The typical individual with an impulse-control disorder begins to feel an increasing tension when presented with the "trigger" stimuli. Emotions continue to build and grow until the individual can no longer resist or control the impulse. He or she engages in the behavior (commits the act) and then experiences gratification, pleasure, and a release of tension. Guilt, remorse, or regret may or may not be felt after the impulse has been acted on.

Impulse-control disorders are named for the impulse that is related to the specific problem. Box 25-2 lists five types of impulse-control disorders. Although all types involve some form of aggression, the impulse-control problems encountered by health care workers most often relate to clients with intermittent explosive disorder.

The main feature of intermittent explosive disorder is a failure to resist aggressive impulses that result in the destruction of property or assault of another individual. "There is some evidence that the neurotransmitter serotonin may play a role in this disorder" (AllPsych, 2007). Persons with intermittent explosive disorder have frequent angry outbursts that are out of proportion to the stressor. For example, an individual may strike the teller at the bank for making him wait in line too long, whereas other people would sigh and continue to wait quietly for their turn.

Because these aggressive behaviors place others at risk for harm, people with these disorders often have difficulty with interpersonal, work, and social relationships. Intermittent explosive disorders more commonly occur in males and usually appear during late adolescence through early adulthood.

ADJUSTMENT DISORDERS

The problems associated with coping with a new set of stressors can be overwhelming for any of us. The discomfort of adjusting from one situation to another can lead to certain mental health problems. **Adjustment disorders** are emotional or behavioral problems that develop in response to an identifiable source.

Persons with adjustment disorders have difficulty adapting to a new situation. These individuals become overwhelmed with the changes required of them during stressful times. Their distress is so great that it

---

Box 25-2 *Impulse-Control Disorders*

INTERMITTENT EXPLOSIVE DISORDER
Repeated failures to resist acting on aggressive impulses, resulting in assaultive or destructive behaviors

KLEPTOMANIA
Repeated failure to resist the impulse to steal objects when they are not needed for personal use or survival

PATHOLOGICAL GAMBLING
Repeated episodes of maladaptive betting, wagering, playing games of chance, or gambling

PYROMANIA
Repeated behavioral pattern of starting fires for pleasure, relief of tension, or gratification

TRICHOTILLOMANIA
Repeated behavioral pattern of pulling out one's hair that results in noticeable loss of hair

Modified from American Psychiatric Association: *Diagnostic and statistical manual of mental disorders,* ed 4, text revision, Washington, DC, 2000, The Association.

Box 25-3 *Types of Adjustment Disorders*

1. Adjustment disorder with depressed mood
2. Adjustment disorder with anxiety
3. Adjustment disorder with mixed anxiety and depressed mood
4. Adjustment disorder with disturbance of conduct
5. Adjustment disorder with disturbed emotions and conduct

interferes with their activities of daily living. The stressor may be a single event (e.g., leaving a romantic relationship), continuous (e.g., living in a crime-filled neighborhood), or repeated (e.g., ongoing marital problems). Whatever the cause, the individual has difficulty coping effectively.

Adjustment disorders are also classified by their most frequent symptoms. The five subtypes are listed in Box 25-3.

By definition, an adjustment disorder lasts no longer than 6 months after the stressor or stressors have stopped. Adjustment disorders are common, with most of us experiencing at least one episode during our lives. Fortunately human beings are adaptable, and most individuals learn to effectively cope with change. However, suicide attempts occur more frequently in persons who are having trouble adjusting to new situations. Do not forget that anger, aggression, or hostility can be present in any individual.

GUIDELINES FOR INTERVENTION

It is important to keep in mind that diagnoses are only labels. You are working with individuals, real people with real problems. Therapeutic interventions should always focus on the person, rather than on the diagnosis.

ASSESSING ANGER AND AGGRESSION

The first step in controlling aggressive behaviors is to assess the client's potential for engaging in inappropriate behaviors. Approach the client slowly and calmly. Stay an arm's length away, and monitor the client for signs of losing control. Obtain a mental status assessment as soon as possible after admission. Use therapeutic communication skills to help clients feel at ease. Work to establish trust, and let clients know that they are respected, even when angry.

Mental Status Assessment

Basic mental status examinations can be performed by any astute observer. During the mental status assessment, observe the client's **general appearance** and note the state of dress, cleanliness, and use of cosmetics or jewelry. Be sure to observe the client's **activity** and behaviors. Many times the clues to violence are being communicated nonverbally. Health care providers need to be alert enough to receive the messages. What about the client's **attitude?** Are interactions friendly and co-operative or resistive and hostile? Listen for the quality, rate, and amount of **verbal communications** in the client's speech. Pay particular attention to the individual's **mood, affect (emotional expressions), perceptions, and thoughts.** Have the client describe his or her mood at the time. Listen to the client's conversation for form and content. Does he or she speak logically, with a flow of ideas that are easily followed? What is the problem according to the client? Is the client's **judgment** or **insight** clear and easy to follow, or does it follow a twisted path of fuzzy explanations for past inappropriate behaviors? Is the client's **reliability** intact (does he or she give accurate information)?

Psychosocial Assessment

Next, perform a psychosocial assessment. Find out which internal or external **stressors** are present in the client's life. Which **coping skills** are being used to adapt to the stressors? Encourage the client to tell you about important **relationships** and how they are affecting the situation. Do not forget the **cultural, spiritual,** and **occupational** areas of the client's life. Is he or she a member of a specific cultural group, organized religion, or occupation? Is there a **value** and **belief system** that the individual feels is valuable, desirable, or worth following? Observe the client's **reactions** and **behaviors** during the interview. His or her reactions, behaviors, and **attitudes** during this time offer many clues concerning the potential for aggression or violent behaviors. Remember, the key to effective intervention begins with assessments. Assess clients often, and report new behaviors. Share your findings with other members of the health care team. Troubleshooting is always an easier task than controlling a full-blown violent reaction. Possible nursing diagnoses for aggressive behaviors are listed in Box 25-4.

THERAPEUTIC INTERVENTIONS

Therapeutic interventions for clients with anger and aggression focus on two basic areas: the client and the caregiver. Interventions for aggressive or potentially aggressive client behaviors occur on three levels (Table 25-3).

Level one interventions focus on the **prevention** of violence. The goal of level one interventions (the best intervention for aggression) is to establish and maintain a trusting therapeutic relationship with clear and honest communications. This is accomplished using a number of simple communication strategies.

Call the client and any family members by name. No one likes to be an anonymous face in the crowd. Explain what is happening, the reason for any delays, and why testing is needed. Most important, listen actively, with your whole body, not just your ears. Communicate your concern nonverbally while listening. Maintain

Box 25-4 *NANDA-I Nursing Diagnoses Related to Anger and Aggression*

Anxiety
Behavior, risk-prone health*
Coping, ineffective individual
Denial, ineffective
Family processes, interrupted
Fear
Hopelessness
Noncompliance
Powerlessness
Self-mutilation, risk for
Situational chronic, low
Social interaction, impaired
Violence, risk for other-directed
Violence, risk for self-directed

Data from NANDA International: *NANDA-I nursing diagnoses: definitions and classification, 2007-2008,* Philadelphia, 2007, NANDA International.
NANDA-I, NANDA International.
*Primary nursing diagnoses for anger and aggression.

Table 25-3 *Levels of Intervention With Anger*

LEVEL	GOAL
Level one—Prevent violence	Establish and maintain a trusting therapeutic relationship.
Level two—Protect	Protect the client and others from potential harm.
Level three—Control violence	Client is out of control. Protect client and others through seclusion, restraints, and intramuscular (IM) medication.

good eye contact while leaning forward slightly to communicate your interest. Give the client time to respond. Concentrate on the message he or she is trying to communicate to you. Paraphrase the problem to make sure that you have a good understanding of the client's point of view. Finally, help identify the emotions associated with the problem and explore appropriate options. Refer to Box 25-5 for an effective communication strategy.

Level one interventions should be practiced routinely as preventive measures. They are also appropriate for clients who are in the "trigger stage" of the assault cycle. "The majority of difficult patients are motivated by fear" (Childers, 2003). Very often just the caring concern of someone who is willing to really listen is enough to prevent anger from turning into aggression or violence.

Level two interventions focus on protecting the client and others from potential harm. These interventions are used when level one interventions are ineffective and signs of trouble are beginning to brew (see Case Study 25-1). Learn to recognize the verbal and physical signs of impending violence.

Interventions during level two include measures to maintain a safe environment. Take charge with a calm,

Box 25-5 *Communicating With Angry Clients*

First, take a deep breath. Become calm, and introduce yourself to the client. Speak slowly, and do the following:
1. Listen actively. Use active listening skills to communicate interest in helping the client. Allow the client to define the problem that is causing the anger or aggression.
2. Identify emotions. Try to understand what is causing the problem and why the client is reacting with anger. Ask yourself what the client may be feeling and verbalize it. "You must be feeling pretty ..." or "How do you feel about that?" allows the client to identify and discuss his or her emotions or problems.
3. Explore options. Help the client to regain some sense of control by brainstorming possible solutions to his or her problems. You may not be able to solve the problems, but you can assist the client in finding his or her own solutions.
4. Offer positive comments. Increase self-esteem by finding something the client does well and complimenting him or her. Many clients and their loved ones feel helpless, and the reassuring words of a concerned caregiver can provide great comfort.

 Case Study 25-1

Randy, a hot-tempered 24-year-old man well known to the clinic staff, visits the clinic for weekly dressing changes for his right eye. Today he arrives seething with anger because his girlfriend just broke off their relationship.

"That _____! Just because we had a little fight, she can't stand to be with me now. You women are all alike. I could punch you out right now and feel just fine," he snarls through clenched teeth as he glares into your eyes.

"You sound pretty upset. Tell me about it," you calmly reply. As Randy tells you about his relationship with his ex-girlfriend, you can see him becoming angrier by the moment. He begins to pound his fists on the table and stomp around the room. You signal for other staff members who are keeping an eye on the situation to be prepared to help, but so far, Randy is acting out by ranting and raving. No damage is being done, and no person is in danger of harm.

After a few moments you reply, "Randy, I understand your anger, but stomping around is not appropriate. Let's take a couple of minutes to cool off, then maybe together we can think of some way to help deal with this problem." Because you remained calm, quiet, and prepared, Randy responded to your request and took a few minutes to regain his composure.

• How do you think Randy would have reacted if he had been approached by three staff members during his ranting?

but firm, attitude. Allow clients to act out as long as they limit their behaviors to verbal assaults and harmless physical movements. Assure clients that they have a right to express angry feelings but not to impose them on others. Gently, but firmly, set limits on the

---

SAMPLE CLIENT CARE PLAN 25-1

Risk for Violence

ASSESSMENT *History.* Bruce, a 15-year-old boy, has been sent to the mental health unit for psychiatric evaluation by the local police. Since age 13 he has been arrested several times for vandalism, drug possession, and menacing. His parents are cooperative but "feel helpless." His older sister is living away from home because she refuses "to be exposed to his violent behaviors."

Current Findings. An unkempt, sullen adolescent boy with tattoos on each knuckle of the right hand. Head is shaved in a pattern. Smoking cigarettes despite the "no smoking" sign posted on the wall.

Multidisciplinary Diagnosis	*Planning/Goals*
Risk for other-directed violence	Bruce will demonstrate absence of aggressive or hostile threats or behaviors by October 10.

Therapeutic Interventions

Intervention	Rationale	Team Member
1. Approach Bruce with respect; avoid judging.	Adolescents need acceptance from adults as much as they need direction.	All
2. Orient to unit routine and policies; give clear, specific rules and the consequences for breaking them.	Assists Bruce until he is able to gain internal control over his aggressive behaviors.	Nsg
3. Assess for warning signs of increasing anger.	Behavioral changes often indicate an aggressive reaction; good assessment skills prevent injury to client and others.	All
4. Assess past acts of aggression, and determine the potential seriousness of present actions.	Knowledge of previous patterns of violence helps assess Bruce's tolerance for current stresses.	All
5. Demonstrate acceptance of the painful feelings underlying Bruce's behaviors.	Helps to encourage Bruce's self-worth even though his behaviors are unacceptable.	All
6. Use open-ended questions; avoid asking "why."	"Why" questions call for an explanation or defensive reaction; open-ended questions help explore feelings, thoughts, and reactions.	All
7. Contract with Bruce for "no violence" while on unit.	Protects others from injury; encourages him to be responsible for his own actions.	
8. Teach stress management and problem-solving techniques.	Redirects energy created by anxiety and anger into healthier responses.	Psy, Nsg

Evaluation

By September 15, Bruce no longer required daily time-out sessions. By October 2, Bruce was able to identify one source of his anger.

❓ CRITICAL THINKING QUESTIONS

1. What purpose does active listening serve when working with angry clients?

2. What caregiver behaviors demonstrate respect for a sullen teen such as Bruce?

A complete client care plan includes several other diagnoses and interventions.
Nsg, Nursing staff; *Psy*, psychologist.

---

client's behaviors by suggesting that the client take a time-out, a cooling-off period. If it appears that the time-out is not effective, offer prn medication. Only after all other measures have been tried are level three interventions implemented. "Nonviolent physical control and restraint should be used only as a last resort" (Stuart and Laraia, 2005).

The last level of therapeutic measures **(level three interventions)** is reserved for those clients who are out of control (crisis stage of the assault cycle). Clients who are out of control fight, bite, kick, scratch, spit, and throw things. They are verbally abusive or physically aggressive. Without intervention, both clients and care providers are at an increased risk for injury. Few clients reach this stage if level one and two interventions were

effective. However, for those who are engaging in violent behaviors, three interventions are available: seclusion, restraints, and intramuscular (IM) medication.

A point to remember here is that using restraints and seclusion as interventions for the control of assaultive behaviors must be planned ahead. Both strategies involve federal and state laws, institutional policies, and special procedures. Study the procedures for applying restraints and placing clients in seclusion. This information is also available in any nursing fundamentals text. Remember to monitor the condition of the restrained client at least every 15 minutes, and use other, less drastic measures as soon as the client has regained behavioral control. Sample Client Care Plan 25-1 offers suggestions for addressing aggressive behavior.

Table 25-4 *Client Education Plan: Modifying Impulsive Behavior*

CONTENT	INSTRUCTIONAL ACTIVITIES	EVALUATION
Describe characteristics and consequences of impulsive behavior.	Select a situation in which impulsive behavior occurred. Ask the patient to describe what happened. Provide the patient with paper and a pen. Instruct the patient to keep a diary of impulsive actions, including a description of events before and after the incident.	Patient will identify and describe an impulsive incident. Patient will maintain a diary of impulsive behaviors. Patient will explore the causes and consequences of impulsive behavior.
Describe behaviors characteristic of interpersonal anxiety. Relate anxiety to impulsive behavior.	Discuss the diary with the patient. Assist the patient to identify interpersonal anxiety related to impulsive behavior.	Patient will connect feelings of interpersonal anxiety with impulsive behavior.
Explain stress reduction techniques.	Describe the stress response. Demonstrate relaxation exercises. Assist the patient to return the demonstration.	Patient will perform relaxation exercises when signs of anxiety appear.
Identify alternative responses to anxiety-producing situations.	Using situations from the diary, and knowledge of relaxation exercises, assist the patient to list possible alternative responses.	Patient will identify at least two alternative responses to each anxiety-producing situation.
Practice using alternative responses to anxiety-producing situations.	Role play each of the identified alternative behaviors. Discuss the feelings associated with impulsive behavior and the alternatives.	Patient will describe the relationship between behavior and feelings. Patient will select and perform anxiety-reducing behaviors.

From Keltner NL, Schwecke LH, Bostrom CE: *Psychiatric nursing*, ed 5, St. Louis, 2007, Mosby.

Think About 25-1

There are several techniques for managing your own anger:
1. **Vent your feelings.** Yell, scream, shout, but do it in a safe place.
2. **Change your focus.** Distract yourself for a moment—listen to the radio, take a walk. Move your energies from the anger to another topic. Playing with a pet is a great tranquilizer. Even counting to 10 can be very effective.
3. **Use your anger constructively.** Take the energy that is used to be angry and do something else with it. Clean the house. Organize the junk drawer. Exercise. Meditate.
4. **Discuss** your anger with those involved. Talking it out (after you are calm) lets people know what is on your mind and how you feel. Discussion also offers opportunities for personal learning and developing more therapeutic behaviors.
5. **Forgive** those with whom you are angry. If harsh words were exchanged, apologize. Apologies are free; they are not a sign of weakness, and they communicate a willingness to cooperate in the future. Forgiveness is an underused therapeutic tool.
6. **Relax.** Take slow, deep breaths, and tell your body to relax and become calm. Remember the effects of our stress neurochemicals? Emotional responses have a strong impact on the physical body. Smile. It requires the use of fewer muscles and promotes positive reactions in yourself and others.

Once the assaultive event has subsided and the client is willing to discuss the problem, begin to enlist his or her help to modify the inappropriate behaviors. Table 25-4 offers an example of an educational plan for controlling impulsive, aggressive behaviors.

Interventions for caregivers focus on learning to effectively control your own feelings of anger. Even the most therapeutic care provider experiences anger. Learning to cope with personal feelings of anger and aggression allows us to be more successful in working with the angry emotions of others (see Think About 25-1).

Practice your ability to cope with feelings and reactions at home and at work. As you improve, you will find yourself becoming more effective when working with the emotional responses of others.

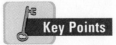

Key Points

- Anger is a normal emotional response to a perceived threat, frustration, or distressing event.
- Anger serves as a coping mechanism, a motivator, or an opportunity for learning.
- Aggression or hostile behaviors are angry feelings and impulses that are converted into action.
- Aggressive behaviors become inappropriate when they affect other people or their possessions.

- Assertiveness is the ability to directly express one's feelings or needs in a way that respects the rights of other people and retains the individual's dignity.
- Gender violence, which is the abuse of members of one gender by members of another, is seen in many cultural and social settings.
- The expression of anger occurs throughout the life cycle.
- Today aggression and violence are worldwide concerns.
- Theories about the nature of aggression fall into one of three basic models: biological, psychosocial, and sociocultural.
- Assaults are aggressive behaviors that violate others' person or properties.
- Assault and violence occur in a predictable pattern of emotional responses called the assault cycle.
- Stages of the assault cycle are the trigger stage, the escalation stage, the crisis stage, the recovery stage, and the depression stage.

- The DSM-IV-TR lists three categories of disorders relating to aggressive behaviors: conduct disorders, impulse-control disorders, and adjustment disorders.
- The first step in controlling aggression is to assess the client's potential for engaging in inappropriate behaviors.
- Interventions for aggressive or potentially aggressive behaviors are divided into three levels: preventing violence, protecting the client and others, and secluding or restraining the out-of-control client.
- Learning to cope with your own feelings of anger or aggression allows you to be more successful in working with the emotions of others.

evolve Be sure to visit the companion Evolve site at http://evolve.elsevier.com/Morrison-Valfre/ for additional online resources.

26 Outward-Focused Emotions: Violence

evolve http://evolve.elsevier.com/Morrison-Valfre/

Objectives

Upon completion of this chapter, the student will be able to:

1. Consider how violence influences the members of a society.
2. Explain three groups of theories that attempt to explain the cause of violence.
3. Describe six characteristics of a dysfunctional family.
4. Illustrate three consequences of abuse during pregnancy.
5. Identify two examples of abuse or neglect for each age-group throughout the life cycle.
6. Outline the essential features of posttraumatic stress disorder and rape-trauma syndrome.
7. Discuss special assessments for suspected victims of violence.
8. Describe three nursing interventions for helping clients recover from violence.
9. Explain how self-awareness can lead to a decrease in violent, abusive, or exploitive behaviors.

Key Terms

abuse (p. 281)
aggression (p. 281)
agitation (p. 281)
battering (p. 283)
domestic violence (p. 283)
emotional abuse (p. 284)
exploitation (ĔK-sploi-TĀ-shən) (p. 281)
forensic evidence (p. 291)
homicides (p. 289)
incest (p. 288)
machismo (mə-CHĔZ-mō) (p. 282)
neglect (p. 281)
physical abuse (p. 286)
pornography (p. 284)
prostitution (p. 284)
rape (p. 290)
sexual abuse (p. 286)
shaken baby syndrome (p. 286)
violence (p. 281)

Aggressive, violent, and exploitive behaviors occur throughout the animal kingdom. Many animals battle violently for the right to mate and pass on their genes. Starlings exploit other birds by laying their single egg in another nest. There is a goal with animal aggression—to procure food, to mate, or to establish dominance. Animals' use of violence is predictable and

useful. They seldom risk injuring themselves just to be violent. Aggressive characteristics are also present in human beings, but they are expressed differently.

Human beings engage in aggressive or violent behaviors for a variety of reasons. In some instances, motives are clear and understandable. In others, however, all we are left with are uneasy questions. Human reactions exist on a continuum ranging from calm to violent (Figure 26-1).

To discuss violence, one must be familiar with its related terms. **Agitation** describes behavior that is verbally or physically offensive. **Aggression** is a forceful attitude or action that is expressed physically, symbolically, or verbally. **Abuse** is the intentional misuse of someone or something that results in harm, injury, or trauma. Abuse can take place in the form of active harm or passive neglect. **Violence** is defined as an outburst of physical force that abuses, injures, or harms another person or object. **Neglect** is harm to another's health or welfare through a failure to provide for basic needs or by placing the individual's health or welfare at unreasonable risk. Neglect often occurs in the more vulnerable members of society, such as children and elders. **Exploitation** refers to the use of an individual for selfish purposes, profit, or gain. Children who must labor with no time for study or play are examples of exploited individuals. Each of these terms describes some type of physical or psychological activity that is socially unacceptable.

The purpose of this chapter is twofold: (1) to help you understand the many ways in which violence is present in society and (2) to provide you with the tools to effectively assess, intervene in, reduce, and prevent aggressive incidents.

SOCIAL FACTORS AND VIOLENCE

No one is certain exactly why violence occurs. We do know, however, that violent acts and their consequences are increasing with alarming frequency. Violence is a major cause of death and disability in most industrialized countries. For example, the murder rate in the United States climbed from 17 murders per 100,000 people in 1970 to an alarming 27 murders per 100,000 by 1991. By 1999, the rate had dropped to 15 homicides per

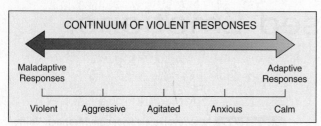

FIGURE **26-1** Continuum of violent responses.

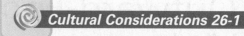

In some poverty-stricken countries, children as young as 4 years are forced to work in the rug mills and other manufacturing businesses. Many labor long hours in miserable working conditions for little pay. If a child does not work fast enough or has the courage to complain, he or she is physically punished. Children who are too outspoken about the poor working conditions have been known to "disappear."

100,000, but by 2002 it was again on the rise with 16 murders per 100,000 people. The United States still has the highest murder rate of all the "civilized countries" in the world. Finland and Hungary claim the sad distinction of having the highest number of suicides in the industrialized countries (U.S. Census Bureau, 2007).

These statistics mean that you will likely encounter victims of violence—as clients, parents of clients, friends, and relatives. Nurses and other health care providers accept and care for all people, but this philosophy also comes with the risk for violence. Therefore it is important to learn as much as possible about the problems and solutions related to the use of violence in society today.

Several cultural and social factors affect violence. Many societies promote the use of aggressive behaviors through beliefs, customs, and rituals. "The American culture of violence is reflected in the history, attitudes, belief systems, and coping styles of the population in dealing with conflicts, frustration, and the quest for wealth and power" (Schacter and Sienfield, 1994). In cultures in which the resources are scarce, violent acts become a way of life (see Cultural Considerations 26-1).

Aggressive and violent acts are found in every group in society, and it appears that poverty plays a role in the development of aggressive behaviors. In many societies, productive and financially rewarding work is expected from most adults, especially men. A lack of fulfilling work often leads to poverty, frustration, and, in many cases, violence. To illustrate, the unemployment rate for young minority men in the United States is "close to 50%. This group also has the highest rate of violence" (Stanhope and Lancaster, 2008).

THEORIES OF VIOLENCE

Several theories attempt to explain the nature of violence. The **psychiatric/mental illness model** views violence as a mental illness. Both victim and abuser are considered mentally disturbed. Recent evidence, however, has found that the incidence of mental illness is no greater in batterers or their victims than the rest of the population.

The **social learning theory** states that aggressive and violent behaviors are learned through role modeling others in the environment. Aggression is believed to be a learned behavior based on the values, attitudes, and actions of role models within the individual's environment.

Sociological theories credit environmental and social factors as causes for violence. Environmental factors, such as overcrowding, lack of adequate housing, and poor hygiene, can increase the incidence of aggression. The social factors of unemployment, poverty, crime, drug abuse, and isolation are believed to be related to violent acts.

Anthropological theories, which are based in the study of humans' social history, explain violence and aggression as the result of cultural patterns, social organizations, or sexual differences. Because some cultures encourage the use of aggressive behaviors, their citizens learn to interact and cope aggressively. In other cultures, equality and harmony are stressed. Male and female roles are less defined in cooperative cultures than they are in cultures with hierarchies or degrees of power.

Finally, the **feminist theories** use the concept of "machismo" to explain the occurrence of violence against women. Machismo is defined as compulsive masculinity. Feminist theories state that males are socialized throughout childhood to behave more aggressively and violently. By the time boys have reached adolescence, they are preoccupied with physical strength, athletic prowess, and attempts to demonstrate daring, violent, or aggressive behaviors. Men who have a high degree of machismo demonstrate certain social, behavioral, and sexual attitudes. Machismo is a strong influence on male behavior in many countries.

These theories do not imply that every man with a high level of machismo abuses other people. They do, however, remind us that the potential for abuse lies within the machismo belief system (Box 26-1).

Dr. Sherry Turkle, a psychologist who studies cyberspace, believes that computers will change the way people think about themselves and their role in society. Her particular fear is "that young people will succumb to the temptation to leave 'real life' behind for the ever-so-much more controllable realm of cyberspace" ("Sessions With a Cybershrink," 1996). As more people become members of the computer network society, the number of "real," face-to-face relationships decreases. In these times of public isolation and anxiety over so many social forces, people are turning more and more to the Internet's chat rooms or other information

Box 26-1 | *Characteristics of a Person With Machismo*

Has an attitude of male pride
Engages in thrill-seeking behaviors
Employs competition as his guiding principle
Is egocentric (self-centered)
Is unable to express emotions except anger and rage
Dislikes being gentle or vulnerable
Values sexual virility
Displays sexist attitudes
    Treats women as objects or commodities
    Sees women as objects of conquest
    Insists on being dominant to girls and women
    Holds to unwritten law that infidelity by a woman
        must be avenged
    Unable to cooperate with women
    Agrees to sexual use and abuse of women
Glorifies war and violence, supports the use of military
    force
Enjoys contact sports
Uses aggression to physically solve problems

Box 26-2 | *Characteristics of Dysfunctional Families*

Family members are self-centered.
Authority is inconsistent or lacking; parents feel they
    cannot control children.
Roles are not clearly defined; it is unclear who is the
    parent, who is the child.
Members are unable to meet own or others' needs,
    but each expects needs to be met.
Individualism is not encouraged; autonomy and trust
    are lacking.
No common goals can be identified; focus is on the
    present only.
Family appears chaotic, disorganized; no one is really
    aware of what is happening in the family.
Communications are cold and indifferent; family members
    feel pain and desperation; humor, caring, empathy,
    intimacy are absent; no clear communications exist.
Conflict is viewed as negative and is expressed through
    power struggles and sexual aggression.
Family may confuse violence with caring.
Family boundaries are rigid; threatened when outsiders
    try to enter group; family members are socially
    isolated; parents often married young and have few
    parenting skills.
Family violence is present.

highways in search of social interaction and supportive relationships.

Social connectedness is more than just an obligation or a desire—it fills the basic human need to belong. Social relationships are important elements in preventing aggression and violence. The lack of supportive relationships has been linked to many negative consequences, including mental illness, crime, and suicide.

ABUSE, NEGLECT, AND EXPLOITATION WITHIN THE FAMILY

For far too long, physical abuse and emotional abuse within the family have remained unspoken issues. Traditionally victims suffer in silence, unable to seek help for fear of being revealed as less than a real person. Today, communities are working to provide care and counseling for abused and exploited people. Family violence comes in several forms.

DOMESTIC VIOLENCE

In Western society, the idea that "a man's home is his castle" has been inviolate. This principle has historically meant that the home is a private place. "What goes on inside one's home is nobody else's business" still remains a popular attitude today, even if activities endanger family members.

Domestic violence describes abuse and battering within a family. Battering is a term that describes repeated physical abuse of someone, usually a woman, child, or elder. Victims of violent or abusive acts often suffer from posttraumatic stress disorder (discussed later in this chapter).

Accurate statistics on the incidence of domestic violence are unavailable because very few victims are willing to share their experiences. In 1994, only 40% of assaults were reported. Today, those numbers have not improved. It is estimated that one American woman out of every two will be physically abused at some time in her life by the man with whom she lives. The Bureau of Justice National Crime Survey states that a woman is beaten in her home every 15 seconds (Statman, 1995). Studies conducted by the March of Dimes indicate that 1 of every 12 pregnant women suffers physical abuse (battering) during pregnancy.

A functional family unit is described by what it does (processes) to achieve its goals. These processes include clear and supportive communications among all family members, conflict resolution, the setting of goals, and the use of resources inside and outside the family (Potter and Perry, 2009). A dysfunctional family is described by its inability or unwillingness to fulfill its basic functions. Box 26-2 lists several characteristics of a dysfunctional family. Not all dysfunctional families have an element of abuse, but the inability of a family to meet the needs of its members greatly increases the opportunity for aggressive or violent behaviors.

The family is considered a social unit that is entitled to privacy and freedom from intrusion. Unfortunately, this doctrine has allowed untold numbers of women and children (and occasionally men) to suffer at the hands of their "loved ones." Violence within the family occurs in several ways, as Case Study 26-1 describes. Common forms include physical, emotional, or sexual abuse and neglect of partners, children, and elderly members.

At first they were small arguments, but soon they grew all out of proportion and he was screaming. He began by "correcting" her, then it was directions about how to do it "the right way." When she forgot or refused, he tormented her by repeatedly reminding her of how stupid and worthless she was—how nobody would have her but him. He was relentless in his destruction of her self-esteem and confidence, but he never hit her.

GENDER ABUSE

No woman enters a relationship with the intent of becoming a battered partner, but wife beating is still considered an accepted part of marriage in many groups. Even in societies where domestic violence is condemned, individuals have their own attitudes, personal agendas, and faults that may cause conflict within the family. The notion that "all is fair in love and war" promotes the idea that marriage is a private relationship and the legal system should stay out of the picture—even when the picture includes assault, abuse, or injury.

There is no "typical" abused woman, but the victims of violence do have some characteristics in common (see Think About 26-1). Perhaps the most common trait is a trusting nature. Many women were raised to be nonaggressive and traditional. They were brought up to believe that the man is master and protector of the household. These women, in turn, often feel that submission is the way to "please your man." The problem is that most abusive partners cannot be pleased.

When abuse occurs, guilt, anger, and terror shatter a woman's self-esteem. She suffers in silence, knowing that the consequences will be severe if she seeks help. Once a woman is battered, a vicious cycle of violence is soon established. Table 26-1 describes the cycle of domestic violence.

Abuser (batterer) behaviors have several characteristics. The profile of a typical abuser includes poor emotional control, a superior attitude toward women, a history of substance abuse, high levels of jealousy and insecurity, and the use of threats, punishment, and physical violence to control another's behavior. This profile may easily be the picture of a client, client's partner, parent, mate, neighbor, friend, or loved one. Early recognition of the characteristics of potential violence allows for interventions that are more effective. Box 26-3 lists several early signs of a potential abuser.

ABUSE DURING PREGNANCY

Pregnancy should be a time of great joy and anticipation, but for some women, pregnancy only increases their chances of being abused. It is difficult to believe that fathers would intentionally harm the mother of their children, but trauma is the leading cause of

Characteristics of victims:
  Feels captive in the system (family, group, community)
  Blames self for problems leading to abuse
  Has low self-esteem; views self as unworthy
  Feels helpless and powerless to change situation
  Is financially, emotionally, or physically dependent on abuser
  Is depressed, unable to see a future without abuse
* How many persons do you know who demonstrate these characteristics?
* What interventions would you choose for a client who feels like a victim?

maternal death during pregnancy. Statistics on prenatal violence are difficult to gather. Studies in public prenatal clinics reveal that more than 15% of clients are physically abused during the pregnancy, and about 60% of the women questioned had suffered two or more assaults, indicating that episodes of abuse were recurrent. The frequency and severity of abuse, as well as the potential for homicide, are significantly increased for white women. In addition, abused women of all races were twice as likely to postpone beginning prenatal care until the third trimester of pregnancy, too late to prevent or treat many problems.

The effects of abuse during pregnancy can be devastating. The frequency of low-birth-weight infants and preterm deliveries is almost doubled in women who have a history of abuse during pregnancy (Hockenberry and others, 2007). Because the mother is afraid to seek help, she often delays her entry into the health care system, thus denying both herself and her developing child the benefit of adequate prenatal care.

CHILD ABUSE

Unfortunately, the most vulnerable individuals in society, our children, are often the most abused. Child abuse occurs in many cultures and in many different manners (see Cultural Considerations 26-2).

Child pornography (writings, pictures, or other messages pertaining to children that are intended to sexually arouse), child prostitution (selling of sexual favors by children), and child sexual abuse exist all over the world. In Brazil alone, it has been estimated that between 250,000 and 500,000 children are involved in the sex trade. The numbers are even greater in Asia with more than one-half million child prostitutes in Thailand. Most of them are girls under the age of 16 years, but in Sri Lanka, many child prostitutes are boys who cater to older men.

Many children are sold into prostitution with the belief that they will not be infected with human immune deficiency virus (HIV) or other sexually transmitted diseases. Sadly, however, this is not the

Table 26-1 | *Cycle of Domestic Violence*

ABUSER	VICTIM
I. TENSION BUILDING	
He has excessively high expectations of her.	She is nurturing, is compliant, and tries to please him.
He blames her for anything that goes wrong.	She denies the seriousness of their problems.
He does not try to control his behaviors.	She feels she can control his behaviors.
He is aware of his inappropriate behaviors but does not admit it.	She tries to alter his behavior to stay safe.
	She tries to prevent his anger.
Verbal abuse and minor physical abuse increase.	She blames external factors: alcohol, work.
Afraid she will leave, he gets more possessive to keep her captive.	She takes minor abuse but does not feel she deserves it.
He gets frantic and more controlling.	She gets scared and tries to hide (withdrawal).
He misinterprets her withdrawal as rejection.	She may call for help as the tension becomes unbearable.
II. SERIOUS BATTERING INCIDENT	
The trigger event is an internal or external event or substance.	In cases of long-term battering, she may provoke it just to get it over with.
The battering usually occurs in private.	She may call for help if she is afraid of being killed.
He will threaten more harm if she tries to get help (police, medical).	Her initial reactions are shock, disbelief, and denial.
He tries to justify his behaviors but does not understand what happens.	Fearing more abuse if police come, she may plead for them not to arrest him.
He minimizes the severity of the abuse.	She is anxious, ashamed, humiliated, sleepless, fatigued, depressed.
His stress is relieved.	She may not seek help for injuries for a day or more and lies about the cause of injuries.
III. HONEYMOON	
He is loving, charming, begging for forgiveness, making promises.	She sees his loving behaviors as the real person and tries to make up.
He truly believes he will never abuse again.	She wants to believe it will never happen again.
He feels that he taught her a lesson and she will not "act up."	She feels that if she stays, he will get help; the thought of leaving makes her feel guilty.
He preys on her guilt to keep her trapped.	She believes in the permanency of the relationship and gets trapped.

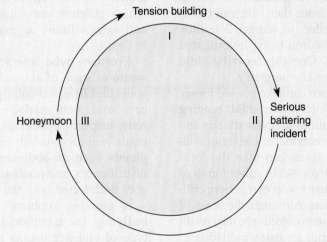

case. The Children's Rights Protection Center in Thailand claims that the AIDS rate among Thai child prostitutes is now greater than 50%.

Children are also bought, sold, and exploited as objects of trade. They are purchased cheaply in one country and sold for a handsome profit in another. Young girls from the Philippines are imported to Japan for prostitution in a business that makes more than 1 million dollars per day. Many gypsy children are forced into begging, often bringing in hundreds of dollars each day while under complete control of their abusers.

In some societies, female infants are undesirable. Girls commonly receive less food, attention, or education than their brothers. For example, according to the World Bank, the death rate for young girls in India outnumbers the death rate for young boys by more than 300,000 deaths per year. The majority of orphans in China are girls. After reviewing these facts, it is easy to understand why child abuse and neglect are important issues of our time.

Spanking was, and still is in several countries, a main form of discipline for children. Unfortunately,

Box 26-3 | *Early Signs of an Abusive Personality*

1. A push for a quick involvement
2. Jealously controlling
3. Unrealistic expectations
4. Isolates partner from family, friends
5. Blames others for own problems and mistakes
6. Makes others responsible for his or her feelings
7. Hypersensitive, easily insulted
8. Cruel to animals and children
9. "Playful" use of force during sex
10. Verbal abuse
11. Enforces rigid sex roles
12. Sudden mood swings
13. History of past batterings
14. Threatens violence

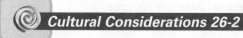

Cultural Considerations 26-2

The following is a popular saying in the red light district of Bangkok, where children are forced into prostitution:

"At 10 you are a woman.
At 20 you are an old woman.
And at 30 you are dead."

spanking and other forms of physical punishment teach children that power and violence are approved coping mechanisms. Today the countries of Sweden, Finland, Norway, Austria, and Switzerland, in an effort to curb the growing rates of child abuse, prohibit all forms of physical punishment in schools and homes. Most other industrialized countries, except the United States, South Africa, and parts of Australia and Canada, have banned physical punishment in schools.

Child abuse went almost unrecognized in the United States until the early 1960s. Since then, the number of reported incidents has swelled to almost 2 million with more than 3 million children being investigated (U.S. Census Bureau, 2007). One can see why child abuse has been called a national emergency.

The mistreatment of children can take several forms. **Physical abuse** is inflicted injury to a child, ranging from minor bruises and lacerations to severe trauma and death. **Sexual abuse** is the intentional engaging of children in sexual acts. Sexual abuse can take the form of rape, incest, fondling, intercourse, or other forms of sexual contact. **Emotional abuse** involves rejection, criticism, terrorizing, and isolation. Although the scars of this type of abuse are seldom seen objectively, they result in deep and penetrating wounds for many individuals.

Neglect is the failure to provide the necessities of life. Physical neglect is the failure to provide a child's basic needs, such as food, clothing, shelter, and a safe environment. Emotional neglect is characterized by a lack of parent-child attachment. Medical care neglect is the refusal to seek treatment when it is needed. Delays in treatment are common in abused children. A rare form of child abuse, called Munchausen's syndrome by proxy, occurs when caretakers simulate or create the signs and symptoms of illness in the child in order to receive attention from health care providers.

Abuse or neglect occurs during every stage of childhood. In infancy, the **shaken baby syndrome** should be suspected in every infant with unexplained or vague injuries. Shaken baby syndrome is defined as

vigorous shaking of an infant that leads to whiplash-induced bleeding within the brain with no external signs of head trauma. This syndrome is difficult to diagnose because of the lack of physical evidence and the parents' refusal to discuss the situation.

Every health care provider must be alert for the possibility of a "shaken baby" whenever there is a history of unexplained lethargy, fussiness, or irritability in an infant. Seizures or swelling in the head demands immediate investigation. Because the incidence of shaken baby syndrome is increasing, efforts must be made to educate parents and community members about the importance of handling the youngest members of our society with gentleness and care.

Children are victimized more often than adults. Types of violent behaviors associated with abused children include pandemic aggression, in which the majority of children are assaulted; acute aggression, in which children are abused, neglected, or exploited; and extraordinary aggression, which usually results in death.

Everyone who interacts with children should be aware of signs of abuse. When a child has bruises or welts that fit a particular pattern, such as a belt buckle or a hand, teeth marks, or burns from a cigar or cigarette, suspect physical abuse. Children who have been sexually abused usually have general, nonspecific complaints such as abdominal pain, bed-wetting, sleep disturbances, and phobias. However, the abuse usually goes undetected until the child discloses the abuse.

A growing problem seen in today's schools is **bullying,** the intentional tormenting of others. This type of violence begins in childhood and can extent into adulthood. A recent study by the National Education Association found that "83% of girls and 79% of boys reported experiencing harassment in schools" (Curriculum Review, 2007).

The victims of bullying are chosen because they are different in some way. They may be big or small for their age, overweight or underweight, belong to a different ethnic group or religion, disabled, or sensitive, anxious, or insecure. Signs of being bullied begin with a change in behavior. The individual becomes withdrawn, preoccupied, and anxious. That leads to depressed moods and recurring somatic symptoms. Headaches and stomachaches, especially in the morning before school, are common. The child does not want to ride the bus or interact with other children.

Box 26-4 *Examples of Bullying Behaviors*

PHYSICAL BULLYING
Choking, hitting, kicking, punching, pushing, tripping

VERBAL BULLYING
Hate talk, mocking, starting rumors, taunting, teasing, threatening

EXCLUSION FROM ACTIVITIES
Encouraging others to stay away from him or her, physically barring attendance

Torn or missing clothing and big after-school appetites are also clues. Some people who are bulled become **reactive** and lash out, often in destructive or hurtful manners.

Bullies need to feel powerful, so they select their targets from those who can be easily intimidated. Often they will blame the victims for the abuse. If repeated frequently enough, the victims accept that blame and begin hold themselves responsible for the abuse.

Bullying behaviors can be physical or verbal. They can involve harassment or exclusion from activities. Box 26-4 lists examples of bullying behaviors. Motives for bullying are unclear, but research suggests that bullies have a strong need to be in control. They are quick to anger and find it easy to use aggressive behaviors when their self-image is threatened. Bullying has its roots in childhood and, unless adults intervene early and effectively, it can escalate to more seriously violent behaviors.

"Adolescents who are involved in bullying, both as victims and as perpetrators, experience poor psychosocial and emotional adjustment, difficulty making friends, and increased loneliness" (Saluja and others, 2006). Victim reactions range from anxiety and avoidance to extreme fear and physical symptoms of illness. "When a child frequently complains of headaches, abdominal pain, or sleeping difficulties but no physical cause can be found, suspect that bullying is occurring" (RN, 2003). The best way to stop bullying is for responsible adults to recognize when it occurs and intervene early.

ADOLESCENT ABUSE

The incidence of abuse in adolescence is greater than once thought. Recent studies have reported that the rate of abuse for adolescents surpasses that of younger children. Abuse of adolescents is often the most overlooked type of family violence. For this reason, abused teens are less likely to receive needed services and counseling.

Adolescence is a time of emotional development, but not all teens have severe mood swings, periods of depression, or suicidal thoughts. Too often, these signs of possible abuse go unnoticed by adults. At other times, they are recognized as natural outcomes of adolescent misbehavior. "He or she had it coming" is still a widely held attitude when it comes to abusing adolescents.

Abused adolescents often have significant health risks. Emotional disorders often result from a history of insecurity and self-survival. The incidences of eating disorders, substance abuse problems, delinquent behaviors, posttraumatic stress disorders (PTSDs), and suicide attempts are increased in adolescents who are abused. Premature sexual activity is common. All too often, it leads to unwanted pregnancies, sexually transmitted diseases, and AIDS. Worse yet, adolescent abuse can result in fatal accidents, murder, and suicide, the three leading causes of death for all adolescents. One in four violent crimes is committed by adolescents.

Girls are more likely to be abused than boys. Women who were repeatedly abused in childhood are three times more likely to be abused as adults (RN, 2002). Boys are more likely to suffer abuse outside the home by peers and others. Individuals "who resort to acts of violence as adolescents are often the same people who end up in the nation's criminal system as adults" (Wood, 1999). Sadly, studies have shown that many adults who were physically disciplined as children approve of the use of physical force for controlling another person's behavior.

Adolescents are abused by parents, siblings, and persons outside the family. The most common form of violence within the home occurs between siblings. Violence between brothers and sisters is so common that it is often considered to be "normal" behavior because parents take it for granted that "kids will be kids" and tend to ignore it. Yet this type of violence can have long-lasting effects.

Children learn to exploit and victimize each other during the early school years. By the teen years, the use of violence can become interwoven with daily activities. Peer pressure is great during adolescence. Those who are different suffer the consequences at the hands of their own peers. Adolescents often receive the most severe abuse, the kind that results in serious disability or death (see Case Study 26-2).

Often, however, the signs of family mistreatment are vague. A history of abuse is frequently found in teens who are runaways, homeless, or incarcerated (in jail or prison). The blossoming problems of teen violence and abuse can be prevented if health care providers are willing to invest their best therapeutic efforts into these "forgotten clients."

ELDER ABUSE

As the number of older people grows, the potential for their maltreatment or neglect increases. Each year more than 1 million elderly persons are victims of abuse or mistreatment, but only one in five cases is reported. More than 5% of crimes involving victims occur in the elderly population (U.S. Census Bureau, 2007).

Vulnerable older adults include those with chronic or disabling illnesses, aged individuals, and those who

Case Study 26-2

Pete is a quiet, thoughtful, and charming young man whose intelligence shines through his sarcastic and tough demeanor. At 17 years old, he is well developed and equipped to cope on the streets of Chicago. Pete is also the leader of a street gang and does not hesitate to use violence.

Pete comes from a family with two older brothers and a younger sister. In his early years, it was common to see his mother and father arguing and hitting each other. By the time Pete was 6 years old, his older brother had shot a neighbor and was "doing time." Throughout his childhood, Pete frequently vented his frustrations on his younger sister by hitting, pinching, and spitting on her.

At 8 years old, Pete was initiated into his brother's gang. By 10, his intelligence and creativity had earned him the nickname of "the brain." By 14 years old, he was destined for leadership. Today, at 17 years, Pete sits in a hospital bed with three bullet holes in his body. His bruised and pregnant girlfriend sits at his side. As soon as he can walk again, he plans to "make a little visit and even the score" with the guys he believes are responsible for his attack.

- Can you see any learned patterns of behavior in this family?
- What do you think could have been done to prevent this situation from occurring?

---

are poor or have few resources. The typical victim of elder abuse is an older woman who is living with a relative and is physically or mentally impaired. She has a history of unexplained bruises or injuries, burns in unusual places, sexually transmitted disease, or poor personal hygiene. She may experience extreme mood swings, be depressed, be fearful, and be extremely concerned about the cost of health care. Many times the families of abused elders "health care shop," miss appointments, and change health care providers frequently.

Family members are the most frequent abusers of elderly people. The demands placed on caregivers often influence the development of abuse. Violence can erupt when caregivers feel stressed, pressured, or frustrated. In addition, many people who abuse their elders are coping with current substance-related or mental health problems themselves.

Neglect and exploitation are also common among the elderly population. Neglect can take the form of not providing food, health care, or aids such as dentures, glasses, or hearing aids. Older adults who are unable to walk can suffer from long periods of isolation or abandonment. Neglect also includes deliberate efforts to cause emotional distress, such as threatening harm or withholding important information.

Exploitation of elderly individuals is often financial in nature. They are a favorite target for cons or extortionists. Many times, older adults are forced to sign over their properties, their pensions, or other assets. Elderly people may be denied the right to vote or to make their own decisions. On some occasions, they are placed in nursing homes without their consent.

Today, many states have passed laws that require reporting of abusive incidents. Each health care provider can go a long way toward preventing elder abuse by recognizing the signs and symptoms of abuse. Become familiar with the laws governing mandatory reporting of abuse, and work to prevent violence in all settings. It is every person's responsibility to protect the aging members of society.

SEXUAL ABUSE

A particularly devastating form of abuse is sexual abuse, the unwanted sexual attentions of another. When sexual activities or intercourse occurs between members of the same family (other than the parents) it is called incest. Sexual violence has strong and lasting consequences for the victims. Children who are sexually abused suffer from a wide spectrum of mental health disorders, ranging from chronic headaches to depression, posttraumatic stress disorders, and severe personality disorders.

Sexually abused adults are most often women. Most sexual assaults are made by women's partners. The most violent form of sexual assault, rape, often occurs more frequently in relationships associated with other forms of physical aggression. Episodes of battering often include sexual and physical attacks—a deadly combination for many maltreated women.

Sexual abuse in elderly people, especially women, occurs with all-too-common frequency. Because sexual mistreatment of elderly individuals is still a taboo subject, it often goes unrecognized by health care providers. Clues to the presence of sexual abuse in the elderly population include complaints of pain, itching, or soreness in the genital area; bruises or other evidence of injury around the genital area or elsewhere on the body; difficulty in walking, sitting, or moving; the presence of unexplained venereal disease or genital infections; and stained, torn, or bloody underclothing.

Health care providers, especially nurses, should routinely assess all clients for a history of abuse or victimization and report any suspicious signs or behaviors to supervisors and required authorities. An individual's well-being is worth the effort.

ABUSE, NEGLECT, AND EXPLOITATION WITHIN THE COMMUNITY

Aggressive and violent behaviors are fast becoming a common way of coping with problems. Violence against innocent bystanders continues to increase as more people approve of its use or turn a blind eye to its occurrence. No statistic can accurately record the number of violent acts that occur (U.S. Census Bureau, 2007).

VIOLENCE, TRAUMA, AND CRIME

People use violence against each other in many ways, in both legal and illegal manners. Today's society is confronted with a steady diet of violent behaviors. Although most **homicides** (taking the life of another person) are committed by family members or friends, a surprising number of them occur at the hands of complete strangers. Robbery has become common in most communities, and an unsettling trend of murder in the workplace is rising. Car theft and drive-by crimes are increasing. Children are being kidnapped with greater frequency, and the incidence of violent crimes by and against children and adolescents continues to soar.

Acts of violence are becoming commonly accepted in society. Radio, television, and the Internet surround people with examples of violence. Our children are soaked in tales of aggressive actions from the time they are first exposed to cartoons. Studies by television's cable network group have revealed that over half of the programs on television are violent or aggressive in nature (*Teen Health and the Media,* no date). In most programs, the victims are not hurt and the aggressor is seldom caught or punished. This steady diet has resulted in children who are more willing to solve their problems with the use of violence than with critical thinking or problem solving.

Acts of violence on television pale in comparison with those that occur in real life (Figure 26-2). Daily newspapers and radio and television news programs announce a litany of the day's violent activities. People listen, shake their heads, and then continue with their own lives, unaware that they may be the next victims.

Violence breeds physical and emotional pain for its victims. The basic needs of trust and autonomy (control) are threatened when one is involved with violence. Victims react with anger, fear, denial, and shame. The well-meaning comments of friends and loved ones may even imply fault. Many victims of violence harbor feelings of unworthiness and contamination. Relationships with family and friends may become disturbed as victims attempt to put the pieces of their lives back together.

Crime is a natural vehicle for violence. Many crimes are committed on impulse, whereas others are well planned. Crime may or may not involve physical aggression and violence, but the impact of being victimized by crime leaves deep emotional scars on most individuals.

GROUP ABUSE

Throughout history people have chosen certain groups of people to define as being different from themselves. Individuals within these groups may be kind and gentle, but association with the group stigmatizes them as "one of those people." This label somehow justifies the aggressive and violent reactions of persons who view the group members with hostility. Excellent examples of this twisted line of thinking can be found

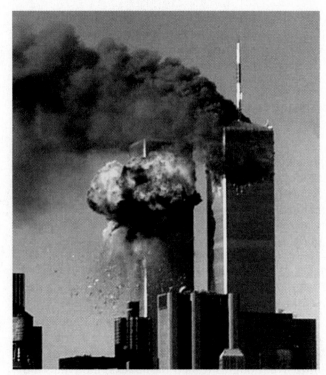

FIGURE **26-2** Violence against a society.

throughout history and in the "ethnic cleansing" that occurs in many countries.

Aggression against certain groups also exists in more subtle ways. Admission to many schools and academic institutions often depends on belonging to the "right group." Job requirements may be structured to attract only a certain kind of applicant, and running for a political office can be done only if one "fits in." These forms of aggression against members of certain groups are all quiet, subtle, and usually unspoken, but they still influence the lives of many good people.

MENTAL HEALTH DISORDERS RELATING TO VIOLENCE

Crisis is a part of every violent act. One's usual coping skills are ineffective when dealing with the effects of a violent act. To recover from an act of violence, new coping behaviors must be found and then applied. The victims of violence suffer through a number of emotional and behavioral experiences that can take months or even years to resolve. Putting one's life back together after a violent act involves many changes that take place over time (Table 26-2). The process of recovery from violence is influenced by the severity of the trauma, the resources of the victim, and the help and treatment received immediately following the traumatic event.

Aggressive and violent behaviors are a part of numerous mental health disorders; however, the *Diagnostic and Statistical Manual of Mental Disorders*

(DSM-IV-TR) defines only one clinical syndrome as directly related to violence: posttraumatic stress disorder. **Rape-trauma syndrome** is a related nursing diagnosis that encompasses the essentials of care for the victims of this violent experience.

POSTTRAUMATIC STRESS DISORDER

"The essential feature of posttraumatic stress disorder (PTSD) is the development of characteristic symptoms following exposure to extreme traumatic stressors" (American Psychiatric Association, 2000). PTSD clearly relates to an actual traumatic event that was outside the realm of common human experience. Examples include war, military combat, violent assault, rape, torture, burglary, natural disasters, terrorist activities, fires, bombings, sudden destruction of one's home, and witnessing the assault, injury, or death of a loved one.

Typically, people with PTSD persistently relive the traumatic event through intrusive thoughts or distressing dreams. Intense fear, horror, and hopelessness are experienced as individuals struggle to rid themselves of their memories. The sudden arrival of these intrusive thoughts (called **flashbacks**) motivates individuals with PTSD to avoid any stimuli associated with the traumatic event. Emotional responses become blunted except for those related directly to the violent event. This psychological numbing effectively shuts out the outside world until the person is exposed to an event, item, or situation that triggers some aspect of the traumatic event. For survivors of war, just watching television can precipitate flashbacks and stress reactions.

People suffering from PTSD feel removed and detached from other people, even those they love. The ability to feel emotions is reduced, especially those associated with love, intimacy, and sexuality. Often persons with PTSD believe that their lives will be short and wonder why they survived when others did not.

RAPE-TRAUMA SYNDROME

Rape is an act of sexual violence by one person against another. Although rape may involve sexual behaviors, it is an act of power that aims to cause pain at the most intimate level of one's being. Forced sexual attentions are a violation of one's person, whether they occur at the hands of a stranger or a loved one.

A woman may be raped at any age, but the ages of 15 to 24 years are associated with the highest risk. Rape is an underreported crime, with estimates of one woman in three being raped at some time during her life. Although not as common, the incidence of men being raped by other men is rising, but it is rarely reported (Keltner, Schwecke, and Bostrom, 2007).

Many victims of rape realize that they have lived through the experience but wish they had died. Body injuries may be minor or severe. Some individuals may have been tortured or injured during or shortly after the rape episode. A threat on the life of the victim or the promise to return may have been made.

Survivors of sexual assaults feel severely violated. Feelings of anger, frustration, loss of control, fear, shame, and guilt haunt the victims of these violent acts. Following the rape, most individuals feel the need to retreat to a safe place, clean themselves thoroughly, and remove all reminders of the event. To do this, however, destroys most of the evidence that is useful in apprehending the offender.

Recovery from being the victim of a rape follows the same steps as the stages of recovery from other violent acts (Table 26-2). Immediately following the incident, the individual becomes disorganized, then attempts to adjust are made, and finally the experience is integrated into her life. The greater the force or brutality, the greater psychological harm and recovery time. Many individuals do not report the assaults to the police. They carry their burden alone and suffer a silent rape-trauma syndrome.

Table 26-2 | *Stages of Recovery From Violence*

STAGE OF RECOVERY	TIME FRAME	EMOTIONS, BEHAVIORS
Impact: disorganization	Minutes to days	Initial reactions: crying, confusion, denial, disbelief, fear, hysteria, helplessness, shock; may have physical responses, eating or sleeping disturbances; may be calm with others and then react in private
Recoil: struggle to adapt	Weeks to months	Slowly becomes aware of impact of event on his or her life; immediate danger is past, but emotional stress remains; may plan for revenge; tries to resume daily routines; needs to discuss details of violent event; may become dependent; needs much emotional support
Reorganization: reconstruction	Months to years	Emotions fade, but event is not forgotten; reviews event with "Why me?" questions; justifies own actions, then gains sense of control over life; grieves over losses; may experience lingering emotions, nightmares; realizes that life will always be different as result of violence; eventually integrates memories and learns to live with reasonable sense of safety and security; may develop mental health problems if reorganization is not successful

Data from Keltner NL, Schwecke LH, Bostrom CE: *Psychiatric nursing*, ed 7, St. Louis, 2005, Mosby.

Nurses may be the first health care providers with whom a rape victim interacts. Strong support, gentle understanding, and nonjudgmental acceptance have a powerful influence on how well the victim copes with and successfully recovers from this violent assault. Because rape is a reportable crime, evidence must be gathered, with the victim's permission. Nurses should make sure to follow the same protocol every time they care for a client who has been raped. Evidence that has been gathered carefully and good documentation are important tools if the case is taken to court.

THERAPEUTIC INTERVENTIONS

When working with the victims of violence, there are two major goals. The first and longest-reaching goal is to prevent violence from occurring. The second goal revolves around early recognition and treatment for violated individuals.

Working with abused or victimized clients on a regular basis requires special education and training. Some health care providers become rape counselors or advocates for abused and exploited clients. However, every caregiver can apply special measures to care for the individuals who have the misfortune to become victims of violence.

SPECIAL ASSESSMENTS

Whenever a suspected victim of violence enters the health care system, be it the emergency department or clinic, special attention is required. The first priority of care is to ensure the client's safety, but the preservation of evidence also is extremely important.

Forensic evidence is information that is gathered for legal purposes. It is the evidence that helps find and convict perpetrators of violent acts. When violence is suspected, the caregiver's most effective tools are accurate observations, precise documentation, and notification of the appropriate authorities. By law, health care providers are required to report these incidences to the police. Although the law does not require victims of rape to report it, all evidence is important and must be gathered carefully.

When assessing a client who has been a victim of violence, first obtain his or her consent. Then document the size, shape, color, and pattern of any wounds, bruises, scars, or other marks. The skin records evidence well. Human bite marks leave a history. Look for them on the ears, nose, nipples, armpits, back, and genitals. Rings, belt buckles, and other items leave telltale marks behind when they are used as weapons. Other physical signs that may indicate violence or abuse include odd marks on the skin, hyperactive reflexes, and poor eye contact. Child abuse or neglect is not always easy to spot. Table 26-3 lists

numerous signs and symptoms of child abuse and neglect.

Caregivers, especially nurses, must know how to assess suspicious injuries and describe their findings objectively. Figure 26-3 (p. 293) offers an example of an abuse assessment documentation form. Document objective evidence as accurately as possible. Do not guess or draw conclusions about the cause of any injury. If the client is a rape victim, all specimens should be labeled and saved for analysis. It is wiser to err on the side of gathering too much information rather than not enough.

TREATING VICTIMS OF VIOLENCE

Remember, the first priority of care for every victim of violence is to ensure safety and security. Once a client feels safe, other therapeutic interventions are more easily implemented.

Do not leave the client alone. Many victims believe that their abusers may attempt to hurt them again, even when they are seeking help. Explain all procedures simply, and ensure cooperation before proceeding. Allow the client to maintain as much control as possible.

The care plan is developed based on the individual client, the type of abuse, and the resources available. Nursing diagnoses are chosen according to identified problems. Refer to Box 26-5 (p. 293) for a list of possible nursing diagnoses.

It is important to remember that each diagnosis has many interventions and the selection depends on each client's particular circumstances. However, all clients who have been abused, exploited, or neglected have certain care needs in common (see Sample Client Care Plan 26-1, p. 294).

Aggressive and violent actions are often seen in clients who are diagnosed with a mental illness. Treatment consists of assessing risk factors, developing interventions to reduce aggressive reactions, and helping clients learn more effective coping skills. Clients are often prescribed medications to help control aggressive and violent behaviors (Table 26-4).

PREVENTING VIOLENCE IN YOUR LIFE

Given the statistics, it is likely that each of us will be exposed to violence at some time during our lives. As members of the health care profession, the odds of being involved in some type of violence are increasing. Health care providers are less immune to acts of violence than they were in the past. It is important to remain aware that violence can erupt in any client situation.

When interacting with clients, watch for signs of growing anxiety, frustration, or agitation and then intervene quickly to prevent problems from escalating. Refer back to Figure 26-1. Trust your own judgment or

Table 26-3 *Signs and Symptoms of Child Abuse and Neglect*

CATEGORY	CHILD'S APPEARANCE	CHILD'S BEHAVIOR	CARETAKER'S BEHAVIOR
Physical abuse	**Bruises and welts:** on face, lips, or mouth; in various stages of healing; on large areas of torso, back, buttocks, or thighs; in unusual patterns, clustered, or reflective of instrument used to inflict them; on several surface areas **Burns:** cigar or cigarette burns; glovelike or socklike burns or doughnut-shaped burns on buttocks or genital indicating immersion in hot liquid; rope burns on arms, legs, neck, or torso; patterned burns that show shape of item (iron, grill, etc.) used **Fractures:** skull, jaw, or nasal fractures; spiral fractures of arms or legs; fractures in various states of healing; multiple fractures; any fracture in child under 2 yr **Lacerations and abrasions:** to mouth, lip, gums, or eye; genitals **Human bite marks**	Wary of physical contact with adults Apprehensive when other children cry Demonstrates extremes in behavior (e.g., aggressiveness or withdrawal) Seems frightened of parents Reports injury by parents	Has history of abuse as child Uses harsh discipline Offers illogical, unconvincing, contradictory, or no explanation of child's injury Seems unconcerned about child Significantly misperceives child (e.g., sees him or her as bad, evil, a monster) Psychotic or psychopathic Misuses alcohol or other drugs Attempts to conceal child's injury or to protect identity of person responsible
Neglect	Consistently dirty, unwashed, hungry, or inappropriately dressed Without supervision for extended time or when engaged in dangerous activities Constantly tired or listless Has unattended physical problems or lacks routine medical care Is exploited, overworked, or kept from attending school Has been abandoned	Engages in delinquent acts (e.g., vandalism, drinking, prostitution, drug use) Begs or steals food Rarely attends school	Misuses alcohol or other drugs Maintains chaotic home life Shows evidence of apathy or futility Mentally ill or of diminished intelligence Has long-term chronic illnesses Has history of neglect as child
Sexual abuse	Has torn, stained, or bloody underclothing Is experiencing pain or itching in genital area Has bruises or bleeding in external genitals, vagina, or anal regions Has venereal disease Has swollen or red cervix, vulva, or perineum Has semen on mouth or genitals or on clothing Is pregnant	Appears withdrawn or engages in fantasy or infantile behavior Has poor peer relationships	Extremely protective or jealous of child Encourages child to engage in prostitution or sexual acts in presence of caretaker
Emotional maltreatment	Emotional maltreatment, often less overt than other forms of child abuse and neglect; indicated by behaviors of child and caretaker	Unwilling to participate in physical activities Engages in delinquent acts or runs away States he or she has been sexually assaulted Appears overly compliant, passive, undemanding Extremely aggressive, demanding, or rageful Shows overly adaptive behaviors, either inappropriately adult (e.g., parents other children) or inappropriately infantile (e.g., rocks constantly, sucks thumb, is enuretic) Lags in physical, emotional, and intellectual development Attempts suicide	Has been sexually abused as child Experiencing marital difficulties Misuses alcohol or other drugs Frequently absent from home Blames or belittles child Cold and rejecting Withholds love Treats siblings unequally Seems unconcerned about child's problem

Modified from *Interdisciplinary glossary on child abuse and neglect: legal, medical, social work terms,* DHHS Pub No 80-30137, Washington, DC, 1980, U.S. Department of Health and Human Services.

1. Have you **ever** been emotionally or physically abused by your partner or someone important to you?   Yes ☐ No ☐

2. **WITHIN THE LAST YEAR,**
   have you been hit, slapped, kicked, or otherwise physically hurt by someone?   Yes ☐ No ☐

   If YES, by whom?_____Total number of times_____

3. Since you've been pregnant, were you hit, slapped, kicked, or otherwise
   physically hurt by someone?   Yes ☐ No ☐

   If YES, by whom?_____Total number of times_____

**MARK THE AREA OF INJURY ON THE BODY MAP, SCORE EACH
INCIDENT ACCORDING TO THE FOLLOWING SCALE:**

SCORE

1 = Threats of abuse including use of a weapon   _____

2 = Slapping, pushing; no injuries and/or lasting pain   _____

3 = Punching, kicking, bruises, cuts, and/or continuing pain   _____

4 = Beating up, severe contusions, burns, broken bones   _____

5 = Head injury, internal injury, permanent injury   _____

6 = Use of weapon; wound from weapon   _____

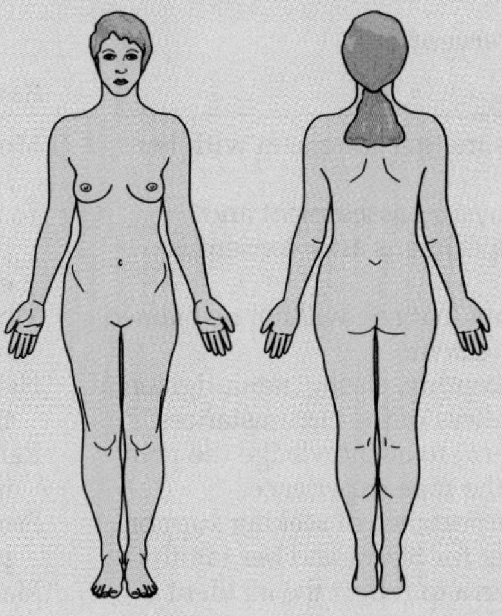

If any of the descriptions for the higher number apply, use the higher number.

4. **WITHIN THE LAST YEAR,**
   Has anyone forced you to have sexual activities?   Yes ☐ No ☐

   If YES, by whom?_____Total number of times_____

5. Are you afraid of your partner or anyone you listed above?   Yes ☐ No ☐

FIGURE **26-3** Abuse assessment screen.

gut-level feelings, and seek assistance from other care providers when needed.

Prevent yourself from becoming victimized by clients or their family members by enforcing your professional boundaries (see the discussion of helping boundaries in Chapter 11) and working within your legal and ethical parameters. The goal of providing emotional/mental health care is to assist clients in successfully coping with their problems. Remembering who "owns" the problem allows care providers to remain therapeutic without becoming victimized.

Work to prevent violence in your life. Contact the sponsors of violent programs on television; write

| Box 26-5 | **NANDA-I Nursing Diagnoses Related to Violence** |

Anxiety	Rape-trauma syndrome
Behavior, risk-prone health*	Self-esteem disturbance,
Coping, ineffective	situational low/chronic
Denial, ineffective	low
Family processes,	Social interaction, impaired
interrupted	Violence, risk for other-
Fear	directed
Hopelessness	Violence, risk for
Powerlessness	self-directed

Data from NANDA International: *NANDA-I nursing diagnoses: definitions and classification, 2007-2008,* Philadelphia, 2007, NANDA International. *NANDA-I,* NANDA International.
*Primary nursing diagnosis for violence.

SAMPLE CLIENT CARE PLAN 26-1

Rape-Trauma Syndrome

ASSESSMENT *History.* Sierra is a 19-year-old college student who lives at home. Three weeks ago she met Ben, a road maintenance worker who was visiting a mutual friend. After a short visit, Sierra said she was going to the club for her workout. Ben offered to drive her because he was going in the same direction. Sierra accepted, saying that she had to stop at her house first to change clothes.

On arrival, Sierra left the car and walked into the house. She was surprised to see Ben following her and asked him to wait in the car. Later that day Sierra's mother found her beaten and tied to her bed.
Current Findings. A stuporous young woman, lying in the fetal position. Numerous bruises and abrasions are noted on the face, both wrists, legs, and feet. Mother is at the bedside.

Multidisciplinary Diagnosis	*Planning/Goals*
Rape-trauma syndrome related to recent sexual attack and injury	Sierra will be free of medical or physical complications of rape trauma.
	Sierra will establish a therapeutic alliance with the primary nurse by October 21.

Therapeutic Interventions

Intervention	Rationale	Team Member
1. Allow Sierra's mother to remain with her at all times.	Mother has historically provided safety and security for Sierra.	Nsg
2. Assist with physical assessment and gathering of specimens after consent is obtained.	To assess the extent of her physical injuries, psychological trauma; to gather forensic evidence.	Nsg
3. Let Sierra know that she will not be blamed for the rape incident.	Violated persons often feel they will be held responsible for encouraging the assault.	Nsg, Psy
4. Convey an accepting, caring, nonjudgmental attitude regardless of the circumstances.	Helps to establish therapeutic communications and builds trust.	All
5. Encourage Sierra to acknowledge the pain and anger of the rape experience.	Releasing painful emotions lessens their intensity and power.	Psy, Nsg
6. Explain the importance of seeking support and counseling for Sierra and her family.	Provides emotional support during the process of returning to "normal."	Psy, Nsg
7. Encourage Sierra to report the incident to the police.	May help to prevent other occurrences; may help to bring the perpetrator to justice.	Psy, Nsg
8. Make referrals to rape crisis center, family counselors (with permission).	Long-term emotional support will help Sierra and her family effectively adapt.	Soc Svc

Evaluation

Sierra tested negative for sexually transmitted diseases 3 weeks after the incident. Following 2 weeks of emotional support and encouragement, Sierra attended her first crisis support group.

? CRITICAL THINKING QUESTIONS

1. What can be done to promote feelings of safety in Sierra?

2. Why is long-term counseling important with rape-trauma victims?

A complete client care plan includes several other diagnoses and interventions.
Nsg, Nursing staff; *Psy,* psychologist; *Soc Svc,* social services.

Table 26-4 | **Medications Used to Manage Aggression**

DRUG CLASS	EXAMPLE	CARE IMPLICATIONS
Atypical antipsychotics	Clozapine, risperidone	Can only be given by mouth
Beta-adrenergic blockers	Propranolol, nadolol, metoprolol, pindolol	Frequent side effects
Antianxiety agents	Buspirone, lorazepam, benzodiazepines	For short-term use only
Anticonvulsants	Valproic acid, divalproex sodium	Frequent side effects; interacts with other anticonvulsants, sedatives, and other medication

companies and protest. Support legislative actions that are designed to reduce violence. Volunteer at shelters, crisis hot lines, or support groups. Educate those who will listen about the effects of violence on children. Volunteer to teach a program on problem solving at local preschools.

Learn to recognize aggression and violence in your personal thoughts, attitudes, and responses. Become aware of how you cope with feelings of anger, frustration, and aggression. Practice developing more effective methods for working with your emotions. Howard Zinn, in his book *You Can't Be Neutral on a Moving Train* (1994), titled the epilogue "The Possibility of Hope." In it, he states that "small acts, when multiplied by millions of people, can transform the world." The small acts of nurses and other health care providers help to nourish the human connections that weave us together. Perhaps we can make a difference in relation to violence—if we are all willing to try.

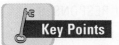

Key Points

- Violence is a major cause of death and disability in most countries.
- Theories that attempt to explain the nature of violence include the psychiatric/mental illness model, social learning theories, sociological theories, anthropological theories, and feminist theories.
- Characteristics of a dysfunctional family include self-centered members, authority that is inconsistent or lacking, no clearly defined roles, and members who are unable to meet their own or others' needs. Individualism is not encouraged. No common goals are identified. Communications are cold and indifferent. Conflict is perceived as negative, family boundaries are rigid, and family violence occurs.
- Battering is a term that describes ongoing physical abuse of someone, usually a woman, child, or elder.
- Trauma is the leading cause of maternal death during pregnancy. Low-birth-weight infants and preterm deliveries are almost doubled in women who have a history of abuse during pregnancy. Inadequate prenatal care is common.
- Since the early 1960s, the number of reported incidents of child abuse or neglect has increased dramatically.
- Adolescent abuse is often an overlooked type of violence.
- Each year more than 1 million elderly persons are victims of abuse or mistreatment.
- Throughout history people have chosen certain groups of people to define as being different and therefore deserving of aggressive behaviors.
- The process of recovery from violence is influenced by the severity of the trauma, the resources of the victim, and the help and treatment received by the victim immediately following the traumatic event.
- The essential feature of posttraumatic stress disorder (PTSD) is the development of characteristic symptoms following exposure to an extreme traumatic stressor.
- Rape is an act of sexual violence by one person against another that involves the use of power.
- Two major health care goals for victims of violence are to prevent violence from occurring and to provide early recognition and treatment for the violated individuals.
- The first priority of care for every victim of violence is to ensure safety and security. Explain all procedures simply, and ensure cooperation. Allow the client to maintain as much control as possible.
- Special assessments for a client who has been involved in violence include documenting the size, shape, color, and pattern of any wounds, bruises, scars, or other marks and looking for human bites on the ears, nose, nipples, armpits, back, and genitals.
- By law, health care providers are required to report incidences of suspected or actual abuse or neglect.
- Work to prevent violence in your life by contacting the sponsors of violent programs on television and protesting. Support legislative actions designed to reduce violence. Volunteer and educate about the effects of violence on children.

---

evolve   Be sure to visit the companion Evolve site at http://evolve.elsevier.com/Morrison-Valfre/ for additional online resources.

27 Inward-Focused Emotions: Suicide

Objectives

Upon completion of this chapter, the student will be able to:

1. Explain the range of self-protective behavioral responses.
2. Discuss three myths about suicidal behaviors.
3. Identify two cultural or social factors that relate to suicide.
4. Examine four categories of motivation for attempting suicide.
5. Explain how suicide affects family members and friends.
6. Describe three theories that attempt to explain the causes of suicide.
7. Discuss the occurrence of suicide throughout each life cycle.
8. Outline the process for assessing the suicidal potential of a client.
9. Choose three therapeutic goals and interventions for clients with suicidal behaviors.

Key Terms

ambivalence (ăm-BĬV-ə-lĕnts) (p. 299)
direct self-destructive behaviors (p. 296)
indirect self-destructive behaviors (p. 296)
parasuicidal (pair-ə-SOO-ĭ-sīd-əl) behaviors (p. 303)
passive suicide (p. 302)
rational suicide (p. 298)
self-injuries (p. 297)
suicidal attempts (p. 303)
suicidal gestures (p. 303)
suicidal ideation (p. 303)
suicidal threats (p. 303)
suicide (p. 296)
suicide precautions (p. 304)
suicidology (SOO-ĭ-sīd-ŌL-ə-jē) (p. 300)

Suicide is the action of intentionally taking one's own life. In England, suicide historically was considered an offense against the king. During the 1930s, many people in the United States committed suicide after the stock market crash that began the Great Depression in 1929. During World War II, Japanese kamikaze pilots intentionally sacrificed their lives for political and religious principles. In some societies, suicide is acceptable, but Western societies generally consider suicide as an immoral act committed by desperate or mentally ill individuals.

Suicide has historically served as a solution to life's great obstacles. Today we struggle with the dilemmas of rational suicide, freedom of choice, and physician-assisted suicide. Discussions about the morality or legality of suicide will grow and fade, but the ending of life by one's own hands continues to occur as people struggle for control over their situations.

CONTINUUM OF BEHAVIORAL RESPONSES

According to Maslow's hierarchy of needs, safety and security are basic requirements for life. Individuals behave in many ways to secure these needs. Some people respond with behaviors that promote growth, whereas others begin a journey to self-destruction. Behaviors that are adaptive and help the individual to cope result in a greater understanding and acceptance of oneself. However, maladaptive self-protective responses, if not changed, can eventually lead to self-destruction. Figure 27-1 illustrates the continuum of self-protective responses.

Self-destructive behaviors are classified as direct or indirect. Direct self-destructive behaviors are any form of active suicidal behavior, such as threats, gestures, or attempts to end one's life. In this case, the individual intends to commit suicide. Although he or she may waver between wanting to live and longing to die, the behaviors communicate an active wish to die.

Many more people, however, engage in indirect self-destructive behaviors, which are more subtle responses to self-protection. Indirect self-destructive behaviors are described as any behaviors or actions that may result in harm to the individual's well-being or death. In this case, people have no actual intention of ending their lives. They may be unaware of the potential for self-harm when engaging in harmful activities and deny the possibility of danger when confronted. Examples of indirect self-destructive behaviors include substance abuse, engaging in inappropriate or dangerous activities, and an unwillingness to change negative thoughts and actions. Because many of these behaviors are legal or socially accepted, people do not realize their potential for harm.

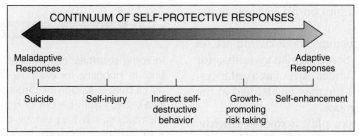

FIGURE **27-1** Continuum of self-protective responses.

Table 27-1 | *Myths and Facts About Suicide*

MYTH	FACT
People who talk about it will not commit suicide.	Most people communicate their intent.
One does not need to take a suicide threat seriously.	Every threat of suicide is serious.
A failed suicide attempt is manipulative behavior.	Manipulation is usually not a factor.
People who are really serious about suicide give no clues.	Many people communicate warnings of their intent by tidying up their affairs, giving away possessions, or being preoccupied with death.
It is harmful to discuss the subject of suicide with clients.	Most suicidal persons need acceptance and emotional support; discussing the topic demonstrates interest and concern.
Only psychotic or depressed people commit suicide.	Depression is a high risk factor for suicide, but not all suicidal persons are depressed. Mental illness is a risk factor for suicide.
Suicide occurs only in the lower socioeconomic classes, the poor.	Although poverty is a risk factor, suicide occurs in all socioeconomic classes.
Young children never commit suicide.	Suicidal behavior is the leading cause of psychiatric hospitalization for young children. Suicide can occur in children as young as 4 years of age.
When people show signs of an improved mood, the threat of suicide is over.	Depressed people often show improved moods, attitude, and behaviors before their deaths because the decision to commit suicide has been made.

Modified from Fortinash KM, Holoday-Worret PA: *Psychiatric mental health nursing*, ed 4, St. Louis, 2008, Mosby.

As the continuum of self-protective responses (see Figure 27-1) moves more toward maladaptive behaviors, indirect self-destructive behaviors progress to active attempts to injure oneself. **Self-injuries** reaffirm to individuals that they are still alive. Pain serves as a reminder of their connection with the body and its physical world. The last and ultimate maladaptive self-protective response is *suicide*, the ending of one's own life. Suicide is a complex and emotional issue, but it is one with which health care providers must cope. Although overt suicidal attempts receive the most attention, individuals who engage in indirect self-destructive behaviors carry risks as great as those individuals who actually attempt to end their lives.

MYTHS ABOUT SUICIDE

Many half-truths and misconceptions about suicide continue to exist despite educational efforts to promote accurate understanding. Although suicide has always been present in a society, little effort has been made to understand its nature until the beginning of the twentieth century. Today, many false ideas about suicide still exist. Table 27-1 explains several of these myths and offers facts to more accurately reflect the nature of suicide.

IMPACT OF SUICIDE ON SOCIETY

More than 1000 suicides occur throughout the world every day. Suicide is the eleventh leading cause of death in the United States and the third leading cause of death among people ages 15 to 24 (Centers for Disease Control and Prevention [CDC], 2005). Sadly, the suicide rate for children ages 10 to 14 has doubled since 1980. Twenty percent of all suicides occur in white men older than 65 years. The true number of persons who end their own lives is unknown because many motor vehicle accidents and other mishaps are actually intentions to commit suicide. For this reason, it is important for nurses and other health care providers to be well versed in recognizing and intervening with clients who are suicidal.

CULTURAL FACTORS

No one knows exactly why a person chooses suicide, but many cultural, social, and individual factors have an influence. The laws, customs, beliefs, values, and norms of a culture usually include a view of suicide. In some cultures, such as ancient Japan, suicide is considered an honorable atonement for transgressions committed during one's life. When a pharaoh king of Egypt died, it was an expected custom for the widow(s) to commit suicide and join him on his journey across the heavens.

Religious beliefs and customs have an impact on the incidence of suicide. Some Christian faiths, for example, forbid suicide under any circumstances, whereas the taking of one's life may be justified in the beliefs of other religious groups.

Customs and rituals may play a role in suicide. The "evil eye" or voodoo practiced by Caribbean islanders is very real for the victim of the curse. In these societies, suicide is not a surprising outcome for an individual who has been hexed or cursed.

Hungary routinely comes in first in the World Health Organization's statistics on suicide (see Cultural Considerations 27-1). Since 1993, with their cultural upheaval, Russia and the Baltic republics have surpassed Hungary in the number of suicides. Providers of health care must remember that people hold strongly to their cultural beliefs and practices. An awareness of a cultural group's attitude about suicide may someday help prevent the suicide of a clients.

SOCIAL FACTORS

Many social influences affect the incidence of suicide. Chief among them is a sense of social isolation felt by members of fast-paced, goal-oriented societies. Family and community support systems have dwindled as mobility, politics, and finances shift people away from the safety and security of family and friends. The support of kind neighbors and friends has been replaced by the generic, ready-made support of massive and complicated governmental systems. Crime and other aggressive actions force people to mistrust the intentions of others and barricade themselves behind locked doors and secured communities, but the price of security is paid with isolation and its ensuing sense of hopelessness.

An inability to meet basic needs has a strong influence on the occurrence of suicide. Since the emptying of state psychiatric hospitals, the number of homeless people has swelled. It is now estimated that persons with mental illnesses make up more than one third of the homeless population. The risk for suicide, for both healthy and mentally troubled individuals, skyrockets when one is unable to meet food, shelter, and clothing needs. Poverty and homelessness lead to depression and hopelessness. Suicide becomes an acceptable alternative when one is continually hungry, cold, ill, or living in fear.

The availability of weapons, especially firearms, is a significant factor in relation to suicide. In countries where the ownership of guns is prohibited, suicide rates are lower. To illustrate, in the United Kingdom, owning a handgun is illegal. According to the U.S. Census Bureau (2006), the suicide rate for England and Wales was 6.7 people per 100,000. In the United States, where gun ownership is hotly debated and defended, the rate is 31.3 suicides per 100,000 persons. The availability of firearms is reflected in a country's statistics on violence and suicide (see Think About 27-1).

 Cultural Considerations 27-1

In some societies, suicide is an accepted, centuries-old tradition. In Hungary, for example, villages dwindle as their residents choose suicide over the uncertainty of living an isolated, lonely life. When people in Hungary "get fed up, they hang themselves, cut their wrists, or swallow pesticides, just like their fathers and grandfathers did," states Dr. Jorge Ulloa, a psychiatrist who runs a suicide clinic near Budapest.

 Think About 27-1

Statistics show that gun-related injuries and deaths in the United States increase in households with firearms.
• Do you think that gun ownership should be controlled? Why or why not?
• If so, how should that be accomplished?

One's state of health influences suicidal considerations. Losses associated with old age can lead to depression and feelings of futility. Why struggle when tomorrow is a sad repeat of today? Suicide rates climb as age, infirmity, and illness take their toll.

The appearance of human immunodeficiency virus (HIV) and acquired immunodeficiency syndrome (AIDS) has had a profound influence on the suicide rates in many countries. In the United States, the death-with-dignity philosophy has influenced many AIDS sufferers to choose the time and place of their passing. This form of suicide is called rational suicide because the choice to end one's life was made freely and rationally with a sound mind.

Other social factors play a role in suicides. Higher suicide rates are seen in survivors of natural disasters or severe acts of aggression, such as ethnic cleansing. Veterans of combat (Figure 27-2) and those with posttraumatic stress disorder (PTSD) suffer higher suicide rates than the general population. The number, availability, and kind of community-based resources for health promotion and treatment influence a society's mental as well as physical health. Without these resources and the support they offer, the stresses of life can overwhelm a society's citizens. Be aware of the social changes in this world. Hidden among them are clues to caring for clients who are thinking of ending their lives.

DYNAMICS OF SUICIDE

The act of attempting suicide has a profound impact on the lives of individuals, families, friends, and communities. When many suicides occur, a whole society becomes affected. Because human beings dynamically

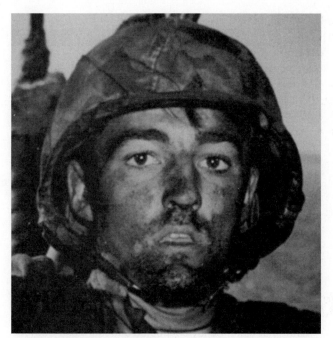

FIGURE **27-2** Combat veterans are at risk for suicide.

function in several realms or dimensions at any given time, it is important to consider suicide from a holistic point of view.

CHARACTERISTICS OF SUICIDE

Suicide is an act of **individual meaning.** The actual reasons for choosing such a final course of action are never known to anyone but the individual. However, it is likely that more than one motive drives a person to suicide.

In the **physical** dimension, thoughts of suicide produce many of the same biochemical changes in the body as depression. Chronic fatigue and vague complaints are common in both depressed and suicidal individuals. Often suicidal persons will not eat, drink, or rest enough to maintain required energy levels. Recent studies have suggested a link between low serum cholesterol levels and suicide attempts in men. Methods of choice for committing suicide differ by gender. Men prefer to rely on firearms, hanging, or drowning, whereas women prefer to overdose with pills or to inhale carbon monoxide.

The **emotional** dimension of functioning for the suicidal person is filled with feelings of ambivalence, anger, aggression, guilt, helplessness, and hopelessness. **Ambivalence** is a state in which an individual experiences conflicting feelings, attitudes, or drives. For the suicidal person, the struggle is between self-preservation (life) and self-destruction (death). Often, suicidal individuals threaten or attempt suicide and then behaviorally act out their feelings of ambivalence by seeking treatment.

Anger and aggression are turned inward in suicidal persons. Fears of being abandoned or rejected add to the dynamics. Many persons who feel trapped in frustrating relationships commonly react with rage that becomes self-directed and harmful.

Guilt can also lead to suicide. Suicidal individuals often shoulder the guilt of the world. They feel sinful and carry around the belief that they must have done something very wrong to deserve their misfortunes. Often personal guilt is exaggerated until the only way to make up for one's transgressions is to offer the final sacrifice—the self.

For the suicidal individual, the emotional dimension is marked by overwhelming feelings of helplessness and hopelessness. Nothing works out the way it was expected. The individual becomes unable to function emotionally. Life is bleak and hopeless as its meaning and purpose slip from one's control. Self-esteem sinks to an all-time low.

In the **intellectual** dimension, intense emotional suffering leads to distorted thinking and self-defeating thoughts. The self becomes devalued and worth little. Everything is glum and depressing, which leads individuals to a negative and pessimistic view of the future. One's self-talk becomes self-defeating, which soon leads to negative behaviors. Thinking is self-centered rather than oriented toward solving problems. Why continue when the future looks so bleak?

The **social** dimension of functioning includes one's views of others. Many suicidal individuals depend on the frequent feedback of others to reaffirm their self-worth. Self-esteem is very low in suicidal people. Their feelings of inferiority, of being less than others, interfere with social relationships and lead to the isolation and loneliness that accompany suicide.

In the last area, the **spiritual** dimension, suicidal individuals grapple with the cultural, religious, and ethical dilemmas associated with one's own demise. Many respond by blaming other people, their society, or their religious practices. Others "make their peace" with the spiritual sides of themselves and experience a spiritual calm and serenity before committing suicide. Some people believe they will be reunited with loved ones in a new life after leaving this reality.

CATEGORIES OF MOTIVATION

People are motivated to take their own lives for many reasons. All suicide victims, however, seem to share two major viewpoints. The first is a deep, inner disturbance of hopelessness, despair, poor self-esteem, and feelings of being trapped. The other is described as a logic whereby suicidal individuals consider the act as a way of relieving themselves of the miseries of this life and connecting with a sense of immortality or a life beyond the one they are leaving behind.

There are several categories of motivation for suicide (Box 27-1). The first motive is called "a cry for help." Most commonly, suicidal persons bounce between the wish to live and the need to die. They feel

■

Box 27-1 *Motivations for Suicide*

Cry for help
Refusal to accept a diminished quality, style,
or pace of life
Need to affirm the soul
To relieve distress
Preoccupied with suicide

 Case Study 27-1

Sandy was young, alone, pregnant, and scared. She knew she was not welcome at home because her father told her when she left for college, "If you get into trouble, don't come crying to me. You'll have to take care of it by yourself."

Her boyfriend, who swore his love and devotion, denied that he was the father of her baby and then left town. Even her new friends deserted her when they heard she was pregnant. Now the school officials were asking about her plans.

In desperation, Sandy sought to terminate the pregnancy but found that she was "too far along." She decided there was only one course of action that could end her troubles. She really did not want to die, but there seemed to be no other way out. The thought of facing life alone with a new baby was more than she could tolerate.

As she made her final plans, a feeling of calm came over Sandy. She would handle the situation in her own way. At least this way, she rationalized, "I am in control. I am the one who will do something about this."

Later that night, Sandy connected a rubber hose from the exhaust system to the interior of her car, rolled up all the windows, and sat quietly with the motor running. The next morning, when her body was discovered, she held a small note in her hand. It said, "Daddy, I took care of it myself. Love, Sandy."

• What do you think motivated Sandy to commit suicide?
• Why did she feel that this was her only or best course of action?
• If Sandy had come to you for help, what could you have done?

trapped in a situation from which they see no other escape. Killing oneself is an effort to break out and take control and to do something about one's life. These individuals are communicating their need for the kind of help that will radically change their lives and alter their present existence. Case Study 27-1 illustrates this type of motivation.

The second motive for considering suicide is the refusal to accept a diminished quality, style, or pace of life. This motive causes persons to commit rational suicide. They assess their situation in a clear and unemotional manner, consider all the options, and then decide to take steps that will end their lives. Decisions and plans are made logically with little or no emotion. The decision to commit suicide is seen as a logical one. An example would be the 80-year-old man who kills his 78-year-old blind and bedridden wife and then ends his own life after making all the arrangements for their funerals and property settlements.

The third motivation centers around the need to affirm one's soul. These persons believe that there are values more important than life. Suicide is a way of fulfilling one's existence. The 18-year-old who takes his life one summer evening when everything is going well and the future is bright may be searching for that fulfillment.

The fourth motive for suicidal behavior is to relieve distress related to situations that threaten the intactness of a person. The 70-year-old businessman with prostate cancer who chooses suicide over potentially life-prolonging surgery is an example of this type of motivation.

Last are those individuals who are preoccupied with suicide. They derive comfort knowing that they will control the time and circumstances of their death. These people are usually unwilling to accept life on any terms but their own. They set conditions for living and refuse to continue with life unless it is on their terms. Often suicide is the only form of real control they feel they have.

When working with suicidal clients, remember that no matter what the motivation, each individual is experiencing deep discomfort and very low self-esteem. Compassion and understanding become valuable therapeutic tools when working with suicidal clients.

THEORIES ABOUT SUICIDE

Because suicide is an end result, it is difficult to understand all the factors that lead up to one's decision to end his or her life. The study of the nature of suicide is called **suicidology**. Several theories attempt to explain the causes of suicidal behavior.

The **psychoanalytical** theory states that all humans have the instinct for life and death within them. Suicidal persons experience much ambivalence between wanting to live and wanting to die. Anger turns inward, and when stressful life events activate their death wish, suicide becomes an option.

Sociological theory considers the relationship between the number of suicides and the social conditions of an area. These theorists believe that suicide rates are affected by group support (or the lack of it), social changes, regulations, religion, legal sanctions or limitations, and philosophical beliefs. In short, the sociological theories consider the impact of social factors on the occurrence of suicide.

Last is the **interpersonal** theory, developed by H. S. Sullivan. Suicide is viewed as the outcome of a failure to work with or resolve interpersonal conflicts.

These three theories form much of the foundation for further studies into the nature of suicide. However, ongoing research into the psychobiological nature of the human being is revealing new information about suicide and its motivations.

New Biological Evidence

Depression, anxiety, and impulsive behaviors are common in suicidal individuals. Because scientists are now able to study the structure and functions of the living human brain, new connections between physical and behavioral activities are being rapidly discovered.

Anxiety and depression are often the forerunners of suicidal thoughts. Researchers have demonstrated that when certain chemicals in the brain (neurotransmitters) are not in balance, people have difficulty regulating their moods. For example, irregularities in a certain neurotransmitter pattern, called the **serotonin system,** have been found in depressed and suicidal persons. These findings have implications for health care providers. As our understanding of the dynamics of suicide grows, so does our ability to recognize the potential for suicide and effectively intervene.

EFFECTS OF SUICIDE ON OTHERS

Suicide, like natural death, has a strong effect on those left behind. Following the suicide, the lives of the survivors can be filled with questions, anger, sadness, shame, guilt, and health problems. "The death of a spouse by suicide has the potential of severely compromising the psychological well-being of the surviving marital partner" (Constantino and others, 2002). The grieving process is further complicated by social attitudes about taking one's own life.

Survivor Guilt

Because of the emotions attached to suicide, the loss of a loved one through suicide is considered a much more stressful event than the grief reaction to a natural death. Guilt is a main response because survivors often think they could have done something to prevent the suicide. Guilt may also stem from unexpressed anger toward the deceased person for abandoning family and friends. Depression, PTSD with flashbacks, and somatic complaints are the common problems of most suicide survivors. Impaired immune system functioning may accompany the emotional disturbances.

Anger may be expressed as "agonized questioning" that helps the survivors cope with their emotional turmoil and disorganization. Some may hide their resentment, anger, and rage, turning it into depression. Children often feel responsible for the suicide. Unless they receive much love, support, guidance, and permission to be angry, depression or other behavioral problems may develop.

Socially, the stigma of suicide is soon felt. Forced interactions with health care providers, the police, or the media soon after death can bring home the feelings of rejection that are often experienced by the family members of suicide victims. Friends and relatives, unsure of how to help, withdraw or do nothing. This reaction limits the social contact and support that are so needed after the suicide of a loved one. The survivors of a suicide victim may also withdraw from social interactions to protect themselves from the gossip and intrusion of inconsiderate others. Thus begins a cycle of guilt, withdrawal, and blame between the survivors of a suicide and others in their world. With support and understanding, survivors eventually recover and accept the fact that the responsibility for the suicide rests with the individual who committed it and not with those who are left behind.

Health care providers are not immune to the effects of suicide. When a client, especially an inpatient, commits suicide, staff members and other clients may experience guilt, anger, or helplessness. Both clients and staff members need to grieve and express the emotions that follow a suicide. Often other clients on the unit will express anger at the staff, act out, or become self-destructive. Sharing emotions about the suicide allows both staff and clients the opportunity to express themselves and cope with the experience. The survivors of suicide, no matter who they are, must grieve and learn to heal.

SUICIDE THROUGHOUT THE LIFE CYCLE

Attempts to end one's life occur in every age-group. Although the motivations for suicide may vary with the developmental level, the act remains the same: an effort to die. Understanding how suicide is used at different developmental levels is important. Recognition and treatment of the problems underlying suicidal behaviors are much more effective when begun early.

SUICIDE AND CHILDREN

Although depression is usually a component of suicide, with children it may be different. Some experts believe that suicide in children is most often the result of family conflict or disruption. Children learn by exposure. The children of depressed mothers think about and attempt suicide more often than those of emotionally healthy mothers. Children commit suicide as a cry for help, to change their situations, or to act out a sincere wish to die. Children with existing mental health problems, such as conduct disorders, attention-deficit/hyperactivity disorders, or psychoses, are at a greater risk for committing suicide than other children. Because they are impulsive, suicides in children are usually not planned. Often the loss of a parent triggers suicidal behaviors in children who were not encouraged to grieve. Because very young children cannot understand the concept of death as a permanent state, their wishes to join their lost parent may lead to suicidal behaviors.

The **key** to recognizing the signs of suicidal intent lies in **a change in the child's behavior.** Any child whose attitudes, behaviors, or habits change dramatically in a short time, especially following a stressful event or situation, is a candidate for suicide.

SUICIDE AND ADOLESCENTS

The rate of adolescent suicide has risen dramatically in the past 30 years. The suicide rates for adolescents and young adults "have tripled in the last four decades" (Kresnow and others, 2002). Presently, suicide accounts for almost 13% of all deaths in 15- to 24-year-olds (CDC, 2005). Young men are the most affected by violence and suicide in adolescence. Statistics may not accurately reflect the actual number of adolescent suicides because many suicidal deaths are listed as accidental.

During adolescence, any long-standing family or social problems may continue to worsen as the difficulties of growing up are experienced. If coping skills or resources are insufficient, adolescents, especially those with low self-esteem, may consider suicide as an option for solving their problems. Adolescents commit suicide when they feel there is no other way out of their problems. They see their problems as genuinely unsolvable, now or in the future.

Many factors come into play in adolescent suicide. Depression, poor impulse control, and emotional isolation are related to suicide in adolescents. Dysfunctional or disrupted family interactions, such as divorce or separation of parents, can devastate many teens. Adolescents with anorexia nervosa have higher rates of suicide. In fact, many theorists believe that anorexia is a slow attempt at suicide.

Social problems with peers, the use of drugs or alcohol, and a lack of consistent relationships also add to the risk for suicide. When the environment lacks security or presents dangers, many teens feel that their lives will be short and they will not live until adulthood. The outlook for the future holds little promise with this attitude.

The incidence of suicidal behaviors is also increased in children and adolescents who suffer from chronic disease. Children and adolescents with immune-mediated (type 1) diabetes, for example, have a higher risk for suicide than healthy individuals. Those diabetics who actually try to commit suicide often do so by some method relating to their diabetes, such as overdosing on insulin. Health care providers should routinely assess every client (including those with medical diagnoses or problems) for the presence of suicidal thoughts. Become aware of the risk factors that can play an important role in an individual's choice to commit suicide (Box 27-2).

SUICIDE AND ADULTS

Suicide is a significant problem in adulthood, especially for white men. Women attempt suicide three times more frequently than men, but men are more successful at completing the act. In 25- to 34-year-old men, suicide ranks as the second leading cause of death (U.S. Census Bureau, 2006).

In young adults, suicide occurs when individuals are unable to cope with the pressures of adulthood. Some experience problems with interpersonal relationships, whereas others lack personal resources and are poor, hungry, or unemployed. All, however, are dissatisfied with their lives.

Loneliness is a factor in adult suicides. The loss of a family member or significant relationship, whether through divorce or death, increases the risk for suicide. In addition, certain professions and occupations are associated with higher rates of suicide.

Most adult suicides can be prevented if the clues are uncovered early enough. Do not hesitate to ask clients if they ever think about suicide. The answer to that question may offer an opportunity to help save an individual's life.

SUICIDE AND OLDER ADULTS

As age increases, so does the rate of suicide. Many studies reveal that the incidence of suicide increases with age. The actual number is difficult to determine because only active suicides are counted. Many older adults choose to commit a passive suicide by refusing to eat, drink, or cooperate with care.

The causes and risk factors of suicide in elderly people are poorly understood. Although many elderly

---

Box 27-2 | *Risk Factors for Suicide*

Abuse, neglect, exploitation
Academic pressures, school problems
Accident prone
Chronic or terminal illness, disability, HIV/AIDS
Dysfunctional family relationships
Family or self history of anxiety, depression
History of alcoholism and/or substance abuse
Inadequate child-rearing practices
Loss of parent or significant other
Low socioeconomic status, poverty, or homelessness
Male gender, unmarried, unemployed
Member of certain religious cults
Mental health problems*
Negative outlook for future
Previous suicide attempts*
Profession/occupation: police officer, firefighter, air traffic controller, physician, psychiatrist, college student, dentist
Social isolation, lack of social support
Stressful or unhappy personal relationships

HIV, Human immunodeficiency virus; *AIDS,* acquired immunodeficiency syndrome.
*Highest risk for suicide.

individuals who commit suicide have had contact with a health care professional within the month before their deaths, their risk was not identified or treated.

Older adults tend not to communicate their intentions unless directly asked; thus suicidal attempts in older adults are more successful. One out of every two suicide attempts in the elderly population results in death. These sobering statements must alert every care provider to perform a suicidal risk assessment for all older adults.

Most older adults view the timing of death in one of three ways—God controlled, physician and individual controlled, or controlled by the individual alone. Older males have the highest suicide rates within the elderly population (Stanhope and Lancaster, 2008). Risk factors for suicide in elderly people are advanced age, male gender, low socioeconomic status, chronic pain or illness, and fear of becoming dependent or helpless. A lack of relationships appears to be a driving force behind many suicides. Other researchers believe that intolerable life circumstances are the main motives for suicides in the elderly population.

Social attitudes about elder suicide differ. Some people think that all suicides in elderly people are irrational decisions, based in depression or physical illness. They believe aggressive interventions are always required. Others view elder suicide as the last rational decision, the last act of control over one's life.

The concept of **rational suicide** in the United States is "at odds with the legal system," but in other countries, such as the Netherlands, suicide is an acceptable way to achieve "death with dignity." It may seem that the important questions and issues surrounding the control of one's own death are issues for philosophers and medical ethicists; however, health care providers will be addressing many of these questions in daily practice.

Some nonsuicidal behaviors are the result of inward-focused emotions. Behaviors such as repeated **cutting** and **scratching** produce the pain that reminds many mentally troubled individuals that they are still alive.

THERAPEUTIC INTERVENTIONS

Thoughts about suicide can be described on several levels. **Suicidal ideation** is described as thoughts or fantasies that are expressed but have no definite intent. Ideas may be expressed directly or symbolically. **Suicidal threats** are verbal or written expressions of the intent to take one's life, but they are without actions. As the seriousness increases, **suicidal gestures** may be observed. These are suicidal actions that result in little or no injury but communicate a message of suicidal intent. **Parasuicidal behaviors** are unsuccessful attempts and gestures associated with a low likelihood of success. **Suicidal attempts** are serious self-directed

actions that are intended to do harm or end life. The last level is completed suicide, the successful attempt to end one's life. Motivation for the successful suicide may be conscious or unconscious.

Suicide is a serious public health threat. Prevention is thus the most important health care action for all our clients, especially for those who may be suicidal. Preventing a suicide from occurring means saving a life. Prevention requires a knowledge of the dynamics of suicide and the ability to recognize the potential for suicidal actions in every client. The nursing (therapeutic) process is an excellent tool for working with clients who may be considering suicide.

ASSESSMENT OF SUICIDAL POTENTIAL

Because suicide is becoming so prevalent, it is important to evaluate **every** client for its potential. To accomplish this, first assess the **risk factors** for the age of the client. Then **ask** the client directly if he or she has any thoughts relating to suicide. Asking clients will not encourage them to take any suicidal actions. On the contrary, it gives them permission to discuss their feelings and attitudes. Box 27-3 offers a list of questions for assessing suicidal intentions. Not every question may be appropriate for every client, but a series of questions such as these will usually bring out expressions of suicidal thoughts if they are present.

Hospitalization may be required for the client's safety and protection if he or she feels unable to control suicidal behaviors. Suicidal intentions can exist with any medical or psychiatric diagnosis. Clients who are depressed must be carefully monitored for expressions of hopelessness. Table 27-2 lists the basic components of a suicide assessment. Do not hesitate to use

---

| **Box 27-3** | *Questions That Assess the Potential for Suicide* |

"What has been the most difficult moment for you in the recent past?"
"Have things been so bad that you have thought about escaping? If so, how?"
"Are there times when death seems like an attractive option to you?"
"Have you thought of harming or killing yourself?"
"If you were to harm yourself, how would you do it?"
"Do you have access to the items you would need to carry out your plan? (This includes a gun, medications, a rope, an enclosed garage.)"
"Have you thought about or attempted to harm yourself in the past?"
"What has kept you from harming yourself thus far?"
"What might keep you from harming yourself in the future?"
"Do you think you can control your behavior and refrain from acting on your thoughts or impulses?" is the **most important question** to ask.

Table 27-2 *Suicide Assessment*

ASSESSMENT	DESCRIPTION
Suicide ideation (thoughts)	Client talks about wanting to be dead, imagines AIDS or other serious illness, seems gloomy, brooding.
History of suicide attempts*	Client has tried to end own life before; there may be family history of suicide.
Present suicide plan	The more detailed a suicide plan, the more likely it will be carried out.
Availability of items to carry out plan	What guns, rifles, knives, or other weapons are available? How difficult is it to obtain such items?
Substance use or abuse	Suicide rates are higher in people who abuse alcohol or other chemical substances.
Level of despair	Ask about the future; when despair is high, hope is low.
Ability to control own behavior	Inpatient hospitalization is indicated for individuals who are unable to control their suicidal impulses.

AIDS, Acquired immunodeficiency syndrome.
*Highest risk.

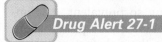

Drug Alert 27-1

Many medications can cause changes in mood. Much publicity has been given to the drug fluoxetine hydrochloride (Prozac), an *antidepressant* that has been reported to cause violent and suicidal reactions in some individuals.

The side effects of certain *steroids* (e.g., prednisolone) have been known to cause elation and feelings of well-being in some individuals. The same drug, administered to others, can result in severe depression and suicidal thoughts.

Elderly persons who are taking potent analgesics (pain medications) are at a high risk for feelings of depression.

Obtain a drug and medication history for every client. Sometimes something as simple as discontinuing or changing a medication can lift spirits and decrease suicidal thoughts.

Box 27-4 *NANDA-I Nursing Diagnoses Related to Suicide*

Anxiety
Behavior, risk-prone health
Body image, disturbed
Coping, ineffective
Denial, ineffective
Grieving, complicated
Hopelessness
Pain, chronic
Powerlessness
Self-esteem, chronic low
Self-mutilation, risk for
Social interaction, impaired
Spiritual distress
Violence, risk for self-directed

Data from NANDA International: *NANDA-I nursing diagnoses: definitions and classification, 2007-2008,* Philadelphia, 2007, NANDA International. *NANDA-I,* NANDA International.

this data-gathering tool whenever problems with the client's emotional state are suspected.

When used as part of a health history, the suicide assessment will yield valuable information about the client's suicidal intentions (if any) along with numerous clues about the individual. Drug Alert 27-1 also offers an important reminder. Nursing diagnoses for suicidal persons are based on each client's identified problems and needs (Box 27-4).

THERAPEUTIC INTERVENTIONS FOR SUICIDAL CLIENTS

The first priority for the care of suicidal clients is **protection** from harm. The client must be physically prevented from actively attempting suicide. If the risks are so high that a serious attempt may be made, suicide precautions are implemented. These precautions are standard interventions to prevent a suicide attempt from occurring. They are listed in Box 27-5. Clients with strong suicidal intents may require constant observation. Constant observation is a staff member keeping the client "in full view at all times" (Billings, 2001).

One of the most important therapeutic interventions (after ensuring safety) with suicidal persons is to establish rapport with the client. Many suicidal

people are alone. Most have little self-esteem. These individuals are distressed and experiencing enormous emotional reactions, but they will usually agree to make a **no self-harm contract** (a promise not to engage in self-destructive behaviors) with their caregivers (Stuart and Laraia, 2005). Establishing a therapeutic relationship with a health care provider is important for clients. The focused communications and concerned actions of caregivers help suicidal individuals to feel self-worth. With the encouragement and advocacy of their caregivers, many suicidal clients are able to develop more effective strategies for living satisfying lives. Sample Client Care Plan 27-1 illustrates a client care plan for an individual who may be suicidal.

Suicide and its associated effects are problems in today's society. Many of us will be or have been touched by the suicide of a loved one or friend. It is our duty and responsibility as health care providers to protect our clients, even from themselves, when we must. Hopefully, through our efforts, the tide of senseless loss of life can be turned, and choices will be made looking toward life instead of away from it.

Box 27-5 | *Suicide Precautions*

Protect client from harming himself or herself.	Refrain from criticizing.
Determine if client has specific suicide plan.	Facilitate discussion of factors or events that precipitated the suicidal thoughts.
Determine history of suicide attempts.	
Make a no-suicide contract.	Facilitate support of client by family and friends.
Remove dangerous items from the environment.	Instruct client and significant others in signs, symptoms, and basic physiology of depression.
Place client in least restrictive environment that allows for necessary level of observation.	
Place client in room with protective window coverings, as appropriate.	Instruct family that suicidal risk increases for severely depressed clients as they begin to feel better.
Observe closely during suicidal crisis.	Instruct family on possible warning signs or pleas for help client may use.
Escort client during off-ward activities, as appropriate.	Refer client to psychiatrist, as needed.
Demonstrate concern about client's welfare.	

Modified from Bulechek GM, Butcher HK, McCloskey Dochterman JC: *Nursing interventions classification (NIC),* ed 5, St. Louis, 2008, Mosby.

SAMPLE CLIENT CARE PLAN 27-1

Self-Directed Violence

ASSESSMENT *History.* Joe, a 19-year-old man, recently lost his best friend in an auto accident. For several weeks, he has been saying that he should have been killed instead of his friend. In the past 2 weeks, Joe has refused to work, eat, or engage in any social activities. Yesterday he bought a gun.

Current Findings. A depressed-looking young man sitting between two worried parents. Grooming is unkempt; shirt and denims are ragged and dirty. He volunteers no information but states, "It's not worth it" to the nurse. After obtaining the history from parents, Joe was admitted to the unit for assessment and observation.

Multidisciplinary Diagnosis	Planning/Goals
Risk for self-directed violence related to loss of significant other	Joe will refrain from making any suicidal gestures or attempts during his inpatient stay.
	Joe will discuss his feelings of loss by August 28.

Therapeutic Interventions

Intervention	Rationale	Team Member
1. Establish contact and rapport.	Open communication and trust must be established before work can begin.	All
2. Establish a no self-harm contract as soon as possible.	Helps prevent Joe from acting impulsively.	Psy, Nsg
3. Implement necessary suicide precautions; watch closely.	Protects Joe from self-injury or death.	All
4. Evaluate and document Joe's suicide potential at least twice daily.	Helps assess for changes in seriousness of client's intent.	Psy, Nsg
5. Help Joe identify and discuss sources of distress.	Increases awareness of feelings; helps to plan effective interventions.	All
6. Offer emotional support and acceptance.	Encourages Joe to think more highly of himself; helps develop self-worth.	All
7. Involve Joe and his family in the treatment plan.	Promotes active decision making; provides emotional support and resources.	All
8. Explore coping strategies that worked in the past.	Helps Joe to apply successful coping mechanisms to prevent problems.	All

Evaluation

During the course of hospitalization, Joe made no attempts at suicide. By August 18, Joe was able to share his sorrow and anger with the unit chaplain.

⁇ CRITICAL THINKING QUESTIONS

1. What do you think are the benefits/disadvantages of a "no self-harm contract"?

2. How does the staff offer emotional support and acceptance to Joe when he refuses to verbally communicate?

A complete client care plan includes several other diagnoses and interventions.
Psy, Psychologist; *Nsg,* nursing staff.

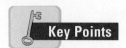
Key Points

- Suicide is the action of intentionally taking one's own life.
- Many misconceptions about suicide continue to exist despite efforts to promote an accurate understanding of the problem.
- Many cultural, social, and individual factors influence the occurrence of suicide.
- The act of suicide has a profound impact on the lives of individuals, families, friends, and communities.
- Thoughts and actions directed at self-destruction affect every dimension of human functioning.
- There are several categories of motivation for suicide, including a cry for help, a refusal to accept a diminished quality of life, a need to affirm one's soul, an attempt to relieve the distress related to situations that threaten the intactness of a person, and an act of those who are preoccupied with suicide.
- Theories that attempt to explain the causes of suicidal behavior include the psychoanalytical theory, sociological theory, and interpersonal theory.
- New connections between physical and behavioral activities are being rapidly discovered.

- After the suicide of a loved one, the lives of the survivors can be plagued with anger, sadness, shame, guilt, health problems, and agonizing questions.
- Some experts believe that suicide in children is most often the result of family conflict or disruption.
- Adolescents commit suicide when they feel there is no other way out of their problems.
- Adult women attempt suicide three times more frequently than men, but men are more successful at completing the act.
- The incidence of suicide in older adults continues to increase with age.
- Prevention is the most important therapeutic action for clients who may be suicidal.
- Because suicide is becoming so prevalent, it is important for nurses to assess every client for its potential.
- The first priority for the care of clients who may be suicidal is protection from harm.
- With encouragement and the advocacy of their care providers, many suicidal clients are able to develop effective strategies for living more satisfying lives.

evolve Be sure to visit the companion Evolve site at http://evolve.elsevier.com/Morrison-Valfre/ for additional online resources.

Objectives

Upon completion of this chapter, the student will be able to:

1. Define five terms relating to substance use and treatment.
2. Explain how chemical dependency affects persons from different age-groups.
3. Describe four serious consequences of substance abuse.
4. Classify four categories of abused substances, and give an example from each group.
5. Identify three reasons why inhalants are abused by adolescents and young adults.
6. Describe the three stages or phases of becoming addicted.
7. Compare the three criteria for the diagnosis of a substance-related disorder.
8. Explain what is meant by the term *relapse*.
9. Plan at least four interventions for clients who are diagnosed with substance-related disorders.

Key Terms

abstinence (p. 308)
abused substances (p. 307)
addiction (p. 308)
alcohol (p. 310)
alcoholism (p. 308)
amphetamines (ăm-FĔT-ə-mēnz) (p. 312)
caffeine (p. 311)
cannabis (KĂN-ə-bĭs) (p. 312)
cocaine (p. 311)
crack (p. 312)
designer drugs (p. 312)
detoxification (p. 317)
disulfiram (dī-SŬL-fĭ-răm) **(Antabuse)** (p. 317)
dual diagnosis (p. 309)
habituation (hə-BĬCH-oo-ā-shən) (p. 308)
hallucinogens (hă-LOO-sĭ-nō-jĕnz) (p. 312)
heroin (HAIR-ō-ĭn) (p. 311)
inhalants (p. 313)
intoxication (p. 314)
methadone (MĔTH-ə-dōn) (p. 317)
narcotics (năr-KŎT-ĭkz) (p. 310)
nicotine (NĬK-ə-tēn) (p. 314)
phencyclidine (fēn-SĬ-klĭ-dēn) **(PCP)** (p. 312)
relapse (p. 317)
substance (p. 307)
substance (drug) abuse (p. 308)
substance (chemical) dependency (p. 308)

substance use (p. 307)
tolerance (p. 314)

The practice of using substances to make one feel better is as old as humans themselves. Even animals have been seen eating certain plants that change their behaviors. Alcohol has played a role in many cultures throughout recorded time. Various drugs, potions, solutions, and formulas have been developed as humans attempted to cope with the problems of disease and illness.

Drugs have also played a role in political history. For example, the Opium Wars of the nineteenth century between China and Britain and the drug movement of the 1970s in the United States changed the course of history. Even today, we are struggling with political and social events that relate to drugs and other illicit substances (see Cultural Considerations 28-1).

The world of substance use and abuse is always changing. As health care providers become familiar with current chemical fads, new and more potent drugs are introduced. The focus of this chapter is to provide an understanding of substance use, abuse, and addiction; its effects on society; and the current interventions used to treat and educate clients with substance-related problems.

VOCABULARY OF TERMS

To communicate about substance-related disorders, an understanding of terms is necessary. Several terms describe addictive disorders. A substance is defined as a "drug of abuse, a medication, or a toxin" (American Psychiatric Association, 2000). Substances are also called chemicals, drugs, or toxins. Substance use is the ingesting (eating, drinking, injecting, or inhaling) of any chemical that affects the body. This includes legal, illegal, and medicinal substances. Abused substances are those chemicals that alter the individual's perception by affecting the central nervous system (CNS). They are often called **mind-altering drugs** because of their ability to enhance or depress moods or emotions.

Substance (drug) abuse is culturally and socially defined. In some cultures, the use of certain drugs is

Today, in the drug-producing countries of Central and South America, the growing of cocaine plants is the only means of making a living for many poor farmers. Prices for coca leaves far outstrip the money paid for corn, wheat, or other agricultural products. When officials spray or otherwise destroy their crops, many men, women, and children suffer from hunger and malnutrition as a consequence.

• What do you think could be done to outlaw drugs and prevent the starvation of farmers at the same time?

expected in order to fulfill religious obligations or some other culturally defined duty. In other societies, the use of the same substance is considered illegal or immoral. In the United States, Canada, Great Britain, and other industrialized societies, for example, laws define which substances are socially approved and legal and those that are illegal. In other cultures, the use of substances that are labeled illegal in the industrialized countries is acceptable and even provides economic opportunities. A broad but workable definition of substance (drug) abuse is the "excessive use of a substance that differs from societal norms" (Keltner, Schwecke, and Bostrom, 2007). No matter which culture, however, when the use of a substance falls outside society's definition of approved use, a drug problem exists.

Drug or chemical habituation occurs when an individual depends on a substance to provide pleasure or relief. Substance (chemical) dependency occurs when a user must take his or her usual dose of the drug to prevent the onset of withdrawal signs and symptoms. When the dependence on the substance is physical, the term addiction is used. The term alcoholism describes an addiction to alcohol. Today, the term substance or chemical dependency is preferred for describing addictions. Abstinence occurs when an addicted individual is not using an addictive substance.

ROLE OF CHEMICALS IN SOCIETY

Chemical substances are important in modern societies. Without them, we would be unable to produce food, fight disease, or develop products that allow us to live comfortably. The use of different chemical substances has increasingly become a part of everyday life.

Children are unconsciously taught to solve problems by using substances. The physician prescribes a medicine to help a family member recover from an illness, and the child learns that drugs can be beneficial. Children observe their parents taking pills or drinking beverages that change their actions and unconsciously register approval of those behaviors.

We are constantly bombarded with encouragement to ingest chemicals in advertisements on television, radio, and the Internet. Commercials routinely encourage us to cope with constipation, heartburn, or allergies by taking drugs. Many of society's athletes and role models freely admit to using body-enhancing chemicals. No wonder so many people, young and old, must cope with the problems of chemical use today.

SUBSTANCE USE AND AGE

The use of chemical substances occurs throughout the life cycle, from the fetus to the elderly individual. Even the growing life protected within the mother's uterus is not safe from the effects of chemicals. It is estimated that 20% of pregnant women still use alcohol during pregnancy despite huge educational efforts about the effects of alcohol on the fetus.

There are no safe drugs for pregnant women. Every chemical ingested by a pregnant woman poses a potential danger to her unborn child, especially during the first trimester of pregnancy, when the developing fetus is highly sensitive. Chemicals taken during pregnancy can seriously interfere with normal fetal growth and development. They may also alter the placenta itself or interfere with its ability to perform its life-promoting functions.

A sad but common example of the effects of maternal drug use can be seen in infants and children with **fetal alcohol syndrome (FAS)**—the result of excessive alcohol use during pregnancy. FAS affects an estimated 1 child per 1000 live births ("Fetal Alcohol Syndrome," 2003). In countries in which the intake of alcohol is high, the incidence of FAS is greater.

Children with FAS are smaller at birth, have small heads (microcephaly), and fail to develop normally. Figure 28-1 illustrates the physical effects on the child of a chronically alcoholic mother. The less obvious effects include CNS deficits, various degrees of mental retardation and hyperactivity, irritability, and poor feeding habits. These children also have slow rates of growth, developmental delays, behavioral problems, intellectual impairment, poor judgment, and certain facial characteristics common to the children of alcoholic mothers.

Infants who were exposed to **cocaine** in utero have sleeping and eating problems, unusual levels of irritability, and high-pitched cries. Other syndromes and developmental problems result from the use of different drugs, but all drugs have one thing in common: pregnancy and substance use do not mix.

Children who live with substance-abusing parents are at increased risk for injuries and developing drug problems themselves. Research has demonstrated that most children of parents who use both legal and illegal chemicals do poorly in school, have difficulty controlling their emotions, and exhibit low self-esteem. Many of these children repeat the cycle of substance use and

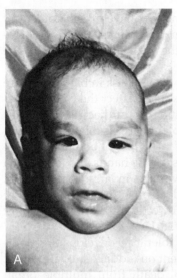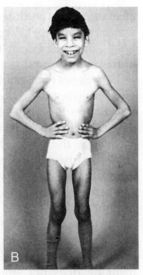

FIGURE **28-1** Fetal alcohol syndrome (FAS). Child of chronically alcoholic mother, diagnosed at birth with FAS. Although he was raised his entire life in one excellent foster home and participated in various remediation programs, he continues to have an IQ around 45 (more severe retardation than most FAS children), with accompanying hyperactivity and distractibility.

child abuse when they reach adulthood. Some choose alcoholic or drug-abusing spouses.

Children abuse substances too, but often the substances are legal and easily available. The 9-year-old who demands cola drinks every day demonstrates the same signs of a caffeine addiction as an adult. The 8-year-old boy who has grown up with beer in the house can become an alcoholic just as quickly as his adult counterpart. The number of admissions of children younger than 12 years old to substance treatment units is increasing. This reminds us that drug abuse problems really do exist among our children.

Adolescent substance use, abuse, and dependence are becoming an ever-increasing problem. Alcohol is the most frequently abused drug of adolescents. High school seniors have experimented with alcohol, cigarettes, marijuana, cocaine, hallucinogens, and designer drugs, such as ecstasy. For people in the 15- to 24-year-old age-group, alcohol-related accidents are the leading cause of death.

Because of their developmental levels, teens are encouraged to explore the adult world, but their ability to exercise sound judgment is still limited. Adolescents experiment with a variety of attitudes, behaviors, and lifestyles, and often substance use becomes a part of that experimentation. The younger an individual begins to use substances, the more likely that abuse problems will occur later in life.

Adolescents have various patterns of substance abuse. They may experiment by using drugs on a few occasions. They may use substances (usually alcohol, tobacco, or marijuana) in recreational ways, in social settings for the purpose of relaxation or intoxication. If actual addiction occurs, teens are likely to become

involved in illegal activities, such as drug trafficking, prostitution, or criminal behaviors.

In adults, substance abuse is common, with about 10% of the adult population regularly abusing alcohol. This statistic is low because episodes of frequent binge drinking are not documented. Substance use and abuse occur most commonly between 18 and 35 years of age, but significant numbers of older adults abuse alcohol and prescription medications.

Older adults are not immune to substance-related problems, but their substance use is often misdiagnosed or treated inappropriately. Older drinkers and elderly persons who misuse drugs are often isolated within their social groups or families. Although the incidence of substance abuse in older adults is unknown, more than 40% of all drug reactions occur in persons older than 65 years. This fact should alert health care providers to the possibility of substance abuse in every older client.

Substances for abuse vary according to ethnic group. For example, the use of cocaine is higher among blacks. Whites and Hispanics prefer alcohol. Drug use also varies with the location. For example, drug use in the United States is highest in the West and lowest in the North Central region.

SCOPE OF THE PROBLEM TODAY

The abuse of chemical substances presents many problems for people in today's society. Alcohol abuse and drug abuse have an impact on every citizen, in both financial terms and human costs. There are more women using street drugs during pregnancy than available drug treatment programs can accommodate. Infants who have been exposed to cocaine and other drugs are filling health and foster care systems as the children of addicted parents are born. Millions of children with alcoholic parents live in the United States today. Children of problem drinkers also have three times the risk for serious injury as children of nondrinking parents.

Substance use and dependence cost society dearly. The suicide rate for 15- to 24-year-olds accounts for almost 13% of all deaths in that age-group (Centers for Disease Control and Prevention [CDC], 2007). The use of alcohol and drugs often results in trauma, violence, and mental health problems. Alcohol-related motor vehicle accidents are one of the leading causes of death among people younger than 45 years. Many deaths attributed to falls, drowning, and burns are often related to alcohol and drug use.

Society's homeless and mentally ill people often use and abuse chemicals. Homeless persons with alcohol, drug, or mental disorders are one of the most disadvantaged and underserved groups in the United States. People with serious mental illness who also are addicted to or use chemicals are said to have a **dual diagnosis**. It is estimated as many as 75% of the mentally ill population have a dual diagnosis.

CATEGORIES OF ABUSED SUBSTANCES

Every chemical has the potential for abuse. For example, the current concern over the effectiveness of antibiotic drugs stems from a form of abuse. As people routinely insisted on being treated with antibiotics for illnesses that did not actually require them, the microorganisms the antibiotics were designed to kill grew stronger and increasingly resistant. The repeated abuse of antibiotics has resulted in serious consequences for us all. Not all abused substances are illegal. In this text, however, the discussion of abused substances is limited to those that are currently considered illicit or harmful.

CHEMICALS OF ABUSE

The most popular substance of abuse in the United States and most developed countries is alcohol. Other substances increase and decrease in popularity, but the fact that more than 10% of the adult population in the United States abuses alcohol has remained constant for more than 20 years.

Alcohol has been used since the beginning of recorded time. The effects of different alcoholic beverages are caused by the presence of ethanol (ETOH), a chemical that results from the fermentation of yeast and grains, malts, or fruits. "Hard liquor," such as whiskey, brandy, gin, and vodka, is derived from distilled spirits, whereas beer and wine are not. The process of distillation increases the alcohol content of the beverage. To illustrate, one shot of distilled alcohol, 5 ounces of wine, and 12 ounces of beer all contain ½ ounce of alcohol.

Many people think of alcohol as a stimulant because they feel relaxation, alertness, and pleasure when they drink. Actually, these feelings are caused by the depressant effects of alcohol on the CNS. Once swallowed, alcohol is rapidly diffused to all the body's organ systems. Because of its high solubility in water, alcohol collects in organs that have a high content of water (brain, heart, liver, gastrointestinal tract). Alcohol is metabolized in the liver and excreted by the kidneys and lungs.

Low doses of alcohol cause a rise in blood pressure and pulse, but large doses can affect the pumping action of the heart, resulting in cardiac dysrhythmias (irregularities). Surface blood vessels dilate, producing flushing of the skin and rapid loss of body heat. Alcohol also causes numbness of the hands and feet, which creates a false sense of warmth. In large doses, alcohol can actually reduce body temperature. The effects of alcohol on the CNS are directly related to the amount (dose) consumed (Table 28-1).

With continued use, tolerance develops and individuals become dependent on (addicted to) alcohol. If drinking does not stop, death from multiple organ failure (especially the liver) results, usually after a series of assorted chronic health problems.

Narcotics are central nervous system (CNS) depressants. They occur naturally, semisynthetically, and synthetically. Some natural narcotics have been altered to make new artificially produced (synthetic) drugs. Natural narcotics are opium and its principal ingredient, morphine, which is used for medicinal purposes. These substances are often called **opioids** or **opiates** and are obtained by milking a flower called *Papaver somniferum*, the opium poppy.

The use of opium was documented 4000 years before Hippocrates, and it continues to be a commonly used substance in many countries today. Before the 1900s, opium was readily available in the United States and a common ingredient in many patent medicines. Today there is little opium use in the United States as a result of the restrictive laws governing the drug.

Opium is found in several forms. The fluid scraped from the base of the poppy flower and rolled into dark brown chunks is called raw opium (Figure 28-2). Processed opium can appear as a fine white powder.

Table 28-1 *Effects of Alcohol on the Nervous System*

BLOOD ALCOHOL CONTENT	APPROXIMATE NUMBER OF DRINKS*	CENTRAL NERVOUS SYSTEM (BEHAVIORAL) RESPONSES
0.05%	1 or 2 (½-1 oz of alcohol)	Thought, restraint, judgment slowed; more socially at ease; reaction time slowed; unable to do complicated tasks
0.10%	3 or 4 (1½ oz of alcohol)	Voluntary motor actions clumsy; depth perception altered; reaction time to stimuli slowed; eye movement and focus affected; judgment and control continue to decrease; legal limit for driving
0.20%	5 or more (≥2½ oz of alcohol)	Entire motor area of brain depressed; may want to lie down; staggers; loses conscious control of reason; easily angered; may weep, shout, fight
0.30%	6 or more (≥3 oz of alcohol)	Acts confused; may be in a stupor; unresponsive to most external stimuli; losing ability to control involuntary responses; decreased heart rate, blood pressure, respiratory rate
0.40%-0.50%	7 or more (≥3½ oz of alcohol)	Comatose; medulla severely depressed; death from respiratory failure; death can occur with 0.40% if blood alcohol rises too rapidly; blood alcohol level of 0.50% is fatal without immediate medical attention

*Consumed within a 4-hr period.

The semisynthetic narcotics include heroin, hydromorphone, and thebaine derivatives. The Bayer Company of Germany first marketed heroin in 1898 as a new pain reliever. In the United States heroin was legally available to the public until the passage of the Harrison Narcotic Act of 1914.

Pure heroin is a white, bitter-tasting powder that is usually put into solution and injected. Today potent forms of heroin are available. Some are so strong that they need only to be smoked or inhaled to produce the same effect as injecting. Street heroin is found in colors ranging from white to dark brown depending on the additives. An especially potent form, called **black tar heroin,** has become available throughout the United States (Figure 28-3). This crudely processed form of heroin is manufactured in Mexico and may contain as much as 80% impurities. It is most commonly diluted and injected. The signs and symptoms of heroin use, overdose, and withdrawal are listed in Table 28-2.

Stimulants are another group of commonly abused substances. They include caffeine, cocaine, and certain prescription drugs, such as amphetamines, appetite suppressants, and methylphenidate (Ritalin).

Caffeine is found in every supermarket. It is the main active ingredient in coffee, black teas, most cola drinks, and other bottled beverages. Caffeine stimulates the nervous system, relieving fatigue and increasing alertness and the body's metabolic rate. In large amounts, it can produce tremors, tachycardia, nervousness, and insomnia. The most prominent withdrawal symptom from caffeine is headache.

Cocaine is a potent natural stimulant. For centuries, the natives of the South American Andes Mountains chewed the weakly psychoactive leaves of the coca plant to relieve fatigue and hunger. Today coca is grown, processed into cocaine, and shipped to many countries throughout the world.

Cocaine is available "on the street" as a white, crystalline powder that is commonly contaminated with local anesthetics or sugar. It is either injected or "snorted" by inhaling. Cocaine produces an immediate rush of energy, vigor, and feelings of well-being that last less than 1 hour. The intense pleasurable feelings

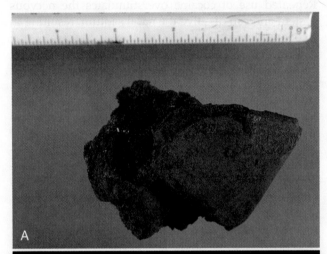

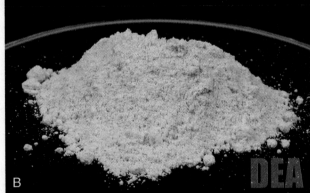

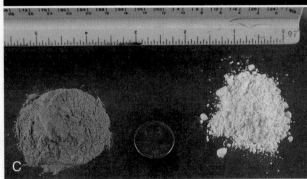

FIGURE **28-2** **A,** Poppy. **B,** Opium.

FIGURE **28-3** **A,** Black tar heroin. **B,** Heroin powder. **C,** Asian heroin.

Table 28-2 *Signs and Symptoms of Heroin Use, Overdose, and Withdrawal*

HEROIN USE	HEROIN OVERDOSE	HEROIN WITHDRAWAL
Constricted pupils	Shallow respirations	Watery eyes
Depression		Runny nose
Drowsiness	Clammy skin	Sweating
Euphoria (feelings of great well-being)	Convulsions Coma	Muscle cramps Loss of appetite, nausea
Nausea		Chills
Respiratory depression		Tremors
		Panic

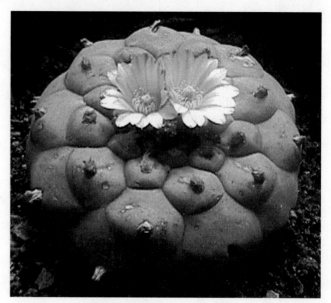

FIGURE **28-4** Peyote cactus.

can lead to a mental dependency that can ultimately destroy one's life as more and higher doses are used. Repeated use of cocaine overstimulates the nervous system and can dissolve the nasal septum, resulting in a collapsed nose.

Crack is a type of processed cocaine. Combining cocaine with ammonia or baking soda and heating it removes the hydrochloride molecule and produces chips or chunks of highly addicting cocaine, called rocks. These are usually vaporized in a pipe or smoked with tobacco or marijuana. Because of its concentrated form, crack reaches the brain immediately and produces a more intense but shorter-lasting high. Tolerance and addiction to the drug develop quickly as users chase the feeling of that first, intense experience.

Amphetamines were originally pharmaceutically manufactured medicines to treat depression, narcolepsy, hyperactivity in children, and obesity. Amphetamines were initially sold without a prescription in inhalers and diet pills. Today, they are available only by prescription, but many are illegally manufactured. They are strong stimulants with addictive properties.

The **hallucinogens**, the last category of abused chemicals, are natural and synthetic substances that alter one's perception of reality. The active ingredient of the peyote cactus, mescaline, has been used in the religious ceremonies of certain American Indians for many years (Figure 28-4).

Lysergic acid diethylamide **(LSD),** an ergot fungus, was discovered by accident in the 1940s, but the introduction of laboratory-designed hallucinogens in the United States did not occur until the early 1970s. Today, they are commonly available. Most doses are taken orally or inhaled, and they are frequently contaminated. These hallucinogens vary in onset, duration of action, and potency, but all produce a sense of altered reality.

Phencyclidine (PCP) was originally developed for use as an animal tranquilizer. When taken by humans, it produces mild depression with low doses and a schizophrenic-like reaction with higher amounts. PCP is a dangerous drug because it causes people to behave in unpredictable, often violent, ways (Table 28-3).

Users of hallucinogens experience everything from profound mind-expanding experiences to "bad trips" in which dangerous behavioral reactions occur. The mind-altering effects of hallucinogens include a heightened awareness of reality; distortions in time, space, and body image; feelings of depersonalization; and the loss of a sense of reality. **Flashbacks,** which are a return to the psychedelic experience after the drug has worn off, can occur with the use of hallucinogens. The repeated use of hallucinogens can lead to various mental health problems.

Cannabis (marijuana) is a term applied to the hemp plant, *Cannabis sativa,* which grows wild in many tropical and temperate climates all over the world. The hemp plant has been used for centuries by many cultures in folk remedies and other medicines. Historically, it is used to treat pain, decreased appetite, muscle and gastrointestinal tract spasms, asthma, and depression. It has also been used as an antibiotic and a topical anesthetic. Commercially, rope, clothing, and paper are made from hemp (marijuana) (see Think About 28-1).

Cannabis is available in several forms. The dried tops and leaves are called **marijuana.** Hashish **(hash)** is the dried resin that seeps from the top and leaves, and **hash oil** is the distilled oil of hashish. All are usually smoked, but they may also be eaten.

Marijuana and other cannabis products produce a sense of well-being and relaxation. They alter time perception and affect short-term memory and concentration. Motivation, especially for distasteful tasks, may be decreased. Frequently, an increase in hunger occurs. Large doses can result in feelings of anxiety and paranoia. There are no proven withdrawal signs or symptoms, but anxious moods, irritability, and sleep disturbances have been reported.

Designer drugs are substances "created by underground chemists who alter the molecular structures

Table 28-3 *Signs and Symptoms of PCP Use*

PHYSICAL SIGNS AND SYMPTOMS	PSYCHOLOGICAL SIGNS AND SYMPTOMS
Increased blood pressure	Belligerence (wants to fight)
Increased temperature	Bizarre behaviors
Muscle rigidity, ataxia (uncoordinated, staggering)	Hallucinations
Repeated jerking	Impaired (poor) judgment
Agitated movements	Impulsive behaviors
Vertical and horizontal nystagmus (eye tremors)	Paranoia
	Unpredictable behaviors

PCP, Phencyclidine.

? Think About 28-1

For years, debate about the legalization of marijuana has taken place. Advocates cite numerous commercial and medicinal properties of the substance. They feel that keeping it illegal prevents many medical advances from being made and commercial products (e.g., paper, cloth, oil) from being developed. Those who disagree state that legalization will lead to increased use.
- What do you think should be done?
- What is your rationale for this position?

of existing drugs" (Hess and DeBoer, 2002). Today designer drugs, such as MDMA **(ecstasy), STP,** and **"ice,"** are easily available in all areas of the United States. The designer drug called ecstasy is fast becoming the preferred recreational drug of teens and young adults because it allows its users to "party" for long periods of time. Taking this drug, however, can have severe consequences. Because the drug suppresses the need to drink, eat, and sleep, it promotes severe dehydration and physical exhaustion. The leading cause of death among ecstasy users is **hyperthermia,** a dangerously high body temperature. Kidney or liver failure can result, even after one dose.

MEDICATIONS

Many chemicals that were developed to save lives and ease suffering have the potential for being abused. For example, almost all the opium arriving in the United States today is broken down into its most useful alkaloids, morphine and codeine. These substances are then refined into powerful pain-relieving medications (narcotic analgesics). They are available in the United States only with the prescription of a licensed physician, dentist, or nurse practitioner, but they remain a source of abuse.

Morphine is one of the most effective painkillers available. It is marketed as a white powder or in solution for injection. It is administered by injection under the direction of a licensed health care practitioner.

Hydromorphone and the thebaine derivatives are semisynthetic narcotics made from opium. Hydromorphone is commonly called Dilaudid. It is used as an analgesic and is produced in liquid or tablet form. It is shorter acting, more sedating, and up to eight times more powerful than morphine. Although available only by prescription, it is highly sought by addicts. Thebaine derivatives, another opium product, are up to 1000 times more potent than morphine. Because of the danger of overdose, these drugs are used by veterinarians for the care of large animals only.

Commonly abused stimulants include the amphetamines, diet pills, and the appetite suppressants. Methylphenidate (Ritalin), a medication used to treat attention-deficit/hyperactivity disorders, is another often abused stimulant. The signs and symptoms of stimulant use include changes in personality, anxiety, tension, anger, restlessness, and rapid speech and movement.

Laxatives and diuretics are commonly abused by elderly people and people who are trying to lose weight. Individuals with eating disorders or altered body images often use these drugs to keep themselves excessively thin or to atone for an eating binge. Elderly people can develop a dependence on laxatives when they are used too frequently.

The sedative, hypnotic, and antianxiety drug classes are commonly used in ways other than therapeutic. During the 1950s, many people were unknowingly addicted to the drug diazepam (Valium) and other sedatives. The individual who is unable to sleep without hypnotic medications may be abusing sleeping pills, and many people reach for their "nerve pills" when they feel anxious or upset. The importance of obtaining a thorough history of every client's medication use cannot be overemphasized.

INHALANTS

The breathing in of volatile substances or chemical gases (inhalants) has become popular with adolescents and young adults for several reasons: they are legal, inexpensive, and easily available, and they have a rapid onset of effects. Unfortunately, the practice is also associated with significant complications, such as sudden death caused by cardiac dysrhythmia or respiratory depression. The use of inhalants can also result in hyperactive motor responses, loss of coordination, and seizures.

The most commonly inhaled substances are alcohol solvents, gasoline, glue, paint thinner, hairspray, and spray paints. Chemicals less frequently used as inhalants include cleaning fluids, typewriter correction liquids, and spray can propellants.

Inhalants are most often used by adolescents in group settings. Several methods are used to inhale the vapors, such as soaking a rag and then holding it to the nose and mouth. The substance may be inhaled directly from the container **(huffing)** or placed in a bag or other closed container and then inhaled. Soon after inhaling, the individual feels a "high" that is associated with feelings of great well-being (euphoria), excitement, sexual aggressiveness, a lessened sense of right and wrong, and loss of judgment. Signs and symptoms of inhalant intoxication include delusions, hallucinations, anxiety, and confusion. Although no withdrawal syndrome has been recognized, the repeated use of inhalants can result in profound physical and psychosocial harm.

Nicotine is currently a legal inhalant. It is present in all forms of tobacco (cigarettes, chewing tobacco, pipe tobacco, cigars, snuff) and certain medications (nicotine patch, nicotine gum). It produces relaxation, increases alertness, and helps to relieve feelings of hunger. Nicotine is frequently used as a method to control body weight.

Although its popularity is declining, tobacco is still a commonly used substance. Tobacco is either smoked or held between the gum and lip and absorbed through the mucous membranes of the mouth. It is never swallowed because of its toxic effects. Tobacco is addictive, and its continued use is associated with many health complications. Recently in the United States, Canada, and other industrialized countries, a movement to restrict the sales and use of tobacco products (especially to children and teens) has arisen.

There are many substances that have the potential for abuse. Some clients may be addicted to more than one substance. Many practice binge drinking, in which short periods of ingestion are followed by periods of abstinence. For these reasons, it is important to obtain an accurate history of every client's substance use patterns.

CHARACTERISTICS OF SUBSTANCE USE AND ABUSE

It is important to remember the differences between substance use and abuse. Some people can use various chemicals to change the way they feel, but the use does not affect their ability to perform the activities of daily life. This is substance **use.** Substance **abuse,** however, occurs when use of the chemical becomes more important than the activities of daily living.

The causes of substance abuse are unknown, but several theories have attempted to explain why people use mind-altering chemicals. Biological theories state that variations among ethnic groups offer genetic and biochemical explanations for substance abuse. Theories relating to psychological factors explore the roles of personality and emotional problems as causes. Environmental theories concentrate on the individual, the family, and the sociocultural surroundings in which substance abuse takes place.

STAGES OF ADDICTION

Many individuals use alcohol, tobacco, or other chemicals and function very well. Those who move from use to dependency (addiction) follow a fairly predictable course. During the **early stage,** individuals are able to use and enjoy their chosen substance. A desire to repeat the first pleasurable experience leads to a frequent pattern of use. One begins to prefer being "high" to other activities.

Soon a habit of excessive use develops as the individual begins to ignore responsibilities and obligations. The person may deny that a problem exists, ignore others' comments, lie to cover up the activity, or conceal the problem by sneaking drinks or doses. During these periods, the individual may also become intoxicated.

Intoxication is defined as a state of maladaptive behavioral or psychological changes resulting from exposure to certain chemicals. Intoxicated people are frequently belligerent (looking for a fight or an argument) and have wide emotional swings. They often lack sound judgment, and their critical thinking ability is reduced. Commonly, they will stagger or show other signs of impaired motor abilities. The actual picture of an intoxicated individual varies greatly. Psychological effects are based on the person's expectations of what the chemical will do and the environment in which the substance is taken.

During the **middle** (crucial) **stage** of addiction, the intoxicating episodes increase as the body attempts to compensate by adapting to the substance. Tolerance develops as increased amounts of the chemical are needed to produce the same effects that one dose once produced. **Physical tolerance** occurs when the body has adjusted to living and functioning with the substance in its system. **Psychological tolerance** develops when individuals feel that they cannot function without the use of their chosen chemical.

By the time one has progressed to the **chronic** (late) **stage,** tolerance for the chemical is usually quite high. The need for the substance now leads to a loss of control over one's behavior. Without the chemical, life is miserable. Daily living becomes a nightmare, and all waking effort and energy are focused on obtaining and using the now required substance. Case Study 28-1 offers a vivid example.

CRITERIA FOR DIAGNOSIS

For a substance-related disorder to be diagnosed, individuals must meet certain criteria. The pattern of substance use must be disabling and lead to significant impaired functioning and distress. The individual must demonstrate signs of tolerance, withdrawal, and dependence (American Psychiatric Association, 2000).

CLINICAL PRESENTATION

Unlike physical illness, there is no classic presentation of a substance abuser. Each person has a unique variety of signs and symptoms, depending on chemical use

Case Study 28-1

Ernie's father was 15 years old when Ernie was born. His mother, who was 14 years old, gave custody to the father after the first 6 months of Ernie's life. To keep Ernie quiet during his infant and toddler years, his father would blow marijuana smoke into his face. It worked. Ernie would sleep for hours while his father partied.

By the time Ernie was 5 years old, he was drinking beer. At 8 years, he graduated to vodka, gin, and tequila. By 10 years old, Ernie was mixing alcohol with cocaine. School became impossible, so he dropped out at 12 years old. By the time he was 14 years old, Ernie was hustling drugs and trying to sell the sexual favors of three neighborhood girls.

Where is Ernie today? Fortunately, he overdosed one evening when he was about 17 years old. The nurse in the emergency department, recognizing the potential in this young man, took the time to tell him that he had choices. Ernie listened. His detoxification was painful. His recovery was slow and difficult, but he persisted, knowing there was something more in life than a fog of consciousness.

Today, despite several setbacks, Ernie has been clean for more than 10 years. He is a college graduate, happily married, and the father of two boys. The strongest thing he drinks now is orange juice.
• How do you think the nurse made an impact on Ernie's life?

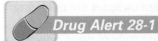

Drug Alert 28-1

Remember, elderly persons are at risk for becoming drug dependent. When an older adult becomes less social and begins to isolate himself or herself, suspect a problem with drugs. The usual drugs of abuse in the elderly population are pain medications and drug combinations.

Have your elderly clients bring all their medications to you in a paper bag. These medications should include all over-the-counter and herbal preparations. In this way, an accurate assessment of their medication use can be obtained. Do not forget to ask about alcohol use, especially in combination with their medications.

and individual characteristics. However, because substance abuse affects every body system, there are some common indicators, such as alterations in neurological functioning or appearance, that can help with the assessment and monitoring of clients. Refer to Tables 28-1 through 28-3 for specific signs and symptoms.

GUIDELINES FOR INTERVENTION

The three most commonly abused types of drugs are alcohol and sedative-alcohol combinations; opiate narcotics, chiefly heroin; and stimulants, chiefly cocaine and amphetamines.

The costs and consequences of substance abuse are high. As individuals progress with their drug abuse, their world narrows as they become isolated from occupational and community relationships (see Drug Alert 28-1).

Absenteeism from work, unpaid bills, and job loss frequently result when chemical use is out of control. Involvement with the legal system can occur. Some people deplete their financial resources to obtain their substances. Accidents, trauma, crime, domestic violence, child abuse, prostitution, suicide, disease, and the loss of safe communities are associated with substance abuse. Therefore it is important for all health care providers to be alert to the possibility of substance-related problems in every client.

ASSESSMENT

The physical examination, client history, and emotional assessment should focus on the following aspects:
• **Central nervous system:** Assess for orientation, level of consciousness, balance, gait, and ability to follow instructions.
• **Head and neck:** Examine eyes, and check pupils and sclera (whites) of the eyes. Note ruddy or pale complexion, distended neck veins, or petechiae (small red dots) on the face. Observe for evidence of injections under the tongue, and inspect the area between the gums and lips.
• **Chest:** Do not forget to take vital signs. Count pulse and respirations for a full minute. Palpate pedal and radial pulses. Observe for any difficulty in breathing. Auscultate the heart for irregular rates or rhythms. Listen to the breath sounds, and note any abnormal sounds.
• **Abdomen:** Inspect the size, shape, and contours of the abdomen. Auscultate all four quadrants, and count the bowel sounds. Check for ascites (water in the abdomen), distention, or enlarged organs. Look for bruising, petechiae, and other signs of bleeding. Have the client describe the color and consistency of stool.
• **Skin:** Observe and document the size, location, and characteristics of any skin lesions or marks. Check for needle marks on the client's arms, fingers, legs, and toes. Note the skin turgor and muscle mass of the arms and legs.
• **Nutritional status:** Many chemically dependent persons do not eat regularly and are at risk for malnutrition. Observe the client's body build and appearance. Ask the client to list everything he or she ate yesterday and tell you how the meals were prepared. Ask if there have been any recent appetite or weight changes. Inspect the client's skin color, hair, and fingernails. If the client lives alone or is homeless, find out how food is obtained on a daily basis.

The psychosocial assessment includes the following:
- **General appearance:** Is the client tidy or unkempt? Note the client's manner and style of dress, jewelry, makeup, hairstyle, and body marks (e.g., tattoos, symbolic scars).
- **Behaviors:** Note rate of speech, motor activity, and interactions during the interview. Observe for signs of memory loss, difficulty following directions, and problems with communication.
- **Emotional state:** Watch for signs of depression, emotional instability (mood swings), suspiciousness, anger, agitation, self-pity, or jealousy. Ask clients if they have ever had a hallucination, a blackout (period of time during which the user cannot remember events), any violent impulses, or suicidal ideas.
- **Social support:** Have clients identify the most important people in their lives. Are these people willing to become involved in treatment with the client? If possible, observe how clients interact with their family and friends. Remember that family members may also need support and treatment.
- **Motivation:** Obtain a description of the chemicals currently being used: how often, how much, when was last dose? When did use begin? What (if anything) has been tried to decrease or stop using the chemical? Describe clients' history of treatment for substance-related or emotional problems. Ask what motivated them to seek treatment now. Is the court, the job, or the family insisting on treatment, or are they seeking relief from the problems associated with the chemical use? The motivation level of clients plays an important part in recovery.
- **Diagnostic tests:** Diagnostic testing usually includes standard blood and urine examinations. A complete blood count (CBC), urinalysis, and chemistry panel is done to assess for organ damage. Frequently tests for hepatitis, human immunodeficiency virus (HIV), tuberculosis (TB), and other infectious diseases are performed. Clients are also assessed for nutritional or bleeding problems. Other diagnostic tests, such as a computed tomography (CT) scan, magnetic resonance imaging (MRI), x-ray films, or an electroencephalogram (EEG), may also be ordered.

TREATMENTS AND THERAPIES

The treatment of substance-related disorders continues to change and grow. Consequently, a broad range of approaches is available today. Most treatment programs are based on a certain philosophy, although they may offer many different types of therapy.

The **disease model** of treatment states that substance abuse is a disease and should be treated as such. Substance abuse has acute and chronic signs and symptoms, a certain pattern of progression, and physical pathological conditions associated with continued use. Two types of treatment programs based on the disease model are the 12-step programs and residential treatment programs.

The first **12-step program** was a self-help, group-centered program developed by two alcoholics in 1935. The 12-step process involves admitting one's powerlessness to control drug use and then seeking help from a higher power through prayer or meditation, moral inventories, confessing wrongs, asking for forgiveness, and carrying the message to others. The first 12-step program was Alcoholics Anonymous (AA). Many other 12-step programs are based on this model and revised to fit the beliefs of the population they serve. Box 28-1 offers a general listing of self-help groups available in many countries throughout the world. Self-help groups can be very effective when the individual wants them to be.

The **medical model** considers addictions from a public health, chronic and acute infectious disease perspective. The biopsychosocial framework for treating clients is a medical model that attempts to explain substance

---

Box 28-1 *Self-Help Groups for Recovering Abusers*

Alcoholics Anonymous—For individuals recovering from alcoholism; founded in 1935

Al-Anon—For families of alcoholics

Alateen—For 12- to 20-year-olds who are affected by someone else's drinking problem

Association of Recovering Motorcyclists—Support group for motorcyclists recovering from alcohol or drug addiction

Calix Society—Catholic alcoholics who maintain sobriety through participation in AA

Christian Addiction Rehabilitation Association—Provides support and ministry to individuals with addictions

Cocaine Anonymous—For those recovering from cocaine addiction; a 12-step program

Drug-Anon Focus—For families and friends of persons addicted to mind-altering drugs; a 12-step program

Drugs Anonymous—For individuals addicted to drugs; a 12-step program

Dual Disorders Anonymous—For people with both alcohol or drug addiction and mental or emotional disorders; a 12-step program

Families Anonymous—For parents, relatives, and friends of drug addicts

Gay AA—Provides support for gay and lesbian alcoholics

Impaired Physician Program—Provides assistance to physicians and their spouses who have problems with alcohol, drugs, or codependence

International Nurses Anonymous—For nurses, nursing students, and former nurses who are involved in a 12-step recovery program

Naranon—Provides assistance to drug-dependent individuals and their families

Narcotics Anonymous—For individuals recovering from drug abuse; a 12-step program

Rational Recovery Systems—Uses rational emotive therapy (vs. a spiritual approach) to assist people in their recovery from substance abuse

Data from Keltner NL, Schwecke LH, Bostrom CE: *Psychiatric nursing*, ed 5, St. Louis, 2007, Mosby.

abuse. New understanding of neurotransmitters and other biochemical activities of the brain is leading to the development of medications that may someday help people cope with their chemical dependencies.

Psychiatric models view substance abuse as an expression of an underlying emotional conflict or mental disorder. Several therapies are based on this framework.

Sociocultural models state that substance abuse can be treated by changing an individual's environment and teaching people how to develop new responses to their current environments. This view has led to the establishment of long-term residential treatment programs and therapeutic communities.

Regardless of the type of substance used, the goals of care remain the same. The first step in treatment is for the individual to **recognize the need for help. Denial** is a strong part of most substance-related disorders. For any treatment to be effective, the client must be truly willing to work toward living without his or her addiction.

Before treatment of the addiction can actually begin, many persons must first go through detoxification, the process of withdrawing from a substance under medical supervision. Clients who are addicted to opium, narcotics, alcohol, or sedatives are often hospitalized because of potentially fatal complications, such as seizures and respiratory and cardiac problems. Sometimes medications, such as phenobarbital, Dilantin, and Valium, are given to ease physical discomforts and prevent complications. Methadone (drug used to treat heroin addiction) has been administered to ease the effects of withdrawing from heroin, but methadone itself is addicting, and it is difficult to "detox" from methadone.

Once clients are physically free from their addictions (practicing abstinence), the focus turns to uncovering and treating existing emotional or mental health problems. The incidence of psychiatric disorders is very high in substance users. Anxiety and depression are often found in clients with substance-abuse problems. These disorders must also be treated if the individual is to remain drug free.

The last, and perhaps the most difficult, goal of treatment is to assist individuals in changing their behaviors. Individual psychotherapy is very effective for clients with certain dependencies (cocaine addictions), but it is expensive and unavailable to many people. Group therapy can offer peer support from individuals "who have been there." It also offers people the opportunity to experiment with and explore their new, drug-free behaviors.

Medications are prescribed with extreme care. Two specific medications used in the care of substance-addicted clients are methadone and disulfiram (Antabuse). Methadone is a chemical relative of heroin. Taken orally once each day, it prevents the symptoms of withdrawal and helps to stabilize the lives of these substance abusers. Another form of methadone, called levo-alpha-acetylmethadol (LAAM), has been developed. It requires that a dose be taken only once every 72 hours.

Disulfiram (Antabuse) is a medication taken daily by nonpracticing (dry) alcoholics. It causes very unpleasant physical reactions when combined with alcohol, including intense headache, flushing, nausea, vomiting, low blood pressure, and blurred vision. It is prescribed as a preventive measure to help reduce the desire for alcohol. It is very important to thoroughly research each of these medications and routinely monitor your clients for therapeutic and adverse reactions to these chemicals.

RELAPSE

Long-term recovery is often marked by periods of relapse. Relapse is the recurrence of substance-abusing behaviors after a significant period of abstinence. In other words, the client returns to "using" after being "dry" for a period of time. Not only do people return to the chemical-abusing behaviors, but also they readopt the psychological and emotional mind-set that brought about the abuse in the first place. Many treatment therapies and programs concentrate on preventing and treating relapses. Remember that clients who have relapsed feel many distressing emotions. True therapeutic care is given when these clients are accepted and respected, even when they are the least accepting and respecting of themselves. Remember, you are a therapeutic agent. Case Study 28-2 illustrates this point.

 Case Study 28-2

Rex had been in treatment so many times that he stopped counting. It seemed that he would relapse about 2 weeks following each discharge from the inpatient treatment program. One evening after an especially tough detox he was chatting with the nurse on duty. Knowing that Rex was an intelligent man when sober, the nurse acted upon an idea—she pulled the medical record and showed Rex his laboratory work. She discussed the meaning of each liver function test and the damage his alcohol and drug use was doing to his body. But she emphasized that the liver had remarkable healing abilities and it could repair itself even when 50% of it was damaged. It was all there, in black and white, and the decision was his. There was still time if he acted, but soon his liver would be beyond repair. Rex left the conversation deep in thought.

The next day the nurse made sure to discuss all the support that was available to Rex. More pondering.

Soon thereafter Rex was discharged. Weeks elapsed and no Rex. The holiday season was in full swing, and the staff prepared for Rex's admission. Instead they received a Christmas card telling them that he was still clean—and they have received a card with the same message each year since 1998.

NURSING PROCESS

An important intervention for clients with substance-related problems is to act as a therapeutic agent. Practice effective listening skills to gain an understanding of who the client really is. Use your knowledge of the therapeutic relationship to establish trust and cooperation. Learn to act as a role model, quietly demonstrating problem solving and other effective coping skills. Be willing to look beyond the addiction to see the person.

Nursing diagnoses that relate to clients with substance abuse problems are based on identified problems and goals. Box 28-2 lists several possible diagnoses.

Sample Client Care Plan 28-1 presents the diagnosis of ineffective coping.

Although the actual care for each client is individually planned, certain key nursing actions are common to all substance-dependent clients (Box 28-3).

Caring for clients with substance-related problems is challenging and frustrating. Nurses and other caregivers are in valuable positions to influence their clients' well-being. Demonstrations of respect, acceptance, and concern can offer many clients the connection that

---

SAMPLE CLIENT CARE PLAN 28-1

Ineffective Coping

ASSESSMENT *History.* Mary is a 34-year-old housewife with three children and a husband who works long hours. Two years ago, she complained of feeling jittery and tense to her physician. He prescribed a mild sedative, which Mary took religiously every evening before bed. Lately, she has begun to take her "nerve pill" during the day and uses alcohol to help "stabilize" her. She is being admitted for evaluation and treatment after her husband found her unconscious on the sofa yesterday.

Current Findings. A well-groomed woman with a flattened speech. Mary answers questions when asked but volunteers no information. She states that she does not belong here because she is not really addicted to anything and resents "being treated like a drugger."

Multidisciplinary Diagnosis	*Planning/Goals*
Ineffective coping related to increasing use of sedatives and alcohol	Mary will abstain from using all mood-altering chemicals for 6 weeks. Mary will identify and seek help for at least three problems by May 1.

Therapeutic Interventions

Intervention	Rationale	Team Members
1. Confront Mary with her substance-abusing actions and their consequences and assist her with identifying the problem.	Denial is very common with persons who have a substance-related problem; identifying problems is the first step toward change.	Psy, Nsg
2. Encourage Mary to agree to participate in the treatment program.	Therapeutic interventions are not effective unless the client wants to cooperate.	All
3. Work with Mary to develop a written contract for behavioral changes.	A personal commitment enhances the likelihood of success.	Psy, Nsg
4. Assist Mary in identifying and adopting more effective coping behaviors.	This encourages problem solving and the use of more effective behaviors.	Nsg, Psy
5. Assess the social support systems available for Mary.	Supportive significant others are often unavailable for substance abusers.	Nsg, Soc Svc
6. Educate Mary and her family about chemical abuse and resources for help.	Knowledge helps Mary and her family cope more successfully with problems.	Nsg, Soc Svc
7. Refer Mary to a Treatment Center, and provide support until Mary is involved in the program.	Specialized drug treatment programs are likely to be more effective if clients are willing to participate.	Soc Svc

Evaluation

During her entire stay, Mary remained chemical free but expressed many discomforts. Mary was able to identify her drug-using behaviors during her stay but refused to participate in an outpatient treatment program.

❓ **CRITICAL THINKING** QUESTIONS

1. How would the staff confront Mary without making her defensive?

2. What can be done to improve Mary's willingness to participate in treatment?

A complete client care plan includes several other diagnoses and interventions.
Psy, Psychologist; *Nsg,* nursing staff; *Soc Svc,* social services.

Box 28-2 | NANDA-I Nursing Diagnoses Related to Substance Abuse

Anxiety
Communication, impaired verbal
Coping, ineffective community
Coping, ineffective
Denial, ineffective
Family processes, dysfunctional: alcoholism
Hopelessness*
Injury, risk for
Loneliness, risk for
Noncompliance (specify)
Powerlessness
Sexuality pattern, ineffective
Social isolation
Spiritual distress*
Trauma, risk for
Violence, risk for other-directed
Violence, risk for self-directed

Data from NANDA International: *NANDA-I nursing diagnoses: definitions and classification, 2007-2008,* Philadelphia, 2007, NANDA International. *NANDA-I,* NANDA International.
*Primary nursing diagnoses for substance abuse.

Box 28-3 | Key Interventions for Abuse and Dependence Problems

Meet physical needs during detoxification; this intervention is very important.
Address the physiological problems resulting from substance dependence in the same manner as these needs would be met in any person.
Monitor the effects of the therapies that may be prescribed to control the substance use.
Teach clients about the disease and its progression.
Focus on clients' strengths, and help clients build on them.
Help clients problem solve the dilemmas they fear.
Encourage focus on the present and the future, not on the past.
Behave toward clients in a consistent manner, confronting them in a nonjudgmental, nonpunitive manner if they break the rules of the treatment setting.
Assist clients' families by encouraging them to become involved in group counseling.

encourages them to work toward freedom from their chemicals. Personalized approaches allow for discussions about diet, health, problem solving, and other health concerns. Drug therapists work with clients to develop long-term strategies for coping with their dependency. Clients are offered opportunities for learning, changing, and developing new and more effective skills for living. Work to become familiar with the subject of substance abuse. Learn as much as you can because you will be caring for clients whose problems are related to the use of chemical substances.

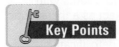

Key Points

- Substance use is the ingesting of any chemical that affects the body.
- Abused substances alter the individual's perception by affecting the central nervous system. They are often called mind-altering drugs because of their ability to enhance or depress mood and emotions.
- Every chemical ingested by a pregnant woman poses a potential danger to her unborn child.
- Children who live with substance-abusing parents are at high risk for injuries and for developing drug problems themselves.
- Adolescent substance use, abuse, and dependence are becoming an ever-increasing problem.
- In adults, substance abuse is common. Substance abuse occurs most commonly between 18 and 35 years of age.
- A significant number of older adults use alcohol and prescription medications.
- Children of problem drinkers have three times the risk for serious injury. Cocaine-exposed and other drug-exposed infants are filling health and foster care.
- Alcohol-related motor vehicle accidents are one of the leading causes of death among people under 45 years of age. Deaths from falls, drowning, and burns may all be related to substance use.
- Many homeless and mentally ill people use and abuse chemicals.
- Abused substances include alcohol, diet pills, coffee, tea, marijuana, cocaine, hallucinogens, inhalants, nicotine, opioids, phencyclidine (PCP), sedatives, hypnotics, and antianxiety drugs.
- Many medications have the potential for being abused.
- The use of inhalants has become popular with adolescents and young adults because they are legal, inexpensive, and easily available and have a rapid onset. Significant complications include cardiac dysrhythmia or respiratory depression.
- Substance abuse occurs when the use of the chemical becomes more important in the individual's life than the activities of daily living.
- The movement from use to dependency (addiction) follows a predictable course. In the early stage, use progresses to excessive use. During the middle stage, intoxication progresses to tolerance. In the chronic (late) stage, tolerance progresses to loss of control, dependence, and addiction.
- For a substance-related disorder to be diagnosed, the pattern of substance use must be disabling and lead to significant impaired functioning and distress, and the individual must demonstrate the signs of tolerance, withdrawal, and dependence.
- The assessment of clients with substance-related problems should include a thorough history and physical examination.
- Detoxification is the process of withdrawing a substance under medical supervision. Relapse is the recurrence of the substance-abusing behaviors after a significant period of abstinence.

- The most important intervention for clients with substance-related problems is to act as a therapeutic agent. Other interventions are designed to meet physical needs, especially during detoxification; monitor effects of therapies; teach about the disease and its progression; help clients problem solve; and encourage the client's family and significant others to become involved.

evolve Be sure to visit the companion Evolve site at http://evolve.elsevier.com/Morrison-Valfre/ for additional online resources.

29 Sexual Disorders

Objectives

Upon completion of this chapter, the student will be able to:

1. Describe the continuum (range) of sexual responses.
2. Explain how self-awareness affects the care of clients with psychosexual problems.
3. Illustrate how sexuality is expressed through each life stage.
4. Describe four modes of sexual expression.
5. Examine three possible theories relating to sexual problems.
6. Compare the difference between a sexual dysfunction and a sexual disorder.
7. Define paraphilia, and list three examples of paraphiliac behaviors.
8. List four specific signs of a sexual addiction.
9. Apply the nursing process to the care of a client with a psychosexual problem.
10. Explain the importance of human immune deficiency virus/acquired immunodeficiency syndrome (HIV/AIDS) counseling for every client with a psychosexual problem.

Key Terms

bisexuals (p. 326)
dyspareunia (DĬS-pə-ROO-nē-ə) (p. 327)
erotic (p. 324)
exhibitionism (ĔG-zĭ-BĬSH-ə-nĭz-əm) (p. 328)
gay (p. 325)
gender identity (p. 322)
gender perception (p. 322)
gender role (p. 322)
heterosexual (p. 324)
homosexuality (p. 325)
lesbian (p. 325)
paraphilias (pair-ə-FIL-ē-əs) (p. 328)
pedophilia (p. 328)
prostitution (p. 321)
sexual addiction (p. 328)
sexual disorders (p. 327)
sexual dysfunction (p. 327)
sexual masochism (MĀS-ə-kĭz-əm) (p. 328)
sexual orientation (p. 322)
sexual sadism (SĀ-dĭz-əm) (p. 328)
sexuality (p. 322)
transsexualism (p. 328)
transvestism (trăns-VĔS-tĭz-əm) (p. 326)
vaginismus (VĂJ-ĭ-NĬZ-məs) (p. 327)
voyeurism (VOI-ĕr-ĭz-əm) (p. 328)

According to Maslow's hierarchy of human needs, sex ranks as a basic physiological need. Humans, like most other creatures, have strong sexual drives; but unlike other creatures, human sexual expression is defined by the social customs, norms, and laws of society. A number of terms are used when discussing sex, and several are listed in Box 29-1.

People express their sexuality through a variety of thoughts, attitudes, and behaviors. Sexuality is important in every dimension of functioning. The physical dimension of sexuality includes anatomy and physiology—the characteristics that physically define us as men or women. Sexuality in the emotional and intellectual dimensions encompasses our thoughts, beliefs, and values about sexuality. The social dimension of functioning is associated with sexuality. Interactions with others may range from the intimacy of sexual intercourse, to discussions of sexual attitudes with trusted friends, to passing feelings generated by attractive strangers. Sexuality and its expressions are social in nature.

Cultures have an impact on sexuality. All societies have laws, rules, or customs that regulate sexual behavior. Attitudes, beliefs, and rituals help define what is appropriate sexually. Religious institutions have a strong impact on views of what is right or wrong sexual behavior. In some cultures, the sexual act is considered a religious ritual, with taboos and regulations governing the experience. Evidence of the practice of religious **prostitution** (the selling of sexual services in exchange for [spiritual] gain) dates as far back as 5000 years ago. Cultural attitudes, beliefs, and behaviors toward sexuality and its expressions have changed throughout the years, and they will continue to change in the future (see Cultural Considerations 29-1).

CONTINUUM OF SEXUAL RESPONSES

Even experts have difficulty agreeing on what is normal sexual behavior. For years, the norm was defined as a married man and woman who engaged in sexual relations in order to procreate (have children). Today a wider range of sexual behaviors is considered socially acceptable.

Sexual behaviors can be viewed as occurring along a continuum (Figure 29-1). At the adaptive end of the

| Box 29-1 | *Terms Relating to Sexuality* |

Human **sexuality** is the combination of physical, chemical, psychological, and functional characteristics that are expressed by one's gender identity and sexual behaviors.

Sexuality comprises one's:

Gender identity: The physical makeup of an individual

Gender perception: A view of one's maleness or femaleness

Gender role: Cultural and social obligations relating to one's gender

Sexual orientation: Gender to which one is romantically attracted

From Stuart GW, Laraia MT: *Principles and practice of psychiatric nursing,* ed 8, St. Louis, 2005, Mosby.

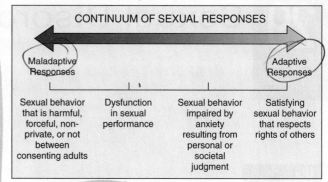

FIGURE **29-1** Continuum of sexual responses.

Cultural Considerations 29-1

Margaret Mead, in her book titled *Growing Up in Samoa,* describes children with few sexual restraints. Although sexual play and experimentation are accepted methods of expression, the pregnancy rate of the islanders is no greater than that among other populations.

In Malaysia, children born out of marriage are common. It is the custom for the father to quietly provide for the child's welfare.

Think About 29-1

- What is your definition of "normal" sexuality?
- How does your view compare with the views of a relative, a friend, and a classmate?
- What is your opinion of those who practice different means of sexual expression?
- How do you think your personal beliefs and opinions affect your interactions with clients?

spectrum lie satisfying sexual behaviors that respect the rights and wishes of others. As the continuum moves toward maladaptive, sexual behaviors become impaired or dysfunctional. The opposite end of the continuum is marked by sexual actions that are harmful to self or others in some manner.

Perhaps a useful definition of adaptive or healthy sexual responses is sexuality that meets the following conditions (Coleman-Kennedy and Pendley, 2002):

1. Between two consenting adults
2. Satisfying to both
3. Not forced or coerced
4. Conducted in privacy

Maladaptive or unhealthy sexual responses are those behaviors that do not meet these criteria. They are, in some way or degree, physically or psychologically harmful for the individual or others. Labeling sexual behaviors must be done with caution because judgments are easy to pass on those who behave differently (see Think About 29-1).

SELF-AWARENESS AND SEXUALITY

Because nurses and other health caregivers work with the human condition, each of us must strive to develop an awareness of our own thoughts, attitudes, values, and beliefs toward sexuality and its modes of expression. **One's self-awareness has a strong influence on discussing sexual issues with clients.** Values that may be unconscious to the caregiver are often transmitted

loudly and clearly to clients. Nonverbal messages of disapproval dampen the effectiveness of the therapeutic relationship and all other interventions. Individuals who feel judged are not likely to cooperate with the plan of care.

Developing an awareness of your views about sexuality involves the process of defining and clarifying attitudes and values. Each of us carries a sexual point of view, a way of looking at sexuality. Much of the foundation for this view was established unconsciously during childhood and adolescence as a part of growing up and interacting with others.

Refer to Chapter 3 for the values clarification process. Apply each of the steps to the topic of sexuality. Then think about how your values may affect the care of clients with sexual disorders. Choose your positions, and prize your choices. Know that values are not static. They change as one learns and develops. Remember, when it comes to working with sexually disordered clients, the caregiver's effectiveness is directly related to personal self-awareness and comfort. No client should have to endure the ignorance of his or her health care provider.

SEXUALITY THROUGHOUT THE LIFE CYCLE

The expression of one's sexuality begins at birth and ends with death. Gender differences define roles in society, attitudes about the dynamics of living, relationships with others, and views of who we are. Gender roles develop as new knowledge, attitudes, and behaviors are added to life experiences. A basic knowledge of sexuality throughout the life cycle is important for care providers.

SEXUALITY IN CHILDHOOD

"From the moment of birth, children are treated differently based on their biological sex" (Hockenberry and others, 2007). Female infants are dressed in pink, males in blue. Each is assigned a name, which usually indicates a gender. For example, girls are seldom named Bruce or Joseph, and few boys are addressed as Sarah or Sally. Families treat boys differently from girls, even in infancy. Female infants are seen as delicate. They are handled and spoken to more tenderly, whereas male infants are stimulated by boisterous voices and play involving motor activity.

Young children are unaware that gender is a permanent attribute. Around the age of 2 years, children learn to label themselves according to their gender. Most respond to being called "good girls" or "brave boys" by the adults in their environment. They soon internalize the label of male or female, boy or girl.

By age 3 years, the majority of children can accurately label the gender of other persons, but they still believe that their gender can be changed with time if they want it. By about age 7 years, children understand that one's gender is permanent and will not naturally change. Between 7 and 9 years of age, they learn that one's gender is identified by genital appearance.

Children learn about gender roles in relation to themselves first. Then they apply their learning to members of the same gender. Finally, their knowledge is applied to persons of the opposite gender. By about 3 years of age, children can identify the simpler aspects of gender roles. They know, for example, that boys and girls differ in appearance, toy preference, and choice of activities.

By school age, most children identify with the same-gender parent. School is the time to learn about the expected behaviors associated with each gender role. In the past, this identification involved much stereotyping. Girls could not play certain sports, for example, and boys were discouraged from taking home economics or engaging in other "sissy" activities. Fortunately, this attitude is fading as individual qualities become more important than playing appropriate gender roles.

By the middle elementary school years, children are aware of most aspects of their gender-role stereotypes. Future goals, occupational choices, personality traits, and sexual behaviors are influenced by gender roles that were established early in childhood.

SEXUALITY IN ADOLESCENCE

During the early teen years, close relationships with same-gender peers intensify. "Through these relationships, children learn about the possibility of intimacy between equals and are exposed to peer standards for appropriate sex-role behavior" (Hockenberry and others, 2007). As time passes, adolescents begin to encounter expectations for mature gender-role behavior from both peers and adults.

Although 12-year-olds are intensely involved with same-gender friends, opportunities for mixed-group activities and dating increase. Dating activities in the United States usually begin in the seventh or eighth grade with group social activities, such as dances, picnics, or organized school functions. Group dating moves to double dating, and by the twelfth grade, most adolescents have been on single-pair dates.

Teens have difficulty believing that sex can exist without love, so each boy-girl attachment is seen as "true love." Because adolescence is an emotionally stressful time for most individuals, steady dating can offer some relief from insecurity and loneliness and provide a sense of belonging.

In the United States and other countries, sexual activity among adolescents has become the norm rather than the exception. Most teens begin experimenting with sexual activity through kissing and petting. As adolescents get older, most become sexually active. Many teens have experienced multiple sexual relationships by the time they are 19 years old. Unfortunately, most adolescent girls use ineffective or no contraception at all and most adolescent boys do not use condoms. Because of this practice, the sexually transmitted disease (including human immune deficiency virus/acquired immunodeficiency syndrome [HIV/AIDS]) and pregnancy rates are higher for adolescents than the general population of sexually active adults.

Adolescence is a time of intense searching and learning. Much information related to sexuality is gained from peers and other inexperienced or unknowledgeable persons. Nurses should always be alert for the opportunity to assess and correct, if necessary, adolescents' misconceptions about sexuality and its expressions.

SEXUALITY IN ADULTHOOD

The age of first intercourse has decreased and the age at marriage has increased over the years. As a result, there are more unmarried, sexually active young adults than ever before. Between ages 18 and 24 years, most adults engage in sexual activity with multiple partners and serial relationships. Women tend to be less sexually aggressive than men, who are more likely to seek out and experience sexual relationships with a number of persons. Most young adults are sexually active, but many are now willing to assume responsibility for preventing pregnancy and disease.

Among adults 25 to 59 years of age, relative **monogamy** (the practice of having only one partner) appears to be the norm. Sexuality becomes shared with one special person as many adults commit to marriage and family relationships. However, as divorce rates continue to climb, more adults are involved with multiple sexual partners.

Sexual behaviors during adulthood change to accommodate the situation. After the birth of children, for example, parents are usually less likely to engage in spontaneous sexual expression. The fear of another unplanned pregnancy on a limited income has a strong effect on the sexual behaviors of many adults who are already coping with all they can financially handle.

The sexuality patterns of middle-age adults have recently changed. More women in their 30s and 40s are bearing children and beginning families. Single parenthood is common. Patterns of sexual functioning continue throughout the middle years. As children leave home and menopause occurs, many women experience a feeling of sexual freedom. The fear of pregnancy is over. The couple is once again alone and able to spontaneously interact.

SEXUALITY IN OLDER ADULTHOOD

The typical picture of the older adult as an asexual and uninterested individual is a myth. Nothing could be further from the truth. Older adulthood, for many people, is a time of pursuing one's own interests and desires, including sexuality.

Sexual expression in older adults shifts "from procreation to an emphasis on companionship, sharing, touching, and intimate communication" (Edelman and Mandle, 2006). The closeness, intimacy, and sharing of sexuality become more important than the physical act for most older adults. Sexuality can also be communicated through touching, stroking, or other means of expression when intercourse is not desirable or possible.

Sexuality persists throughout life, and, although sexual activity may decrease in frequency as one ages, established sexual patterns continue. Unfortunately, the sexual expression of older adults meets many cultural and social barriers, attitudes, and expectations. Poor health, medications, disabilities, and the normal aging process influence one's sexual behaviors, but sexuality is a basic need that will be with us until we die.

SEXUALITY AND DISABILITY

Many permanently disabled persons are able to enjoy rich and satisfying sexual lives with some adaptation. People with spinal cord injuries, for example, can still be lovers, partners, and parents. Any condition that affects well-being, mobility, or self-esteem has an impact on sexuality and its expressions. Health problems such as diabetes, arthritis, cancer, and cardiovascular disease can affect one's sexuality. However, these conditions only affect the expression of sexuality, not one's sexuality itself.

Men and women who are disabled learn to adapt to their conditions. Most must also cope with negative attitudes and stigmas toward disabled people. People with disabilities have the exact same needs as the rest of the population. Remember, everyone is an individual first; some of us just happen to be different. Improving the quality of life for people with disabilities involves changing the social attitudes that limit the disabled population.

MODES OF SEXUAL EXPRESSION

An individual's sexual attraction to others is one's sexual orientation, or sexual preference. In 1948, one of the first researchers into human sexual responses (A.C. Kinsey) developed a scale of human sexual preference, ranging from exclusively heterosexual to exclusively homosexual (Figure 29-2). He stated that most people were not exclusively one or the other because many had experienced both heterosexual and homosexual expressions of sexuality (Kinsey, Pomeroy, and Martin, 1953). Today, several modes of sexual expression are practiced (Table 29-1).

HETEROSEXUALITY

Persons who express their sexuality with members of the opposite gender are called **heterosexual**. Heterosexual relationships are the foundation for bearing children and family. Today, however, it is common to encounter families with homosexual or bisexual parents.

Historically, heterosexual relationships have been the norm—the culturally and socially acceptable form of coupling. However, variations of the man-woman relationship have existed throughout history. For example, in ancient Greece it was customary for men to regard the women they married as useful for having children and taking care of household affairs. The social, emotional, and **erotic** (sexually desiring) needs of husbands were filled by other men, especially adolescent boys. In this culture, both heterosexuality

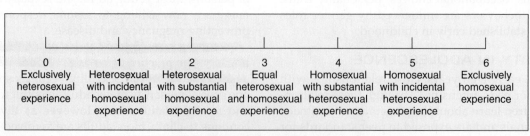

FIGURE **29-2** Kinsey's rating scale of sexual preference.

and homosexuality were considered socially appropriate expressions of sexuality. History is filled with examples of sexual restrictions and permissions, but it appears that heterosexual relationships are here to stay because biology still requires a male and a female to produce the next generation of human beings.

HOMOSEXUALITY

The sexual desire or preference for members of one's own gender is known as **homosexuality**. People who prefer homosexuality are often referred to as **gay** (applies to both genders) or **lesbian** (applies to female homosexuals). Historically, same-gender relationships have been around as long as opposite-gender relationships, but cultural and social attitudes toward them have changed as history has evolved.

One's sexual orientation is established in late childhood and continues to develop through adulthood. For adolescents who are homosexual, adolescence is a particularly difficult time because, in addition to the average developmental tasks, these individuals are faced with "their own unique issues of identity formation" (Hockenberry and others, 2007). The process of establishing an integrated or complete identity as a homosexual is known as **coming out,** and it occurs in predictable stages (Table 29-2).

Table 29-1 | *Modes of Sexual Expression*

TERM	DEFINITION
Heterosexuality	Sexual desire or preference for members of opposite gender
Homosexuality	Sexual desire or preference for members of same gender
Bisexuality	Sexual desire or preference for members of both genders
Transvestism	Practice of receiving sexual satisfaction from dressing in clothes of opposite gender; also called cross-dressing
Paraphilia	Sexual preference for or obsession with objects or situations that are not normally arousing; considered socially undesirable behaviors or disorders

Historically, homosexuality has been considered a maladaptive mode of sexual expression. However, many studies have revealed that homosexuals commonly function as well with their love relationships as heterosexual persons. Studies of homosexual couples (Bell and Weinberg, 1978) found that homosexual relationships or behaviors tend to fall into one of five categories: close-coupled, open-coupled, functional, dysfunctional, and asexual.

Close-coupled relationships are akin to a married couple. Each individual looks to the other for emotional and sexual satisfaction. These couples spend the majority of their evenings at home and do not seek sexual experiences outside the relationship. They are less likely to visit gay bars, and they report few sexual problems. Couples in this type of homosexual relationship are usually well adjusted and more accepting than average individuals.

Open-coupled relationships consist of two persons living together while continuing to have sexual experiences with others. These couples are less committed to their primary relationship and seek the company of a larger circle of homosexual friends. They visit gay baths and bars and report higher levels of sexual activity than close-coupled homosexuals.

The third type of homosexual relationship is called **functional.** These persons have no special sexual partner, and they are usually not interested in finding one. Their lives are organized around sexual activity, and they report a greater number of sexual partners than any other group. Many are unconcerned with homosexuality and are openly involved in the gay community. Both open-coupled and functional homosexuals are at high risk for contracting sexually transmitted diseases.

Dysfunctional homosexuals have a number of worries and problems. They regret their sexual orientation and are often more unhappy, depressed, or paranoid. Although they try, dysfunctional homosexuals have great difficulty in establishing a permanent relationship. Problems can extend to other areas of their lives as evidenced by the high number of mental health

Table 29-2 | *Identity Formation Process of Gay Adolescents*

APPROXIMATE AGE/STAGE	STEPS IN PROCESS	DESCRIPTION
Childhood to early adolescence	Identity awareness	Becomes aware of feeling differently about stereotyped gender activities; feels discomfort with gender stereotypes and the expected behaviors that accompany them
Middle to late adolescence (about age 17 yr in boys, 18 yr in girls)	Identity recognition	Discomfort with gender-role behaviors increases as attraction to same-gender persons begins to emerge; begins to feel that he or she is probably homosexual; period of identity confusion, isolation, depression, and great discomfort
Early to middle 20s	Identity assumption	Acknowledges homosexual identity; begins to experiment with sexuality; socializes within homosexual community and subculture
Mid-20s and beyond	Commitment	Individuals assume homosexual lifestyle; state to themselves and world that they are homosexual; give themselves permission to be who they are

problems and crime rates in this group. Many are receiving long-term mental health care.

Last is the category called **asexual.** Individuals in this group feel sexually unattractive, lonely, and unhappy with themselves. They report few sexual partners, little sexual experience, and low levels of sexual activity. Because they are not likely to visit gay bars or other gathering places, much of their time is spent alone. Mental health problems are often present.

It appears that both homosexual and heterosexual behavior styles have much in common. Homosexuality is now receiving acceptance as a mode of sexual expression, but many health care providers still carry attitudes and stereotypes that can interfere with the care provided to gay and lesbian clients. We must all work to develop the self-awareness that enhances our therapeutic effectiveness, especially with persons of different sexual orientations. Case Study 29-1 illustrates this point.

BISEXUALITY

Persons who are attracted to and engage in sexual activities with members of both genders are known as bisexuals. These individuals identify themselves as bisexual as compared with homosexuals or heterosexuals. Little research has been done on bisexuals because they do not receive the research attention that is focused on homosexuals or heterosexuals. Most bisexual individuals appear to be as well adjusted as

those who prefer other modes of sexual expression, but they are at high risk for contracting HIV/AIDS and other sexually transmitted diseases.

TRANSVESTISM

Transvestism is commonly referred to as crossdressing. It is defined as sexual excitement from wearing the clothing of the opposite gender. Two types of transvestism are usually practiced. In the first, a man is aroused by a certain article of clothing, such as shoes or undergarments. With the second type, the individual dresses completely in women's clothing (Figure 29-3). The typical transvestite is a married man with children who is rather secretive about his cross-dressing. He is heterosexual, and his behaviors are usually accepted by his wife. Although few reliable statistics are available, transvestism may be more common than once thought.

THEORIES RELATING TO PSYCHOSEXUAL VARIATIONS

Although no one understands exactly why an individual prefers a certain mode of sexual expression, many theories and explanations have been offered.

Biological theories explain sexual variations as differences in chromosomes, the genetic material that determines hereditary traits. Some studies have "suggested that homosexuality may be inherited from the maternal side of the family through the X chromosome" (Stuart and Laraia, 2001). Some researchers suggest a correlation between brain structure and sexual orientation, whereas others are pursuing the notion that hormones wire the brain for sexual orientation

Case Study 29-1

It is evening in a busy medical-surgical unit. You have just received notice that a 42-year-old man, Jim S., is being admitted for injuries suffered in a motor vehicle accident. Because of the severity of his injuries, the physician has ordered that he be visited by immediate family only.

Jim is admitted to the unit and made comfortable. As you glance around for family members who accompanied him from the emergency department, you see only one youngish-looking gentleman, peering anxiously at your client. "I'm sorry, but immediate family only is allowed in here," you say politely, as you usher him out the door.

Later that evening, Jim begins to respond. He keeps calling out for "my love, J.J." and asking you where J.J. is, so loudly that you are sure everyone on the floor can hear. Finally, Jim quiets down only after he extracts a promise from you to find J.J. Exhausted, you agree, hoping she would somehow arrive and help to keep this man quiet.

As you open the door to leave the room, the youngish-looking man from earlier in the evening almost falls through to the floor. With tears in his eyes, he glares intently at you but says nothing. Quietly you ask if his name could possibly be J.J.

• What is the lesson to be learned from this case study?
• How could this experience help you to be more sensitive and therapeutic?

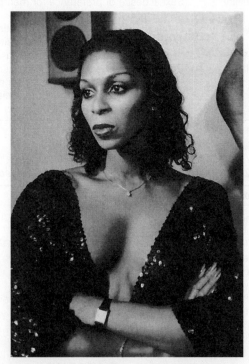

FIGURE **29-3** Male transvestite.

during the prenatal period. Researchers (Dessens and others, 1999) have found that certain anticonvulsant medications alter the hormone levels of developing fetuses and lead to disturbances in gender orientation.

Psychoanalytical theories as proposed by Freud and his followers consider sexual variations (other than heterosexuality) as behaviors with neurotic or psychopathic motivations (Fortinash and Holoday-Worret, 2008). Problems arise early in life because of the child's Oedipus/Electra complex, in which children experience sexual feelings for the opposite-gender parent and resent the same-gender parent. According to this theory, persons with different sexual behaviors also exhibit problems in other areas of their lives. Aspects of the psychoanalytical point of view have been criticized for being male oriented and viewing women as inferior. Little scientific evidence has been found to justify Freud's psychoanalytical view of sexual orientation.

Finally, the **behavioral theories** consider the various modes of sexual expression as learned, measurable responses. The learning theory states that individuals are introduced to a certain sexual variation by an accidental experience that is sexually stimulating. When other sexual experiences lead to feelings of inadequacy, the "pleasurable accident" experience encourages continued use of the sexual variation. Behavioral theorists also believe that the sexual behaviors of adults in the child's environment have a strong influence on sexual preferences and behaviors. Significant emotional, adjustment, and mental health problems are common in adults who were sexually abused as children.

PSYCHOSEXUAL DISORDERS

Because knowledge of human sexuality is still evolving, a broad definition of psychosexual problems is needed. Sexual disorders are those problems that cause distress and impaired functioning in an individual or others who are exposed to the sexual behavior. These disorders include problems with sexual functions, gender identity disorders, and socially inappropriate or illegal methods of sexual expression.

SEXUAL DYSFUNCTION

The average person experiences four stages of sexual excitement and pleasure: appetite, excitement, orgasm, and resolution. A sexual dysfunction is a disturbance anywhere during these four stages of the sexual response cycle (American Psychiatric Association, 2000). Its definition also includes any discomfort or pain associated with sexual intercourse. Sexual dysfunctions may be lifelong or acquired after a period of normal functioning. They may be limited by certain situations, partners, or types of stimulation, or they may be generalized to every sexual experience. The causes are often related to psychological distresses, medication or illicit drug use, and many physical conditions. Arthritis, diabetes, and chronic illness can result in various sexual dysfunctions or alterations in sexual desire. Impaired hormonal functioning and neurological problems can also lead to difficulties with sexual functioning. Problems with relationships or unrealistic attitudes about sex may also contribute. Table 29-3 describes the most common sexual dysfunctions in men and women. Many

Table 29-3 *DSM-IV-TR Classification of Sexual Dysfunctions*

CLASSIFICATION	DISORDER	DESCRIPTION
Sexual desire disorders	Hypoactive sexual desire disorder	Absence of sexual fantasies and desire for sexual activity
	Sexual aversion disorder	Active avoidance of sexual contact with partner; reacts to sexual opportunity with anxiety, fear, or disgust
Sexual arousal disorders	Female sexual arousal disorder	Inability to attain or maintain sexual excitement during sexual activity; has little sexual arousal
	Male erectile disorder	Inability to attain or maintain adequate erection during sexual activity
Orgasmic disorders	Female/male orgasmic disorder	Delay in or absence of orgasm following normal excitement
	Premature ejaculation	Ejaculation that occurs with minimal stimulation before person wishes it to occur
Sexual pain disorders	Dyspareunia	Pain associated with sexual intercourse; may occur in both females and males
	Vaginismus	Persistent involuntary contractions of muscles around vagina when penetration is attempted
Sexual dysfunction caused by medical condition	Dependent on medical diagnoses	Significant sexual problems caused by direct effects of medical condition
Substance-induced sexual dysfunction	Dependent on substance used	Significant sexual problems caused by direct physical effects of substance

Modified from American Psychiatric Association: *Diagnostic and statistical manual of mental disorders, ed 4,* text revision, Washington, DC, 2000, The Association.

Box 29-2 *DSM-IV-TR Description of Paraphilias*

EXHIBITIONISM

Exhibitionism is exposure of one's genitals to unsuspecting person(s) followed by sexual arousal

FETISHISM

Fetishism is utilization of objects (e.g., panties, rubber sheeting) for purposes of sexual arousal

FROTTEURISM

Frotteurism is rubbing up against nonconsenting persons to heighten sexual arousal

PEDOPHILIA

Pedophilia is fondling and/or other types of sexual activities with prepubescent child (usually under age 13 years and having not yet developed secondary sex characteristics)

SEXUAL MASOCHISM

Sexual masochism is sexual arousal achieved by being receiver of pain (either physical or emotional), humiliation, or being made to suffer

SEXUAL SADISM

Sexual sadism is sexual arousal achieved by infliction of pain (either physical or emotional) or humiliation onto another person

TRANSVESTIC FETISHISM

Transvestic fetishism is the act of cross-dressing (heterosexual men wearing female clothing) to achieve sexual arousal

VOYEURISM

Voyeurism is Sexual arousal achieved by observing unsuspecting persons who are naked, in act of disrobing, or engaging in sexual activity ("peeping Tom")

PARAPHILIA NOS (Not Otherwise Specified)

These disorders do not meet criteria for aforementioned categories:

Telephone scatologia: Obscene phone calling; "900" sex lines

Necrophilia: Sexual activity with corpses

Partialism: Exclusive focus on particular body part for sexual arousal

Zoophilia: Sexual activity involving participation with animals (bestiality)

Coprophilia: Sexual arousal by contact with feces

Klismaphilia: Sexual arousal generated by use of enemas

Urophilia: Sexual arousal by contact with urine

Ephebophilia: Fondling and/or other types of sexual activities with pubescent children who are developing secondary sex characteristics (e.g., pubic hair, breasts); these children are usually between ages 13 and 18 years

Paraphilic coercive disorder: Rape; aggressive sexual assault involving act of sexual intercourse against one's will and without consent

Modified from American Psychiatric Association: *Diagnostic and statistical manual of mental disorders*, ed 4, text revision, Washington, DC, 2000, The Association.

sexual dysfunctions are treatable, so clients are referred to their physicians.

PARAPHILIAS

The paraphilias are a group of sexual variations that depart from society's traditional and acceptable modes of seeking sexual gratification. When the word *paraphilia* is taken apart, the suffix *philia* means "an attraction to." When used to describe a specific behavior, the descriptive term replaces the prefix *para*. For example, pedophilia refers to a person who is sexually attracted to children (*pedo*, meaning "child"). Several of these behaviors, such as exhibitionism, pedophilia, and voyeurism, are considered illegal in some countries, including the United States. Others are harmless when practiced in private with other consenting adults. Box 29-2 names and briefly describes the more common paraphilias.

GENDER IDENTITY DISORDER

One of the first things an individual develops is a gender identity, the knowledge that one is a boy or a girl. When there is an inconsistency between the child's biological gender and his or her gender identity, a gender identity disorder is usually diagnosed.

Children with gender identity disorder are unhappy with their own gender. They want to eliminate their sexual characteristics and trade them for those of the opposite gender. Many truly believe they were born into the wrong body and reject expectations and behaviors associated with their biological gender. Older children often fail to develop same-gender relationships in school, leading to isolation and loneliness. Adolescents and adults with gender identity disorder commonly find that their desire to be another gender interferes with work and social relationships. Separation anxiety disorders are common in children with gender identity disorder, and mental health problems are often seen in both parents and children.

Transsexualism is the persistent desire to become a member of the opposite gender. Transsexuals are discontented with their biological gender. Some actually become an opposite-gender person to fit their gender identity. This is accomplished by a series of psychological counseling, hormonal treatments, and major surgeries. Because decisions made by the individual are irreversible, the process of changing one's sexual identity is deliberately prolonged and can take as long as 2 years.

SEXUAL ADDICTION

A sexual addiction is a progressive and chronic addiction characterized by patterns of compulsive sexual behavior despite negative consequences. It impairs social and work relationships, destroys marriages, and increases the risk for HIV/AIDS. "As many as 20 million people in the United States are affected by sexual addiction" (Coleman-Kennedy and Pendley, 2002).

Healthy sexuality is a mutual energy exchange between two consenting individuals. Sexual addictions, however, are characterized by an obsessive need for self-gratification. Each act is without emotion, and partners may be forced into submission. "The sex addict uses sex as a coping mechanism for emotional turmoil" (Coleman-Kennedy and Pendley, 2002).

Sexual addicts usually have a dysfunctional history with their primary caregiver. There may also be a history of abuse, neglect, or abandonment. The addict fails to develop adequate communication skills, which develops into low self-worth and a fear of intimacy. The sex act becomes a way to gain power over another person and control over one's anxiety. This leads to many health, social, occupational, and legal problems.

Sexual addicts, like people with substance addictions, experience tolerance. More and more sexual encounters are needed to relieve the emotional pain. The specific signs of sexual addiction are listed in Box 29-3.

THERAPEUTIC INTERVENTIONS

Treatment for sexual problems depends on the cause, the distressing signs and symptoms, and the type of disorder. Group or individual therapy may help clients explore their emotions, behaviors, and coping mechanisms. Behavioral therapies, such as positive reinforcement or aversive therapy, focus on changing or managing sexual behaviors in a more acceptable way. Hormonal drug therapy is sometimes employed to reduce sexual drives (see Drug Alert 29-1).

Environmental controls for sexually undesirable behaviors include incarceration (prison or jail). The individual is removed from society and may or may not be accepted into a special program for sexual offenders while in prison.

Most clients with sexual problems are treated on an outpatient basis. In some states, they must register as sex offenders and keep authorities informed of their whereabouts at all times. Health care providers in all settings work with problems of sexuality in relation to clients and their surgical procedures or medical conditions.

An important point to remember is that if you are uncomfortable with any aspect of a client's sexuality, your professional judgment and behaviors could be affected. Some psychosexual problems are complex and require the skills of specially educated nurses or sexual therapists. Discuss the situation with your supervisor because the goal is still to provide the client with the best possible care. As with other clients, therapeutic interventions remain the same: accept, assess, intervene, and educate.

PSYCHOSEXUAL ASSESSMENT

Sexuality is a sensitive topic for most persons. For this reason, be aware of the client's level of comfort when assessing sexual functioning. Barriers to obtaining a sexual history also lie with the nurse or other care provider. They include inadequate training, embarrassment, and a fear of offending the client (Warner, Rowe, and Whipple, 1999). Hopefully, both client and caregiver will establish enough trust in the therapeutic relationship to honestly share information.

NURSING PROCESS

Nursing diagnoses for psychosexual disorders are based on each client's identified problems. The primary nursing diagnoses for problems with sexuality are sexual dysfunction and ineffective sexuality pattern. Other nursing diagnoses are selected to help to enhance the client's physical, emotional, social, and spiritual functioning, and several are listed in Box 29-4.

The quality of care for clients with psychosexual problems depends on each caregiver's abilities to remain nonjudgmental and accepting of his or her clients. The team treatment approach is usually more effective in treating individuals with sexual problems because it helps to maintain objectivity and prevents any one member from becoming too involved in a client's treatment. Sample Client Care Plan 29-1 describes treatment for a client with a sexual dysfunction.

 Drug Alert 29-1

Hormones that reduce the sexual drive have many side effects. Be familiar with each medication, and remember to monitor clients routinely for any unusual symptoms.

Many medications prescribed for various medical problems can cause sexual problems. Examples include the following:
- Antihypertensives
- Antidepressants, anticonvulsants, and other psychotropic medications
- Medications used for problems of the stomach and small intestine, pain-relieving medications

A complete and accurate history should include an assessment of each client's medication (including over-the-counter and street drugs) history and current use.

Box 29-3 *Signs of Sexual Addiction*

1. Out-of-control sexual behaviors
2. Behaviors continue despite severe consequences
3. Inability to stop
4. Persistently engages in high-risk behaviors
5. Ongoing attempts to limit or stop behaviors
6. Sexual behavior: the primary coping strategy
7. Seeks increased sexual encounters (tolerance)
8. Experiences severe mood changes around sexual activity
9. Excessive time spent in obtaining sex, being sexual, or recovering from sexual experiences
10. Reduces or eliminates important social, occupational, and recreational activities

Box 29-4 *NANDA-I Nursing Diagnoses Related to Sexual Disorders*

Anxiety
Coping, ineffective community
Coping, ineffective
Denial, ineffective
Injury, risk for
Noncompliance (specify)
Sexual dysfunction*
Sexuality pattern, ineffective
Violence, risk for other-directed
Violence, risk for self-directed

Data from NANDA International: *NANDA-I nursing diagnoses and classification, 2007-2008,* Philadelphia, 2007, The Association.
NANDA-I, NANDA International.
*Primary nursing diagnosis for sexual disorders.

Assessment and treatment are only two important functions of client care. Advocacy and education are also important in relation to providing effective care for clients with sexual difficulties. Advocacy allows care providers to provide an atmosphere of acceptance where clients feel safe in discussing sexuality. It also encourages us to discover our prejudices and refine our own professional and personal values about sexuality.

Perhaps most important is our ability to educate, to share information that could spell the difference between life and death for people. Education about the prevention of HIV/AIDS and other sexually transmitted diseases, appropriate methods of preventing unwanted pregnancies, and various means of sexual expression are

---

SAMPLE CLIENT CARE PLAN 29-1

Sexual Dysfunction

ASSESSMENT *History.* Brian, a 31-year-old man, has been treated for chronic depression for the past 2 years. Since his medications were changed 3 months ago, Brian has been complaining of a lack of sexual interest. He has been married for approximately 10 months, and his wife is "worried."
Current Findings. An anxious-appearing man. General appearance, speech, motor activity, and interactions are appropriate. Brian describes his problem as a "growing lack of interest" and fears that it will interfere with his marriage.

Multidisciplinary Diagnosis	*Planning/Goals*
Ineffective role performance related to treatment for depression	Brian and therapist will identify the medications he is taking and list four side effects of each medication by April 10. Brian's anxiety will decrease from level 3 to level 2 by April 15 as he works to solve his problems.

Therapeutic Interventions

Intervention	Rationale	Team Member
1. Assess degree of sexual frustration and dysfunction; begin with less personal statements.	Builds trust and rapport; helps determine extent of problems and plan effective therapeutic interventions.	Psy, Nsg
2. Reassure that symptoms are troubling but not unique.	Provides reassurance that no physical problems exist.	Nsg
3. Develop a list of every medication (including over-the-counter drugs) that Brian is currently taking.	Certain medications, or combinations of medications, can lead to changes in sexual functioning.	Nsg, Psy
4. Consult with physician for possible dosage regulation of Brian's medications.	Adjustment of dosages may decrease or correct the problem.	Nsg, Psy
5. Educate Brian about each medication's effects on sexual functioning.	Learning to recognize side effects early lessens their intensity and offers opportunities for early interventions.	Nsg
6. Refer Brian and his wife for sexual counseling.	Increases knowledge regarding sexuality and its expressions.	Psy

Evaluation

Brian listed each medication and demonstrated great interest in learning about side effects. Brian reported a decrease in his level of anxiety as his knowledge of his medications and their effects grew.

? **CRITICAL THINKING** QUESTIONS

1. How comfortable are you in obtaining a sexual history?

2. How does learning about the side effects of his medications reassure Brian?

A complete client care plan includes several other diagnoses and interventions.
Psy, Psychologist; *Nsg,* nursing staff.

within the realm of nursing. If we are to save a population from the ravages of HIV/AIDS, sexual abuse, and mental illness, all health care providers should teach about sexuality at every opportunity. It is up to us in the helping professions to care for us all.

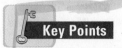

Key Points

- Human sexuality is the combination of physical, chemical, psychological, and functional characteristics that are expressed by one's gender identity and sexual behaviors.
- Sexual behaviors occur along a continuum. At the adaptive end of the spectrum are satisfying sexual behaviors that respect the rights of others. As the continuum moves toward maladaptive, sexual behaviors become impaired or dysfunctional.
- Healthy sexual responses occur between two consenting adults. They are satisfying to both, are not forced or coerced, and are conducted in privacy.
- The expression of one's sexuality begins at birth and ends with death.
- Many permanently disabled persons are able to enjoy rich and satisfying sexual lives with adaptation.
- Persons who express their sexuality with members of the opposite gender are known as heterosexual.
- The sexual desire or preference for members of one's own gender is known as homosexuality.
- Persons who engage in sexual activities with members of both genders are known as bisexuals.
- Transvestism, referred to as cross-dressing, is defined as the practice of wearing the clothing of the opposite gender for sexual excitement.
- Theories that attempt to explain why an individual prefers a certain mode of sexual expression include biological, psychoanalytical, and behavioral viewpoints.
- Sexual disorders are those problems that cause distress and impaired functioning in an individual or others who are exposed to the sexual behavior.

- A sexual dysfunction is a disturbance anywhere in the sexual response cycle and includes any discomfort or pain associated with sexual intercourse.
- Problems with sexual expression can be caused by medication or illicit drug use and many physical conditions.
- The paraphilias are a group of sexual behaviors considered socially undesirable.
- A gender identity disorder is an inconsistency between a child's biological gender and his or her gender identity.
- Transsexualism is the persistent desire to become a member of the opposite gender.
- A sexual addiction is a progressive and chronic addiction characterized by patterns of compulsive sexual behavior despite negative consequences.
- Treatment of sexual problems depends on the cause, distressing signs or symptoms, and type of disorder.
- If a care provider is uncomfortable with any aspect of a client's sexuality, his or her professional judgment and behaviors may be affected.
- Be sensitive to the client's level of comfort when assessing sexual functioning.
- The quality of care for clients with psychosexual problems depends on care providers' abilities to remain nonjudgmental and accepting of the client.
- Assessment, treatment, advocacy, and education are important therapeutic activities in relation to caring for clients with sexual difficulties.
- Education about prevention of HIV/AIDS and other sexually transmitted diseases and appropriate methods of preventing unwanted pregnancies is an important health care responsibility.

---

evolve   Be sure to visit the companion Evolve site at http://evolve.elsevier.com/Morrison-Valfre/ for additional online resources.

30 Personality Disorders

Objectives

Upon completion of this chapter, the student will be able to:

1. Explain the continuum of social responses.
2. Describe how personality develops throughout the life cycle.
3. Compare four theories relating to the development of personality disorders.
4. Discuss four characteristics of a personality disorder.
5. Explain the meaning of the term *dual diagnosis.*
6. Classify 10 types of personality disorders and their most significant associated behaviors.
7. Describe the main goal of therapy for clients with personality disorders.
8. Compare four classes of drugs used to treat clients with personality disorders.
9. Plan nursing diagnoses and therapeutic interventions for a client with a personality disorder.

Key Terms

antisocial personality (p. 337)
avoidant personality (p. 339)
borderline personality (p. 338)
deceit (dĭ-SĔT) (p. 337)
dependent personality (p. 339)
dual diagnosis (p. 339)
gregarious (grĭ-GAIR-ē-ə s) (p. 332)
histrionic (HĬS-trē-ŎN-ĭk) **personality** (p. 338)
ideas of reference (p. 336)
impulsivity (p. 338)
manipulation (p. 337)
narcissistic (NĂR-sĭ-SĬS-tĭk) **personality** (p. 338)
object constancy (p. 333)
obsessive-compulsive personality (p. 339)
paranoia (PAĪR-ə-NŌY-ə) (p. 336)
personality (p. 332)
personality disorders (p. 335)
psychopath (p. 334)
schizoid (SKĬT-sōyd) **personality** (p. 336)
schizotypal (SKĬT-sō-TĪ-pəl) **personality** (p. 336)
splitting (p. 340)
temperament (p. 384)

The social realm of functioning is a vital part of being human. People are **gregarious** (sociable and in need of the company of others). Although some individuals are able to live in isolation, the vast majority of us need interactions with other people throughout our lives.

During childhood, individuals establish their personalities. **Personality** is defined as the composite of behavioral traits and attitudes that identify one as an individual. Personality is the unique pattern of thoughts, attitudes, values, and behaviors each individual develops to adapt to a particular environment and its standards. In short, our personalities define who we are.

To find satisfaction in life, people establish relationships with other people. Some relationships assume a special degree of closeness and sharing that becomes important. These relationships develop intimacy, as another person becomes significant in one's life.

Developing intimate relationships requires a willingness to reveal the private side of oneself: the emotions, beliefs, attitudes, dreams, and anxieties that describe one's personal nature. Most people are able to develop and sustain their social relationships. Families are established, maintained, and transformed. Relationships outside the family grow and fade as individuals interact and life progresses. For many individuals, however, the intimacy of important relationships is not achieved because of lifelong patterns of maladaptive thoughts, social responses, and behaviors.

CONTINUUM OF SOCIAL RESPONSES

Interactions with others (social responses) range from autonomy to the disordered behaviors of manipulation, intimidation, aggression, and hysteria. Highly functional people move freely along the continuum, recognizing and balancing their needs for intimacy with their needs for solitude. Those with ineffective behaviors cope with feelings of dependence, loneliness, and the need to withdraw from others. Individuals with personality problems struggle to define and meet their social needs (Figure 30-1).

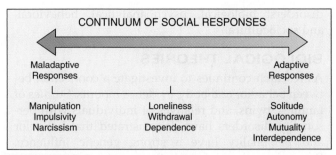

FIGURE **30-1** Continuum of social responses.

PERSONALITY THROUGHOUT THE LIFE CYCLE

Personalities are unique patterns of being that are shaped and influenced throughout life. One's personality becomes established early in childhood and is molded through experience. Personality expresses the emotional, intellectual, social, and spiritual realms of an individual. A basic understanding of personality and the factors that influence its development helps health care providers assess and plan for more effective and therapeutic care.

PERSONALITY IN CHILDHOOD

Infants do not see themselves as separate beings until about 18 months (Hockenberry and others, 2007). The majority of infants experience their environments as warm, nurturing, and unconditionally accepting. When the infant's needs for food, comfort, safety, and socialization are consistently met, a sense of trust and self-worth develops. Infants who are denied love and nurturing have difficulties in forming and maintaining significant relationships in adulthood because they have not learned to trust in others.

With toddlers, much of the personality is still fluid, changeable, and undefined. As children age, the personality gradually takes shape. Between 18 months and 3 years, toddlers begin to learn to separate from their caregivers and explore the world about them. During this time, they develop a sense of object constancy, which is the knowledge that a loved person or object continues to exist, even though it is out of sight. For example, a child learns that his toys are still there in the toy chest, even though he or she cannot see them at this time.

Toddlers often seek out their parents for support, encouragement, and approval. If responses to their independent exploratory behaviors are positive, children build a solid sense of self and develop the capacity for interacting successfully with others. Most researchers believe that, once established, personality traits and temperament are consistent, stable, and generally predictable.

Feelings of morality begin to develop between 6 and 10 years. These years are marked by a preoccupation with self, a strong sense of right and wrong, and peer interactions. Trust grows into the capacity for empathy (understanding the feelings and behaviors of others). This is an important ingredient for later relationships. Thinking (intellectual development) moves from here and now to thoughts of the future, from concrete to abstract. The focus of fantasies changes from imagined objects to real ones, and the use of fantasy becomes a primary way of coping with anxiety.

During the early school years, children learn about cooperation, competition, and compromise. Peer relationships assume more importance, and approval from persons outside the family is sought. Conflicts with parents begin to occur in later childhood as the child's search for independence is tempered by the parents' limits on behavior. "During this period, a supportive environment that encourages the budding sense of self fosters development of a positive, adaptive self-concept" (Stuart and Laraia, 2005). Without support and encouragement, children's needs for guidance and approval go unmet, and this helps set the stage for numerous problems later in life.

PERSONALITY IN ADOLESCENCE

By the time an individual reaches the teen years, the personality is well established. Relationships with others (especially peers) help adolescents assert their independence from parents. Best friend relationships offer chances for sharing, clarifying values, and learning about the differences in people. These relationships become very interdependent and often include efforts to exclude others. Within their peer group, adolescents support each other in their struggles to assert themselves and cope with the distresses of becoming adults.

As adolescents grow, their relationships expand to include members of the opposite gender. Sexual issues produce anxiety as teens struggle to assume a sexual identity. Sexual activity is experimental and spontaneous. Struggles continue over autonomy within the family. By the early 20s, most have weathered the emotional ups and downs of adolescence and emerge with identities that can carry them into adulthood.

PERSONALITY IN ADULTHOOD

By young adulthood, most persons are self-sufficient, making decisions, and involved in give-and-take relationships. Occupational choices are made. Families may be started. Self-awareness grows as individuals learn the balance between personal independence and meeting the needs of others. Sensitivity to and an acceptance of the feelings of other persons are critical characteristics of mature relationships in adulthood.

By middle adulthood, most persons are comfortable enough with themselves and their personalities to encourage independence in others. Relationships with friends and significant others grow and evolve. Demands on time and resources change as children mature, and many middle-age adults enjoy new freedoms to pursue their own wishes.

Many experts believe that, once established, the personality remains stable and constant. However, adulthood offers opportunities for individuals to look within and decide which aspects of their personality they wish to keep and develop and which aspects they would like to change. People are dynamic, always in physical or psychological motion, and change does occur—even within one's "well-established" personality.

PERSONALITY IN OLDER ADULTHOOD

Older adults must cope with loss and change. Old friends are lost. Family members move away. Occupational careers end, and friendships from the workplace fade as time passes.

The personality, however, remains intact as individuals age. Life takes on a deeper meaning as personal accomplishments and contributions to society are reviewed. Older adults with strong, integrated personalities are able to cope with losses by maintaining what independence they can and accepting their limitations. Strength of personality carries them through life's rougher times.

An important reminder about older adults is that **a sudden change in personality is not a normal sign of aging.** By older adulthood, the personality is deeply entrenched. Patterns of thinking and behaving remain intact until death. Do not assume that a personality change in an older adult is normal. Changes in emotional control, responses, and levels of interest must be investigated. Many physical and biochemical problems first appear as subtle changes in personality. The majority of sudden-onset personality changes in older adults are caused by physical problems, such as drug reactions or illness. Alert investigations by nurses and all health care providers can often spell the difference between functional living and dementia.

THEORIES RELATING TO PERSONALITY DISORDERS

Interest in disordered personalities dates back to the time of the ancient Greeks. During the Middle Ages, individuals who behaved in unusual ways were thought to be possessed by evil spirits. The term **psychopath** was introduced in 1891 to describe a gross disturbance in social behavior with no impairment in mental state. Today, the differences between normal personality and a personality disorder are being hotly debated, but clear definitions are rarely found in nature, and mental disorders are no exception.

It is difficult to tell the exact point at which a blood pressure reading becomes abnormal. It is just as difficult to establish the point at which a normal personality becomes a disordered one. Theories of personality development and disorder have been developed to help understand the complex nature of human beings. Currently there are four general theories of personality

disorders: biological, psychoanalytical, behavioral, and sociocultural.

BIOLOGICAL THEORIES

As research continues to investigate a connection between behavior and body, evidence mounts. Studies of families, twins, and relatives of individuals with personality disorders have demonstrated that behavior and personality have a strong genetic influence. Researchers have found that one's **temperament** (the biological bases that underlie moods, energy levels, and attitudes) is genetically linked. Several studies of twins raised in separate environments have shown a remarkable consistency in temperament when tested.

Cardiovascular responses, brain wave tracings, and brain dysfunctions have been studied as possible causes of personality disorders (Marshall and Cooke, 1999). Other biological evidence is beginning to establish a neurophysical basis for the behaviors seen in individuals with personality disorders. For example, abnormalities in certain neurotransmitters, such as dopamine and serotonin, are linked to maladaptive behaviors. Brain imaging studies suggest a possible physical basis for the failure to appreciate the emotional significance of words and images. In other words, the brain mechanism that connects emotions and intellect may be missing or inefficient in persons with personality disorders. As studies into the biobehavioral connection are conducted, new developments will influence the treatment of persons with problem personalities (see Think About 30-1).

PSYCHOANALYTICAL THEORIES

According to psychoanalytical theories, infants begin to discover the nature of "good/bad" and "love/hate" as the superego grows. If the mother responds in ways that cause frustration, distress, or pain, the child will have difficulty finding the proper fit between aggression and love. Certain patterns of parental responses, ranging from overinvolvement to neglect, prevent the

 Think About 30-1

The defense "not guilty due to mental incompetence" has been used in many cases of murder and other crimes. Arguments in favor of this defense state that many individuals with diagnosed personality disorders did not know what they were doing at the time of the crime and therefore should not be held responsible for their actions.

Arguments in favor of abolishing the mental illness defense state that an individual is always responsible for his or her actions, no matter what the mental state.

• What do you think about the "mental illness" defense?
• How should people be held accountable for their behaviors?

child from developing a strong sense of self and balance among the three forces of the personality (ego, id, superego).

BEHAVIORAL THEORIES

Theorists from the behavioral school of thought see personality disorders as the result of conditioned responses caused by previous events. The separation-individuation theory states that the average 1- to 3-year-old is able to achieve object constancy. Personality disorders occur in persons who are not able to hold a consistent, stable image of the mother when she is absent. This results in fears that range from abandonment and separation to a complete loss of connection with others. Other behaviorists view personality disorders as the result of unmet needs during critical developmental periods.

SOCIOCULTURAL THEORIES

Sociocultural theories find the causes of personality disorders embedded in one's culture and society. One researcher (Paris, 1998) demonstrated that "a lack of social structure, **normlessness,** and a lack of available social roles are risks for the development of personality disorders." Numerous cultural expectations are seen to influence the use of adaptive or maladaptive behaviors. Cultural Considerations 30-1 offers an interesting historical enigma.

Sociocultural theorists believe that the foundation for personality disorders is built on society's social and cultural stresses. Many social stressors can lead to difficulties with relationships. Family instability, divorce, and mobility often isolate people from those they love. Traditions that once bound people together are no longer practiced, adding to the sense of isolation. Rates of violent crime and aggression force us to seclude ourselves from each other for protection. Unemployment, homelessness, and acquired immunodeficiency syndrome (AIDS) add to the powerlessness felt by many people.

 Cultural Considerations 30-1

In some cultures, individuals with personality disorders are considered gifted or connected to spirits. The wife of Russia's last czar, Alexandra, was highly criticized for associating with a monk named Rasputin, a man with a supposed "connection to God." Because of concern for her hemophiliac son's health, she sought his guidance. Rasputin would spend his days in the company of priests, royalty, and generals, but nights were spent in drunken sexual parties with prostitutes and other street people.

While the czar was at the front with the troops, Rasputin met his demise. For his unusual behaviors and profound influences on Alexandra, he was poisoned and then shot, beaten, and thrown into a river by a group of noblemen. Rasputin is a compelling historic example of a man with a personality disorder.

PERSONALITY DISORDERS

Personality disorders are defined as long-standing, maladaptive patterns of behaving and relating. All personality disorders are characterized by continual difficulties with interpersonal relations. Many individuals have maladaptive behaviors but are not diagnosed as mentally ill because their actions do not deviate from or go beyond the limits of society's expectations.

The most important criterion for a personality disorder is that behaviors are "inflexible and maladaptive and cause significant functional impairment or subjective distress" (American Psychiatric Association, 2000). The rigid, ineffective behavior patterns must occur throughout a broad range of occupational, social, and personal situations. The onset of the maladaptive patterns can be traced back to childhood or adolescence, and no medical or other mental health problem can account for them. Box 30-1 describes the common characteristics of personality disorders. Study it well because clients with these problems are often encountered in health care situations.

The *Diagnostic and Statistical Manual of Mental Disorders* (DSM-IV-TR) has classified 10 separate personality disorders. For the sake of discussion, personality disorders are grouped into three clusters based on similar

Box 30-1 *Characteristics of Personality Disorders*

COGNITION (INTELLECT, PERCEPTION, VIEW)
Impaired self-perceptions: Distorted picture of self; tends to hate or idealize self
Impaired thought processes: Thinking concrete, difficulty abstracting; impaired concentration, memory; poor attention span
Impaired reality testing: Distorts and confuses inner and outer reality; projects own feelings onto others
Impaired judgment: Ability to problem solve is impaired; does not understand consequences of behaviors; does not learn from past behaviors

AFFECT (EMOTIONAL RESPONSES, MOOD)
Impaired stimulus barrier: Unable to filter out or regulate incoming sensory stimuli; easily excited; responds excessively to noise or light; easily agitated; anger escalates rapidly

CHARACTERISTIC MOODS
Dysphoric feelings, depression; abandonment when significant others are absent; emptiness; fear; guilt; rage

INTERPERSONAL FUNCTIONING (SOCIAL RESPONSES)
Impaired object relations: Has rigid and inflexible patterns of relating to others; has difficulty with intimate relationships
Poor impulse control: Has uncontrollable pressures to act on internal urges; copes with internal pain by acting out
Examples of acting-out behaviors: verbal and physical aggression, attacks on things or others, physical abuse; psychological abuse; manipulation; inappropriate sexual behaviors, casual sex; suicide attempts

behaviors: eccentric, erratic, and fearful. Table 30-1 lists the main feature of each disorder. Remember that individuals can exhibit behaviors from different clusters because human beings seldom fit neatly into any category. Many individuals also abuse drugs or alcohol or suffer from other mental health problems.

ECCENTRIC CLUSTER

The eccentric cluster is characterized by odd or strange behaviors. Persons with problems in this cluster (group A) find it difficult to relate to others or socialize comfortably. Often they live in isolation and interact only when necessary. Diagnoses in this cluster include paranoid, schizoid, and schizotypal disorders.

Paranoia is a suspicious system of thinking that includes delusions of persecution and grandeur. Individuals with a paranoid personality disorder have developed a pattern of behaviors marked by suspiciousness and mistrust. They automatically assume that everyone is out to harm, deceive, or exploit them. Loyal and trustworthy friends are often questioned for hostile intentions. The search for hidden meanings can turn a casual remark into a conflict. Sharing information or

becoming close to someone is avoided because it may provide ammunition that may be used against them. Individuals with paranoid personality disorders are constantly alert for harmful intentions from other persons and are quick to counterattack if they feel wronged or slighted. Often a minor event arouses intense hostility and aggression.

These people are very short tempered and unwilling to forgive even the slightest error. Feelings of tenderness or respect are nonexistent. Many suffer from pathological (extreme) jealousy and often accuse their significant others of secretly having sexual relationships. Problem solving is difficult, and high anxiety levels keep these individuals resistant to change. Paranoid personality disorders are diagnosed in up to 2.5% of the population. Men are diagnosed more often than women, and substance abuse is common. Ten to thirty percent of psychiatric inpatients are diagnosed with paranoid personality disorders (Fortinash and Holoday-Worret, 2008).

Schizoid and schizotypal personality disorders are marked by an inability to develop and maintain relationships with other people. Individuals with schizoid personality disorder lack the desire or willingness to become involved in close relationships. They are society's "loners" who prefer solitary activities and their own company. These people are emotionally restricted and unable to take pleasure in activities, friendships, or social relationships. Often individuals communicate emotional detachment. There is a coldness and lack of concern for others. Sexual experiences hold little interest. Schizoid personality disorders are slightly more common in men and families with an already diagnosed member.

Persons with schizotypal personality disorder have the same interaction pattern of avoiding people as schizoid personalities, but behaviors here are characterized by distortions and eccentricities (odd, strange, or peculiar actions). These individuals often have ideas of reference (incorrect perceptions of causal events as having great or significant meaning), and they commonly find special, personal messages in everyday events.

Schizotypal people are often superstitious or believe in the paranormal (events outside human understanding). Many think they have special powers to foretell events or read people's minds. Some claim to have magical control over others and to be able to make people do their bidding just by wishing or thinking about it. These persons commonly experience perceptual alterations, such as sensing that there is another person present (when there is not). Speech is often loose and vague, but it can be understood. Often they will use words in odd combinations or unusual ways.

As with the other disorders in the eccentric cluster, schizotypal personalities are marked by suspiciousness and paranoid ideation, the idea that people are

Table 30-1	*Clusters of Personality Disorders*
CLUSTER/DISORDER	**MAIN CHARACTERISTIC**
A: ECCENTRIC	
Paranoid	Distrust and suspiciousness; sees others' motives as malevolent (intend to do harm)—may interact in odd or distant ways—may have bizarre ideas about their illness
Schizoid	Detachment from social relationships; emotional expression is restricted
Schizotypal	Acute discomfort with close relationships; sensory distortions; odd behaviors, thinking, and speech
B: ERRATIC	
Antisocial	Disregards/violates rights of others
Borderline	Unstable self-image, affect, and interpersonal relationships
Histrionic	Excessive emotional expression and attention-seeking behaviors
Narcissistic	Grandiose, no empathy, needs to be admired
C: FEARFUL	
Avoidant	Social distress, feelings of inadequacy, oversensitivity
Dependent	Excessive need to be cared for, resulting in clinging, submissive behaviors
Obsessive-compulsive	Preoccupation with control, orderliness, and perfectionism

Modified from American Psychiatric Association: *Diagnostic and statistical manual of mental disorders,* ed 4, text revision, Washington, DC, 2000, The Association.

"out to get them," to undermine their efforts or do them harm. Emotional expressions **(affect)** are usually inappropriate or restricted. Because of unusual mannerisms, style of dress or grooming, and inattention to appropriate social behaviors, these individuals are considered odd or eccentric. They have problems relating to other people and are very anxious in social situations. They have few, if any, friends because they feel different and just do not "fit in" with others. As many as 50% also have signs of major depression. Schizotypal personality disorders are diagnosed more frequently in men.

ERRATIC CLUSTER

The main characteristic for the group of disorders called the erratic cluster is dramatic behavior. Each disorder in this cluster (group B) is associated with a dramatic quality in the way in which these individuals live and conduct their lives. The erratic cluster consists of four separate disorders: antisocial, borderline, histrionic, and narcissistic.

One of our most pressing mental health problems today is people who have antisocial personality disorders. "The central feature of antisocial personality disorder is a pervasive pattern of disregard for and violation of the rights of others" (American Psychiatric Association, 2000). These persons are often referred to as psychopaths or sociopaths because they rely on deceit and manipulation to get their way. Deceit is lying. It is the act of representing as true something that is known to be false. Manipulation is controlling others for one's own purposes by influencing them in unfair or false ways.

The hallmark of psychopaths is a **lack of conscience.** Psychopaths use charm, manipulation, intimidation, and violence to control others and satisfy their own selfish needs. They have a stunning lack of conscience and no feelings for others. Because of these traits, it is important for care providers to remain alert for these behaviors and investigate sources other than the client when performing assessments. Case Study 30-1 describes an antisocial personality.

Antisocial personality disorders are rooted in childhood. Some children have trouble controlling their impulses so they become disruptive and develop antisocial ways of coping. Many of these maladaptive behaviors can be seen as early as 4 years of age.

Children with **conduct disorders** usually express their distress by being aggressive to animals and people. They deceive, lie, steal, destroy property, and break important rules. Many become bullies in school. They are impulsive and quick to anger, and they have no regard for others. If the child is seen by mental health care providers at this time, a conduct disorder is usually diagnosed.

During adolescence, maladaptive behaviors become well established. Truancies from school, open disregard for rules, and thrill-seeking behaviors often get these teens into trouble with authorities and the law. Fighting and physical and verbal abuses are common in adolescents with antisocial personalities.

By adulthood, psychopaths are usually adept at manipulating and deceiving others. They gain money, power, or influence at the expense of others and feel no guilt. They lie, cheat, con others, and malinger (pretend to be ill) to achieve their goals. However, they are unable to plan ahead and act because they are too impulsive. Decisions are made with no thought to the consequences. Often they are able to inflict great pain and suffering and feel **no** remorse or **guilt.**

Individuals with antisocial personality disorders (psychopaths) are often charming. They are glib and clever conversationalists complete with compliments and entertaining statements. An inflated view of their own importance makes them the center of attention and justifies living by different rules.

Psychopaths have a remarkable ability to rationalize their own actions. That, coupled with a lack of guilt

 Case Study 30-1

Rusty was the younger of two boys born to an older, loving couple. As a child, he was always in some type of trouble. When he was about 7 years old, he broke his femur (upper leg) and was required to wear a cast from his chest to his knees for 6 weeks. Although his mother checked on him frequently, he managed mobility. One day Rusty walked out of the house and was seen propelling his encased hips and legs down the street, disinterested in the fact that he could have harmed himself.

By 12 years old, Rusty was self-centered, demanding, and intolerant of his parents' wishes. He often threatened to burn the house down or kill the dog when he did not get his way. Soon his father was bailing him out of jail for various minor offenses, such as stealing. His parents, unable to control him and afraid for their safety, allowed him free run of the house.

At 18 years old, Rusty joined the Army. By 19 years of age, he had received a general discharge for not following orders. Much to his parents' dismay, Rusty returned home and announced that he would attend the local college. By this time, however, he was deeply involved with cocaine, alcohol, and a crowd of thrill seekers. His arrest record continued to grow.

One night at a party, Rusty strangled the homeowner's pedigreed Siamese cat. The owner became angry and threatened to have him arrested. Rusty coldly looked into the homeowner's eyes, pulled a gun, and fired.

Later, when asked why he did it, he calmly replied, "What else could I do? That guy was in my face, and his stupid cat was in my way. I didn't hurt him bad."

• What are your reactions to Rusty's behaviors?
• How would your feelings affect the care of the client?
• Do you think anything could have prevented this event? If so, what?

and empathy, allows them to shrug off any responsibility for their behaviors. Their emotions are shallow, and their behaviors are impulsive. Their need for excitement often involves breaking rules.

Individuals who are psychopathic have a "hair trigger" on their emotions. They can fire off with very little cause. However, when they are violent, it is "cold," without the intense emotional arousal that others experience. There is little remorse, and victims are often blamed for being weak, stupid, or in the wrong place.

Men are more affected by antisocial personality disorders than women. Commonly, they fail to become self-supporting and spend years being impoverished, homeless, or institutionalized. They may abuse chemicals. Psychopaths constitute a large portion of the populations in prisons and psychiatric institutions.

A borderline personality disorder can be summarized as a pattern of instability in mood, thinking, self-image, behavior, and personal relationships. Intense fears of being abandoned motivate these persons to avoid being alone. Relationships with others are marked by rapid shifts from adoring and idealizing to devaluing and cruel punishment. These extreme shifts are also seen in the area of self-image. Sudden, dramatic changes in career plans, values, types of friends, and even sexual identities are characteristic of these individuals.

Impulsivity, acting without forethought or regard to the consequences, is a feature of personality disorders. Persons with borderline personality disorders may gamble, abuse food or drugs, engage in unsafe sex with multiple partners, spend money irresponsibly, and engage in self-mutilating or suicidal behaviors. Cutting, burning, pulling out hair, or scratching oneself is very common. Of these individuals, 8% to 10% actually commit suicide.

Although people with borderline personality disorders experience chronic feelings of emptiness, they commonly express intense anger and frequent displays of aggression or temper. Moods are unstable. Emotions range from great joy to deep depression and change within minutes or hours. They express inappropriate anger and have difficulty controlling their aggression. These individuals become easily bored, so they are always busy. During stressful times, they may develop paranoid delusions and feelings of depersonalization (loss of contact with the self).

The most important feature of histrionic and narcissistic personality disorders is attention-seeking behaviors. Individuals with these disorders are often highly emotional and self-centered. They feel inadequate and unappreciated when they are not the center of attention.

Histrionic personality disorder is a pattern of excessive emotional expression accompanied by attention-seeking behaviors. Histrionic persons may be flashy or dramatic in style of dress, mannerisms, and speech in order to draw attention to themselves. They are emotionally shallow and often live in a romantic fantasy world.

A narcissistic personality disorder is characterized by a pattern of grandiosity and the need to be admired. These individuals believe they are special, unique, or extra important. They crave admiration and have unrealistically inflated beliefs about their accomplishments. They can become extremely angry if criticized or outshone by others. Often, they fantasize about unlimited money, power, or love. They take advantage of and exploit others without guilt or remorse. Case Study 30-2 illustrates such behaviors.

It is interesting to note that more women are diagnosed with histrionic personality disorder, whereas 50% to 75% of persons diagnosed with narcissistic personality disorder are men (Fortinash and Holoday-Worret, 2008).

Individuals with personality disorders are often the perpetrators of violence in our culture. Children who were bullies commonly grow up to abuse their partners. Individuals who had problems with anger and impulse control as children become unable to express themselves appropriately as adults. Teens with histories of being "difficult" or "temperamental" often engage in illegal activities. Even within the criminal population, psychopaths stand out because their antisocial and illegal activities are more varied and frequent than those of other criminals. They tend to try every type of crime and then wonder what all the fuss is about when they are caught.

 Case Study 30-2

The only reason he was sitting there in the counselor's office was because she threatened him with divorce. He knew the counselor would see things his way. After all, she was only a woman, one who could not function without him (although she effectively managed a large business with many employees and he did not work). As the session progressed, the counselor learned about her many inadequacies. She was expected to return from work to cook, clean, and tend to his needs. No matter how hard she tried, she was unable to live up to "his standards." One of his complaints was about her smoking—not because she was hurting herself, but because of the inconvenience it would cause him if she should become ill and unable to care for him.

In response, his wife assured him that he would never be burdened with caring for her. He reached to slap her, but she avoided his blow and walked out of the room, slamming the door behind her. He looked at the counselor and said, "Why is she doing this to me?"

- What kind of insight does this person demonstrate?
- Do you think this person believes he has a problem? Why or why not?

FEARFUL CLUSTER

The common characteristic of the fearful cluster (group C) is anxiety. The three personality disorders in this cluster are avoidant, dependent, and obsessive-compulsive. Each disorder is related to certain expressions of anxiety.

In avoidant personality disorder, anxiety is related to a fear of rejection and humiliation. To prevent possible rejection, individuals narrow their interests to a small range of activities. They have a minimal support system because they are so afraid of the reactions of others. Their tension does not allow for new friends who may be critical, so they withdraw into a world of isolation and self-pity. These people "are hypersensitive to criticism, but they have the capacity to develop appropriate relationships if they feel safe and accepted" (Ward, 2004). Often individuals with avoidant personality disorders also suffer from general anxiety, depression, or hypochondria.

The anxiety of a dependent personality disorder is associated with separation and abandonment. People with this problem carry a deep fear of rejection, which expresses itself as the need to be cared for. To avoid turning people away, they become overcooperative and docile. They do not make demands or disagree with others. When alone, they feel helpless and will go to great lengths to find someone to care for them.

Individuals with dependent personality disorder refuse to be responsible for their own actions. They are unwilling to begin a task alone, take any independent actions, or assume responsibility for daily living activities. Feelings of worthlessness often motivate them to seek out overprotective, dominating, or abusive relationships.

Dependent personality disorder is one of the most commonly diagnosed personality disorders. Men and women are equally diagnosed, although some studies show a higher incidence in women. Cultural factors must be considered before a diagnosis is made because many societies consider certain dependent roles as appropriate.

Persons with obsessive-compulsive personality disorder focus their anxiety on uncertainty about the future. They are extremely orderly and so preoccupied with details that they actually accomplish very little. Delegating tasks to others is impossible because no one "can do it as well." These individuals are devoted to work, have few leisure activities, and are consumed by the need for perfection. About two thirds of compulsive personalities are men.

DUAL DIAGNOSIS

Many individuals with personality disorders also suffer from substance abuse or other mental health problems. They are categorized as having a dual diagnosis. Substance abuse problems occur as individuals attempt to cope by using alcohol or street drugs. Many dual-diagnosed persons are also homeless, unemployed, or involved in legal troubles. Numerous mental health care facilities have units dedicated to clients with dual diagnoses. Those who care for such clients must be aware of the multiple problems involved with dual diagnosis clients. Thorough assessments and careful planning are necessary to address the problems present in this population. Issues of housing, employment, and socialization, as well as treatment for substance abuse and mental illness, must be considered. The multidisciplinary treatment team uses many resources in the care of these individuals.

THERAPEUTIC INTERVENTIONS

People with personality disorders have disturbed self-images. They lack the ability to have successful relationships. Their range of emotions is inappropriate, and impulse control is poor. The way in which they perceive themselves, others, and the world is quite different from cultural norms.

The treatment for individuals with personality disorders is complex because these individuals have extremely diverse treatment needs, and no single treatment is appropriate for every client. Unfortunately, many do not seek treatment or refuse to accept it when it is recommended because of their history of conflict and basic mistrust of others.

TREATMENT AND THERAPY

Persons with personality disorders may have significant impairments in functioning, but they seldom present for treatment because they are usually unable to recognize their problems. When they do cooperate, a combination of various psychotherapies and medications is used only after all physical causes are ruled out.

At one time, it was thought that personality disorders were untreatable because the personality was fixed by adulthood. We now know that people continue to change throughout life. Most individuals with personality disorders "are now considered treatable, although the degree of improvement may vary" (Gale, 1999). Treatment decisions are guided by the client's presenting symptoms, complaints, and problems.

A number of different psychotherapies are selected to treat clients with personality disorders. Types of psychotherapy that have been used with success include psychodynamic, cognitive, behavioral, group, and family therapy. Cure is not the goal of therapy. Care providers "can hope only to make patients more aware of how their habits affect their lives, modifying their behavior enough so that a personality disorder becomes a more adaptive personality type or style" ("Personality Disorders," 1996).

Medications are used with great caution in the treatment of people with personality disorders. They are

| Table 30-2 | *Drugs Used to Treat Personality Disorders* | |

CLASS	EXAMPLE	COMMON SIDE EFFECTS
Antianxiety agents	Ativan, Valium, BuSpar	Monitor kidney function; side effects are usually minimal; fatigue, sedation, dizziness, and orthostatic hypotension (a drop in blood pressure on standing); long-term use can result in dependence.
Antidepressants	Elavil, Prozac	Side effects vary according to class but include dry mouth, nausea, vomiting, constipation, diarrhea, anorexia, differences in taste; headache, changes in alertness, tremor, dizziness, weakness, fatigue, increased sweating, sexual dysfunction; visual disturbances, urinary disturbances (see Chapter 7).
Anticonvulsants	Dilantin, phenobarbital, Tegretol	Bone marrow depression is most serious; gastrointestinal (GI) symptoms; gingival hyperplasia (gum tissue growth); slurred speech, confusion.
Antipsychotics	Haldol, Thorazine	Extrapyramidal side effects (EPSEs) characterized by abnormal movements; dry mouth, blurred vision, photophobia (sensitivity to bright light), tachycardia, and hypotension (see Chapter 7).
Lithium	Eskalith, Lithane	Mild side effects are fine hand tremor, increased thirst and urination, nausea, anorexia, and diarrhea or constipation. Serious side effects of lithium include vomiting, extreme hand tremor, sedation, muscle weakness, and dizziness. Monitor and assess clients frequently for therapeutic responses and the many side effects of these medications.

Drug Alert 30-1

People taking psychotropic medications often use herbal preparations to treat common symptoms, such as headaches, insomnia, and fatigue. The use of both at the same time can lead to unpleasant drug-herb interactions such as the following:

Herb	When Taken With:	Can Cause:
Ginseng	MAOI antidepressants	Headache, tremors, mania
Kava-kava	Alprazolam (Xanax)	Lethargy, disorientation
St. John's wort	MAOI antidepressants	Toxicity
	SSRI antidepressants	Serotonin syndrome: agitation, confusion, flushing, sweating, tremors
Valerian root	Fluoxetine (Prozac)	A delirium-like state

MAOI, Monoamine oxidase inhibitor; *SSRI,* selective serotonin reuptake inhibitor.

prescribed to help relieve some of the distressing symptoms associated with these disorders. Most psychotherapeutic medications are prescribed in limited amounts for short periods because their effectiveness in treating personality disorders is still under investigation (Ward, 2004) (Table 30-2).

Nurses must exercise great care when administering medications to individuals with personality disorders. A thorough drug history, including herbs and street drugs, is needed (see Drug Alert 30-1).

Compliance must be monitored frequently, and safeguards to prevent or reduce the risk for suicide must be in place. If the client is being treated on an outpatient basis, the amount of any prescribed medication must never be large enough to allow a successful suicide.

Also, be alert to the fact that suicidal clients will hoard their medications until they have a lethal dose on hand. Do not hesitate to assess every medicated client for suicidal thoughts or plans. Finally, be familiar with each class of drugs and their side effects. The prudent nurse does not wait to research a medication until a client must take one.

NURSING (THERAPEUTIC) PROCESS

The goals of care for clients with personality disorders are twofold: (1) to help clients identify and then become responsible for their own behaviors and (2) to assist clients in developing satisfactory interpersonal relationships.

The assessment of every client should include a mental status examination, but for the client with a personality disorder, this is extremely important. A nursing history and observation of client behaviors will reveal how individuals cope with interpersonal relationships and the many aspects of daily life.

The therapeutic relationship is begun at this time, so it is important to remain nonjudgmental. Remember, however, that many clients use manipulation, charm, or other subtle behaviors to achieve their purposes. They often use a technique called **splitting**, emotionally dividing the staff by complimenting one group and degrading another. Consistent limit setting and reinforcement help clients to define their limits, but care providers must keep in mind their own therapeutic boundaries and communicate with each other frequently.

SAMPLE CLIENT CARE PLAN 30-1

Personality Disorders

ASSESSMENT *History.* Sophie was 6 years of age when her parents divorced after years of fighting and abuse. Sophie, her mother, and her older brother, Sam, were forced to find shelter in a small hotel room. Shortly after moving in, her mother began to leave Sophie alone for long periods. Once Sophie set the room on fire. Another time she strangled the neighbor's canary. On one occasion, she was molested by a drunken visitor.

At 13 years old Sophie dropped out of school and began living in the streets. Occasionally she would return home. *Current Findings.* Today 19-year-old Sophie has been admitted to the medical unit for recovery from repeated attempts to "cut herself apart." She is suicidal and angry, and she has difficulty in identifying her actions and their consequences.

Multidisciplinary Diagnosis	*Planning/Goals*
Risk for self-directed violence related to feelings of abandonment, depression, and worthlessness	Sophie will verbally identify the emotions associated with her self-destructive activities by August 15. Sophie will not engage in self-destructive behaviors during her inpatient stay.

Therapeutic Interventions

Intervention	Rationale	Team Member
1. Inform Sophie that self-harm is not acceptable behavior while she is here.	Setting limits lets her know which behaviors will not be tolerated.	All
2. Have Sophie sign a no-harm contract.	Offers objective data of agreed-on behaviors.	Nsg
3. Establish trust and rapport with Sophie.	Allows Sophie to identify current behaviors and explore new ones within an atmosphere of safety and trust.	All
4. Institute suicide precautions; monitor continuously if acting out.	Provides safety, prevents self-harm, encourages therapeutic relationships.	All
5. Assess skin on arms and legs daily for new wounds or signs of trauma.	To monitor for further evidence of self-harm behaviors.	Nsg

Evaluation

Sophie expressed relief at knowing limits are set on her behaviors 2 days after admission. During the first week, Sophie was able to identify her emotions after a dispute with another client.

? CRITICAL THINKING QUESTIONS

1. What interventions could help Sophie learn about "cause and effect" relating to her behaviors?

2. What purpose do you think "acting out" serves for Sophie?

A complete client care plan includes several other diagnoses and interventions.
Nsg, Nursing staff.

Possible nursing diagnoses relating to personality disorders are listed in Box 30-2. Short-term goals are based on each individual's assessed problems. They usually focus on the discomforts or ineffective behaviors associated with daily living activities.

Clients with personality disorders often have several problems at once. The most important ones are identified and linked to the appropriate multidisciplinary and nursing diagnoses. Interventions and evaluations are developed for each diagnosis based on the individual client. Sample Client Care Plan 30-1 describes the care for an individual with a personality disorder. Caring for these clients can be a challenge, but the process can promote growth in both client and caregiver when they are willing to work together.

Box 30-2 *NANDA-I Nursing Diagnoses Related to Personality Disorder*

Anxiety
Behavior, risk-prone health
Coping, compromised family
Coping, ineffective
Identity, disturbed personal
Loneliness, risk for
Noncompliance
Role performance, ineffective
Self-esteem, chronic low
Self-mutilation, risk for
Social interaction, impaired
Violence, risk for other-directed

Data from NANDA International: *NANDA nursing diagnoses: definitions and classification, 2007-2008,* Philadelphia, 2007, NANDA International. *NANDA-I,* NANDA International.

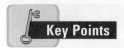

Key Points

- Personality is the composite of behavioral traits and attitudes that identifies one as an individual.
- The social responses of humans can range from autonomy and interdependence to the ineffective, disordered behaviors of manipulation, intimidation, aggression, and hysteria.
- The human personality is shaped and influenced throughout life.
- Currently there are four general theories of personality: biological, psychoanalytical, behavioral, and sociocultural.
- Personality disorders are defined as long-standing, maladaptive patterns of behaving and relating to others.
- The eccentric cluster (group A) of personality disorders is characterized by odd or strange behaviors and includes the paranoid, schizoid, and schizotypal personality disorders.
- The erratic cluster (group B) is characterized by dramatic behaviors and consists of antisocial, borderline, histrionic, and narcissistic personality disorders.
- The fearful cluster (group C) of personality disorders is characterized by anxiety and includes the avoidant, dependent, and obsessive-compulsive personality disorders.

- Individuals with personality disorders who are also suffering from drug abuse or some other form of mental illness are categorized as having a dual diagnosis.
- People with personality disorders may have significant impairments, but they seldom present for treatment because they are unable to recognize their problems.
- Types of psychotherapy that have been used with success for different personality disorders include psychodynamic, cognitive, behavioral, and group therapy.
- Medications are used with great caution in the treatment of people with personality disorders to help relieve the distressing symptoms associated with these disorders.
- The goals of care for clients with personality disorders are to help clients identify and then become responsible for their own behaviors and to assist clients in developing satisfactory interpersonal relationships.

evolve Be sure to visit the companion Evolve site at http://evolve.elsevier.com/Morrison-Valfre/ for additional online resources.

Objectives

Upon completion of this chapter, the student will be able to:

1. Compare the differences between a psychosis and other mental health disorders.
2. Describe the continuum of neurobiological responses.
3. Outline the signs and symptoms of psychosis in childhood, adolescence, and adulthood.
4. Discuss three theories relating to the causes of schizophrenia and other psychoses.
5. Compare and contrast four subtypes of schizophrenia.
6. Describe the signs, symptoms, and behaviors exhibited by a person with schizophrenia.
7. Outline the main pharmacological treatments and mental health therapies for persons with schizophrenia.
8. Apply the therapeutic process to clients suffering from schizophrenia or another psychosis.
9. Plan three nursing responsibilities related to antipsychotic medications.

Key Terms

agnosia (ăg-NŌ-zhə) (p. 347)
akathisia (ĂK-ə-THĒ-zhə) (p. 351)
akinesia (Ā-kĭ-NĒ-zhə) (p. 352)
alexithymia (ə-LĔK-sĭ-THĬ-mē-ə) (p. 349)
anhedonia (ĂN-hĭ-DŌ-nē-ə) (p. 349)
apathy (p. 349)
bradykinesia (BRĂD-ē-kĭ-NĒ-zhə) (p. 352)
delusions (p. 347)
derealization (dē-RĒ-əl-ĭ-ZĀ-shən) (p. 347)
dyskinesia (DĬS-kĭ-NĒ-zhə) (p. 353)
dystonia (dĭs-TŌ-nē-ə) (p. 353)
extrapyramidal (ĔKS-trə-pĭ-RĂM-ĭ-dəl) **side effects (EPSEs)** (p. 351)
hallucinations (hə-LOO-sĭ-NĀ-shənz) (p. 347)
ideas of reference (p. 347)
illusions (p. 347)
laryngeal-pharyngeal (lə-RĬN-jē-əl fə-RĬN-jē-lə) **dystonia** (p. 353)
negative symptoms (p. 349)
neuroleptic malignant (NOOR-ō-LĔP-tĭk mə-LĬG-nənt) **syndrome (NMS)** (p. 353)
oculogyric (ŎK-yoo-lō-JĪ-rĭk) **crisis** (p. 353)
perseveration (pĕr-SĔV-ər-Ā-shən) (p. 347)
positive symptoms (p. 349)
poverty of thought (p. 347)
psychosis (sī-KŌ-sĭs) (p. 343)

schizophrenia (SKĬT-sō-FRĒ-nē-ə) (p. 343)
tardive (TĂR-dĭv) **dyskinesia** (p. 354)
torticollis (TŌR-tĭ-KŎL-ĭs) (p. 353)

To function effectively in society, individuals must be able to process information and adapt to countless internal and external stimuli. Information is tested or validated through interactions with people and the environment. The result is a logical flow of thoughts and actions that allow us to function effectively.

Most people with mental health problems are able to think and act logically, even when their behaviors are maladaptive. However, for a certain group of people, reality is distorted and disturbed. These individuals suffer from a psychosis: the inability to recognize reality, relate to others, or cope with life's demands.

The most common psychosis is schizophrenia, a group of related disorders characterized by disordered thinking, perceptions, and behaviors. Other psychotic disorders include **brief psychotic disorder, delusional disorder,** and **psychoses related to medical conditions or drug use.** All these diagnoses involve the individual's perception of reality. Because individuals with psychotic behaviors are often encountered in general health care settings, care providers who can recognize and intervene appropriately with these clients are more effective than those who work in ignorance.

CONTINUUM OF NEUROBIOLOGICAL RESPONSES

Highly adaptable persons are able to integrate all aspects of human functioning into a workable framework for coping with the world. In other words, the physical, emotional, intellectual, social, and spiritual realms work in combination and allow individuals to function effectively.

The ability to function, change, and adapt is influenced by certain physical brain functions, their connections, and their chemical messengers. In psychiatry, these interactions are called **neurobiological functions.** They can be viewed as existing along a continuum of behavioral responses ranging from highly adaptive, effective responses to maladaptive, even destructive behaviors (Figure 31-1).

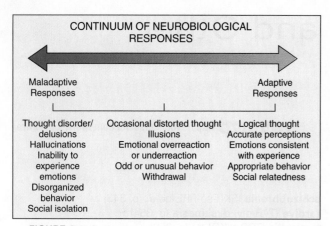

FIGURE **31-1** Continuum of neurobiological responses.

When everything is functioning in harmony, people are able to successfully adapt to their environments. They use logical thought, have clear perceptions, and are able to socially relate in appropriate ways. This state of functioning represents the adaptive end of the neurobiological continuum.

People who do not adapt as well are placed at the middle of the spectrum. These persons function within reality, but they may have emotional overreactions, distorted thoughts, or odd behaviors. Many will never seek mental health services because their behaviors are not recognized as problems. Individuals at the maladaptive end of the spectrum are disorganized in their thought, emotions, and social behaviors.

PSYCHOSES THROUGHOUT THE LIFE CYCLE

As human beings grow and develop, they integrate new information into their knowledge stores. Infants begin to unify information at birth, and the process continues throughout life. Because of certain physical, social, or environmental factors, some individuals have difficulty in relating to new information. Although most cases of psychoses are encountered primarily in late adolescence or adulthood, some do begin in childhood. An awareness of the early signs of possible psychosis assists both client and care provider in providing early interventions.

PSYCHOSES IN CHILDHOOD

Children learn about their worlds through observation and experience. As senses develop, infants become interested in the world around them. By 10 months, children have developed a wide range of complex behaviors and interactions with their caregivers. At 2 years of age, they begin to integrate emotional and behavioral patterns, and by 4 years of age, they have a rich and complex fantasy life.

Also at this time, children are beginning to discover their intellectual side. Basic personalities emerge, and social experiences become important. During the

school years, relationships and experiences are combined into the personality as children engage in more complex activities and behaviors.

For some children, however, processing or combining information is a near-impossible task. Infants with failure to thrive syndromes have slowed physical growth because of an inability to integrate the physical, emotional, and sensorimotor realms of functioning (Hockenberry and others, 2007). Most often, this problem is related to neglect, environmental problems, or severe family stress. Whatever the cause, children with failure to thrive do not have a consistent opportunity to experience the activities and conditions for normal growth and development.

Psychotic disorders can occur in children as young as 5 years old. The actual cause of childhood schizophrenia is unknown, but three risk factors have been identified:

1. *Genetic influences.* Studies have found that schizophrenia and other psychoses occur more often in families who have parents, siblings, or other relatives with schizophrenia.
2. *Complications during pregnancy or birth.* Exposure to the influenza virus during the second trimester of pregnancy has been linked to some cases of schizophrenia (Schultz and Andreasen, 1999).
3. *Biochemical imbalances.* Problems with a neurotransmitter, dopamine, upset the normal neurochemical system (Stuart and Laraia, 2005), so the child perceives and acts differently.

Signs, symptoms, and behaviors of schizophrenic children vary considerably depending on the child's age, developmental stage, quality of previous experiences, and coping mechanisms. A core of behaviors generally indicates these children's increasing lack of contact with reality and withdrawal into a world of their own. There is an impaired ability to process visual information, regulate attention, and sort out incoming information. The child's affect (behavioral display of emotions) changes. Impaired interpersonal relationships and language or communication disturbances arise. Schizophrenia involves every area of functioning, so the child has problems with motor control, emotional control and expression, perception and understanding, thinking logically, and communicating effectively.

PSYCHOSES IN ADOLESCENCE

The unpredictable, up-and-down behaviors of adolescence are intensified in teens with schizophrenia or other psychotic problems. Whereas the average teen is in contact with reality, the adolescent with schizophrenia is not. Even before the onset of a full-blown psychosis, family members may note certain changes in behavior. Poor hygiene and grooming habits are most noticeable. Strange, vague speech and a lack of interest soon lead to social withdrawal. Odd behaviors, such as hoarding food or talking to oneself,

Case Study 31-1

Rob was a model child, cooperative, pleasant, and enjoyable—until he turned 17 years old. It all seemed to start when he began a campaign to see every science fiction movie ever made. Soon he was speaking an "interplanetary space language" that no one but he could understand.

About 6 months into his outer space–oriented lifestyle, Rob quit school and began to spend his days "attending intergalactic conferences of great minds." His family became worried when Rob refused to bathe or change his clothes for weeks at a time. Often they would enter the room to find Rob arguing animatedly with the lamp or listening with interest to the wall. When an outburst of unprovoked anger resulted in injuries to his younger sister, the family sought counseling.

- What do you think is the family's first priority with Rob?
- What do you think the mental health care team's first priority would be?
- What signs do you think would indicate a need for an inpatient psychiatric setting?

occur. Thoughts and beliefs may be bizarre. Unusual superstitions, the belief that one is able to read others' minds **(telepathy),** and ideas that one is remotely controlled by others are common. Self-injury and destructive behaviors often begin in adolescence with these teens. Case Study 31-1 describes an adolescent with a psychotic disorder.

Most psychotic adolescents are first treated in the inpatient setting, where their behaviors can be assessed, monitored, and controlled. Therapeutic interventions focus on decreasing acute symptoms and behaviors, improving relationships with significant others through family therapy, and educating client and family about the illness and its management.

PSYCHOSES IN ADULTHOOD

The onset of acute symptoms most often occurs in men during the middle 20s, whereas women usually do not present with symptoms until the late 20s. Men endure their symptoms longer than women before seeking help. With continued treatment, one third of schizophrenic persons improve. Without treatment, one third improve; and with or without treatment, one third progress into a chronic downhill course.

The prognosis (long-term outlook) for schizophrenic individuals is better if adaptive interpersonal relationships, school performance, and work histories were present before the onset of symptoms. The outlook is also better for women. On the average, men with schizophrenia respond less well to treatment, have higher relapse rates, and spend more time in inpatient settings.

Families with schizophrenic members face enormous demands. Because the length of institutional stays has sharply decreased, many individuals with schizophrenia return to the home while still psychotic, thus requiring constant observation and support. This places great strain on family resources. Social and occupational activities of caretakers are limited by the demands of the illness. The ability to communicate with the schizophrenic family member is limited. Family members, especially parents, struggle with guilt and frustration as they attempt to understand "why." Parents suffer the grief of losing a normal child and then must cope with the stigma of having a child who is "mentally ill." Brothers and sisters are strongly affected by their sibling's behaviors. They must also cope with the question of "Could it happen to me?" Then there are the repeated role changes that occur with each hospitalization and each return home. Most families have difficulties because of the enormous amount of energy required to cope with a psychotic family member.

PSYCHOSES IN OLDER ADULTHOOD

Historically, schizophrenia is seldom diagnosed in elderly people. However, there is "growing acceptance of the concept that schizophrenia can have its first onset in people in their 40s and 50s" (Peck, 2002). Older adults with schizophrenia or another psychosis have long-standing problems. Many suffer from the irreversible side effects of long-term antipsychotic drug use in addition to other chronic medical problems.

Often the hallucinations and delusions of younger years decrease or even disappear. Many older persons with schizophrenia become more withdrawn or paranoid. They are frequently homeless. Fortunate elderly individuals with schizophrenia may spend the remainder of their days in long-term care facilities (see Case Study 31-2).

An important reminder: **The acute onset of psychotic behavior in any elderly client must be investigated.** Older clients who lose contact with reality, experience impaired interpersonal relationships, suddenly have difficulty communicating, or experience great emotional changes may be experiencing some physical or biochemical change. Changes in electrolyte balances, reactions to medications, drug interactions, and nutritional deficiencies can cause signs, symptoms, and behaviors that appear psychotic. The causes of most acute-onset psychoses in older adults are related to physical problems.

THEORIES RELATING TO PSYCHOSES

"Schizophrenia is a condition that exists in all cultures and socioeconomic groups" (Fortinash and Holoday-Worret, 2008). The first theory of psychosis was that those not in contact with reality were possessed by demons, spirits, or devils. Evidence of this belief is found in early Chinese, Egyptian, Greek, and Hebrew

Case Study 31-2

Vern had been a resident of the psychiatric unit for as long as anyone could remember. He was admitted in the late 1950s as a young man. All anyone knew about him was his name. He was too delusional to give any clear information. He had served in the Navy but was discharged because of violent behaviors. By the time he was admitted here, he was quite subdued due to large doses of Haldol and Thorazine.

The years passed, and every time an attempt was made to wean him from his high doses of psychotropic drugs, Vern became belligerent and tried to hit everyone around him. Decreasing his medications was out of the question. Today, Vern is old—we do not know how old—and he now suffers from **tardive dyskinesia.** His tongue sticks out when he is not grinding his teeth or puffing his cheeks. He constantly smacks his lips and blinks his eyes. His face contorts into an ever-changing series of grimaces, giving him an unusual appearance. He is no longer violent unless provoked and spends his days in his room interacting with his voices in a language only he can understand.

Cultural Considerations 31-1

In India, a man with schizophrenia is often considered a "wise man" because of his ability to speak with spirits. He is usually honored and sought out for his advice.

In Haiti, many people believe that humans can communicate with spirits and deities (gods) and have religious ceremonies to induce spirit possession. The group considers being possessed not as a shameful experience, but a privilege. Psychotic persons are believed to be victims of the "evil eye," called *maldyok,* or to be possessed by supernatural beings. Their behavior is tolerated by members of the community, but they are expected to consult native healers "who treat with amulets, packets of herbs and spices, liquids, baths, powders, rubbing, and massage" (Giger and Davidhizar, 2008).

---

writings. Cultural Considerations 31-1 offers an interesting insight.

The possession theory existed until the nineteenth century, when the work of two psychiatrists began to define schizophrenic behaviors. Emile Kraepelin (1856-1926) described the syndrome of hallucinations and delusions seen in persons with schizophrenia. In 1911 a Swiss psychiatrist (Hans Bleuler, 1857-1939) coined the word *schizophrenia* (meaning, "to split the mind") to describe the disconnection between the intellectual and emotional aspects of a personality. Today, confusion about the term exists because the public often uses the word to describe someone with multiple personalities.

Once, psychoses were thought to be the result of faulty parent-child interactions or failure of the ego (part of the psyche that maintains conscious contact with reality) to combine the drives of the id (the unconscious, pleasure seeking part of the psyche) with reality. Today, scientific evidence points to possible physical causes for psychotic behaviors. Other theories that attempt to explain schizophrenia focus on psychosocial and sociocultural factors. A brief explanation of each theory group helps in the understanding of clients with psychotic disorders.

BIOLOGICAL THEORIES

Evidence for viewing schizophrenia as a brain disorder is building. Studies of fetal development have demonstrated that, in persons with schizophrenia, cell connections in the area of the brain that coordinates thinking and motivation have trouble communicating with other brain areas. Neurochemical production and transmission problems are being investigated as having a possible role in the development of schizophrenia.

Research with identical twins found that schizophrenic twins develop differently by the age of 5 years (Torry and others, 1994). Such data have led to the development of the **genetic/heredity model** as an explanation of schizophrenia.

The **stress/disease/trauma model** looks at the effects of stress on the individual, especially during the prenatal period. Immune reactions to viral infections during pregnancy and severe malnutrition during pregnancy have been shown to contribute to the development of schizophrenia in the children, especially the girls, of these mothers. Complications occurring during birth, such as prolonged labor, difficult birth, or umbilical cord prolapse, have been related to the development of schizophrenia. Cocaine use and other drug use during pregnancy have been linked to schizotypal behaviors in the children of users.

Because of the many refinements in brain-imaging technology, scientists have been able to pinpoint certain parts of the brain that are different in schizophrenic people. Other studies found that certain chemical messengers (neurotransmitters) are altered in persons with schizophrenia (NIMH, 2007). The neurotransmitters serotonin, norepinephrine, and dopamine have been implicated as possible causes of schizophrenia. Theories developed from this type of research are called **neurochemical models.**

OTHER THEORIES

Some theories see schizophrenia as resulting from certain environmental or social factors. **Psychological models** view schizophrenia as being caused by a basic character flaw combined with poor family relationships. Overprotective, anxious mothers; cold, uncaring fathers; and couples who "stayed together for the sake of the children" were implicated. The child's failure to accomplish a developmental task, such as trust or intimacy, was also thought to be related to schizophrenia.

Sociocultural theories consider the effects of environment on the development of psychoses. Poverty, homelessness, unstable families, and cultural differences all

Table 31-1	*Subtypes of Schizophrenia*

SUBTYPE	DESCRIPTION
Catatonic	Characterized by marked psychomotor problems: immobility or excessive activity with no purpose; odd movements, rigid posture, stereotyped movements, echopraxia (mimics movements of others); may be extremely negative or mute, echolalia (echoes others' speech), automatic obedience; may suffer from malnutrition, dehydration, exhaustion; prognosis is fair.
Disorganized	Disordered thinking, speech, and behavior; affect is flat or inappropriate; primitive, uninhibited behaviors, unusual mannerisms, distorted facial expressions, giggles or cries out; loosely organized hallucinations, delusions; withdrawn, socially inept; unable to perform activities of daily living; onset is early, prognosis is poor.
Paranoid	Organized delusions of grandeur or persecution, auditory hallucinations; high anxiety levels, guarded, suspicious, aloof, hostile, angry, can be violent or suicidal; onset is late, prognosis is good with treatment.
Undifferentiated	Does not meet criteria for other subtypes; disorganized speech, behavior; hallucinations, delusions, negative symptoms; prognosis is fair.
Residual	Has had at least one acute episode of schizophrenia, is free of acute psychosis but still has negative symptoms of withdrawal, emotional changes, disorganized thinking, and odd behaviors; schizophrenia present for many years; time is limited between acute episodes; prognosis is poor.

have been suggested as causative factors. Some researchers believe that individuals become psychotic as a way of coping with life. Although environmental and social factors may influence the development of psychoses, evidence for a neurobiological cause of psychosis is becoming more and more convincing.

PSYCHOTIC DISORDERS

SCHIZOPHRENIA

Schizophrenia affects about 1% of the world's population. In the United States, that is about 2.5 million people. Although it occurs in every socioeconomic class, it is found more commonly in lower socioeconomic levels. An estimated 10% to 15% of homeless people are schizophrenic (Herbert, 1998). Because of the intense discomfort associated with the disorder, as many as 10% of all schizophrenic individuals commit suicide.

The costs of treating schizophrenia are enormous—in terms of lost productivity, continued medical care, and social maintenance. In this day of scarce mental health resources, millions of dollars are spent in treatment for this disorder. The costs in terms of distress and suffering cannot even be estimated.

Subtypes of Schizophrenia

Because schizophrenia is a cluster of related behaviors, it can be classified into different groups based on the clinical picture. Although many persons have symptoms of more than one cluster, diagnosis is made based on the most prominent symptoms or behaviors. The five subtypes of schizophrenia are **catatonic, disorganized, paranoid, undifferentiated,** and **residual.** Table 31-1 explains each subtype and its characteristics.

Signs, Symptoms, and Behaviors

The main characteristic of psychotic disorders is loss of contact with reality to the point where functioning is grossly impaired. Although each individual behaves

uniquely, many appear to share certain basic symptoms. Table 31-2 describes the signs and symptoms of schizophrenia in each area of function.

The physical appearance of individuals with schizophrenia is one of an unkempt person. Focus on inner matters prevents them from routinely seeking out food or shelter. Personal hygiene is often poor, and body images are distorted. Motor activity ranges from agitated to immobile.

The signs and symptoms of schizophrenia affect **perception,** the way that one views the world. Individuals suffer from **hallucinations,** which are false sensory inputs with no external stimuli. Hallucinations may take the form of smells, sounds, tastes, sight, touch, or feelings of altered internal workings of the body. **Illusions** (false perceptions of real stimuli) and **agnosia** (an inability to recognize familiar objects or people) are common.

In the **cognitive** (intellectual) area of functioning, persons with schizophrenia have problems with attention, memory, and use of language. Thinking may involve **delusions,** fixed false ideas that are not based in reality; **ideas of reference,** the idea that people or the media are talking about oneself; and **derealization,** a loss of ego boundaries with an inability to tell where one's body ends and the environment begins.

Language difficulties involve incorrect usage. The speech of persons with schizophrenia includes a number of unusual characteristics: **clang associations, concrete thinking, echolalia, flight of ideas, loose associations, ideas of reference, mutism, pressured speech, neologisms, verbigeration,** and **word salad.** Table 31-3 explains each term and provides an example of each communication difficulty.

Thought processes in people with schizophrenia vary widely, from contact with reality to fantasy thinking. Negative experiences are remembered more than positive ones. Individuals may demonstrate **perseveration,** the repeating of the same idea in response to different questions, or **poverty of thought,** a lack of ability to produce new thoughts or follow a train of

Table 31-2 *Clinical Symptoms of Schizophrenia*

PERCEPTUAL	INTELLECTUAL	EMOTIONAL	BEHAVIORAL	SOCIAL
Hallucinations: May be commanding; content matches delusions 1. Auditory: May be commanding; content matches delusions 2. Visual 3. Tactile: For example, may feel surrounded by spider webs 4. Olfactory and gustatory: May refuse to eat because food smells or tastes bad **Illusions:** False perceptions because of misinterpretations of real objects **Altered internal sensations:** 1. Formication: Sensation of worms crawling around inside 2. Chill: Feeling of chills in the marrow of one's bones **Agnosia:** Failure to recognize familiar environmental stimuli such as sounds or objects seen or felt; sometimes called "negative hallucinations" **Distortion of body image:** Relating to size, facial expression, activity, detail, exaggeration or diminution of body parts **Negative self-perception:** Relating to ability and Competence	**Delusions:** Unusual ideas, not reality based: 1. Omnipotence 2. Persecution 3. Control **Derealization:** Loss of ego boundaries; cannot tell where own body ends and environment begins; feeling that the world around one is not real **Ideas of reference:** Notion that other people or the media are talking to or about one **Errors in recall of memory:** Caused by incorrect categorization **Difficulty sustaining attention:** 1. Unable to complete tasks 2. Errors of omission **Incorrect use of language:** 1. Neologisms (invented words) 2. Incoherence, verbigeration 3. Echolalia, word salad 4. Concrete, restricted vocabulary 5. Poor comprehension 6. Loose associations **Flight of ideas:** Abrupt change of topic in a rapid flow of speech	**Labile affect:** Range of emotions: 1. Apathy, dulled response 2. Flattened affect 3. Reduced responsiveness 4. Exaggerated euphoria 5. Rage **Inappropriate affect:** Laughing at sad events, crying over joyous ones **Disruption in limbic functioning:** Inability to screen out disruptive stimuli and loss of voluntary control of response	**Little impulse control:** 1. Sudden scream as a protest of frustration 2. Self-mutilation, to substitute physical for emotional pain 3. Injury to a body part believed to be offensive 4. Responds to command hallucinations **Inability to cope with depression:** 1. Depressed client has a 50% risk for suicide 2. Frequent ups and downs in one who has insight 3. Lack of social support to help **Inability to manage anger:** Anger and lack of impulse control lead to violence: verbal aggression, destruction of property, injury, homicide **Substance abuse:** Dulls painful psychological symptoms **Noncompliance with medication:** May feel it is not needed or has too many side effects	**Poor peer relationships:** 1. Few friends, as a child or teen 2. Preference for solitude **Low interest in hobbies and activities:** 1. Daydreamer 2. Not functioning well in social or occupational areas 3. Preoccupied and detached 4. Behavioral autism **Loss of interest in appearance:** 1. Careless grooming 2. Introversion **Not competitive in sports or academics:** 1. Poor adjustment to school 2. Withdrawal from activities **May suffer from:** 1. Attention deficit–hyperactivity disorder 2. Somatic symptoms

Modified from Fortinash KM, Holoday-Worret PA: *Psychiatric mental health nursing*, ed 4, St. Louis, 2008, Mosby.

| Table 31-3 | *Speech Disturbances in Schizophrenia* |

SPEECH PROBLEM	DESCRIPTION
Clang associations	Repeating words or phrases that sound alike or substituting a word that sounds like the appropriate word *Example:* "Honey, money, sunny" or "I need some honey to buy the paper"
Concrete thinking	Inability to consider the abstract meaning of a phrase; frequently tested by having clients interpret proverbs *Example:* "A stitch in time saves nine" may mean "sew the holes in your clothes" to a schizophrenic person
Echolalia	Repeating words of another after one has stopped talking *Example:* Nurse: "How is your day going?" Client: "Day going, day going, day going."
Flight of ideas	Rapid change in topics with a rapid flow of speech *Example:* "The sky is blue. The dog is dead, and I have two eyes."
Ideas of reference	The belief that some events have special personal meaning *Example:* "The United States is sending satellites into space so that they can spy on me."
Loose associations	Thinking characterized by speech that moves from one unrelated idea to another *Example:* "I'm hungry, but the desert has no rain so it's cold outside."
Mutism	Refusal to speak
Neologisms	Words or expression invented by the individual *Example:* "The ispy is not happy when the fulgari is green."
Verbigeration	Purposeless repetition of phrases Example: Client repeats for days: "Prepare to launch the orbiter."
Pressured speech	Rapid, forced speech *Example:* "I must prepare. There's no time to waste. Can't talk now."
Word salad	A random, jumbled set of words that have no connection or relationship to each other *Example:* "Hot happies are spying on me but no men love short feet."

thought. People with chronic schizophrenia have little insight into their problems. Often their judgment is impaired. Usually there is a general decline in intellectual abilities as the disorder progresses.

In the **emotional** realm, persons with schizophrenia experience a range of inappropriate emotions. Affect, the outward expression of one's emotions, is described as blunted, flat, inappropriate, or labile. Other emotional responses include alexithymia, a difficulty in identifying and describing emotions; apathy, a lack of concern, interest, or feelings; and anhedonia, the inability (or decreased ability) to experience pleasure in life.

Behaviorally, individuals with schizophrenia display little impulse control and an inability to manage anger. They may injure themselves and others or act in response to hallucinations commanding them to do something. A lack of energy or motivation (**avolition**) often leads to poor performance at work or school, unemployment, and homelessness. The inability to cope with depression, added to a lack of social supports, leads to a high risk for suicide. Many refuse to comply with treatment by not taking their medications. Others abuse alcohol and street drugs. These dual-diagnosis individuals present many challenging health care situations.

Socially, schizophrenic persons are unable to establish or maintain relationships with others. Self-esteem is low, and gender identity confusion may exist. They have few friends and little interest in hobbies or other activities. Social behaviors are often inappropriate. Many prefer to be alone because of hallucinations or feelings of paranoia. The few family and social relationships that do exist usually follow a rocky course. Refer to Table 31-2, and review the description of symptoms in schizophrenia.

The characteristic symptoms of schizophrenia also fall into two broad categories: positive and negative symptoms. Positive symptoms relate to maladaptive thoughts and behaviors. They include hallucinations, speech problems, and bizarre behaviors. Negative symptoms relate to the lack of adaptive mechanisms. They include flat affect, poor grooming, withdrawal, and poverty of speech. Mental health care team members commonly refer to the symptoms of schizophrenia by using the terms *positive* and *negative* symptoms.

Most terms used to describe schizophrenic behaviors are not a part of everyday vocabulary. For this reason, it is important to focus more on accurately describing clients' behaviors, communications, and interactions than finding the best label. If you are not sure of the meaning of the term, do not use it. One good behavioral description is worth many psychiatric terms.

Phases of Becoming Disorganized

The course of schizophrenia is marked by episodes of acute psychosis alternating with periods of relatively normal functioning. The symptoms of schizophrenia must occur for at least 1 year before a diagnostic label is assigned.

The slide into schizophrenia commonly occurs through four stages. The **prodromal phase** begins with withdrawal, a lack of energy, and little motivation. Individuals may appear confused and in a world of their own. They may complain about multiple physical problems or show a new, excessive interest in religion or philosophy. Affect becomes blunted. Ideas and beliefs become odd or unusual. Personal hygiene is ignored. Some individuals become agitated or angry. Speech becomes difficult to follow. These symptoms

? **Think About 31-1**

The prodromal signs and symptoms of schizophrenia often begin in adolescence. As the teen's behavior becomes more bizarre, friends and family become uncomfortable with and afraid of the individual, so they respond by limiting their interactions with him or her.

- What are your feelings and reactions about people who are unable to share reality?
- How do you think you would react to a close friend who was diagnosed with schizophrenia?
- How would you cope with being afraid of someone whose behaviors are out of contact with reality?

can occur during both the prodromal and the residual stages of the disorder (see Think About 31-1).

In the **prepsychotic phase,** individuals are usually quiet, passive, and obedient, and they prefer to be alone. They have few or no friends because of their odd, suspicious, or eccentric behaviors. Hallucinations and delusions may be present, but behaviors are not completely disorganized at this point. Family members may report that they can sense the individual "slipping away" in front of their eyes.

Signs, symptoms, and behaviors during the **acute phase** vary widely but include disturbances in thought, perception, behavior, and emotion. Frequently individuals lose contact with reality and become unable to function even in the most basic ways.

The **residual phase** follows an acute episode. It is marked by a lack of energy, no interest in goal-directed activities, and a negative outlook. Many of the behaviors seen in the prodromal phase are also present during the residual phase.

Following the residual phase is a period of relative **remission.** The ability to manage some basic activities of daily living returns, and the individual experiences some relief from the distresses of psychosis. The course of schizophrenia alternates between acute episodes and periods of decreased symptoms. The outlook for recovery is fair to poor because of the many complex aspects of this disorder.

OTHER PSYCHOSES

Besides schizophrenia, the *Diagnostic and Statistical Manual of Mental Disorders* (DSM-IV-TR) lists other psychoses. A **brief psychotic disorder** is a psychotic disturbance that lasts for more than 1 day but less than 1 month. A **delusional disorder** is characterized by more than 1 month of nonbizarre (reality-based) fixed ideas. A **shared psychotic disorder** is defined as "a disturbance that develops in an individual who is influenced by someone else who has an established delusion with similar content" (American Psychiatric Association, 2000). **Schizoaffective disorder** is diagnosed when depression or mania is also present.

Psychotic behaviors are also related to the abuse of street drugs and several medical conditions. The alert care provider is always observant for changes in client's behavior or affect. Early detection of behavioral changes frequently prevents later complications from occurring.

THERAPEUTIC INTERVENTIONS

Because of impaired judgment and other problems, many individuals with schizophrenia do not receive treatment. Those who do cooperate with treatment are most often cared for by a multidisciplinary mental health team. The core team consists of psychiatrists, nurses, psychologists, and psychiatric social workers. Dietitians, occupational therapists, and spiritual advisors join the team when needed.

Individuals are admitted to an inpatient unit during episodes of acute psychoses, when they are a danger to themselves or others, or for stabilization of disorganized or inappropriate behaviors. The goals of inpatient, short-term care are to **stabilize the client, prevent further decline** in functioning, and **assist the client in coping** with his or her disorder. Long-term goals include psychosocial and vocational rehabilitation. When available, family members are included in the care and education of the client.

TREATMENTS AND THERAPIES

Clients with acute psychoses are treated with a combination of therapies and medications. The multidisciplinary treatment team may recommend "personal therapy, social skills training, vocational rehabilitation, and behavioral therapy. In addition, stress reduction, family education, and early intervention are important in the treatment of schizophrenia" (Kane and McGlashan, 1995). Although psychotherapies may focus on different areas of treatment, each relies on the therapeutic interactions of care providers.

Pharmacological Therapy

Medications used to treat psychoses are called **antipsychotic** or **neuroleptic** drugs. They are listed in Table 31-4.

Antipsychotic drugs slow the central nervous system (CNS). These effects include an emotional quieting, slowed motor responses, and sedation. Antipsychotics exert their influence on the body by interrupting the dopamine (neurotransmitter) pathways in the brain, thus producing a calming effect throughout the entire nervous system. After an antipsychotic drug is taken, hallucinations and delusions decrease, thought processes change, and hyperactivity subsides. Mental clouding clears, and previously withdrawn people begin to socialize.

Antipsychotic drugs interact with many other chemicals. They also have additive effects. When used

Table 31-4 *Drugs Used to Treat Psychosis (Antipsychotics)*

CLASS	EXAMPLES
High-potency antipsychotics	Fluphenazine (Prolixin), haloperidol (Haldol), thiothixene (Navane), trifluoperazine (Stelazine)
Moderate-potency antipsychotics	Loxapine (Loxitane), molindone (Moban), perphenazine (Trilafon)
Low-potency antipsychotics	Chlorpromazine (Thorazine), mesoridazine (Serentil), thioridazine (Mellaril)
Atypicals	Clozapine (Clozaril), olanzapine (Zyprexa), quetiapine (Seroquel), risperidone (Risperdal)

Box 31-1 *Interventions for Clients With Psychotic Disorders*

Maintain health and safety.
Establish a trusting interpersonal relationship.
Confirm the client's identity.
Orient the client to reality.
Assist the client in communication to help the client understand and be understood.
Decrease psychosocial stressors and demanding situations.
Help the client manage anxiety.
Encourage responsibility for self.
Promote compliance with prescribed therapeutic regimen.
Assist with activities of daily living.
Promote social interaction.
Regulate activity levels.
Encourage and praise socially acceptable behaviors.
Encourage family involvement and understanding.
Teach the client to identify stressors and how to recognize, manage, and prevent symptoms.
Educate client and family about side effects and toxic effects of antipsychotic medications.

Modified from Fortinash KM, Holoday-Worret PA: *Psychiatric nursing care plans*, ed 5, St. Louis, 2007, Mosby.

in combination with other drugs, an enhanced effect is produced that increases CNS depression. The side effects and adverse reactions of these medications are numerous and troublesome for the client. In fact, as many as half of the clients who are prescribed antipsychotics do not actually take them or do not take them according to directions because of the side effects. Individuals who abuse alcohol and drugs are more likely to neglect taking their antipsychotic medications. Refer to "Antipsychotic (Neuroleptic) Medications" in Chapter 7 for a discussion of side effects and adverse reactions.

NURSING (THERAPEUTIC) PROCESS

Caring for clients with psychoses requires a team effort. First, a thorough physical and mental assessment is obtained. Histories include a description of the client's most distressing problems and a complete review of systems if the client is able to communicate appropriately. Interpersonal relationships and support systems are also explored when possible.

The mental status examination is performed (see Chapter 9). Risks for violence and suicide are assessed, and a past medication history is taken.

After all data are obtained and organized, both care team and nursing diagnoses are established. Primary nursing diagnoses include **disturbed thought processes, disturbed sensory perception, social isolation, impaired verbal communication,** and **ineffective therapeutic regimen management.** Box 31-1 provides several important general principles for working with schizophrenic and other psychotic clients.

The basic goals of care are to assist clients in controlling their symptoms and achieving the highest possible level of functioning. For this to happen clients and their families must be actively involved in the treatment. The expected outcome is for the client to live, learn, and work at the maximum possible level of success. Short-term goals relate to keeping the client safe, restoring adequate nutritional and rest habits, establishing and maintaining contact with reality, and fostering open communications. Sample Client Care Plan 31-1 describes the care for a client with schizophrenia.

SPECIAL CONSIDERATIONS

Because antipsychotic medications affect the body's nervous system, they are potentially harmful chemicals. Several special assessments, interventions, and evaluations are required for clients who are receiving these powerful chemicals. Some side effects are harmless, and some are uncomfortable. Others are life threatening. The most common side effects of antipsychotic medications are alterations in the CNS and peripheral nervous system functions.

CNS alterations include extrapyramidal side effects (EPSEs), best described as "abnormal involuntary movement disorders [that] develop because of a drug-induced imbalance between two major neurotransmitters, dopamine and acetylcholine, in portions of the brain" (Keltner and Folks, 2005). As many as 75% of clients will experience EPSEs when taking these medications. The low-potency antipsychotics, such as chlorpromazine (Thorazine), are more likely to cause **sedation** and **anticholinergic side effects** (dry mouth, blurred vision, urinary retention). The high-potency antipsychotics, such as haloperidol (Haldol), are less sedating and anticholinergic, but they have an increased risk for **EPSEs.**

Extrapyramidal side effects include akathisia, akinesia, dyskinesia, dystonia, and drug-induced parkinsonism. The most serious side effects are neuroleptic malignant syndrome and tardive dyskinesia. All these symptoms arise from a lack of the neurotransmitter dopamine in the brain and the subsequent blocking of nerve transmissions.

Akathisia is an inability to sit still. Clients experiencing akathisia report that they feel nervous and jittery or

SAMPLE CLIENT CARE PLAN 31-1

Schizophrenia

ASSESSMENT *History.* Terry, a 22-year-old man, was found wandering naked in the streets talking to himself. He seems preoccupied and appears to be listening to voices. Further history is unobtainable because Terry is unable to communicate understandably at this time.

Current Findings. A wild-eyed, unkempt young man who is preoccupied. Clothes are ragged and dirty. Speech is unintelligible; he carries on animated conversations with himself. Since admission, 24 hours ago, Terry has refused to eat, drink, or bathe because "someone is trying to poison" him. He is polite but responds only when addressed. No family or friends can be located.

Multidisciplinary Diagnosis	*Planning/Goals*
Disturbed sensory perception related to social isolation and lack of adequate support systems	Terry will communicate in a logical manner within 15 days after admission. Terry will carry out his activities of daily living independently within 25 days after admission.

Therapeutic Interventions

Intervention	Rationale	Team Member
1. Establish therapeutic relationship; be available, listen actively; do not pass judgment.	Trust must be established if therapy is to be effective.	All
2. Establish and reinforce a daily routine.	Increases security by knowing what to expect; helps refocus on the activities of daily living.	Nsg, All
3. Use clear, direct statements when talking; make sure body language is in keeping with the message being sent.	Unclear or confusing communications can increase Terry's distorted perceptions.	All
4. Intervene with active hallucinations; move Terry to quiet area, focus on reality, assure client that he will be safe, identify needs filled by the hallucination.	Decreases sensory input; helps divert attention to reality, provides reassurance; helps decrease anxiety.	Nsg, All
5. Accept and support Terry's feelings and appropriate expressions of emotion.	Communicating empathy and understanding decreases anxiety.	All
6. Encourage Terry to take his medications routinely.	Medications must be taken regularly to control psychotic symptoms.	Nsg, MD
7. Carefully monitor Terry's response to his medications.	Early recognition prevents serious side effects and complications.	Nsg
8. For discharge planning, explore the possibility of placement in an assisted living home.	A stable and predictable environment decreases acute psychotic episodes.	Soc Svc

Evaluation

Fifteen days after admission, Terry stated he was in control of his hallucinations. Twenty-five days after admission, Terry was independently eating, drinking, and performing his own activities of daily living, but he still required routine encouragement to bathe.

? CRITICAL THINKING QUESTIONS

1. How does a lack of support systems influence Terry's mental illness?

2. How important is a group home for Terry after he is discharged from the inpatient environment?

A complete client care plan includes several other diagnoses and interventions.
Nsg, Nursing staff; *MD,* physician; *Soc Svc,* social services.

have lots of nervous energy. Assaultive behaviors can result if they are forced to remain in one position for even a short time. Many clients stop taking their medications because of these side effects. The best treatment for akathisia is to reduce the dose of antipsychotic medication. Nurses must be careful not to evaluate the signs and symptoms of akathisia as a worsening of the client's psychosis. If a prn antipsychotic drug is administered at this time, it will cause an increase in the client's symptoms.

Akinesia means the absence of movement, both physically and mentally. Actually, clients who are experiencing this unwanted effect demonstrate bradykinesia (slowing of body movements and a diminished mental state). Clients lack spontaneity and do not try to move or speak. They may assume bizarre postures and maintain them for long periods. Here is another case for careful assessment because many of the behaviors associated with EPSEs are very similar to the behaviors for which the clients sought treatment. Astute caregivers who routinely observe their clients' behaviors stand a better chance of distinguishing between drug-induced and psychosis-induced behaviors.

Dyskinesia is characterized by involuntary abnormal skeletal muscle movements. They are usually seen as jerking motions and sometimes seriously interfere with the client's ability to walk and perform other voluntary movements.

Dystonia is impaired muscle tone. Dystonic reactions produce rigidity in the muscles that control gait, posture, and eye movements. When dystonia involves the muscles that control eye movements, the eyes involuntarily roll to the back of the head. This side effect is called oculogyric crisis, and it is a frightening experience for the client. Another unsettling dystonic reaction is torticollis, in which contracted cervical muscles force the neck into a twisted position.

The most serious and potentially life-threatening side effect is laryngeal-pharyngeal dystonia. When the muscles of the throat become rigid, the client begins to gag, choke, and become cyanotic. Respiratory distress and asphyxia result if immediate intervention does not occur. Anticholinergic drugs are used to treat all these reactions.

Drug-induced parkinsonism is a term used to describe a group of symptoms that mimics Parkinson's disease. Tremors, muscle rigidity, and difficulty with voluntary movements are seen in clients with Parkinson's disease and some individuals undergoing antipsychotic drug therapy. Other unwanted CNS effects include seizures, which can occur at any time during therapy. The drug clozapine (Clozaril) appears to be associated with a higher incidence of seizures, so clients taking this medication must be carefully monitored for signs of seizure activity.

Neuroleptic Malignant Syndrome

Neuroleptic malignant syndrome (NMS) is a potentially fatal extrapyramidal side effect of antipsychotic medications. The condition is poorly understood and frequently goes undiagnosed. Death can occur from respiratory failure, kidney failure, aspiration pneumonia, or pulmonary emboli. Although NMS is usually associated with the high-potency antipsychotics, it can occur with many other dopamine-altering drugs.

NMS occurs more often when two or more psychotherapeutic drugs are combined. When lithium is used with a psychotherapeutic drug or depot (oil-based, long-acting) injections are given, clients are assessed frequently for signs of NMS. The development of NMS may occur suddenly after a single dose or after years of drug treatment. It is often associated with other extrapyramidal reactions, such as dystonia and akathisia.

Symptoms of NMS begin with a sudden change in the client's level of consciousness and a rapid onset of rigid muscles. Often there is an associated respiratory difficulty, tremors, and an inability to speak; however,

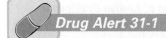

Drug Alert 31-1

Frequently monitor clients taking antipsychotics for:
Sudden change in level of consciousness
Rapid onset of rigid muscles
Respiratory difficulty
Tremors
Inability to speak
Cardinal sign of neuroleptic malignant syndrome (NMS):
   high body temperature (101° to 108° F)
Autonomic nervous system signs and symptoms
   Rapid, labored respirations
   Tachycardia
   Rapid changes in blood pressure
   Increased perspiration (diaphoresis)
   Incontinence
Central nervous system signs and symptoms
   Sudden agitation
   Confusion
   Delirium
   Combativeness
   Rigid posturing
Without intervention, the client's physical **condition declines rapidly.**

the cardinal sign of NMS is a high body temperature. Temperatures can reach as high as 108° F but usually range between 101° and 103° F. The temperatures of all clients receiving psychotherapeutic drugs must be frequently and routinely monitored. Without intervention, the client's physical condition declines rapidly (see Drug Alert 31-1).

Signs of autonomic nervous system dysfunctions are evident in NMS: tachycardia, rapid changes in blood pressure, increased perspiration (diaphoresis), incontinence, and rapid, labored respirations. CNS alterations include sudden agitation, confusion, delirium, combativeness, and rigid posturing. Severe muscle rigidity leads to tissue breakdown, an increased white blood cell count, and possible kidney failure.

No specific treatment exists for NMS. Supportive measures, including intensive respiratory care, are instituted, and all medications that may be implicated in the development of NMS are stopped.

Subclinical (mild) cases of NMS have been reported. Nurses should suspect NMS in any client with signs or symptoms of **pneumonia** or **urinary tract infection.** Clients who have diaphoresis, tachycardia, an elevated white blood cell count, or any muscle rigidity may be experiencing NMS. Sudden changes in consciousness should always be investigated and reported.

Those who care for clients taking psychotherapeutic medication must be aware of the potential for the development of NMS. An action as simple and routine as obtaining vital signs may save the life of a client. Do not hesitate to notify your supervisor or physician if a client develops a sudden fever, changes in blood

---

Box 31-2 *Signs and Symptoms of Tardive Dyskinesia*

Protrusion of the tongue (fly-catcher sign)
Puffing of cheeks or tongue in cheek (bonbon sign)
Grinding of teeth, chewing, lateral jaw movements
Lip smacking, puckering
Grimacing, making faces, tics
Blinking, squinting
Impaired gag reflex (choking, aspiration)*
Shrugging of shoulders
Thrusting of pelvis
Twitching of trunk, legs, and arms
Toe movements, foot tapping
Impaired diaphragmatic movements (breathing
  difficulties)*

*Potentially life threatening.

pressure, sudden changes in alertness, confusion, or altered levels of consciousness.

Tardive Dyskinesia

Tardive dyskinesia is a serious, irreversible side effect of long-term treatment. The word *tardive* means "appearing later." *Dys* means "difficult," and *kinesis* means "movement" in Greek. Therefore the literal translation of "late difficult movement" explains the condition. Tardive dyskinesia is a drug-induced condition that produces involuntary, repeated movements of the muscles of the face, trunk, arms, and legs. Many clients exhibit the signs of tardive dyskinesia after several months or years of drug treatment. Others develop signs and symptoms after discontinuing their medications.

After a period of antipsychotic drug use, the body attempts to compensate for the lack of dopamine by developing extrasensitive receptors in the brain. When the brain is stimulated by dopamine, it overreacts and produces abnormal muscle movements. Elderly people, especially women, and those who have had a stroke are at the greatest risk for developing tardive dyskinesia, but symptoms are most severe in young men.

The signs and symptoms of tardive dyskinesia usually involve the facial muscles first. Box 31-2 lists the major signs and symptoms. Appendix D lists the AIMS assessment tool. People who experience the effects of tardive dyskinesia are frightened at their lack of control. In addition, the sight of a person engaged in these unusual movements and behaviors can be unnerving for care providers. Sensitive, caring staff can help to ease the client's distress.

This condition is difficult to treat, and the effects are persistent. At this time, tardive dyskinesia is considered irreversible except in the very early stages. Nursing measures for tardive dyskinesia include routine assessments and measures to prevent injuries. Clients with impaired gag reflexes may require soft foods. Be sure

oropharyngeal suction devices are readily available. Teach every client and family member how to recognize the signs and symptoms of tardive dyskinesia.

Anticholinergic Effects

Most medications are not effective for the treatment of tardive dyskinesia, but some success has been reported with the drugs bromocriptine (Parlodel), reserpine, and clonazepam (Klonopin). Vitamin E has been found to be effective in reducing symptoms.

Undesired effects of antipsychotic drugs also influence the **peripheral nervous system.** The anticholinergic effects of **dry mouth, blurred vision, urinary retention,** and **photophobia** (sensitivity to bright light) are common, especially during the first few days of therapy. **Tachycardia** is a more serious side effect and can cause sudden death.

Hypotension is another potentially serious anticholinergic side effect. Nurses must protect clients from falls during the first few weeks of therapy because the **hypotensive** response is greatest when clients stand or change positions suddenly. These episodes of low blood pressure cause a rapid heart rate (tachycardia) as the body attempts to adapt to a lower blood pressure. Antipsychotic drugs are contraindicated in clients who have a history of low blood pressure, cardiac irregularities, or heart failure. Table 31-5 lists the major side effects of antipsychotic medications.

Nursing Responsibilities

Nurses have three major responsibilities when caring for clients who are receiving antipsychotic drug therapy. The first relates to drug administration. Nurses should review the desired actions, side effects, and incompatibilities for each medication prescribed. If the drugs are to be administered intramuscularly, choose a large muscle mass and warn the client of a burning sensation on injection. Rotate injection sites. If liquid preparations are ordered, be sure to follow the instructions for dilution. Some neuroleptic drugs cannot be mixed with water, so read the manufacturer's instructions before diluting any liquid medication. **Read all labels carefully.**

Some injectable drugs are water based, and others are oil based. Oil-based medications are never given intravenously. They are intended for intramuscular use only. The drug class called the **phenothiazines** can cause contact dermatitis, so avoid getting these drugs on the skin. Wash your hands after every contact, and wear gloves if you frequently handle phenothiazines.

The second major nursing responsibility relates to monitoring client responses to each medication. During the first 1 to 2 weeks of therapy, assess the client's vital signs every 4 hours, record fluid intake and output, and routinely assess skin condition. Assess frequently for signs or symptoms of side effects.

All care providers must constantly remain vigilant to the occurrence of side effects with each

Table 31-5 *Side Effects of Antipsychotic Drugs and Nursing Care*

SIDE EFFECTS	INTERVENTIONS
PERIPHERAL NERVOUS SYSTEM EFFECTS	
Constipation	Encourage high-fiber diet; increase water intake; give laxatives as ordered.
Dry mouth	Sip of water frequently; provide sugarless hard candies, sugarless gum, and mouth rinses.
Nasal congestion	Give over-the-counter nasal decongestant if approved by physician.
Blurred vision	Advise client to avoid potentially dangerous tasks. Reassure client that normal vision typically returns in a few weeks when tolerance develops. Pilocarpine eyedrops can be used on a short-term basis.
Mydriasis	Advise client to report eye pain immediately.
Photophobia	Advise client to wear sunglasses outdoors.
Hypotension or orthostatic hypotension	Ask client to get out of bed or chair slowly. Client should sit on the side of the bed for 1 full minute while dangling feet, then slowly rise. If hypotension is a problem, measure blood pressure before each dose is given.
Tachycardia	Tachycardia is usually a reflex response to hypotension. When intervention for hypotension (previously described) is effective, reflex tachycardia usually decreases. With clozapine, hold the dose if pulse rate is greater than 140 pulsations per minute.
Urinary retention	Encourage voiding whenever the urge is present. Catheterize for residual fluids. Ask client to monitor urine output and report output to nurse. Older men with benign prostatic hypertrophy are particularly susceptible to urinary retention.
Urinary hesitation	Provide privacy, run water in the sink, or run warm water over the perineum.
Sedation	Help client get up early and get the day started.
Weight gain	Help client order an appropriate diet; diet pills should not be taken.
Agranulocytosis	A high incidence of agranulocytosis (1% to 2%) is associated with clozapine. White blood cell count (WBC) should be performed weekly.
CENTRAL NERVOUS SYSTEM EFFECTS	
Akathisia	Be patient and reassure client who is "jittery" that you understand the need to move. Since akathisia is the chief cause of noncompliance with antipsychotic regimens, switching to a different class of antipsychotic drug may be necessary to achieve compliance.
Dystonias	If a severe reaction such as oculogyric crisis or torticollis occurs, give antiparkinson drug (e.g., benztropine mesylate [Cogentin]) or antihistamine (e.g., diphenhydramine [Benadryl]) immediately, as needed, and offer reassurance. Call the physician at once to obtain an order for intramuscular administration. For less severe dystonias, notify the physician when an order for an antiparkinson drug is warranted.
Drug-induced parkinsonism	Assess for the three major parkinsonism symptoms—tremors, rigidity, and bradykinesia—and report to physician. Antiparkinson drugs may be indicated.
Tardive dyskinesia	Assess for signs by using the abnormal inventory movement scale. Drug holidays may help prevent tardive dyskinesia. Anticholinergic agents will worsen tardive dyskinesia. Young men taking large doses of high-potency antipsychotic drugs (e.g., haloperidol) may be prescribed prophylactic antiparkinson drugs.
Neuroleptic malignant syndrome	Be alert for this **potentially fatal** side effect. Routinely take temperatures and encourage adequate water intake in all clients on a regimen of antipsychotic drugs, and routinely assess for rigidity, tremor, and similar symptoms.
Seizures	Seizures occur in approximately 1% of clients receiving antipsychotic drug treatment. Clozapine causes an even higher rate, up to 5% of clients taking 600 to 900 mg/day. Use seizure precautions. Document and report any seizure activity.

medication prescribed. In addition, nurses thoroughly assess clients before administering any prn drug because a medication will actually worsen symptoms if the nurse is not able to tell a side effect from a behavior. Clients who are receiving antipsychotic drugs are at risk for developing NMS and tardive dyskinesia. Accurate identification of their signs and symptoms early helps prevent permanent problems.

The third nursing responsibility, client and family education, has a direct impact on the client's level of functioning. One of the primary tasks of nurses is to assist clients in coping with their daily living activities.

When the client and family are willing to learn about the client's medications, treatment can be more successful. Box 31-3 lists the most important points of client and family education.

Keep these general guidelines in mind. Get to know the clients for whom you are caring. The more you know about the person, the better you will be able to tell the difference between behaviors that are from the effects of medication and those that belong to the client. Antipsychotic drugs are powerful medications. They demand to be treated with respect and require knowledge from those who receive them and those who work with them.

Box 31-3 *Client and Family Education: Antipsychotic Drugs*

Review the expected benefits and possible side effects of drug therapy with the patient and family. Review extrapyramidal side effects. Because there is no effective treatment for tardive dyskinesia, signs or symptoms should be reported immediately. Fine vermicular (wormlike) movements of the tongue may be the first sign of this side effect.

Instruct client and family to **report any new signs or symptoms.**

Help clients understand that several weeks of drug use may be necessary before a benefit is received.

Instruct clients to swallow extended-release forms whole; do not crush or chew.

Warn clients to avoid driving or operating hazardous equipment and notify the physician if vision changes or sedation occurs.

Instruct client to report signs of agranulocytosis, including sore throat, fever, and malaise. Tell clients to report signs of liver dysfunction, including jaundice, malaise, fever, and right upper quadrant abdominal pain.

These drugs may interfere with the body's ability to regulate temperature. Warn clients to avoid prolonged exposure to extreme temperatures, allow for frequent cooling-off periods when exercising or in hot environments, and dress warmly for exposure to the cold.

Review possible endocrine side effects with client and family. Assess carefully and tactfully for these side effects. Provide emotional support as appropriate. If side effects are intolerable, consult the physician for possible drug or dosage change.

Instruct clients to monitor weight (if possible). If weight gain is a problem, counsel about low-calorie diets. Refer to a dietitian as needed.

Stress the importance of informing all health care providers of all drugs being taken.

Warn clients to avoid over-the-counter drugs unless first approved by the physician.

Caution clients to avoid alcoholic beverages while taking antipsychotics.

Warn diabetic clients that antipsychotics may alter blood glucose levels. Monitor blood glucose levels carefully. Consult the physician about changes in dietary or drug treatment for diabetes.

Tell clients not to discontinue therapy abruptly or without discussion with the physician.

Instruct clients to keep these and all drugs out of the reach of children.

The drugs may produce false-positive pregnancy results. Women who suspect they are pregnant should consult the physician. Women may desire to use contraceptive measures while taking these drugs; counsel as appropriate. As always, pregnant or lactating women should avoid all drugs, if possible.

If additional drugs are prescribed to treat side effects of antipsychotic agents, review their use and side effects with the client and family.

Modified from Clark JK, Queener SF, Karb VB: *Pharmacologic basis of nursing practice,* ed 6, St. Louis, 2000, Mosby.

Caring for persons with psychoses is one of the most challenging areas of mental health. Hospitalization and education are only the beginning steps in a long road toward optimal functioning. Relapse is common. Continued treatment and support are needed for family members and clients alike if we are to cope with the devastating effects of schizophrenia and other serious psychotic mental illnesses.

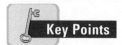

Key Points

- A psychosis is a disorder in which there is an inability to recognize reality, relate to others, or cope with life's demands.
- Neurobiological responses can range from adaptive contact with reality to disorganized thoughts, emotions, and behaviors.
- Although the majority of psychoses are encountered primarily in late adolescence or adulthood, some do present in childhood.
- The actual cause of childhood schizophrenia is unknown, but genetic influences, complications during pregnancy or birth, and biochemical imbalances have been identified as risk factors.
- The average teen is in contact with reality, and the adolescent with schizophrenia is not.

- The onset of acute symptoms most often occurs in men during their middle 20s and women in their late 20s.
- Schizophrenia can have its first onset in people in their 40s and 50s. Older adults with psychosis have long-standing problems. Many suffer from irreversible side effects of long-term antipsychotic drug use as well as other chronic medical problems.
- Today scientific evidence points to possible biological (physical) causes for psychotic behaviors.
- Schizophrenia is a group of related mental health disorders characterized by disordered perceptions, thinking, and behavior.
- The five subtypes of schizophrenia are catatonic, disorganized, paranoid, residual, and undifferentiated.
- Other psychotic disorders include brief psychotic disorder, delusional disorder, and psychoses related to medical conditions or drug use.
- The treatment goals for inpatient, short-term care are to stabilize the client, prevent further decline in functioning, and assist the client in coping with his or her disorder.
- Long-term goals include psychosocial and vocational rehabilitation when possible.
- Clients with acute psychoses are treated with a combination of therapies and medications.
- Antipsychotic drugs, which may take weeks to become effective, help to stabilize behaviors.

- Psychosocial therapies include personal therapy, social skills training, vocational rehabilitation, behavioral therapy, stress reduction, and family education.
- Several special nursing assessments, interventions, and evaluations are required for clients who are receiving powerful antipsychotic medications.

- Nursing responsibilities with antipsychotic medications relate to drug administration, monitoring client responses, and client and family education.

---

evolve Be sure to visit the companion Evolve site at http://evolve.elsevier.com/Morrison-Valfre/ for additional online resources.

Objectives

Upon completion of this chapter, the student will be able to:

1. Explain how deinstitutionalization has affected the delivery of mental health care in the United States.
2. Describe the experience of mental illness from a client's viewpoint.
3. Outline three psychological and three behavioral characteristics of chronic mental illness.
4. Explain how children and adolescents can be affected by chronic mental health problems.
5. Examine the connection between human immunodeficiency virus (HIV)/acquired immunodeficiency syndrome (AIDS) and mental illness.
6. Summarize the care for clients with multiple mental health problems.
7. Discuss three principles of psychiatric rehabilitation.
8. Apply the nursing (therapeutic) process to clients with chronic mental health disorders.
9. Plan seven basic interventions for clients who are chronically mentally disordered.

Key Terms

chemical restraint (p. 359)
chronic mental illness (p. 358)
co-morbidity (KŌ-mŏr-BĬD-ĭ-tē) **(co-occurring)** (p. 363)
exacerbations (ĕg-zăs-ĕr-BĀ-shənz) (p. 358)
psychiatric rehabilitation (p. 364)
remissions (p. 350)

The majority of mental health problems are solved with time and treatment. However, some mental illness follows the individual throughout life. The word **chronic** means long lasting, persistent, or continual. Most chronic mental health problems follow a wavy course, marked by periods of exacerbations and remissions. **Exacerbations** are periods of dysfunction accompanied by an increase in the signs, symptoms, and seriousness of a problem. **Remissions** are times of partial or complete disappearance of symptoms. The course for chronic mental health problems follows this up-and-down pattern.

Many mental health problems are acute. They begin abruptly, increase in intensity, and then subside after a short time. Persons with phobias, anxiety disorders, or depression often respond well to therapeutic interventions and have no further problems. However, for a certain group of individuals, being mentally ill becomes a way of life.

Chronic mental illness is the presence of one or more recurring psychiatric disorders that result in significantly impaired functional abilities. Individuals with chronic mental health problems are often referred to as CMI (chronically mentally ill) or SMI (seriously mentally ill). Many people with chronic mental illness are contributing members of society, struggling to hold onto some degree of mental health. They are also the homeless, the criminals, and the odd neighbors down the street. They are our relatives, our friends, and members of our community.

SCOPE OF MENTAL ILLNESS

Chronic mental disorders are disabling for people in every society and culture. Each year millions of individuals seek help for mental health problems. "Approximately 23% of American adults each year have a diagnosable mental disorder and as many as 5.4% of American adults have a serious mental illness" (Editors, 2003). One in every five families is affected by a severe mental illness in its lifetime (see Think About 32-1).

The estimated costs of treating persons with mental disorders are about 4% of total U.S. direct health care costs. Inpatient stays cost more than 12 billion dollars per year (U.S. Census Bureau, 2006). When the social costs of lost productivity, shortened lives, and implementation of criminal justice are factored in, the total costs are enormous.

The costs in terms of suffering cannot be estimated. Society encourages people to recover from acute mental disorders and resume normal daily activities, but it tends to ignore the needs of those persons who are (and will be) unable to cope independently with life. Chronic mental illness carries social stigmas, and being labeled as "crazy" keeps many people from seeking help.

Individuals with chronic mental health problems have much higher rates of suicide. Because mental illness affects every area of functioning, each chronically mentally troubled person has a unique life experience. Many individuals handle their distressing symptoms

? Think About 32-1

Did you know that in any given year:
52 million adults experience a mental health disorder.
28% seek mental health treatment.
9 million people develop a mental disorder for the first time.
8 million individuals suffer a relapse.
35 million persons have continuing symptoms.
The number of chronically mentally ill persons is relatively stable at about 28% of the total population.

• What possible trends does an analysis of these statistics reveal?

by using alcohol, street drugs, or other chemicals. They must cope with an addiction in addition to their illness. Remember, however, that every CMI individual is a real person who is coping with personal problems plus suffering from the stigmas of being labeled mentally ill.

PUBLIC POLICY AND MENTAL HEALTH

Today, CMI individuals are cared for in the community. Society expects them to provide for their basic needs, protect themselves, and seek help for their problems—all rather complex behaviors. The reality is that most CMI people are unable to meet these expectations.

EFFECTS OF DEINSTITUTIONALIZATION

When antipsychotic medications became available in the 1960s, chemical restraints replaced physical ones. A chemical restraint is a medication that reduces psychotic symptoms and quiets behavior. When major tranquilizers were marketed, people no longer had to be physically controlled. The state psychiatric hospitals began to discharge long-term patients into the community through a practice called deinstitutionalization. The thought was that most people released from the state hospitals could live in the community with the proper support and aftercare. Unfortunately, the aftercare, which was a critical part of the overall plan for providing community psychiatric services, failed to be implemented. Changing political parties and government policies chose to ignore CMI individuals, thinking that everything would eventually work itself out. Today the consequences of our federal mental health policy can be seen in the ever-increasing numbers of homeless persons, prisoners, and county jail inmates.

EXPERIENCE OF CHRONIC MENTAL ILLNESS

What is it like to be CMI? To face each day knowing the struggle ahead? To wonder if this day will bring acceptance and hope or another slide into "madness"?

Persons who face mental illness must cope with problems that are unknown to the rest of us. Individuals are often lumped into a group labeled CMIs and stripped of their identity, dignity, convictions, and feelings. They lack choice, respect, and control, and they are expected to cooperate with therapies that make them feel sick. Case Study 32-1 allows a glimpse into the world of one CMI individual. Hopefully, this true account will serve as a reminder that every client is truly a unique individual and should always be viewed as such.

MEETING BASIC NEEDS

The issues facing the mentally troubled population are the same as those with which the rest of us must cope: adequate food, shelter, and clothing; gainful employment; and access to health care. People with chronic mental illness, however, must strive to meet their needs on a daily basis. Most people with chronic mental illness live with their families. Because their disorders prevent them from planning or logically carrying out an activity, many CMI individuals are homeless, hungry, and unable to care for themselves. They are found everywhere, some chatting amiably with or responding to voices in their heads. In 1999, Torrey and Zdanowicz found that CMI individuals made up one third of the total homeless population, and that figure has not changed much over the years.

Many of our society's mentally ill members are now housed in county jails and prisons, awaiting available beds in the few state institutions that remain. Other mentally ill persons are jailed on "dine-and-dash" charges (eating a restaurant meal they cannot pay for) or as "mercy bookings" just to get them off the streets and provide some basic needs. State prisons are also feeling the increase in mentally ill inmates. It is estimated that up to 25% of inmates in state prisons suffer from mental illness.

The CMI individuals who do manage to provide for their own basic needs must struggle with the labels and expectations of others. Often it is difficult for them to remain employed for long periods because of occasional relapses. As one chronic mental health client put it, "I am an effective, loyal worker for over 90% of the time, but the 10% of the time I have troubles is all that's remembered."

Poverty and mental illness go hand in hand. Although many mentally troubled persons receive some financial assistance, most are unable to plan or use the money wisely. Because about half the population abuses alcohol or drugs, few dollars are spent on life's necessities. Today it is estimated that more than one-quarter million CMI individuals are living on the streets, in public shelters, in jails, and in prisons (Figure 32-1).

ACCESS TO HEALTH CARE

Until the time of community psychiatric care, people with severe or chronic mental health problems were treated (or at least provided with custodial care)

Case Study 32-1

The following case study was modified from the words of Betty Blaska (1991):

You spend the whole first night crying because you don't want to be here. There must be some awful mistake. You are very naive, only 18. You're not yet a CMI (chronically mentally ill). Next day the "staffing" (as they call it) is very intimidating. The hospital's brass are all there, and they just chuckle when you tell them you do not want to stay. They patronize you: "Oh, we think we will just keep you here for a while." You don't know it yet, but you are on the way to becoming a CMI.

The first time you experience dystonia from the drugs they've given you, you are extremely frightened. Your tongue is rigid, and you can't control its movements. You rush to the nurses' station, where they are huddled inside their little cage. No one comes out for fear of contamination. They are puzzled by your presence, but you can't speak because of your tongue's movements. They wait impatiently for you to tell them what is wrong. You wonder what is wrong with them. Can't they see your problem? But no—it's not that they don't see. They don't feel, because you don't count. You are on the way to becoming a CMI.

After your first discharge, you are loaded up on medications, and your follow-up therapist announces that he will not continue with you unless you come in with your family for therapy. But you have eight family members scattered all across the state. And they don't want to come, anyway, because they have been belittled and browbeaten too much already. So the therapist refuses to see you. And he refuses to refill your prescriptions. So you go through withdrawal. And you end up back on the same psych ward. And then they say to you accusingly, "Why did you go off your medicines?" It's then you realize: You're a CMI.

You've been in and out of hospitals, seen numerous mental health professionals (some stranger than you), and been off and on loads of psychoactive drugs, given in doses you complain are too high and in combinations that you complain are too much. And there are the side effects—nausea, diarrhea, dizziness. Vision so bad that you are afraid to cross the street. Drug-induced psychoses so bad you can't leave your bed or look out the window because of the terror you feel. Blood pressure so low that you can't stand for very long and a voice so weak that you can't be heard across a telephone.

Oh great! Now you're without a job. So they send you to a place called Vocational Rehabilitation, where they "help" you get a clerical job. Never mind that you have a degree—or two. You get the clerical job because you are a woman. A woman CMI. But the men CMIs are just as lucky. They get to become janitors! Now you are truly a full-fledged CMI.

- With what labels (stigmas and stereotypes) is this person coping?
- How has reading this case study changed your impressions of the mentally ill experience?

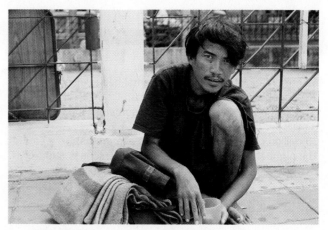

FIGURE **32-1** Homeless man sleeping on the street.

through state programs. With ongoing therapy and medications, many people with chronic mental disorders could return to their communities and function effectively. However, community support was not often available after hospitalization and many individuals once again fell victim to their psychoses.

Only this time the tightened admission policies of most institutions did not allow most of the CMI population back, so they were forced to cope with their disorders the best they could. Other mentally ill persons became involved in the **revolving door syndrome,** a cycle of repeated short hospital admissions and discharges. This in-and-out-of-the-institution behavior is also called **recidivism.**

Today, a new generation of CMI individuals is emerging, known as the young chronically mentally ill. These individuals are young (18 to 35 years old) and severely ill. Most have never sought treatment. Those who do receive treatment commonly refuse to follow therapeutic advice. "They lack internal controls, rarely take psychotropic medications, and exhibit excessive drug and alcohol abuse" (Fortinash and Holoday-Worret, 2008). Many self-medicate to relieve distressing symptoms. **Cocaine** is often used by persons with mood disorders, whereas **alcohol** is more likely to be consumed by schizophrenic individuals. **Heroin** is usually preferred by individuals with conduct disorders. Many young mentally ill individuals are **polysubstance** abusers; that is, they use a variety of different chemical substances, sometimes in combination. Case Study 32-2 illustrates this point

Access to health care is limited in the United States today. Currently as much as 25% of the population has no health insurance (U.S. Census Bureau, 2006). For many who do, mental health services are capped or limited to a certain amount of money per person. Individuals with chronic mental problems are often unable to plan for or manage their health care because of their illness, even if they are fortunate to have some sort of insured coverage. Many refuse shelter or treatment because of their paranoia, believing people will harm them.

Case Study 32-2

Alan's favorite Friday night activity was "getting messed up." During the first year of his marriage, his wife would join him, but she soon realized how bad the stuff was and left him. He kept a job for a while, until his "hobby" got in the way. Tonight, Alan and his buddies have been drinking boiler-makers—beer and whiskey combinations. Soon they decide to have some real fun so they drop two reds (sleeping medication), two whites (a stimulant), and a couple hits of acid (LSD). They settle into comfortable positions under the bridge and pull the newspapers up around their bodies. Soon they are "toasting" as Alan calls it. There is no money for food tomorrow, but that is a long time away and they have the good stuff tonight.

- How would you expect these people to behave while under the influence of these drugs?
- Do you think Alan feels that he needs help? Why?

People with mental health problems also have physical problems. It is estimated that 50% of the mentally ill population suffer from a medical disorder. People with mental illness live an average of 10 to 15 years less than the general population (Farnam and others, 1999).

On the other hand, people who want to receive treatment often find that services are inadequate or unavailable. Even when admitted to an institution, their stay may not be long enough to improve their condition. Outpatient services are the basis for supporting the mentally ill person in the community. However, they may not be available or the individual may refuse treatment. Access to comprehensive mental health care remains a problem today. This is why health care providers must be prepared to recognize and assist those individuals whose only crimes are being too disordered to effectively care for themselves.

CHARACTERISTICS OF CHRONIC MENTAL ILLNESS

Each person's experiences with mental illness are unique. Diagnoses serve only to group and label certain behaviors. The real meaning of being "depressed" or "schizophrenic" is found only within the individual who suffers from the distresses associated with the particular label.

Many mentally troubled persons are labeled with more than one psychiatric diagnosis. Schizophrenic individuals frequently suffer from severe depression after an acute psychotic episode. Suicidal gestures increase as depressed persons begin to stabilize from their medications and see the hopelessness of their situations. Persons with personality disorders may have disturbing phobias or anxiety. However, the experience and suffering of living with these labels are unique to each individual. Certain features are common to all

persons who must live with mental illness. For the sake of discussion, these characteristics are divided into two categories: psychological characteristics and behavioral characteristics.

PSYCHOLOGICAL CHARACTERISTICS

CMI individuals have several intellectual, emotional, social, and spiritual features in common. Intellectually, **altered thought processes** disrupt the ability to think clearly, solve problems, or make plans. Hallucinations, delusions, and obsessive thoughts are unwelcome intrusions that routinely disrupt the flow of reality-based thinking. Fear, mistrust, and paranoia can complicate the picture by presenting problems with daily living activities.

Chronic **low self-esteem** follows the label of mental illness everywhere. The ability to make logical sense out of life is hampered by the many distresses of being mentally ill. Even when one is adapting effectively, the stigma of being odd, crazy, or eccentric is wrapped around each action. Other people feel uncomfortable and avoid interacting, thus reinforcing the differences between "sick" and "well."

Mentally troubled people often see themselves as helpless, ineffective, and incapable of change. The experience of a small success will often prevent them from making any further attempts because they "just know" that they will eventually fail. When the self-concept is that low, it is difficult to convince someone that a brighter future can exist.

Depression is a partner of many mental health disorders, which makes a difficult life even more distressing. Depressive episodes can occur when an individual is coping with stress or in association with a psychotic episode. Even when mentally troubled persons are functioning effectively, depression can be a companion for many of them. Prudent nurses assess each client for the presence of depressive symptoms.

Loneliness is the suffering that results when one is isolated from other people. People need associations, and they suffer when removed from the company of others. Individuals with chronic mental health problems are usually very lonely. Their basic needs for love and belonging go unmet, and they respond by becoming more emotionally paralyzed.

Starved for social interactions, some CMI persons go to great lengths, such as criminal or violent activity, to gain attention. Others withdraw from society, fearing further rejection, and live a life of mistrust and solitude. Those who do have social interactions often are unable to express themselves, make decisions, or adapt to certain social roles. As the distress of attempting to cope socially increases, many find that retreating into their illness is easier than struggling with the complexities of interacting with other people.

Another characteristic of chronic mental illness is **hopelessness,** the catalyst for suicide. The struggle for mental health consumes much energy. Feelings of worthlessness plague self-esteem and lead to depression. Hopelessness brings with it the feeling that there are no solutions to one's problems, that life is destined to remain distressful, and that the only way to relieve the pain is to destroy the sufferer.

BEHAVIORAL CHARACTERISTICS

The nature of one's mental disorder determines the level of disability. Persons who suffer from chronic mental illness often have difficulty with behaviors and activities required for successful living. Impaired judgment, lack of motivation, or altered realities often lead to an inability to perform even the most basic activities. Individuals may lack knowledge of personal grooming habits, table manners, or expected social behaviors. They may have difficulty relating to others. Often they are unable to function socially or occupationally. Assaultive behaviors or criminal activities may be present. The majority of CMI individuals depend on others for their care. Many times, this involves living with family members or in group homes. For those who try to live independently, it all too often means a life of homeless shelters and nameless streets.

An estimated 42 million people worldwide are living with HIV/AIDS. The Centers for Disease Control and Prevention (CDC) estimates that 1,039,000 to 1,185,000 U.S. residents are living with HIV infection (Fleming and others, 2002).

The **sexual behaviors** of chronically mentally disordered persons place them at an increased risk for contracting and sharing sexually transmitted diseases, such as HIV/AIDS. Research into the sexual behaviors of the CMI population revealed that more than half of the clients screened were at a high risk for contracting HIV infection because of drug use and sexual practices. Studies regarding the knowledge of HIV/AIDS and its risk behaviors demonstrated that the CMI participants had less knowledge about AIDS than most public high school students (HIV/AIDS, 2005). Clearly, these individuals need education to prevent the increase of HIV infection, and this is one of the greatest challenges for nurses and health educators today.

Violence is an unfortunate aspect of many chronically mentally troubled people. The inability to solve problems, make sound judgments, or control emotional behaviors makes some individuals a threat to the safety and well-being of others. Family members, especially children, frequently become the targets for anger and aggression. Life within the community becomes difficult for persons who behave violently because these behaviors lead to extensive contact with the criminal justice system. Stays in county jails or prisons do little to address the issues underlying violence. Many potentially dangerous individuals are released back into the community under the banner of self-determination and individual rights (Howd, 1998). Society's response to the problems posed by these individuals reflects the attitude toward people with severe chronic mental illness in general.

SPECIAL POPULATIONS

Chronic mental health problems can begin at any stage in life, but they are usually not noted until early or middle adulthood. Children, adolescents, adults, and elderly people all suffer from the difficulties of chronic mental illness, but each group poses some unique and special problems that affect their abilities to respond to mental health interventions.

CHILDREN AND ADOLESCENTS WITH CHRONIC MENTAL ILLNESS

The seeds of many adult mental health problems are planted in childhood. Some children must learn to cope with psychological impairments early in life. Children with mental retardation (an IQ below 70 with impairments in functioning) have problems with the intellectual and emotional aspects of life. Also, people who are mildly or moderately retarded "are believed to be more susceptible to mental illness" (Fortinash and Holoday-Worret, 2008). Emotional problems, such as anxiety or depression, often accompany the challenges faced by these individuals. Conflicts between expectations and actual abilities may result in the development of a personality disorder or psychosis.

Children with **autism** are in a world of their own. Because they do not develop the ability to respond to and communicate their needs, they remain dependent on others, sometimes throughout their lives. Without the help and care of others, these children could not survive reality.

Health care providers play important roles in the care of autistic individuals and their families. Occupational therapy teams and nurses focus on the skills needed for daily activities. Psychologists and special education teachers measure functional abilities and encourage skill development, and psychiatrists monitor clients' overall progress. All provide emotional support and information.

Childhood **schizophrenia,** although uncommon, does occur and almost always develops into a chronic mental health problem. Children at risk for developing chronic mental health problems include those who have been neglected, have been repeatedly abused or mistreated, and have witnessed or experienced violence. Children with conduct disorders, attention-deficit/hyperactivity disorders, and depression also have a greater risk of developing a chronic mental health disorder.

During adolescence, many maladaptive behaviors become ingrained and new ones are developed. Because all parts of an individual are related, adolescents with chronic physical health problems, such as arthritis, diabetes, and cystic fibrosis, commonly experience psychological problems as well. Teens with diabetes have high rates of depression and suicidal behaviors.

Several chronic mental health problems develop during adolescence. Eating disorders, personality disorders, and schizophrenia can begin during the teenage years. Depression can become a long-standing problem with adolescents who have not learned to cope successfully. The road to chemical dependency most frequently begins in adolescence. The effects of posttraumatic stress can lead teens to stress-reducing but maladaptive behaviors that over time become daily patterns of ineffective functioning.

OLDER ADULTS WITH CHRONIC MENTAL ILLNESS

Elderly people with chronic mental illness fall into two groups: those who have had mental health problems for decades and those diagnosed with a mental disorder after age 50 years. The most common acquired mental health problems in older adulthood are Alzheimer's disease and other dementias. "As many as 20% of elderly persons over the age of 80 suffer from some form of dementia" (Fortinash and Holoday-Worret, 2008). Depression is another frequent chronic mental health problem of older adults, especially if accompanied by sensory losses and communication impairments.

The social epidemic of crack cocaine and other drug use has resulted in a completely new group of primary care providers in the United States: grandparents who must raise a second family, their grandchildren. Because of increased drug abuse, violence, and chronic behavioral problems that leave adult children incapable of raising their children, many older adults have assumed the primary responsibility and care for their grandchildren.

At a time when individuals should be looking forward to personal freedom and decreased responsibilities, the prospect of spending another 15 to 20 years raising more children can be overwhelming. Health care providers work to address the issues of grandparents experiencing the strain of caring for the children of parents with addictions. The mental health of at least two generations depends on timely and supportive health care interventions.

PERSONS WITH MULTIPLE DISORDERS

The word co-morbidity (co-occurring) refers to the presence of two or more mental health disorders. Individuals with a **dual diagnosis** are suffering from two mental health disorders, one of which is usually substance related. The depressed person who uses cocaine is an example. Substance abuse and mental illness result in an interactive process that is seen in physical, psychological, and behavioral patterns that differ from those patterns in persons with only an addiction or serious mental illness.

As many as 75% of individuals with chronic mental illness use or abuse drugs. These people present a significant challenge for treatment because of the complexity of their disorders. The multidisciplinary treatment team seems to be the most promising approach for helping clients with co-occurring disorders cope with their problems in each area of functioning.

PROVIDING CARE FOR CHRONICALLY MENTALLY ILL PEOPLE

People with chronic mental health problems are found everywhere in society. Today, the majority of mental health care is provided within the community, outside the world of the institution. For this reason, most interactions between health care providers and clients usually address some issues or problems relating to mental health.

INPATIENT SETTINGS

Persons with chronic mental health problems are hospitalized only when their behaviors pose a threat to themselves or others. Even then, it is often for only a short time. The most immediate goal of care for clients with exacerbations of their mental health problems is to help them control their behaviors. The average length of stay for mental illness is about 10 days. Inpatient treatment settings for the CMI population include the acute care hospital, psychiatric unit of an acute care facility, state psychiatric institution, and private mental health facility.

State psychiatric institutions still provide care for more than 50% of all psychiatric inpatients. However, stays in all inpatient treatment settings are shorter and readmissions more frequent. The pattern of admission, a short institutional stay, discharge, a short community stay, and readmission (recidivism) remains a problem for both health care professionals and their clients.

Frequently, high levels of stress precipitate acute psychotic behaviors. Table 32-1 lists several common stressors that can trigger acute reactions and thus readmissions to inpatient care settings.

Unfortunately, the justice system is providing inpatient psychiatric care for many CMI individuals. "Today, some 283,800 inmates are identified as having a mental illness. This represents 16% of the inmate population of state and local jails" ("Mental Illness and the Criminal Justice System," 2003). Inmates with mental disorders seldom receive treatment because of inadequate resources of an overburdened system (Box 32-1).

OUTPATIENT SETTINGS

Once an acute psychiatric episode has subsided, many chronically mentally disordered clients are discharged to halfway houses or other group-living environments. Aftercare programs range from partial hospitalization to sheltered living arrangements or home care, depending on the size, economics, and support of the community (see Cultural Considerations 32-1).

Table 32-1 *Common Triggers of Acute Psychotic Episodes*

HEALTH	ENVIRONMENT	ATTITUDES/BEHAVIORS
Poor nutrition	Hostile/critical environment	"Poor me" (low self-concept)
Lack of sleep	Housing difficulties (unsatisfactory housing)	"Hopeless" (lack of self-confidence)
Out of balance circadian rhythms	Pressure to perform (loss of independent living)	"I'm a failure" (loss of motivation to use skills)
Fatigue		"Lack of control" (demoralization)
Infection	Changes in life events, daily patterns of activity	Feeling overpowered by symptoms
Central nervous system drugs	Stress (lack of survival skills)	"No one likes me" (unable to meet spiritual needs)
Impaired reasoning	Interpersonal difficulties	Looks/acts different from others same age, culture
Impaired information processing	Disruptions in interpersonal relationships	Poor social skills
Lack of exercise	Loneliness (social isolation, lack of social support)	Aggressive behavior
Behavioral disorder	Missed environmental cues	Violent behavior
Mood abnormalities	Job pressures (poor occupation skills)	Poor medication management
Moderate to high levels of anxiety	Poor social skills	Poor symptom management
	Poverty	
	Lack of transportation (resources)	

From Stuart GW: *Pocket guide to psychiatric nursing*, ed 6, St. Louis, 2005, Mosby.

Box 32-1 *Prison Inmates With Mental Disorders*

Studies of chronically mentally ill prison inmates revealed several interesting facts about them:
 They received longer sentences.
 They served a high proportion of their sentences.
 They committed five times more staff assaults.
 They broke the rules more often.
 They were more likely to be victimized than inmates who were not mentally ill.

From O'Connor FW, Lovell D, Brown L: Implementing residential treatment for prison inmates with mental illness, *Arch Psychiatr Nurs* 16:232, 2002.

 Cultural Considerations 32-1

When chronic mental health clients are cared for in community group housing situations, make sure to perform a complete cultural assessment. People from different cultures have different points of view about mental illness. Living with people from other cultures requires open communication and a willingness to accept other points of view. These qualities are often difficult to achieve, especially when one is mentally troubled.

Many people with chronic mental illness live with their families, who require much support to cope effectively. In some communities, CMI individuals live with therapeutic families in foster care programs. Unfortunately, more mental health care is needed in settings such as homeless shelters, health clinics for the poor, jails, and prisons.

PSYCHIATRIC REHABILITATION

The concept of psychiatric rehabilitation focuses on assisting individuals with serious mental illness to effectively cope with their life situations. A multidisciplinary approach uses the special talents of physicians, psychologists, nurses, occupational and physical therapists, dietitians, and other specialists.

Each realm of human functioning is addressed during treatment. Physically, clients are assessed for and taught the skills needed to effectively perform the activities of daily living, including proper nutrition, activity, and rest habits. Emotional problems are explored, and clients are taught how to identify their feelings, control their anger, and reach their goals. Intellectually, clients are encouraged to problem solve and set goals. Occupational or vocational training allows individuals the opportunity for employment.

Involvement with psychiatric rehabilitation programs also offers opportunities for people with severe mental illness to meet their often neglected social needs. Many programs provide group therapies and opportunities to learn more socially appropriate behaviors. Some psychiatric rehabilitation programs lend spiritual help in the form of staff members, clergy, or referrals to the religious organization of the client's choice. Unfortunately, too few psychiatric rehabilitation programs exist for the many individuals who truly need them.

THERAPEUTIC INTERVENTIONS

In 1978, the President's Commission on Mental Health recommended that persons with chronic mental disorders be treated in the "least restrictive environment." This was defined as a setting that encouraged the greatest degree of freedom, self-determination, autonomy, dignity, and integrity. However, the concept is not so easily implemented when clients are unable or unwilling to seek out or consent to treatment and the funding for mental health care remains unstable.

Table 32-2	*Basic Interventions: Chronic Mental Illness*

NURSING INTERVENTIONS	RATIONALE
RELATING TO RISK OF DANGER	
Assess risk for harm to self or others.	Ensures safety and prevents violence
Encourage client to notify staff when feeling angry or when destructive thoughts begin.	Helps prevent violence before it actually occurs
Frequently orient client to reality in nonthreatening way.	Reduces risk of violence, decreases client anxiety
SENSORY/PERCEPTUAL ALTERATIONS	
Assess for delusions and hallucinations.	Helps to determine the level of psychosis
Ask client to share the meaning of his or her hallucinations, delusions.	To determine client's point of view and intent
Teach client distraction techniques, such as whistling, clapping hands, telling hallucination to go away when hallucinating.	Offers client strategies for controlling hallucinations
ACTIVITIES OF DAILY LIVING	
Establish a schedule for grooming, eating, sleeping.	Increases self-esteem, encourages responsibility, and helps client appear more socially acceptable
Monitor intake, output, personal hygiene activities.	
COMMUNICATION	
Use active listening; establish trust; encourage conversation; praise attempts to speak clearly and effectively.	Helps to assess client's communication style and patterns; increases understanding of and respect for client
SOCIAL SKILLS	
Encourage good social skills, such as table manners, personal grooming, appropriate communications, behaviors.	Promotes client's acceptability by other persons; increases self-esteem; helps to teach effective social behaviors

Modified from Fortinash KM, Holoday-Worret PA: *Psychiatric mental health nursing,* ed 4, St. Louis, 2007, Mosby.

TREATMENTS AND THERAPIES

Basic goals for chronically disordered mental health clients are to achieve stabilization and maintain the highest possible level of daily functioning. Therapies are designed for the individual based on identified problems, available resources, and the client's willingness to cooperate with the therapeutic regimen. Various individual and group therapies, along with certain medications, are usually recommended by the treatment team after a complete health assessment and consultation with the client.

With support and assistance, many CMI individuals are able to function outside the institution. However, a number of problems or situations can disrupt their stability and trigger an acute psychiatric episode. When hospital stays are shorter and acute episodes occur frequently, individuals bounce between living in the community and the institution. In 1991, the average length of hospitalization for psychiatric problems was 23 days. Today, it is 9 days. Many hospital stays allow even less time for clients to stabilize and begin treatment.

Pharmacological Therapy

Persons with chronic mental disorders are treated with a variety of medications depending on symptoms and distress levels. Antianxiety agents and antidepressants are often prescribed to improve emotional comfort. Antipsychotic (neuroleptic) drugs are prescribed to help control hallucinations and other symptoms of psychosis.

Drug therapy is an important part of treatment. The side effects of many of these medications are uncomfortable, and clients often stop taking them as soon as the acute symptoms subside. Several antipsychotic medications are available in long-acting injectable forms called decanoate. One of the most powerful predictors of medication refusal is one's insight into the illness, and most chronically or severely mentally ill individuals have little insight. Nurses must carefully monitor clients routinely for compliance with medications.

NURSING (THERAPEUTIC) PROCESS

The first step in working with severely mentally disordered clients is to obtain the most complete database possible. Because mental health problems affect every area of functioning, nurses must perform thorough histories and assess clients' physical status, perceptions, and behaviors.

After each member of the treatment team completes his or her assessment, client problems are identified and therapeutic interventions are designed. Nurses focus on helping clients cope with each activity of daily living. Multidisciplinary and nursing diagnoses are chosen and basic interventions are agreed on by the treatment team and (when possible) the client. Nursing diagnoses for CMI clients are selected according to the client's identified problems.

Therapeutic interventions are then designed to help the client solve the identified problems. Although each client requires a unique combination of interventions, several fundamental therapeutic actions apply to all clients. Table 32-2 lists each intervention and its rationale. A care plan for a CMI client is presented in Sample Client Care Plan 32-1.

Care plans for long-term psychiatric clients are adapted to the particular care setting—be it the home,

---

SAMPLE CLIENT CARE PLAN 32-1

Chronic Mental Illness

ASSESSMENT *History.* Tom is a 34-year-old man with a history of at least 11 admissions to psychiatric units of various general hospitals. Today he is being readmitted after he was found wandering the streets arguing with himself and threatening to kill someone else if they "don't stop calling me names." He was medicated with 1 mg of haloperidol (Haldol) intramuscularly in the emergency department.

Current Findings. An unkempt man with a strong body odor and soiled clothing; speech is slow and disjointed; responds verbally without external stimuli. Emotional state (affect) is flat except for verbal responses to hallucinations. Tom states that he is and has been hallucinating for the past 3 days. The hallucinations are auditory; the voices want Tom to kill himself. He thinks they may be right because during the time he is in the community, he feels forced to spy on other people for the FBI and the voices tell him that he is better off dead than being a spy. When asked what made him take to the streets, Tom replied that he thought he could "outwalk the out talk." He has not taken his prescribed medications since he last saw his therapist about 4 weeks ago.

Multidisciplinary Diagnosis	Planning/Goals
Disturbed sensory perception related to impaired perceptions	Tom will seek out a staff member when he begins to hallucinate. Tom will not harm himself or others. Tom will report the absence of auditory hallucinations within 4 days after admission.

Therapeutic Interventions

Intervention	Rationale	Team Member
1. Orient Tom frequently to place, time, current activity.	Presents reality; reminds Tom of this reality.	All
2. Speak slowly; use clear, simple messages.	Helps to increase Tom's understanding, thus decreasing his anxiety.	All
3. Reassure often that he will not be harmed by the voices or other people.	Helps Tom to trust the safety of his environment, presents reality as safe.	All
4. Listen to and accept descriptions of his feelings, hallucinations.	Conveys respect and acceptance of the person and encourages communication.	All
5. Set limits on aggressive behaviors; make a no-harm contract with Tom.	Promotes a safe environment for all clients and staff, helps Tom to be responsible for his own behaviors.	Nsg, All
6. Encourage Tom to take his medications; make copy of the daily medication schedule, and encourage Tom to follow it.	Medications help to control psychotic symptoms, reduce anxiety, improve functioning; developing a daily medication routine in the hospital helps increase compliance after discharge.	Nsg, MD
7. Discharge planning for Tom to return to his foster home.	A stable and predictable environment helps decrease acute psychotic episodes.	Soc Svc

Evaluation

After the fourth day of hospitalization, Tom sought out staff members when he was beginning to hallucinate. With the exception of one acting-out episode, Tom abided by his no-harm contract. Reports of hallucinations have decreased from "continually" on admission to once or twice per week the second week of his stay.

？ **CRITICAL THINKING** QUESTIONS

1. What strategies would help increase Tom's compliance with his medications?

2. What discharge planning does Tom require?

A complete client care plan includes several other diagnoses and interventions.
Nsg, Nursing staff; *MD,* physician; *Soc Svc,* social services.

---

community day center, clinic, or institution. If the mental health care services are well coordinated, care plans move with the client. That is, the care plans established in the institution move to a different care setting when the client does. This method encourages the continuity of care that is so important for coping with severe mental problems.

Once clients return into the community, mental health centers provide them with the ongoing care needed to help them function effectively, but many services are unavailable because of unstable sources of funding. Community mental health centers with strong financial bases are able to provide their clients with services such as medical care, medication supervision, individual and family therapy, crisis intervention services, family support services, skills training, and vocational counseling or training in addition to continued emotional support and encouragement. With long-term support, many individuals with severe mental illness and their families are able to cope with the numerous problems associated with their disorders.

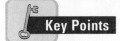

Key Points

- Each person's experiences with mental illness are unique, but most chronic mental health problems are characterized by periods of exacerbations and remissions.
- Chronic mental disorders are disabling for people in every society and culture.
- As a result of deinstitutionalization, many chronically mentally ill individuals are homeless, hungry, and unable to care for themselves.
- Access to comprehensive mental health care remains a problem in the United States today.
- Psychological characteristics of chronically mentally ill persons include altered thought processes, chronic low self-esteem, depression, hopelessness, loneliness, and suicidal behaviors.
- Behavioral characteristics of chronically mentally ill individuals include the inability to perform activities of daily living; being dependent on or living with family; employment difficulties; ineffective independent living; and sexually active, violent, or criminal behaviors.
- Chronic mental health problems can begin at any stage in life, but they are usually not noted until early or middle adulthood.
- The social epidemic of violence, crack cocaine, and other drug use has resulted in a new group of primary care providers: grandparents who are raising their grandchildren.

- Substance abuse and mental illness result in an interactive process that is seen in physical, psychological, and behavioral patterns uniquely different from those of persons with only an addiction or serious mental illness.
- Chronically mentally ill individuals are at a high risk for contracting HIV infection due to current behaviors and past histories.
- Chronically mentally ill persons have little knowledge of HIV/AIDS and its risk behaviors.
- Psychiatric rehabilitation is a multidisciplinary treatment approach that focuses on assisting clients with serious mental illness to cope effectively with their life situations.
- The basic goals for chronically disordered mental health clients are to achieve stabilization and be maintained at their highest level of daily functioning.
- Persons with chronic mental disorders are treated with a variety of medications depending on symptoms and distress levels.
- Nurses focus on helping the chronically mentally ill client cope with each activity of daily living.
- Once returned into the community, chronically mentally ill people require aftercare or rehabilitation services.
- Because all areas of human functioning are deeply interwoven, mental health nursing is a critical component of every nursing situation.
- The mental health of a society depends on the mental health of each of its individual citizens.

---

evolve   Be sure to visit the companion Evolve site at http://evolve.elsevier.com/Morrison-Valfre/ for additional online resources.

33 Challenges for the Future

Objectives

Upon completion of this chapter, the student will be able to:

1. List three challenges that health care providers face in delivering mental health care in the United States.
2. Discuss the characteristics of a typical "old" and "new" homeless person.
3. Explain the purpose of the Americans With Disabilities Act of 1990.
4. Describe the roles, functions, and interactions of the mental health care team.
5. Explain what is meant by "the right of self-determination."
6. Examine three obligations of the therapeutic partnership for the client and the care provider.
7. Describe three expanded roles for nurses who care for mentally ill people.
8. Examine two challenges involved with the change process.
9. Examine the role of the mental health team in providing care for clients with human immunodeficiency virus (HIV)/acquired immunodeficiency syndrome (AIDS).
10. Outline two techniques for coping with information overload.

Key Terms

change process (p. 375)
competent (p. 372)
entrepreneur (ŎN-trə-prə-NOOR) (p. 375)
homelessness (p. 369)
information overload (p. 377)
mental health care team (p. 371)
nurse case managers (p. 374)
psychosocial (psychiatric) rehabilitation (p. 375)

The need for mental health applies to us all. Every person experiences periods of emotional turmoil and crises, and, at some time, we all need a little assistance to help us cope. When one is experiencing physical illness, it produces emotional stresses ranging from indifference to crisis behaviors. With this thought in mind, every person becomes a mental health client in some way because an emotional reaction always follows a physical diagnosis, an uncomfortable procedure, or time spent as a patient. Nurses and other health care providers help provide the nurturing that all clients

(not just those with mental illnesses) need. In addition, they are now challenged to provide that care within ever-changing health care delivery environments.

CHANGES IN MENTAL HEALTH CARE

"Mental disorders rank among the top ten illnesses causing disability—more that 37% worldwide." Other research indicates that "the world's mental health care needs are largely going unmet" (National Institute of Mental Health [NIMH], 2007a). In the United States one in four adults suffers from a diagnosable mental disorder. This means that almost 58 million individuals need help to cope with daily life (NIMH, 2007b).

Health care is undergoing many changes today. Escalating costs in several countries are forcing officials to take a close look at where and how health care funds are spent. In the United States, new patterns of providing health care services are emerging as preferred provider and health maintenance organizations. Social changes, such as an aging population, an over-burdened welfare system, and a cost-conscious U.S. Congress, are all exerting their influences on today's health care system. Men and women are returning from armed conflicts with wounds that change lives. The mental health care so urgently needed is often unavailable—or the veterans do not recognize or admit their mental health difficulties.

The influences of many cultures and new technologies are changing the way we look at health and illness. Today, clients may not speak the same language. Technological advances are opening new areas of exploration, and discoveries about the biochemical nature of humans are challenging the foundations of our thinking.

In 2006, the National Alliance on Mental Illness graded America's mental health care system. The report was based on the most comprehensive survey in 15 years, and it found that "nationally the system is in trouble. Its grade is no better than a D" (NIMH, 2007a). Much work is needed.

The treatment and prevention of mental illness (and other health issues) are caught up in the web of change. As a result, all health care providers will be challenged to deliver effective, cost-accountable care.

This will call for creativity and innovation. Change is a certainty, and adaptability is a key.

CHANGE IN SETTINGS

Until recently, most psychiatric care was limited to the inpatient setting, either a unit at the local community hospital or a long-term care institution. Today, however, most psychiatric long-term care institutions are closed. Those that remain are full, and local emergency departments are becoming havens for those experiencing crisis. Some individuals with acute problems are denied care and told to return when "something happens."

When the large state mental health institutions began to discharge their clients, it was argued that most people could live in the community if they continued to receive medication and aftercare (Torrey, 1998). Many mentally ill persons were transferred to nursing homes and long-term care facilities. Changes in the system that once supported mentally ill clients are now moving them into community health care systems, but the specialized "aftercare" that was promised is commonly not provided.

As a result of the unsupported release, many mentally troubled persons became sick again and eventually homeless. The seriously mentally ill population now constitutes more than one third of the homeless population (Torrey and Zdanowicz, 1999). Jails and prisons have evolved into holding facilities for people with mental problems (Harrington, 1999). Many mentally ill individuals are jailed just to get them off the streets. Others are found living at the fringes of society, sleeping in abandoned buildings, and depending on the generosity of others for food and clothing.

The treatment settings for people with mental illness have changed to follow the clients from the institution to the street, jail, neighborhood clinic, or local physician's office. Mental health care is an important component of overall health. It must be addressed if we are to become capable, adaptable, and functional people. Health care providers must become skilled in assessing and working with clients suffering from mental or emotional disorders, no matter where the setting or what the situation.

HOMELESSNESS

Many families live just "one paycheck away from poverty." They can financially cope for the present; but add one stressor, and the whole situation becomes threatened. It is not uncommon to hear of a working-class family whose father was laid off his job. If work is not found soon, the family becomes unable to make the mortgage payments. Eventually they are forced out of their home onto the streets. Sad as it seems, this scenario has become a reality for many families.

Homelessness means to be without a permanent residence, a place to live. Homelessness means to have every possession you own stuffed into the back of the car (if you are lucky enough to own a car). Homelessness means your children cannot attend school because they have no permanent address, no phone number, and no immunization records.

Historically, homeless people were unmarried, intermittently employed, white male adults with an average age of 50 years. However, they seldom actually slept in the streets because of the availability of cheap hotels, missions, and SROs (sleeping rooms only). A study of Chicago's homeless population in the late 1950s revealed that 25% of the homeless people were receiving Social Security (and trying to live inexpensively), 25% were chronic alcoholics, 20% had a physical disability, 20% had a chronic mental illness, and 10% were maladjusted. These men are the "old homeless," the traditional less fortunate members of society.

During the 1960s and 1970s, the number of homeless people declined in the United States; however, by the early 1980s a growing number of the "new homeless" began to appear, and that number has rapidly increased ever since. Today's homeless people are younger and much poorer than their counterparts of yesterday. Many have no actual shelter, much less a home. The numbers of women, children, and minorities have swelled the ranks of the homeless to significant numbers. Families without a home now make up 38% of the homeless population in a city. "Almost half of the homeless population works, but does not earn enough to pay for housing" (NLCHP, 2007).

Loss of control over the daily events of their own lives leads homeless people toward a loss of self-worth, learned helplessness, and depression. Children who are homeless for any length of time experience serious threats to their current well-being and their future ability to succeed.

The health status of the homeless population, both mental and physical, is poor. The average age of death for a homeless person in the United States is about 50 years. About one third of today's homeless persons are mentally ill. Many of these people were relatively adjusted when they were discharged from an institution, but when their medications ran out and the aftercare was not provided, their psychiatric problems returned. Without adequate support, resources, and encouragement, many chronically mentally ill individuals find it almost impossible to take steps to improve their lives.

Homelessness has become a national tragedy that in some way affects us all. When people cannot find health care for the smaller problems, they wait until immediate attention is required. This practice brings about a high incidence of severe disorders. The trauma of losing one's home, adjusting to life in a shelter or on the street, and struggling for a way out produces symptoms of psychological and emotional distress. Stress disorders are common among the homeless population, even those with previously high levels of functioning.

The children of this subsociety endure hardships that most of us can only imagine. Low-birth-weight babies and infant illness are common. Studies of homeless women in New York City revealed that infant mortality is very high.

If the children survive infancy, they are at risk for double the incidence of respiratory infections and skin ailments, as well as the usual childhood diseases. Parasitic infestations, such as lice or scabies, occur in homeless children much more frequently than in the general population. Homeless children are also affected by poor educational opportunities, anxiety, depression, and behavioral difficulties.

Few homeless children are immunized, fewer are educated, and many live with hunger and chronic malnutrition. Developmental delays, including short attention spans; immature motor, speech, and interpersonal skills; and inappropriate social behaviors, are frequently encountered with homeless children. Poverty, inadequate shelter, lack of access to day care services, and the stresses of having no home all contribute to homeless children's lack of development. For homeless children, childhood is not the happy time of exploration and learning that it should be.

Adolescents are also found in greater numbers among the homeless. Estimates of homeless adolescents are as high as 1.5 million individuals. Many of these are the children of dysfunctional families who are frequently neglected, abused, and exploited. Homeless adolescents are at a much greater risk for hepatitis, AIDS, and other sexually transmitted diseases. Life on the streets leads to high rates of substance abuse, depression, and frequent suicidal attempts. The future holds little promise for a teen without hopes, aspirations, or emotional support.

Adults with chronic mental illness constitute about one third of the homeless population. Their ability to function in daily life is severely limited. Self-care activities, interpersonal relationships, and abilities to work or attend school are compromised for mentally troubled individuals. Financial resources are usually very limited. Many rooming houses that once provided inexpensive shelter have been converted to other uses or destroyed. Publicly financed housing, especially for mentally ill individuals, is difficult to obtain. Given the lack of community mental health services, one can understand why a large number of people with chronic mental illnesses are now wandering the streets of both large and small communities.

When research was conducted to compare mentally ill homeless people with non–mentally ill homeless people, those with severe mental illnesses were similar to their counterparts in age, ethnicity, gender, and extent of substance abuse. However, the homeless mentally ill group was in poorer health, was homeless for longer periods of time, struggled with more barriers to employment, and had less contact with family or friends than the homeless individuals without mental difficulties.

The actual number of homeless persons is difficult to determine, but estimates range from less than 1 million to more than 7 million. Homelessness is a national health problem that must be solved if we are to save a generation from the despair of having no future. Health care problems for the homeless population are monumental, but they can be addressed. As the providers of health care, we must find new ways of working with this population if we are to protect and encourage the health of all people.

THE AMERICANS WITH DISABILITIES ACT

The Americans with Disabilities Act (ADA) of 1990 is a federal statute designed to remove the barriers that prevented qualified people with disabilities from having the same employment opportunities that are available to persons without disabilities. The ADA requires employers to make "reasonable accommodation" for disabled individuals, thus allowing them to perform the essential functions of the job.

Under the ADA guidelines, a person is considered disabled when a physical or mental impairment "substantially limits one or more major life activities" (Equal Employment Opportunity Commission, 1992). A mental impairment is defined by the ADA as "any mental or psychological disorder, such as mental retardation, organic brain syndrome, emotional or mental illness, and specified learning abilities." If the condition substantially limits one's functioning, the person is covered by the ADA. Employers can no longer refuse to hire persons solely because of disability and must make reasonable adjustments for the disabled employee. The implications of this legislation excite and challenge those who work with psychiatric clients.

The intent of the ADA is to tailor the needs of the job to the needs of the disabled individual. However, Congress cannot legislate social change. Only time and successful work experiences with mentally ill employees will remove the stigma of mental illness in the workplace. This is our next challenge: to prepare our clients for gainful employment while convincing employers that people with mental disorders can be reliable employees (see Think About 33-1).

CULTURAL INFLUENCES

The world is shrinking. In the past a person would grow, live, procreate, and die within one community or geographical region. Today, world travelers work in one part of the globe and commute to another area to raise their families. Waves of immigrants move from their homelands in search of a better life. Rapid forms of transportation move thousands of people around the world in a matter of hours instead of days. As more individuals become computer literate and users of the global computer networks, our world will shrink even more. Because of these changes, health care providers will be encountering persons from various cultural backgrounds with greater frequency. Learning to interact effectively and respectfully is a challenge that faces

You are working in a community hospital. Today you find that one of your co-workers who told you that he has a history of mental illness has been assigned to your care team. You have never worked with this person before today.

- What is your initial reaction?
- How do you think this will affect the activities of the workplace?

all the world's citizens, but for health care workers this is especially important.

The mental problems of a culture can have a universal quality. There are some behaviors, such as those associated with depression, that all cultures define as mental health disorders. Other mental health problems may be specifically limited to the members of a certain group. These types of problems are called **culture-bound disorders** because they appear to be related to specific cultures. For example, the Hispanic disorder *susto* is an emotional anxiety that results from "soul loss."

Health, illness, and mental illness are defined differently throughout various cultures. The person who talks to himself may be considered "a nut" in one society and revered as a holy man in another. Their behaviors might be exactly the same, but the social setting in which they take place differs. The point is that mental illness is culturally defined to a large extent. To work effectively with clients from other cultures, health caregivers must discover how clients define mental illness.

As displaced individuals adapt to their new cultures, they combine elements of both the home and the host culture into their daily lives. The result is a unique blend of both worlds, a "third culture." Bicultural clients require a thorough cultural assessment to discover their individual frames of reference (how they view the world). Only then can therapeutic interventions be planned with the expectation of success. An effective therapy in one culture is not always successful when applied in another culture.

As more people emigrate throughout the world, care providers will encounter many clients whose first language is not English. This presents many challenges, especially when a psychiatric component is involved. Even when the client speaks or understands some English, the stresses of illness (and the complexities of a modern health care system) increase anxiety, and clients often attempt to communicate by reverting back to their native language. Many times these communications can be misunderstood and result in poor treatment outcomes. Cultural Considerations 33-1 offers an illustration of poor communication. If mental health care providers are to deliver effective care, we must be aware of the cultural backgrounds of our clients and develop our plans of care with each client's unique

Sam was a white nurse working at an American Indian reservation health center. He frequently monitored the physician's chronically ill clients, did his best to educate all of them about their conditions, and provided emotional support to help them cope with their conditions. Why then, he wondered, did he have such difficulty communicating with his clients?

On the suggestion of his physician, a long-term resident on the reservation, Sam began to look at how his behaviors affected his clients. After finding no real answer there, he consulted a tribal elder with his problem. All that he was told was that "the eyes are the window of the soul." This statement perplexed Sam until he realized that he was "staring down" his clients when he was interacting with them.

Sam was so intent on putting his client education messages across that he repeatedly missed an important nonverbal clue—all his clients avoided direct eye contact and looked downward whenever Sam was instructing them. Once he realized that his problem was a culturally based miscommunication, he revised his method of teaching and changed his eye contact behaviors. His clients began to communicate with him. Sam had learned a valuable lesson: not all people communicate the same way.

- How does Sam's experience affect your interactions with clients?

cultural heritage in mind. Caring for culturally diverse clients is another challenge, because our services are only as effective as they are perceived to be by our clients.

THE MENTAL HEALTH CARE TEAM

Mental illness has a multifaceted nature that includes physical disorders, social factors, psychological issues, and spiritual concerns. To attempt to meet the many client needs and to provide care in both inpatient and community settings, interdisciplinary mental health care teams were introduced. A **mental health care team** is a group of professionally trained specialists who develop and implement comprehensive treatment plans for clients with mental and emotional problems.

TEAM MEMBERS

The ideal composition of an interdisciplinary (also called multidisciplinary) mental health care team is the client, a physician, a psychologist, a nurse, a dietitian, a social worker, a representative of the client's spiritual beliefs (e.g., minister or priest), an occupational therapist, and other specialists as needed. The main function of the team is to coordinate care as the client moves from inpatient to community settings and through the health care system. Refer to Table 2-3 for a description of each team member's role in the health care team.

Interdisciplinary Interactions

Members of the mental health care team communicate frequently because scarce services must be allocated and clients need effective care. Some care teams meet often to monitor client progress, review the client's use of services, and establish treatment goals. Others may interact by phone or e-mail. All work with clients and each other to meet defined goals. To illustrate, nurses who care for hospitalized clients begin discharge planning on admission and communicate with the care team. Discharge planners and social workers communicate with community members who provide services. When clients are ready for discharge, the care team is able to help with a smooth transition back into the community because the interactions of each team member focus on the treatment goals.

MENTAL HEALTH CARE DELIVERY SETTINGS

In the past, mental health care was obtained in the psychiatrist's office or the inpatient setting. Today, mental health care is delivered in three general settings: the institution, the community, or the home. Mental health units in general hospitals and inpatient mental facilities are examples of institutional settings. Mental health specialists are found in many community settings, ranging from prisons and jails to private clinics. Many work in neighborhood clinics or with social service agencies. Mental health home care is frequently delivered through psychiatric nurses and technicians who regularly visit clients in their home environments. Client care and support are the web that helps individuals cope within rapidly changing societies.

CHANGE AND MENTAL HEALTH CLIENTS

Throughout history, mental illnesses have been labeled as being somehow "different" from physical maladies. People with mental illnesses were obviously not in this reality, so why should they care about how they are treated? This attitude prevailed for many centuries. Consequently, persons with mental illnesses were neglected, abused, and confined without hope of improvement.

As new psychiatric theories arose, attitudes toward the mentally ill population changed, but individuals were still viewed as culprits or victims who somehow caused their own problems. During this time, the role of the patient was to be a passive recipient of care. Therapies were designed and delivered without regard to appropriateness, and patients were expected to quietly cooperate. Relationships between clients and care providers ranged from patronizing to adversarial.

Today both the providers and consumers of mental health care are striving to change attitudes and practices. Involving clients in treatment means every party must assume an active role. This interaction involves the building of trust, mutual respect, and acceptance.

COMPETENCY

Are people with mental illness capable of making decisions about proper care and treatment of their problems? Society struggles to balance individual rights with the need to protect its citizens. Meanwhile, our legal system and those who work with mentally ill individuals are often challenged to provide the answer to this complex question.

To be considered competent, an individual must be able to (1) make a choice, (2) understand important information, (3) appreciate one's own situation, and (4) apply reasoning. Studies reveal that mental illness can coexist with competent decision making, but as many as 50% of individuals with mental illness show seriously impaired judgment. Many hospitalized clients with severe symptoms, such as paranoia or disorganized thought, are usually incompetent. Apply the four measures of competence described above when assessing a client's decision-making abilities. It may help solve the dilemma of discerning which clients are able to make reasonable treatment decisions.

The challenge of meeting client needs without violating their rights is especially true for clients with mental health problems. When people were discharged from institutions into their "least restrictive environments," their rights to freedom, autonomy, and self-determination were protected. However, the concept of the least restrictive setting begins to break down when clients are unable to provide the essentials of daily living for themselves and are in need of treatment.

Individuals are not exercising their rights to freedom when they wander the streets aimlessly, out of touch with reality. They are able to determine little for themselves and have virtually no ability to self-direct their lives. In these cases, an institutional setting may prove to be a more beneficial environment.

To implement the concept of the least restrictive treatment environment, mental health care team members assess the available community resources and match their services to the needs and limitations of each client. In today's health care environment, the linking of mentally troubled clients with too few community resources is, and will likely remain, a challenge for us all.

EMPOWERMENT OF CLIENTS

The traditional role of a client was passive. Clients were expected to accept the physician's diagnosis, therapies, and comments without question. They were also expected to be motivated, cooperative, and passive enough to get well. As a result, people became increasingly detached from the responsibility for their own health care and discontented with the system that delivered that care.

Today, people are becoming more responsible and active consumers of health care, but many health care services remain tied to the old models of the passive client. Individuals entering the health care system are beginning to exercise the right of self-determination. They seek out information about their conditions, weigh the pros and cons of each treatment option, and select the ones that best suit them. Because the consumer's role has moved from a passive to an active one, the term **client** becomes more appropriate than the passively connoted term **patient.** Hopefully the relationship between care providers and client develops into a dynamic interchange, with therapeutic goals that are mutually acceptable. This therapeutic partnership, however, involves responsibility.

OBLIGATIONS OF CLIENTS

To receive the most effective care, clients must fulfill certain obligations. These responsibilities are few, but they are important for success of treatment. First, clients must be truthful. Many times people are uncomfortable about sharing personal information. They may expect health care providers to pass judgment on their actions or refuse care. Nevertheless, honest, complete data are essential for planning care. Second, clients have an obligation to be responsible for their own behaviors. Even people who periodically lose contact with reality are capable of assuming some responsibility. Third, clients have an obligation to cooperate with treatment, that is, assuming clients want to "get well." Consumers of mental health services who are willing to assume the obligations of truthfulness, responsibility, and cooperation can play an active role in successful diagnosis and treatment of their problems. Within the therapeutic relationship, care providers also have certain obligations.

OBLIGATIONS OF CARE PROVIDERS

As clients assume certain obligations, so do the care providers who work with them. From the psychiatrist to the technician, each assumes specific responsibilities when working with clients. However, all health care providers share the following obligations.

First and most important, **accept** the client "as is." We do not have to like or approve of any behavior, but the **person** must be accepted as a worthy human being—capable of change. Do not pass judgment. We are here to help—not to conjure up emotionally based opinions.

Second, demonstrate **respect** for clients. Refer to clients by name. Ask permission before entering their living space, if necessary. Show approval for gains made in therapy. Express concern for their well-being, and remember to be polite. All these behaviors demonstrate respect for clients much more clearly than words. Even the most disturbed person responds to respectful care.

Third, **empower** clients. Much mental illness is associated with clients' feelings of lack of control over their lives. Care providers who recognize this can provide small, but frequent, opportunities for decision making and success. As clients choose among various options, they are exercising some control over their environment. Hopefully, decisions gradually move from making choices to solving problems. During the process, each success provides encouragement for the next step and a sense of control.

Fourth, mental health professionals, especially nurses and therapists who work closely with clients, have the added obligation to provide educational opportunities—in short, to **educate.** Unless clients are comatose, they are capable of learning. New knowledge allows people to change. Empowerment education is an intervention that helps mentally troubled clients attain increased control of their lives (Schofield, 1998), and empowered clients are more willing to explore and change their behaviors. Table 33-1 summarizes the obligations of the therapeutic partnership.

Health care providers in the United States are also expected to comply with federal privacy rules. The Health Insurance Portability and Accountability Act of 1996 (HIPAA) provided the first national standards for protecting the privacy of an individual's health information and regulates how personal health information is disclosed and used. The last basic obligation of health care providers is to protect the client's privacy.

Studies have demonstrated that clients who feel they have some control over their situation report fewer symptoms and less discomfort. They have speedier recoveries and are able to participate in the activities of daily living earlier than clients who perceive little or no control. In short, clients need to be active participants in their own care.

PROVIDERS OF CARE

Membership in the health care profession is also changing. Once, only physicians, nurses, and family members provided mental health care. Today, several technicians, assistants, and aides provide many services that were once exclusively within the realm of psychiatry. Because each technician works within a narrow specialty, it becomes the nurse's responsibility to ensure that safe, coordinated health care is being delivered to clients. Nurses need to understand and exercise their roles in coordinating health care.

Table 33-1 *Obligations of the Therapeutic Partnership*

CLIENTS	CARE PROVIDERS
To be truthful	To accept the client as a person capable of change
To be responsible for one's own behaviors	To demonstrate respect and acceptance of the person
To cooperate with treatment	To empower clients
	To educate clients

The services of nursing assistants and patient care technicians (PCTs) are just as important in the mental health setting as they are in acute care. Certified nursing assistants (CNAs) help nurses with client care and treatments. PCTs have advanced CNA training and are relatively new to the health care profession. However, both roles have expanded into the community, where they have met with success.

To illustrate, the Supportive Homemaker Program of Haverhill, Massachusetts, employs mental health supportive home care aides (HCAs) to provide emotional and social support for clients in their homes. The program is designed to serve children who are at risk for abuse or neglect, people who lack family or social support, depressed people, severely ill people, and senile elderly adults.

The program depends on the HCA's abilities. Those who demonstrate an acceptance of others, compassion, cultural awareness, patience, and a gentle sense of humor are selected. Once a modest training period is completed, each HCA is assigned a caseload and a psychiatric nurse coordinator, who provides support and guidance.

With frequent visits, the HCA establishes a relationship with each client. Because they are not threatening, are nonjudgmental, and represent no authority, supportive HCAs provide a reliable relationship that helps to ease the anxiety and apprehension of being alone or unable to cope.

The main function of supportive HCAs is to act as helping individuals. Responsibilities include providing homemaker services, transportation, and instruction. Skills in daily activities, home management, and self-care are taught and reinforced on subsequent visits. The importance of good nutrition and medical care for children is stressed. When teaching is needed, clients are instructed in ways to obtain food, clothing, shelter, and education.

Supportive HCAs encourage clients to use appropriate community resources. They act as advocates by instructing clients about how services can help, assisting them in making contact with specific services, and providing transportation for appointments. The success of these mental health care providers lies not with their academic or political prowess but with one fundamental thought: they are there to care—to help, to make things better.

Other providers of care for mentally troubled people are the psychiatric technicians who are formally trained to provide mental health care in both inpatient and outpatient settings. "Psych techs" were once commonly employed in large state institutions, but as clients were discharged into the community, their numbers became smaller. Today, psychiatric technicians can be found in practice settings ranging from community mental health centers to prisons. As mental health care moves into the community, larger numbers of care providers will be needed.

EXPANDED ROLE FOR NURSES

The profession of nursing has undergone many changes in the past 20 years. The "handmaiden to the physician" model has been replaced by the role of a professional, with all its accompanying rights and obligations. Nurses of today are considered experts in the area of assisting people in coping with the impact of health problems on everyday living. They are guided by each state's nurse practice act and professional standards of care. Appendix A describes psychiatric nursing standards.

Nurses participate fully as members of the treatment team. They also provide education for clients and their significant others and coordinate the activities of various therapeutic interventions and support agencies. Nurses' roles are continuing to evolve, and the challenge every nurse must face is to grow with change.

As mental health care moves into the community, new roles are opening up for nurses. Hospitals no longer employ the majority of nurses because attempts to control costs have decreased the numbers of nurses per institution. Clients are being discharged from acute care facilities earlier and now require nursing services in their homes and communities. Because nurses help people to adjust to and cope with the changes in daily living that result from their illness or condition, they practice in a number of challenging new settings.

For example, nurses play a vital role in centers for homeless people where treatment teams assess each client for medical, psychiatric, and social service needs. The role of the nurse is one of facilitator/advocate who assists clients in gaining access to services. Nurses commonly perform unconventional nursing tasks and must be flexible with treatment plans. Collaboration with the multidisciplinary treatment team and numerous community agencies assists them in referring clients to various resources.

Preventive health care is another main responsibility of these nurses. Routine screening for weight, hypertension, and response to medications allows them many opportunities to instruct clients in more healthful living activities. Weekly lectures and discussions about proper nutrition, sexually transmitted diseases, and current health issues are planned and conducted by nurses. Realistic goals are set to encourage clients to commit to meeting their needs, and much support by all members of the staff helps clients to regain their self-esteem (see Case Study 33-1).

Nurses also collaborate with physicians to plan and implement programs for people with serious mental illness. One such program employs only nurses as case managers because they value continuity of care and are knowledgeable and comfortable with medication management. **Nurse case managers** work with psychiatrists to develop treatment plans tailored to each client's special needs. Clients are encouraged to share their concerns with their nurse case manager, who evaluates the need for psychiatric consultation. Nurses

Case Study 33-1

A 30-year-old man presents to the treatment center complaining of overwhelming feelings of agitation and hostility. During the nurse's initial assessment, the client reveals that he has not been taking his psychotherapeutic medications because they make him too drowsy. "So, this is not an uncommon complaint," the nurse thinks; but on further questioning, the nurse discovers that the client becomes vulnerable to street predators when he sleeps after taking his medication. In fact, the client reveals that he has often been mugged and beaten while sleeping in subways.

At the nurse's request, the client's medications were adjusted. The client agreed to come to the center for daily administration and monitoring. After a few months, his behavior changes were so remarkable that he was able to become reunited with his family. He continues to visit the treatment center daily for support and evaluation.

- How can Maslow's hierarchy of needs be applied to this case?
- How did the nurse's assessment lead to changes in the client's life?

and psychiatrists meet weekly for discussions and decisions about each client's medications, therapies, and referrals.

Nurses in this setting provide intake assessments and referral services, initial and ongoing medication services, supportive counseling, and individual and group education. They act as advocates for clients interacting with family, the legal system, or other parts of the health care system. Because of the nurse case manager's support and guidance, clients with severe mental illnesses are able to function more adequately within their community and costly and unnecessary psychiatric consultations are reduced. The nurse-physician collaborative practice model may prove to be one solution to the challenge of delivering mental health care to clients within their home environments.

Psychosocial (psychiatric) rehabilitation is another area in which nurses are expanding their roles. Evolving as a social model of treatment rather than a medical model, psychosocial rehabilitation is a way of assisting people with mental health problems in readjusting and adapting to life in the community. In these settings, nurses are able to use their full range of skills without the focus being placed on illness or disability. Wellness, wholeness, and the abilities of the individual are emphasized. Vocational, educational, residential, social, and personal adjustment services are offered. Clients are encouraged to exercise freedom of choice and become consciously self-directed. Individual care plans, called "personal service plans," are developed but controlled by clients who identify the goals that are important to them. Resources and support people are chosen by the clients with guidance from the treatment team (referred to as a service delivery team).

Self-help is a fundamental concept of psychosocial rehabilitation. Care team members offer social and vocational coaching, but clients must act for themselves. The belief that all people have the inherent capacity for change and the focus on what the client can do have resulted in some remarkable successes. Nurses who practice within these settings truly work with persons in their environment to maximize wellness.

As health care moves into the community, the need for mental health clinical nurse specialists will continue to grow. Mental health (psychiatric) home care nurses focus on prevention and wellness care. They collaborate with other professionals and serve as the client's advocate within the mental health delivery system. Clients who are facing the crises of illness are assisted with both their physical and emotional difficulties. Because they are able to intervene during the early stages of dysfunction, the services of mental health home care nurses are proving to be successful as well as cost-effective.

One of the most exciting expanded roles for nurses is that of entrepreneur, or self-employed nurse. Today, nurses are establishing their own clinics, acting as health care consultants, and working to provide a variety of health care services to business and industry. Mental health care nurses are involved in businesses that provide services for adults, children, employees, organizations, and public and government agencies. Nurses are accepting the challenge to seek out and create innovative models for the delivery of mental health care services.

MANAGING CHANGE

Because life is a dynamic process, all living things undergo change. Seasons, plants, people, and processes all change. All providers must keep pace with continual changes in health care, new therapies, theories, medications, and more. Therefore it is important to understand the characteristics of change and how to successfully cope and adapt.

Change process is defined as the series of steps that result in a difference. **Change itself is inherently neither good nor bad.** The reactions of the people involved in the process label or judge a change.

People resist change because it implies uncertainty, which brings about a disturbance in the status quo. We all resist change to some extent to maintain our equilibrium and keep things "the way they are." People resist change for several reasons. Although major problems may be present in the current situation, they are known and comfortable. Change brings about discomfort when the status quo is disrupted. Individuals may feel that their self-interests are threatened. They may have inaccurate perceptions about the nature or implications of the changes or become so threatened that they begin to use psychological defense mechanisms to defend their viewpoints. Some people resist

Box 33-1 | *Reasons People Resist Change*

1. Problems are known and comfortable.
2. Change brings about discomfort.
3. Change disrupts the status quo.
4. Individuals feel their self-interests are threatened.
5. Individuals have inaccurate perceptions about the nature or implications of the change.
6. Individuals may believe the changes will not be beneficial.

Table 33-2 | *Coping With Unplanned Change*

NURSING ACTION	COMMENTS
Do not panic.	Remain calm no matter what happens. Keep your own reactions under control by staying in the "thinking" mode. Remember decisions made during high stress are more likely to be ineffective. Stay cool.
Analyze the situation.	Define the problems that are occurring as a result of the change. Assess why the change is happening now, and consider its possible effects. Assess resources and limitations.
Reset priorities.	Determine what needs to be done. List needs in order of importance, and then communicate and act.
Match resources with priorities.	Match what needs to be done with the best available resource. Resources are always limited. Do the best you can with what you have.
Continuously evaluate.	This step is even more important when the change is unplanned. Monitor individuals and groups as they progress through the change process. Monitor the situation's dynamics. Be prepared for the possibility of other changes.

change because they truly believe the changes will not be beneficial (Box 33-1). Dealing effectively with change requires a period of transition and psychological adaptation. Understanding the change process will help both care providers and clients adapt to the continuing process of change.

THE CHANGE PROCESS

There are two basic types of change: **planned** change and **unplanned** change (Morrison, 1993). Planned change is the deliberate effort to make things different within a system. Changes are carefully planned and implemented slowly and deliberately. When done appropriately, planned change meets with minimal hostility and resistance. Planned change is always the ideal, but seldom the reality.

Unplanned change is unexpected, not anticipated, and usually not desired. Change happens whether it is planned or unexpected. In health care settings, unplanned changes are daily occurrences. "Expect the unexpected" is a statement often made by managers and supervisors in the workplace to describe unplanned change.

Whether change is unanticipated or expected, intense reactions are provoked in some people. Although reactions to change are highly individual and can range from simple acceptance to outright hostility, most reactions can be generalized into three categories: anxiety, mistrust, and loss. All these reactions affect mental health clients.

When the comfort of a daily routine is lost, people (especially those with mental health problems) become anxious. Planned changes for these clients must be implemented slowly, in small steps, giving time for adjustment. Unexpected change, however, does not allow for this luxury, and anxiety levels increase.

Mistrust develops when people are unclear about what is happening. Once individuals feel threatened, resistance develops, and an "us versus them" attitude evolves. To keep mistrust at a minimum, maintain open communications with all those involved in the change. Listen to everyone's concerns, and provide what information you can.

Change also involves loss when one gives up old, comfortable attitudes or behaviors. Phrases such as "in the old days" or "the way we used to do it" are expres-

sions associated with loss. Replacing loss with hope by focusing on possible benefits helps people to cope with change, especially if it is unexpected. Hints for coping with unplanned changes are offered in Table 32-2.

Mental health care providers must be especially adept at coping with unexpected changes. Change affects us all, but adaptability, healthy emotional responses, and a willingness to support ourselves and others go a long way toward meeting the challenge of coping successfully with changes in today's busy world.

OTHER CHALLENGES

Life today is filled with a myriad of personal, professional, and social challenges. Personally, we are constantly challenged to move calmly through the struggles of everyday living. Professionally, we are charged with all the obligations and responsibilities of a helping professional, not to mention our duty to the people who become our clients. Socially, we are confronted with many complex relationships and interrelated social problems.

CHALLENGES TO SOCIETY

The social order of many countries is being disrupted by change. Third World countries must cope with the problems of providing the basic necessities of life (food, clothing, shelter) for their citizens. Health care and education are placed lower on the priority list when a country's people are going hungry or are without shelter. Add to this various political disputes, wars, and terrorist activities and one can see why so many challenges to mental health exist throughout the world.

Modern industrial societies usually manage to feed and clothe the majority of their citizens, but numerous social problems remain. Family structures are changing in many societies. This one factor alone spins off new challenges related to child rearing, financial support, role changes, and group interactions. Homeless families are growing, and with homelessness comes the loss of opportunities for appropriate health care and a solid education. Violence is on the upswing because some persons cannot tolerate the stresses of the modern world.

Social problems affecting health care include challenges to immunize children; control the spread of sophisticated new communicable diseases; provide humane care for the ill, infirm, and aged populations; and educate the general population about healthy living practices. Politically, nurses and all people interested in health are challenged to make health care more accessible, delivering primary care in convenient, familiar community settings.

PERSONS WITH AIDS

Individuals with HIV who progress to the next stage of the disease are known as "persons with AIDS," or PWAs. Because of the long incubation period, the changing nature of the virus, and the attitudes of many people, PWAs pose a special challenge for health care providers.

Early detection of HIV infections is important, especially for those who work with mental health clients. Individuals with HIV can have signs of central nervous system damage that may present as a psychiatric illness. Many demonstrate "mental symptoms" before the better known opportunistic infections develop. Clients may have a single complaint or multiple symptoms (Box 33-2). Many of these complaints can be mistaken for mental illness, so each must be carefully investigated.

Homeless youth and chronically mentally ill individuals are at an increased risk for contracting HIV. Lack of judgment and high-risk sexual and substance abuse behaviors make these groups of people especially vulnerable. The incidence of HIV infection is increasing in the 15- to 25-year-old age-group because of the lack of accurate information and the syndrome of "it can't happen to me" so common to many individuals of that age. Community health care providers must meet the challenge to develop new comprehensive knowledge and skills to serve an ever-increasing population of clients with HIV.

INFORMATION OVERLOAD

No single person can keep up with all the new knowledge constantly being generated. **Information overload** is a state of mind in which so many facts have

| Box 33-2 | *Mental Signs and Symptoms of HIV Infection* |

Agitation
Apathy
Confusion
Decreased memory function
Dementia
Emotional changes
Poor appetite
Sleep disturbances
Slowed thinking
Tiredness, lethargy

HIV, Human immunodeficiency virus.

been absorbed that they all become an unrelated jumble of stored information. It is easy to become overwhelmed with information today. More information has become available to the average citizen. In addition, integrated communication systems offer an even greater availability of information. Clients are becoming more informed, and sometimes their information contains inaccuracies or half-truths. Health care providers have the responsibility to be accurately informed and knowledgeable about the health care information each client is receiving.

"But how do I cope with the bombardment of information?" you wonder. Learn something new every day. We cannot be expected to move through our daily activities and spend our remaining hours pondering over the latest facts or theories, but we can commit ourselves to making the effort to discover something we did not know this morning. Strive to learn at least one new piece of information each day. By the end of 1 year, you will have gained much new knowledge.

Be open to new information. Some things that sound silly in one period become reality in another. People said in the 1950s that humans would never walk on the moon. Now space travel is taken for granted. Do not discard information that does not fit into your way of thinking. Keep it tucked away. Sooner or later it will prove itself to be accurate or false.

Learn to think critically. Use logical thinking and the problem-solving process to practice critical thinking skills. Maintain an open mind and a questioning attitude. Realize that knowing how to question and relate information is more important than having many facts at hand. This is one of our great challenges.

THE CHALLENGE TO CARE

People remember the health care workers who cared for them, who listened, who held their hand, and who supported them when times were rough. Caring is the essence of nursing and the power of the health care professions. Do not become so involved in the physical aspects that you forget to nurture the art of caring for people. Scientific evidence is lending new support for the actions that make up the art of caring.

Connections between the mind and body are an intricate network that responds as a whole. Emotions are responses of a whole person, complete with physical and psychological reactions. Certain therapeutic actions, such as touch, have been found to reduce anxiety levels and may play a role in actually boosting the immune system by decreasing the immunosuppressive effects of stress. Therapeutic touch can decrease pain and promote wound healing. The U.S. government has funded research into the effects of therapeutic touch on the immune system's response to stress. Therapeutic emotional interventions are finally receiving scientific attention. We have known all along that caring is a powerful weapon in the search for health and wholeness.

A LOOK TO THE FUTURE

All areas of human functioning are deeply interwoven. Physical illnesses are always accompanied by some level of emotional, intellectual, social, and spiritual distress. The opposite is also true. Therefore "psychiatric" or "mental health" care is a critical component of every therapeutic situation. Caring for the physical body is not enough. For high levels of wellness and adaptation, the whole individual, every aspect of the dynamic being we call "the client," must be considered with every therapeutic action.

Health is defined by the client's criteria for wellness. Care providers emphasize clients' strengths and their abilities to adapt and to change. By working with clients' personal definitions of health, the focus is on their goals, and an understanding of the interactions between them and their complex and changing environments is gained.

Nurses help clients to adjust to the activities of daily living when clients are confronted by health problems. Because of this, they are in the position to shift the focus of health care from one that concentrates on "deficits and deficiencies" to one that considers the possibilities and positive achievements that are within the grasp of each client. This health-oriented point of view allows for successful interventions by concentrating on solutions that draw on clients' strengths and supportive resources.

The health care professions are undergoing change. Because mental distress or illness affects every aspect of a person's life, the care needs of individuals with acute and chronic mental health problems are many. Although issues affecting mental health policies in the United States and elsewhere are being explored, too few resources are available for treating the numerous individuals who require therapeutic care. As a result, nurses and other health care providers must consider every interaction with their clients as an opportunity for encouraging high levels of mental health. If we are to make progress with the social problems of crime, violence, abuse, homelessness, and poverty, we must treat each mentally troubled person as our most important client because the mental health of a society depends on the mental health of each of its individual citizens.

It is an exciting time to be a health care provider. Maintain a positive attitude. Do your best and strive to learn. Numerous challenges await us. Perhaps one of the greatest will be to bring caring into the community that ensures health care services will be available to every individual.

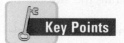
Key Points

- Challenges facing health care providers are escalating costs, sociocultural changes, and advances in technology.
- Treatment settings for people with mental illness have evolved from the institution to the street, jail, neighborhood clinic, community hospital, and local physician's office.
- Historically, homeless people were white male adults who were about 50 years old, unmarried, intermittently employed, and with no permanent residence.
- Today's homeless people are younger and much poorer; and one third of homeless people are families.
- The Americans With Disabilities Act of 1990 states that people with mental health problems have the same opportunity for employment as other people.
- Learning to interact respectfully and effectively with people from different cultures is an important challenge for health care workers.
- The interdisciplinary (multidisciplinary) mental health care team is the client, physician, psychologist, nurse, dietitian, social worker, minister, occupational therapist, and other specialists as needed. The main function is to coordinate care as the client moves from inpatient to community settings and through the health care system.
- The role of client has changed from passive participant to active consumer of health care services.
- To be considered competent, an individual must be able to make a choice, understand important information, appreciate one's own situation, and apply reasoning.
- Clients are obligated to be truthful, responsible, and cooperative with care.
- Care providers are obligated to accept the client "as is," demonstrate respect, empower clients, and educate.
- Today's mental health care providers include certified nursing assistants, home care aides, and psychiatric technicians.
- Expanded roles for nurses include positions in centers for homeless people, collaborating with physicians as case managers, working with psychosocial rehabilitation teams, and meeting the needs of special populations through nurse-owned businesses.

- Change, the process of making something different or becoming different, is inherently neither good nor bad.
- Early detection of HIV infections is especially important because many clients with HIV show signs of central nervous system damage that may present as a psychiatric illness.
- To cope with information overload, develop your critical thinking skills by using logical thinking and the problem-solving process.

- Care providers are in the position to shift the focus of health care from one that concentrates on deficits and deficiencies to one that considers the possibilities and positive achievements that are within the grasp of each client.

evolve   Be sure to visit the companion Evolve site at http://evolve.elsevier.com/Morrison-Valfre/ for additional online resources.

A Standards of Practice for Psychiatric–Mental Health Nursing

STANDARD 1. ASSESSMENT

The psychiatric–mental health registered nurse collects comprehensive health data that is pertinent to the patient's health or situation.

STANDARD 2. DIAGNOSIS

The psychiatric–mental health registered nurse analyzes the assessment data to determine diagnoses or problems, including level of risk.

STANDARD 3. OUTCOMES IDENTIFICATION

The psychiatric–mental health registered nurse identifies expected outcomes for a plan individualized to the patient or to the situation.

STANDARD 4. PLANNING

The psychiatric–mental health registered nurse develops a plan that prescribes strategies and alternatives to attain expected outcomes.

STANDARD 5. IMPLEMENTATION

The psychiatric–mental health registered nurse implements the identified plan.

STANDARD 5A. COORDINATION OF CARE

The psychiatric–mental health registered nurse coordinates care delivery.

STANDARD 5B. HEALTH TEACHING AND HEALTH PROMOTION

The psychiatric–mental health registered nurse employs strategies to promote health and a safe environment.

STANDARD 5C. MILIEU THERAPY

The psychiatric–mental health registered nurse provides, structures, and maintains a safe and therapeutic environment in collaboration with patients, families, and other health care clinicians.

STANDARD 5D. PHARMACOLOGICAL, BIOLOGICAL, AND INTERGRATIVE THERAPIES

The psychiatric–mental health registered nurse incorporates knowledge of pharmacological, biological, and complementary interventions with applied clinical skills to restore the patient's health and prevent further disability.

STANDARD 5E. PRESCRIPTIVE AUTHORITY AND TREATMENT

The psychiatric–mental health advanced practice registered nurse uses prescriptive authority, procedures, referrals, treatments, and therapies in accordance with state and federal laws and regulations.

STANDARD 5F. PSYCHOTHERAPY

The psychiatric–mental health advanced practice registered nurse conducts individual, couples, group, and family psychotherapy using evidence-based psychotherapeutic frameworks and nurse–patient therapeutic relationships.

STANDARD 5G. CONSULTATION

The psychiatric–mental health registered nurse provides consultation to influence the identified plan, enhance the abilities of other clinicians to provide services for patients, and effect change.

STANDARD 6. EVALUATION

The psychiatric–mental health registered nurse evaluates progress toward attainment of expected outcomes.

From American Nurses Association, American Psychiatric Nurses Association, and International Society of Psychiatric-Mental Health Nurses: *Psychiatric-mental health nursing: scope and standards of practice,* Silver Spring, MD, 2007, The Association.

B DSM-IV-TR Classification

NOS = Not Otherwise Specified.

An *x* appearing in a diagnostic code indicates that a specific code number is required.

An ellipsis (…) is used in the names of certain disorders to indicate that the name of a specific mental disorder or general medical condition should be inserted when recording the name (e.g., 293.0 Delirium Due to Hypothyroidism).

If criteria are currently met, one of the following severity specifiers may be noted after the diagnosis:
Mild
Moderate
Severe

If criteria are no longer met, one of the following specifiers may be noted:
In Partial Remission
In Full Remission
Prior History

DISORDERS USUALLY FIRST DIAGNOSED IN INFANCY, CHILDHOOD, OR ADOLESCENCE

Mental Retardation

Learning Disorders

Motor Skills Disorder

Communication Disorders

Pervasive Developmental Disorders

Attention-Deficit and Disruptive Behavior Disorders

Feeding and Eating Disorders of Infancy or Early Childhood

Tic Disorders

Elimination Disorders

Other Disorders of Infancy, Childhood, or Adolescence

DELIRIUM, DEMENTIA, AND AMNESTIC AND OTHER COGNITIVE DISORDERS

Delirium

Dementia

Amnestic Disorders

Other Cognitive Disorders

MENTAL DISORDERS DUE TO A GENERAL MEDICAL CONDITION NOT ELSEWHERE CLASSIFIED

SUBSTANCE-RELATED DISORDERS

Alcohol-Related Disorders
Alcohol Use Disorders
Alcohol-Induced Disorders

Amphetamine (or Amphetamine-Like)–Related Disorders
Amphetamine Use Disorders
Amphetamine-Induced Disorders

Caffeine-Related Disorders
Caffeine-Induced Disorders

Cannabis-Related Disorders
Cannabis Use Disorders
Cannabis-Induced Disorders

Cocaine-Related Disorders
Cocaine Use Disorders
Cocaine-Induced Disorders

Hallucinogen-Related Disorders
Hallucinogen Use Disorders
Hallucinogen-Induced Disorders

Inhalant-Related Disorders
Inhalant Use Disorders
Inhalant-Induced Disorders

From American Psychiatric Association: *Diagnostic and statistical manual of mental disorders*, ed 4, text revision. Washington, DC, 2000, American Psychiatric Association.

Nicotine-Related Disorders
Nicotine Use Disorder
Nicotine-Induced Disorder

Opioid-Related Disorders
Opioid Use Disorders
Opioid-Induced Disorders

Phencyclidine (or Phencyclidine-Like)–Related Disorders
Phencyclidine Use Disorders
Phencyclidine-Induced Disorders

Sedative-, Hypnotic-, or Anxiolytic-Related Disorders
Sedative, Hypnotic, or Anxiolytic Use Disorders
Sedative-, Hypnotic-, or Anxiolytic-Induced Disorders
Polysubstance-Related Disorder

Other (or Unknown) Substance-Related Disorders
Other (or Unknown) Substance Use Disorders
Other (or Unknown) Substance-Induced Disorders

SCHIZOPHRENIA AND OTHER PSYCHOTIC DISORDERS

Other or Unspecified Pattern

MOOD DISORDERS

Depressive Disorders

Bipolar Disorders

ANXIETY DISORDERS

SOMATOFORM DISORDERS

FACTITIOUS DISORDERS

DISSOCIATIVE DISORDERS

SEXUAL AND GENDER IDENTITY DISORDERS
Sexual Dysfunctions

Sexual Arousal Disorders

Orgasmic Disorders

Sexual Pain Disorders

Sexual Dysfunction Due to a General Medical Condition

Paraphilias

Gender Identity Disorders

EATING DISORDERS

SLEEP DISORDERS
Primary Sleep Disorders
Dyssomnias
Parasomnias

Sleep Disorders Related to Another Mental Disorder

Other Sleep Disorders

IMPULSE-CONTROL DISORDERS NOT ELSEWHERE CLASSIFIED

ADJUSTMENT DISORDERS

PERSONALITY DISORDERS

OTHER CONDITIONS THAT MAY BE A FOCUS OF CLINICAL ATTENTION
Psychologic Factors Affecting Medical Condition

Medication-Induced Movement Disorders

Other Medication-Induced Disorder

Relational Problems

Problems Related to Abuse or Neglect

Additional Conditions That May Be a Focus of Clinical Attention

ADDITIONAL CODES

MULTIAXIAL SYSTEM

Other Conditions That May Be a Focus of Clinical Attention

Mental Retardation

C Mental Status Assessment at a Glance

1. Appearance
Manner of dress

_____

Personal grooming

_____

Facial expressions

_____

Posture and gait

_____

2. Speech
Manner of response (frank, evading)

_____

Choice of words (to assess general intelligence, education, levels of function, thought)

_____

Speech disorder

_____

3. Level of consciousness
Level of alertness

_____

Orientation (time, place, person)

_____

4. Attention span
Ability to keep thoughts focused on one topic

_____

Repeat a series of numbers

_____

Serial 7s (ask client to subtract 7 from 100, 7 from 93, and so on)

_____

5. Memory
Immediate memory (ask client to repeat words after 15 minutes)

_____

Recent memory (ask client about yesterday's activities)

_____

Remote memory (ask client about dates of birth, marriage, schooling)

_____

6. Understanding abstract relationships
Understanding of proverbs (concrete or abstract)

_____

Ability to understand similarities (e.g., "How are a bicycle and an automobile alike?")

_____

7. Arithmetic and reading ability
Simple addition, subtraction, multiplication, and division (ask client to make change)

_____

Ability to read newspaper, magazine

_____

8. General information knowledge
Discuss newspaper or magazine article

_____

General information questions (e.g., "How many days in a year? Where does the sun set?")

_____

9. Judgment
Responses to family, work, financial problems

_____

Responses to "What would you do if ...?" questions

_____

10. Emotional status
Ask, "How do you feel today?" or "How do you feel about ...?" questions

_____

Affect (mood)

_____

Current situation and coping behaviors

_____

Modified from Jess LW: Investigating impaired mental status: an assessment guide you can use, _Nursing_ 18(6):42, 1988.

D A Simple Method to Determine Tardive Dyskinesia Symptoms: AIMS Examination Procedure[*]

Patient Identification   _____

Date   _____

1. Observe the client unobtrusively at rest (e.g., in waiting room). (The chair used in this examination should be a hard, firm one without arms.)
2. After observing the client, he or she is rated on a scale according to the severity of symptoms:
   - 0 = none
   - 1 = minimal
   - 2 = mild
   - 3 = moderate
   - 4 = severe
3. Ask the client whether there is anything in his or her mouth (i.e., gum, candy) and, if there is, to please remove it.
4. Ask the client about the current condition of his or her teeth or dentures. Do teeth or dentures bother client now?
_____ 5. Ask the client if any movements in mouth, face, hands, or feet are noticed. If yes, ask to describe and to what extent they currently bother or interfere with activities.

_____ 6. Have client sit in chair with hands on knees, legs slightly apart, and feet flat on floor. (Look at entire body for movements while in this position.)
_____ 7. Ask client to sit with hands hanging unsupported. (Observe hands and other body areas.)
_____ 8. Ask patient to open mouth. (Observe tongue at rest within mouth.) Do this twice.
_____ 9. Ask client to protrude tongue. (Observe abnormalities of tongue movement.) Do this twice.
_____10. Ask client to tap thumb, with each finger, as rapidly as possible for 10 to 15 seconds, separately with right hand, then with left hand. (Observe facial and leg movements.)
_____11. Flex and extend client's left and right arms (one at a time).
_____12. Ask client to stand up. (Observe in profile. Observe all body areas again, hips included.)
_____13. Ask client to extend both arms outstretched in front with palms down. (Observe trunk, legs, and mouth.)
14. Have client walk a few paces, turn, and walk back to chair. (Observe hands and gait.) Do this twice.[†]

_____
From Sandoz Pharmaceuticals, East Hanover, NJ.
*AIMS, Abnormal Involuntary Movement Scale.
†Activated movements.

Chapter 1 The History of Mental Health Care
Suggestion for Further Reading
An excellent text about psychiatric practices through the ages is *The History of Psychiatry*, written by Franz Alexander and Sheldon Selesnick (New York, 1996, The New American Library).

References
Ackerknecht EW: *A short history of medicine*, New York, 1968, The Ronald Press.

Alexander FG, Selesnick ST: *The history of psychiatry*, New York, 1966, The New American Library.

Anderson KN, Anderson LE, Glanze WD, editors: *Mosby's medical, nursing, & allied health dictionary*, ed 7, St Louis, 2006, Mosby.

Dolan J: *History of nursing*, Philadelphia, 1968, WB Saunders.

Donahue MP: *Nursing: the finest art*, ed 2, St Louis, 1996, Mosby.

Harrington SPM: New bedlam: jails—not psychiatric hospitals—now care for the mentally ill indigent, *The Humanist* 59(3):9, 1999.

Kelly LY: *Dimensions of professional nursing*, ed 6, New York, 1991, Pergamon Press.

Keltner NL, Folks DG: *Psychotropic drugs*, ed 4, St Louis, 2005, Mosby.

Morrissey JP, Goldman HH: Cycles of reform in the care of the chronically mentally ill, *Hosp Community Psychiatry* 35(89): 785, 1984.

National Alliance on Mental Illness (NAMI): *Grading the States, A Report on America's Health Care System for Serious Mental Illness*, www.nami.org, 2006.

Taylor CM: *Essentials of psychiatric nursing*, ed 14, St Louis, 1994, Mosby.

Chapter 2 Current Mental Health Care Systems
Suggestion for Further Reading
Your daily newspaper offers discussions about our current health policies, proposed changes to the health care delivery system, proposed and adopted mental health care legislation, and events that shape attitudes toward the mentally and emotionally troubled populations.

References
Haber J and others: *Comprehensive psychiatric nursing*, ed 5, St Louis, 1997, Mosby.

Harrington SPM: New bedlam: jails—not psychiatric hospitals—now care for indigent mentally ill, *The Humanist* 59(3):9, 1999.

Kirkpatrick DC: Mental health care above and below the 49th parallel, *Harvard Mental Health Letter* 15(11):1, 1999.

National Mental Health Association: *National prevention coalition position statement*, no. 9, Alexandria, Va, 1999, The Association.

Procter BD, Dalaker J: Poverty in the United States, 2001. In *Current population reports*, Washington, DC, 2002, U.S. Census Bureau.

Salkever D and others: Assertive community treatment for people with severe mental illness, *Health Serv Res* 34(2):577, 1999.

Sherer RA: Mental health care in the developing world, *Psychiatric Times* 9(1), 2002.

U.S. Surgeon General: *Mental health: a report of the surgeon general*, Washington, DC, 2002, U.S. Government Printing Office.

Walker C: Homeless people and mental health, *Am J Nurs* 98(26), 1998.

Chapter 3 Ethical and Legal Issues
Suggestion for Further Reading
"Document it Right" by Maureen Habel in *Nurse Week* (4[1]: 20-21, 2003) explains the value of legally credible documentation. All caregivers will find this interesting.

References
Edelman CL, Mandle CL: *Health promotion throughout the lifespan*, ed 6, St Louis, 2006, Mosby.

Keltner NL, Schwecke LH, Bostrom CE: *Psychiatric nursing*, ed 5, St Louis, 2007, Mosby.

Loewy EH: Ethical considerations in executing and implementing advanced directives, *Arch Intern Med* 58(4):32, 1998.

Morrison MW: *Professional skills for leadership: foundations of a successful career*, St Louis, 1993, Mosby.

Potter PA, Perry AG: *Fundamentals of nursing: concepts, process, and practice*, ed 7, St Louis, 2009, Mosby.

Stuart GW: *Handbook of psychiatric nursing*, ed 6, St Louis, 2005, Mosby.

Chapter 4 Sociocultural Issues
Suggestion for Further Reading
Pocket Guide to Cultural Health Assessment, ed 3, by CE D'Avanso and EM Geissler (St Louis, 2003, Mosby) is interesting reading and an excellent source of information for many cultural groups. It is highly recommended for all health care providers.

References
D'Avanso CE, Geissler EM: *Pocket guide to cultural health assessment*, ed 3, St Louis, 2003, Mosby.

Edelman CL, Mandle CL: *Health promotion throughout the lifespan*, ed 6, St Louis, 2006, Mosby.

Flaskerud JH: Ethnicity, cultures, and neuropsychiatry, *Issues Ment Health Nurs* 21(1), 2000.

Giger JN, Davidhizar RE: *Transcultural nursing: assessment and intervention*, ed 5, St Louis, 2008, Mosby.

Haber J and others: *Comprehensive psychiatric nursing*, ed 5, St Louis, 1997, Mosby.

Jackson VH: Cultural competency, *Behavioral Health Management* 22(2):21, 2002.

Lipson JG: Afghan refugees in California: mental health issues, *Issues Ment Health Nurs* 14:411, 1993.

Orrell MW: Perceptions of schizophrenia in multi-cultural Britain, *Ethnicity & Health* 20(7):7, 2003.

Rairdan B, Higgs ZR: When your patient is a Hmong refugee, *Am J Nurs* 92(3):52, 1992.

Taylor CM: *Essentials of psychiatric nursing*, ed 14, St Louis, 1994, Mosby.

Chapter 5 Theories and Therapies
Suggestion for Further Reading
Toward a Psychology of Being by Abraham Maslow (New York, 1968, Van Nostrand Reinhold) presents an interesting discussion of the potential we all are capable of achieving.

References
Ader R: *Psychoneuroimmunology*, New York, 1981, Academic Press.

Adler A: *The individual psychology of Alfred Adler: a systematic presentation in selections from his writings*, ed 2, New York, 1964, Harper & Row.

Bandura A: *Social foundations of thought and action: a social cognitive theory*, Englewood Cliffs, NJ, 1986, Prentice-Hall.

Corsini RJ, editor: *Encyclopedia of psychology*, ed 2, New York, 1994, John Wiley & Sons.

Dillon KM, Minchoff B, Baker KH: Positive emotional states and enhancement of the immune system, *Int J Psychiatry Med* 15:13, 1985.

Glasser W: *Reality therapy: a new approach to psychiatry*, New York, 1965, Harper & Row.

Graves, B: Brain therapy study offers hope, *The Oregonian*, 157(52,468):B2, 2007.

Jung CG: *Analytical psychology: its theory and practice*, New York, 1968, Random House.

Maslow AH: *The farthest reaches of human nature*, New York, 1971, Viking Press.

Royce JR, Powell AD: *A theory of personality and individual differences*, Englewood Cliffs, NJ, 1983, Prentice-Hall.

Selye H: *Stress in health and disease*, Toronto, 1976, Butterworth Press.

Skinner BF: Behaviorism at fifty, *Science* 140:951, 1963.

Smoyak S: American psychiatric nursing: history and roles, *AAOHN J* 41(7):316, 1993.

Szasz TS: *The myth of mental illness: foundations of a theory of personal conduct*, ed 2, New York, 1974, Harper & Row.

Wilson HS: The 1990s as the decade of the brain, *Capsules of Community Psychiatric Nursing* 1(1):1, 1994.

Chapter 6 Complementary and Alternative Therapies

Suggestions for Further Reading

A wealth of information about meditation is available through The Center for Mindfulness at the University of Massachusetts (website www.umass.edu/cfm).

References
Beecher H: *Measurement of subjective response*, New York, NY: Oxford University Press, 1959.

Bierman SF: Medical hypnosis, *Adv J Mind-Body Health* 11(1):65, 1995.

Boiron T: *Easy guide to homeopathy*, Newtown Square, PA, 2007.

Glaser G: Eye-catching therapy, *The Oregonian*, 155(52,420):C1, August 23, 2006.

Glower T: Your best alternative, *Health*, 19(6), 2005.

Green S: Chelation therapy: unproven claims and unsound theories, *Quackwatch*, www.quackwatch.org. Accessed June 27, 2007.

ICBS, Inc: *History of aromatherapy* (website): www.holisticonline.com. Accessed June 26, 2007.

Moore S: Meditation. In Corsini RJ, editor: *Encyclopedia of psychology*, ed 2, New York, 1994, John Wiley.

NCCAM: National Center for Complementary and Alternative Medicine: *Energy medicine: an overview*, www.nccam.nil.gov/health. Accessed July 2, 2007.

NCCAM: National Center for Complementary and Alternative Medicine: *Biologically based practices: an overview*, www.nccam.nil.gov/health. Accessed June 26, 2007.

NCCAM: National Center for Complementary and Alternative Medicine: *What is CAM?* www.nccam.nil.gov/health. Accessed May 23, 2007.

Pellegrini N, Ruggeri M: The diffusion and the reason for the use of complementary and alternative medicine among users of mental health services: a systematic review of literature, *Epidemiology Psychiatry Soc* 16(1):35-49, 2007.

Rawlins RP, Williams SR, Beck CK: *Mental health–psychiatric nursing: a holistic life-cycle approach*, ed 3, St Louis, 1993, Mosby.

Sarnat RL: The future is now, *Total Health* 23(2):22, 2001.

Rosenthal N: *Winter blues: SAD—what it is and how to overcome it*, New York, 1993, Guilford Press.

Vaughn D: Doggone helpful, *NurseWeek*, 8(13):20, 2007.

Chapter 7 Psychotherapeutic Drug Therapy

Suggestions for Further Reading

The book titled *Psychotropic Drugs*, fourth edition, by Norman Keltner and David Folks (St Louis, 2005, Mosby), offers a thorough discussion of most medications for mental health problems.

Several websites, such as *www.crescentlife.com* and *www.findarticles.com*, offer a wealth of information about psychiatric drugs.

References
Balon R: Managing compliance, *Psychiatric Times* 19(5):1, 2002.

Finkelman AW: Psychopharmacology: an update for psychiatric home care, *Home Care Provider* 5(5):170, 2000.

Jarboe KS: Treatment nonadherence: causes and potential solutions, *Journal of the American Psychiatric Nurses Association* 8(4):18, 2002.

Keltner NL, Folks DG: *Psychotropic drugs*, ed 4, St Louis, 2005, Mosby.

Keltner NL, Schwecke LH, Bostrom CE: *Psychiatric nursing*, ed 5, St Louis, 2007, Mosby.

Skidmore-Roth L: *Mosby's 2007 nursing drug reference*, St Louis, 2007, Mosby.

Chapter 8 Skills and Principles of Mental Health Care

Suggestions for Further Reading

"Negative Behaviors in Nursing," by Rosanna DeMarco and Susan Roberts (*Am J Nurs* 103[3]:113, 2003), provides sound advice to all caregivers.

References
Chenevert M: *STAT: special techniques in assertiveness training*, ed 4, St Louis, 1994, Mosby.

Giger JN, Davidhizar RE: *Transcultural nursing: assessment and intervention*, ed 5, St Louis, 2008, Mosby.

Glasser W: *Choice theory*, New York, 1998, Harper-Collins.

Kabot-Zinn J: Meditate! … for stress reduction, inner peace … or whatever, *Psychology Today* 26(4):36, 1994.

Keltner NL, Schwecke LH, Bostrom CE: *Psychiatric nursing*, ed 5, St Louis, 2007, Mosby.

Morrison M: *Professional skills for leadership: foundations of a successful career*, St Louis, 1993, Mosby.

Pilette PC, Berck CB, Achber LC: Therapeutic management of helping boundaries, *J Psychosoc Nurs Ment Health Serv* 33:40, 1995.

Sherwood G: The responses of care givers to the experience of suffering. In Starck PL, McGovern JP, editors: *The hidden dimension of illness: human suffering*, New York, 1992, National League for Nursing Press.

Stuart GW, Laraia MT: *Principles and practice of psychiatric nursing*, ed 8, St Louis, 2005, Mosby.

Taylor CM: *Essentials of psychiatric nursing*, ed 14, St Louis, 1994, Mosby.

Chapter 9 Mental Health Assessment Skills

Suggestions for Further Reading

"Asking Questions Effectively," written by Susan Smith (*Nursing 95* 25[3]:83, 1995), offers some excellent hints for improving your interviewing skills.

Internet Mental Health (www.mentalhealth.com) dispenses information, diagnostic tools, news, articles, and editorials about common mental disorders.

References
American Psychiatric Association: *Diagnostic and statistical manual of mental disorders*, ed 4, text revision, Washington, DC, 2000, The Association.

Anderson KN, Anderson LE, Glanze WD: *Mosby's medical, nursing, and allied health dictionary*, ed 7, St Louis, 2006, Mosby.

Forster P: Accurate assessment of short-term suicide risk in a crisis, *Psychiatr Ann* 24:571, 1994.

Keltner NL, Schwecke LH, Bostrom CE: *Psychiatric nursing*, ed 5, St Louis, 2007, Mosby.

National Depressive and Manic-Depressive Association: Patient's cultural background important in diagnosis and treatment, *DMDA Newsletter* 7(3):3, 1995.

Potter PA, Perry AG: *Basic nursing: theory and practice*, ed 7, St Louis, 2009, Mosby.

Stuart GW, Laraia MT: *Principles and practice of psychiatric nursing*, ed 8, St Louis, 2005, Mosby.

Chapter 10 Therapeutic Communication

Suggestion for Further Reading

"Listening," by Elizabeth Hawkin-Walsh (*Am J Nurs* 100[9]:24, 2000), explores the basics of listening and its significance on the delivery of care.

References

Bennett MJ: *Checklist for intercultural communications*, Portland, Ore, 1994, The Intercultural Communication Institute.

Berne E: *Games people play: psychology of human relationships*, New York, 1964a, Grove Press.

Berne E: *Principles of group treatment*, New York, 1964b, Oxford University Press.

Giger JN, Davidhizar RE: *Transcultural nursing: assessment and intervention*, ed 5, St Louis, 2008, Mosby.

Jourard S: *The transparent self*, New York, 1971, Van Nostrand Reinhold.

Rawlins RP, Williams SR, Beck CK: *Mental health–psychiatric nursing: a holistic life-cycle approach*, ed 3, St Louis, 1993, Mosby.

Ruesch J: *Therapeutic communications*, New York, 1961, WW Norton.

Stuart GW, Laraia MT: *Principles and practice of psychiatric nursing*, ed 8, St Louis, 20051, Mosby.

Sundeen SJ and others: *Nurse-client interaction: implementing the nursing process*, ed 6, St Louis, 1998, Mosby.

Taylor CM: *Essentials of psychiatric nursing*, ed 14, St Louis, 1994, Mosby.

University of Dundee Press Release: Dundee professor to advise government, May 17, 1999.

Chapter 11 The Therapeutic Relationship

Suggestion for Further Reading

"Uncool Customers," by Linda Childers (*NurseWeek* 4:22[2], 2003), describes how caregivers can decrease the fears of challenging clients with a respectful, calm demeanor and personal contact.

References

Anderson KN, Anderson LE, Glanze WD: *Mosby's medical, nursing, and allied health dictionary*, ed 7, St Louis, 2006, Mosby.

Dufault K, Martocchio BC: Hope, its spheres and dimensions, *Nurs Clin North Am* 20(2):379, 1985.

Forman L: Medication: reasons and interventions for noncompliance, *J Psychosoc Nurs Ment Health Serv* 31(10):23, 1993.

NSDUH Report: Depression among adults employed full-time, by occupational category, National Survey on Drug Use and Health, October 11, 2007.

Pilette PC, Berck CB, Achber LC: Therapeutic management of helping boundaries, *J Psychosoc Nurs Ment Health Serv* 33:40, 1995.

Stuart GW, Laraia MT: *Principles and practice of psychiatric nursing*, ed 8, St Louis, 2005, Mosby.

Sundeen SJ and others: *Nurse-client interaction*, ed 6, St Louis, 1998, Mosby.

Taylor CM: *Essentials of psychiatric nursing*, ed 14, St Louis, 1994, Mosby.

Travelbee J: *Interpersonal aspects of nursing*, Philadelphia, 1971, FA Davis.

Vellenga BA, Christenson J: Persistent and severely mentally ill clients' perceptions of their mental illness, *Issues Ment Health Nurs* 15:359, 1994.

Chapter 12 The Therapeutic Environment

Suggestion for Further Reading

The popular movie *A Beautiful Mind* with Russell Crowe offers a sensitive and moving portrayal of one man's journey into madness.

References

Breggin PR: *Toxic psychiatry*, New York, 1991, St Martins Press.

Cohen LJ: Psychiatric hospitalization as experience of trauma, *Arch Psychiatr Nurs* 8(2):78, 1994.

Delaney C: Reducing recidivism: medication versus psychosocial rehabilitation, *J Psychosoc Nurs Ment Health Serv* 36(11):28, 1998.

Editors: Federal agency report finds public mental health system in crisis, *Mental Health Weekly*, Oct 21, 2002.

Goren S, Orion R: Space and sanity, *Arch Psychiatr Nurs* 8:237, 1994.

Haber J and others: *Comprehensive psychiatric nursing*, ed 5, St Louis, 1997, Mosby.

Herman NJ: Return to sender: reintegrative stigma-management strategies of ex-psychiatric patients, *Journal of Contemporary Ethnography* 22:295, 1993.

Holmberg SK: Ambient sound levels in a state psychiatric hospital, *Archives of Psychiatric Nursing* 13(3):117, 1999.

Jones M: *The therapeutic community*, New York, 1953, Basic Books.

Joseph-Kinzelman A and others: Clients' perceptions of involuntary hospitalization, *J Psychosoc Nurs Ment Health Serv* 32:11, 1994.

Stuart GW, Laraia MT: *Principles and practice of psychiatric nursing*, ed 8, St Louis, 2005, Mosby.

Wichowski HC, Kubsch S: Improving your patient's compliance, *Nursing 95* 25(1):67, 1995.

Chapter 13 Problems of Childhood

Suggestions for Further Reading

Read your local newspaper daily for 1 week. Note the articles relating to children. What picture do you get of children in your community? What problems in your community are associated with children?

The American Psychological Association (*http://helping.apa.org*) offers interesting information about the prevention of violence in our schools.

References

AACAP Facts for Families: Understanding violent behavior in children and adolescents, *American Academy of Pediatric & Adolescent Psychiatry* 55(3):1, 2001.

AACAP Facts for Families: Children and TV violence, *American Academy of Pediatric & Adolescent Psychiatry* 13(4):1, 1999.

American Psychiatric Association: *Diagnostic and statistical manual of mental disorders*, ed 4, text revision, Washington, DC, 2000, The Association.

Bullying by the numbers, *Curriculum Review* 46(5):11, 2007.

Cowen PS: Crisis child care: implications for family interventions, *J Am Psychiatr Nurs Assoc* 7(6):196, 2001.

Frazier J and others: Treatment of early-onset schizophrenia spectrum disorders (TEOSS): demographics and clinical characteristics, *J Am Acad Child Adolesc Psychiatry* 46(8):979, 2007.

Hagerman RJ: Growth and development. In Hay WH and others: *Current pediatric diagnosis and treatment*, ed 15, Norwalk, Conn, 2001, Appleton & Lange.

Hazel P: Depression in children, *Br Med J* 325(30):229, 2002.

Hockenberry M and others: *Wong's nursing care of infants and children*, ed 8, St Louis, 2007, Mosby.

Mencap study reveals widespread bullying, *Community Care* 1678:6, 2007.

Ogden CL, Tabak CJ: Children and teens told by doctors that they were overweight—US, 1981-2002, *MMWR* 54(34):848, 2005.

Rafferty Y, Shinn M: The impact of homelessness on children, *Am Psychol* 46(11):1170, 1991.

Showers J: "Don't shake the baby": the effectiveness of a prevention program, *Child Abuse Negl* 16(1):11, 1992.

Sourander A and others: What is the early childhood outcome of boys who bully or are bullied in childhood?, *Pediatrics* 120(2):397, 2007.

U.S. Census Bureau: *Poverty in the United States*, Washington, DC, 2001a, U.S. Government Printing Office.

U.S. Census Bureau: *Statistical abstract of the United States: 2007*, ed 126, Washington, DC, 2006, www.census.gov/statab/www/

Chapter 14 Problems of Adolescence
Suggestion for Further Reading
"Tough Girl, Tough Patient," by Cortney Davis (*RN* 65[10]:49, 2002), is an account of one care provider's attempt to reach an abused, culturally different teen.

References
American Psychiatric Association: *Diagnostic and statistical manual of mental disorders*, ed 4, text revision, Washington, DC, 2000, The Association.
Ash K: Teen suicide, *Educ Week* 26(24):13, 2007.
Center for Mental Health Services, *www.nmha.org/infoctr*, 2003.
Clark RB: Psychosocial aspects of pediatrics and psychiatric disorders. In Hay WW and others, editors: *Current pediatric diagnosis and treatment*, ed 15, Norwalk, Conn, 2001, Appleton & Lange.
Hazell P: Depression in children, *Br Med J* 325(7):229, 2002.
Hockenberry M and others: *Wong's nursing care of infants and children*, ed 8, St Louis, 2007, Mosby.
Hogarth CR: *Adolescent psychiatric nursing*, St Louis, 1991, Mosby.
Inmates' kids may fill cells themselves in future, *New York Times*, p 4, April 7, 1999.
Kaplan DW, Mammel KA: Adolescence. In Hay WW and others, editors: *Current pediatric diagnosis and treatment*, ed 15, Norwalk, Conn, 2001, Appleton & Lange.
National Institute of Mental Health: "Eating Disorders: Facts About Eating Disorders and the Search for Solutions." Pub No. 01-4901, www.nimh.nih.gov/publicat/eatingdisorder.cfm. Accessed June 2007.
U.S. Census Bureau: *Statistical abstract of the United States: 2007*, ed 126, Washington, DC, 2006, www.census.gov/statab/www/

Chapter 15 Problems of Adulthood
Suggestion for Further Reading
The "Fact Sheet on Mental Illness" (http://www.mentalhelp.net/poc/ center_index.php?id=72) is filled with interesting data about mental health problems.

References
Bauer J, editor: Despite healthcare visits most women still aren't screened for violence, *RN* 65(3):22, 2002.
Edelman CL, Mandle CL: *Health promotion throughout the lifespan*, ed 6, St Louis, 2006, Mosby.
Foster J: The nurse in a center for the homeless, *Nurs Manage* 23(4):38, 1992.
Kessler RC and others: A methodology for estimating the 12-month prevalence of serious mental illness. In *Mental health United States*, Rockville, Md, 1999, Center for Mental Health Services.
Rawlins RP, Williams SR, Beck CK: *Mental health–psychiatric nursing: a holistic life-cycle approach*, ed 3, St Louis, 1993, Mosby.
Stanhope M, Lancaster J: *Public health nursing: population-centered health care in the community*, ed 7, St Louis, 2008, Mosby.
U.S. Census Bureau: *Statistical abstract of the United States: 2007*, ed 126, Washington, DC, 2006, www.census.gov/statab/www/
U.S. Surgeon General: *Mental health: a report of the surgeon general*, Washington, DC, 2002, U.S. Government Printing Office.

Chapter 16 Problems of Late Adulthood
Suggestion for Further Reading
"A Trio to Treasure: the Elderly, the Nurse, and Music," by MK Kramer (*Geriatr Nurs* 22[4]:191, 2001), describes the benefits of music for older adults and offers a gentle therapeutic tool for holistic care.

References
Burggraf V, Barry R: What the future holds for gerontology, *Nursing* 31(1):52, 2001.
Burke MM, Laramie JA: *Primary care of the older adult: a multidisciplinary approach*, ed 2, St Louis, 2004, Mosby.
Ebersole P, Hess P, Luggen AS: *Towards healthy aging: human needs and nursing response*, ed 7, St Louis, 2007, Mosby.
Edelman CL, Mandle CL: *Health promotion throughout the lifespan*, ed 6, St Louis, 2006, Mosby.
Editors: Can your patient name her drugs? *Nursing 2002* 32(8):34, 2002.
Giger JM, Davidhizar RE: *Transcultural nursing: assessment and intervention*, ed 5, St Louis, 2008, Mosby.
Hogstel MO: *Geropsychiatric nursing*, ed 2, St Louis, 1995, Mosby.
Kramer MK: A trio to treasure: the elderly, the nurse, and music, *Geriatr Nurs* 22(4):191, 2001.
National Center on Elder Abuse: *The 2004 survey of state adult protective services: abuse of adults 60 years of age and older*, Lexington, Ky, 2006, The Center.
Ruholl L: Tips for teaching the elderly, *RN* 66(5):48, 2003.
Wold G: *Basic geriatric nursing*, ed 4, St Louis, 2008, Mosby.

Chapter 17 Cognitive Impairment, Alzheimer's Disease, and Dementia
Suggestion for Further Reading
"Comforting a Confused Patient," by Jessica Hilgers (*Nursing 03* 33[1]:49, 2003), describes several simple but effective care measures for individuals with confusion.

References
Alzheimer's Association of Los Angeles, Riverside and San Bernardino Counties: *Guidelines for Alzheimer's disease: conducting an assessment*, The Association, www.alz.org/professional, Los Angeles, 2007.
Gerstein PS: Delirium, dementia, and amnesia, *EMedicine*, www.emedicine.com, no. 7, 2002.
Gray-Vickery P: Advances in Alzheimer's disease, *Nursing 2002* 32(11):64, 2002.
Henry M: Descending into delirium, *Am J Nurs* 102(3):49, 2002.
Higginbottom E: The misuse of psychotropics in the elderly, *RN* 66(3):67, 2003.
Lang MM: Screening for cognitive impairment in the older adult, *Nurse Pract* 26(11):26, 2001.
National Institute on Aging: Alzheimer's disease, US Department of Health and Human Services, www.nia.nih.gov/Alzheimers, 2007.
Peterson R: *Mayo Clinic on Alzheimer's disease*, Rochester, Minn, 2002, Mayo Health Clinic Information.
Rowe MA: People with dementia who become lost, *Am J Nurs* 103(7):32, 2003.
Sclan S, Kanowski S: Alzheimer's disease: stage-related interventions, *Lippincott's Case Management* 6(2):48, 2001.
Watari K, Gatz M: Dementia: a cross-cultural perspective on risk factors, *Generations*, p 32, Spring 2002.

Chapter 18 Managing Anxiety
Suggestions for Further Reading
A thorough but understandable discussion of anxiety disorders can be found at the Anxiety Disorders Association of America website at www.adaa.org/AnxietyDisorderInfo.
The American Psychiatric Association (*www.psych.org*) provides updated information about anxiety disorders.

References
American Psychiatric Association: *Diagnostic and statistical manual of mental disorders*, ed 4, text revision, Washington, DC, 2000, The Association.
Bulecek GM, Butcher HK, and Dochterman JC: *Nursing interventions classification (NIC)*, ed 5, St. Louis, 2008, Mosby.
Craighead WE, Nemeroff CB, editors: *The Corsini encyclopedia of psychology and behavioral science*, ed 3, New York, 2002, John Wiley & Sons.
Forster P, King J: Traumatic stress reactions and the psychiatric emergency, *Psychiatr Ann* 24:603, 1994.

Fortinash KM, Holoday Worret PA: *Psychiatric nursing care plans*, ed 4, St Louis, 2003, Mosby.

Hockenberry M and others: *Wong's nursing care of infants and children*, ed 8, St Louis, 2007, Mosby.

Hyman SE: A new image for fear and emotion, *Nature* 393(6684):417, 1998.

Bulechek GM, Butcher HK, and Dochterman JC: *Nursing interventions classification (NIC)*, ed 5, St Louis, 2008, Mosby.

Microsoft Encarta Online Encyclopedia: Anxiety, www. encarta.msn.com, 2007.

Stuart GW, Laraia MT: *Principles and practice of psychiatric nursing*, ed 8, St Louis, 2005, Mosby.

Chapter 19 Illness and Hospitalization

Suggestions for Further Reading

"Nurse as Patient: Unmet Needs" by Mary Ballou Rogers (*RN* 66[3]:45, 2003) shares her experience and resultant realization of the unmet needs of individuals undergoing coronary artery bypass surgery.

Nursing Net (www.nursingnet.org) offers interesting suggestions for client care.

References

Anderson KN, Anderson LE, Glanze WD: *Mosby's medical, nursing, and allied health dictionary*, ed 7, St Louis, 2006, Mosby.

Campbell DB, Anderson BJ: Setting behavioral limits, *Am J Nurs* 99(12):40, 1999.

Edelman CL, Mandle CL: *Health promotion through the lifespan*, ed 7, St Louis, 2007, Mosby.

Ferszt GG: Performing a crisis assessment, *Nursing 95* 25(5):88, 1995.

Messinger JA and others: Getting conscious sedation right, *Am J Nurs* 99(12):44, 1999.

Potter PA, Perry AG: *Basic nursing: theory and practice*, ed 7, St Louis, 2009, Mosby.

Chapter 20 Loss and Grief

Suggestions for Further Reading

On Death and Dying by Elisabeth Kübler-Ross (New York, 1969, MacMillan) is the classic work on the dying and grief processes.

"Ethical Concerns in End-of-Life Care" by Colleen Scanlon (*Am J Nurs* 103[1]:31, 2003) explains some of the difficulties associated with advance directives, refusal of treatment, and withholding treatment.

Crisis, Grief, and Healing (www.webhealing.com) offers information and resources for grieving individuals and families.

References

American Psychiatric Association: *Diagnostic and statistical manual of mental disorders*, ed 4, text revision, Washington, DC, 2000, The Association.

Calandra B: A death in the family: helping children cope, *Adv Nurs Pract* 1(3):17, 1993.

Ebersole P, Hess P: *Geriatric nursing and healthy aging*, ed 2, St Louis, 2005, Mosby.

Geissler EM: *Pocket guide to cultural assessment*, ed 3, St Louis, 2003, Mosby.

Giger JM, Davidhizar RE: *Transcultural nursing: assessment and intervention*, ed 5, St Louis, 2008, Mosby.

Glaser B, Strauss A: *Awareness of dying*, Chicago, 1965, Aldine.

Hayes ER and others: Near death: back from beyond, *RN* 61(12):54, 1998.

Hockenberry M and others: *Wong's nursing care of infants and children*, ed 8, St Louis, 2007, Mosby.

Kübler-Ross E: *On death and dying*, New York, 1969, MacMillan.

Lueckenotte AG: *Gerontologic nursing*, ed 2, St louis, 2000, Mosby

Meiner SE, Lueckenotte AG: *Gerontologic nursing*, ed 3, St Louis, 2006, Mosby.

Wilson D, Hockenberry MJ, Wong DL: *Wong's clinical manual of pediatric nursing*, ed 7, St Louis, 2008, Mosby.

Chapter 21 Depression and Other Mood Disorders

Suggestion for Further Reading

"Spotting Depression in Asian Patients" by Phyllis J. Estin (*RN* 62[4]:39, 1999) is an an older, but still excellent reminder of how cultural differences influence the signs and symptoms of depression.

References

American Psychiatric Association: *Diagnostic and statistical manual of mental disorders*, ed 4, text revision, Washington, DC, 2000, The Association.

Hockenberry M and others: *Wong's nursing care of infants and children*, ed 8, St Louis, 2007, Mosby.

Isaacs A: Depression and your patient, *Am J Nurs* 98(7):26, 1998.

Keltner NL, Schwecke LH, Bostrom CE: *Psychiatric nursing*, ed 5, St Louis, 2007, Mosby.

National Institute of Mental Health (NIMH): *Depression: a treatable illness*, Bethesda, 2004, The Association.

NANDA International: *NANDA nursing diagnoses: definitions and classification 2007-2008*, Philadelphia, 2007, North American Nursing Diagnosis Association.

National Depressive and Manic-Depressive Association (NDMDA): *Depression and bipolar illness*, Chicago, 2007, The Association.

Perry BL: A 45-year-old woman with premenstrual dysphoric disorder, *J Am Med Assoc* 281(4):368, 1999.

Rollant PD: *Mosby's review cards: mental health nursing*, St Louis, 1998, Mosby.

Scott S: Biology and mental health: why do women suffer more depression and anxiety? *Maclean's* 111(2):62, 1998.

Stuart GW, Laraia MT: *Principles and practice of psychiatric nursing*, ed 8, St Louis, 2005, Mosby.

Chapter 22 Physical Problems, Psychological Sources

Suggestions for Further Reading

"Illness Without Disease, parts I and II" by Lester Grinspoon (*Harvard Mental Health Letter* 16[3]:1, 1999) offers an excellent description of somatoform disorders and is written for the general public.

"Somatoform Disorder: What It Is and How to Cope." Available at http://familydoctor.org/162.xml.

References

American Psychiatric Association: *Diagnostic and statistical manual of mental disorders*, ed 4, text revision, Washington, DC, 2000, The Association.

Craighead WE, Nemeroff CB, editors: *The Corsini encyclopedia of psychology*, ed 3, New York, 2002, John Wiley & Sons.

Epstein RM, Quill TE, McWhinney IR: Somatization reconsidered: incorporating the patient's experience of illness, *Arch Intern Med* 159(3):215, 1999.

Geissler EM: *Pocket guide to cultural assessment*, ed 3, St Louis, 2003, Mosby.

Giger JN, Davidhizar RE: *Transcultural nursing: assessment and intervention*, ed 5, St Louis, 2008, Mosby.

Holloway KL, Zerbe KJ: Simplified approach to somatization disorder, *Postgrad Med* 108(6):12, 2000.

Kirmayer LJ, Robbins JM, Paris J: Somatoform disorders: personality and the social matrix of somatic distress, *J Abnorm Psychol* 103(1):125, 1994.

Miller MC: Somatization disorder: what is it? *www.intelihealth. com*, 2003.

NANDA International: *NANDA nursing diagnoses: definitions and classification 2007-2008*, Philadelphia, 2007, North American Nursing Diagnosis Association.

Stuart GW: *Handbook of psychiatric nursing*, ed 6, St Louis, 2005, Mosby.

Chapter 23 Eating and Sleeping Disorders

Suggestions for Further Reading

"The Skinny on Eating Disorders" by Kathryn Murphy, (*Nursing Made Incredibly Easy* 5(3):24, 2007) describes the features, diagnosis, and treatment of clients with three types of eating disorders.

The National Eating Disorders Association (www.nationaleating disorders.org) offers help lines, referral networks, support groups, and public information about anorexia and bulimia.

References

American Psychiatric Association: *Diagnostic and statistical manual of mental disorders*, ed 4, text revision, Washington, DC, 2000, The Association.

Crosscope-Happel C, Hutchins DE, and others: Male anorexia: a new focus, *J Ment Health Counseling* 22(4):365, 2000.

Hobson JA, Silvestri L: Parasomnias, *Harvard Mental Health Letter* 15(8):1, 1999.

Hockenberry M and others: *Wong's nursing care of infants and children*, ed 8, St Louis, 2007, Mosby.

Lai KY: Anorexia nervosa in Chinese adolescents: does culture make a difference? *J Adolesc* 23(5):561, 2000.

Mishima K and others: Morning bright light therapy for sleep and behavior disorders in elderly patients with dementia, *Acta Psychiatr Scand* 89(1):1, 1994.

Montgomery L, Haynes LC, Garner LF: An unusual sleep disorder, *RN* 565(4):41, 2002.

NANDA International: *NANDA nursing diagnoses: definitions and classification 2007-2008*, Philadelphia, 2007, North American Nursing Diagnosis Association.

National Institute of Mental Health: "Eating disorders: facts about eating disorders and the search for solutions." Pub No. 01-4901. http://www.nimh.nih.gov/publicat/eatingdisorder.cfm. Accessed August 24, 2007.

National Institute of Mental Health: "Cell networking keeps brain's master clock ticking." *Science Update*, www.nimh.nih.gov/press/masterclockr.cfm. Accessed August 27, 2007.

Potter PA, Perry AG: *Basic nursing: concepts, process, and practice*, ed 7, St Louis, 2009, Mosby.

Shields J: It's never too soon to prevent obesity, *NurseWeek* 8(16):12, 2007.

Travis J: The threat of a piece of pumpkin pie, *Science News* 154(23):367, 1998.

U.S. Census Bureau: *Statistical abstract of the United States: 2007*, ed 126, Washington, DC, 2006, www.census.gov/sata/www/.

Walsh T: Eating disorders: progress and problems, *Science* 280(5368):1387, 1998.

Zaider TI, Johnson JG, Cockell SJ: Psychiatric disorders associated with the onset and persistence of bulimia nervosa and binge eating disorder during adolescence, *J Youth Adolesc* 31(5):319, 2002.

Chapter 24 Dissociative Disorders

Suggestion for Further Reading

This suggestion involves a classic old movie. *Three Faces of Eve* is an old but very accurate portrayal of a woman who suffers from dissociative identity disorder with several interesting and conflicting personalities.

References

American Psychiatric Association: *Diagnostic and statistical manual of mental disorders*, ed 4, text revision, Washington, DC, 2000, The Association.

Fortinash KM, Holoday-Worret PA: *Psychiatric–mental health nursing*, ed 4, St Louis, 2008, Mosby.

Hockenberry M and others: *Wong's nursing care of infants and children*, ed 8, St Louis, 2007, Mosby.

Keltner NL, Schwecke LH, Bostrom CE: *Psychiatric nursing*, ed 5, St Louis, 2007, Mosby.

NANDA International: *NANDA nursing diagnoses: definitions and classification 2007-2008*, Philadelphia, 2007, North American Nursing Diagnosis Association.

National Alliance for the Mentally Ill: *Dissociative disorders*, Arlington, Va 2003, The Alliance.

Shives LR: *Basic concepts in psychiatric–mental health nursing*, ed 6, Philadelphia, 2008, Lippincott.

Stuart GW, Laraia MT: *Principles and practice of psychiatric nursing*, ed 8, St Louis, 2005, Mosby.

Chapter 25 Anger and Aggression

Suggestions for Further Reading

There are many good articles on anger and aggression in various nursing, mental health, and social work journals, such as "Uncool Customers" at www.nurseweek.com.

Mental Help Net at www.mentalhelp.net offers a wide range of information about many mental health problems.

References

All Psych: Intermittent explosive disorder, *http://allpsych.com*, Aug 31, 2007.

American Psychiatric Association: *Diagnostic and statistical manual of mental disorders*, ed 4, text revision, Washington, DC, 2000, The Association.

Childers L: Uncool customers, *NurseWeek* 4(2):22, 2003.

Hockenberry M and others: *Wong's nursing care of infants and children*, ed 8, St Louis, 2007, Mosby.

Keltner NL, Schwecke LH, Bostrom CE: *Psychiatric nursing*, ed 5, St Louis, 2007, Mosby.

Landers A, Jacobs NR, Siegel MA: *Violent relationships: battering and abuse among adults*, ed 7, Wylie, Tex, 1995, Information Plus.

Potter PA, Perry AG: *Basic nursing*, ed 6, St Louis, 2005, Mosby.

Stuart GW, Laraia MT: *Principles and practices of psychiatric nursing*, ed 8, St Louis, 2005, Mosby.

U.S. Census Bureau: *Statistical abstract of the United States: 2007*, ed 126, Washington, DC, 2006, www.census.gov/statab/www/

Chapter 26 Outward-Focused Emotions: Violence

Suggestions for Further Reading

The Battered Woman's Survival Guide, by Jan Berliner Statman (Dallas, 1995, Taylor Publishing), is a must-read for every health care provider. The true stories contained within will give you a realistic and valuable look into the lives of battered women and their children.

A wealth of online trauma resources and support information can be found at David Baldwin's Trauma Info Pages (*www.trauma-pages.com*).

References

Carson VB: *Mental health nursing: the nurse-patient journey*, ed 2, Philadelphia, 2000, WB Saunders.

Editors: Bullying by the numbers, *Curriculum Review* 46(5):11, 2007.

Editors: History repeats when it comes to abuse, *RN* 65(2):18, 2002.

Editors: Is your pediatric patient a victim of bullying? *RN* 66(5):30, 2003.

Hockenberry M and others: *Wong's nursing care of infants and children*, ed 8, St Louis, 2007, Mosby.

Keltner NL, Schwecke LH, Bostrom CE: *Psychiatric nursing*, ed 5, St Louis, 2007, Mosby.

NANDA International: *NANDA nursing diagnoses: definitions and classification 2007-2008*, Philadelphia, 2007, North American Nursing Diagnosis Association.

Potter PA, Perry AG: *Basic nursing*, ed 7, St Louis, 2009, Mosby.

Saluja G and others: Prevalence of and risk factors for depressive symptoms among young adolescents, *Arch Pediatr Adolesc Med* 158(1):760, 2006.

Schacter B, Sienfield J: Personal violence and the culture of violence, *Soc Work* 39(4):347, 1994.

Sessions with a cybershrink: an interview with Sherry Turkle, *Technol Rev* 99(2):41, 1996.

Stanhope M, Lancaster J: *Community and public health nursing,* ed 7, St Louis, 2008, Mosby.

Statman JB: *The battered woman's survival guide: breaking the cycle,* ed 2, Dallas, 1995, Taylor Publishing.

U.S. Census Bureau: *Statistical abstract of the United States: 2007,* ed 126, Washington, DC, 2006, http://ww.census.gov/statab/www/

Wood T: Defusing school violence, *UC Davis Magazine* 17(1):18, 1999.

Zinn H: *You can't be neutral on a moving train: a personal history of our times,* New York, 1994, Beacon Press.

Chapter 27 Inward-Focused Emotions: Suicide
Suggestions for Further Reading

Survivor Guilt: A Self-Help Guide, by Aphrodite Matsakis (Oakland, Calif, 1999, New Harbinger Publications), is written by a posttraumatic stress disorder (PTSD) psychotherapist who shows survivors how to overcome the chronic guilt and other emotional problems associated with the suicide of a friend or loved one. It is highly recommended reading.

Suicide Awareness/Voices of Education *(www.save.org)* is an excellent source for information relating to suicide.

References
Beck E: In gloomy Hungary, suicide takes on a life of its own, *Wall Street Journal* 48(132):A1, 1995.

Billings CV: Close observation of suicidal inpatients, *J Am Psychiatr Nurs Assoc* 7(2):49, 2001.

Center for Disease Control: *Suicide:facts at a glance* (website): www.cdc.gov/injury. Accessed September 9, 2007.

Constantino RE, Sekula LK, Lebish J, Buehner E: Depression and behavioral manifestations of depression in female survivors of suicide and female survivors of abuse, *J Am Psychiatr Nurs Assoc* 8(1):27, 2002.

NANDA International: *NANDA nursing diagnoses: definitions and classification 2007-2008,* Philadelphia, 2007, North American Nursing Diagnosis Association.

Stanhope M, Lancaster J: *Public health nursing, population-centered health care in the community,* ed 7, St Louis, 2008, Mosby.

Stuart GW, Laraia MT: *Principles and practices of psychiatric nursing,* ed 8, St Louis, 2005, Mosby.

U.S. Census Bureau: *Statistical abstract of the United States: 2007,* ed 126, Washington, DC, 2006, www.census.gov/statab/www/

Chapter 28 Substance-Related Disorders
Suggestions for Further Reading

"Ecstasy Overdose," by Dori Rogers (*Nursing 2002* 32[6]:112, 2002), offers an overview of the treatment for clients who have overdosed on the drug.

"Addiction: A Nurse's Story," by James Hastings (American Journal of Nursing, 107[8], 75 describes an occupational hazard for nurses.

The following websites are filled with current information about alcohol and drug abuse:

National Clearinghouse for Alcohol and Drug Information (www. health.org/index.htm)

Alcohol Problems and Solutions at (www.potsdam.edu/alcohol-info/)

References
American Psychiatric Association: *Diagnostic and statistical manual of mental disorders,* ed 4, text revision, Washington, DC, 2000, The Association.

Center for Disease Control: *Suicide: facts at a glance* (website): www.cdc.gov/injury. Accessed September 9, 2007.

Fetal alcohol syndrome: fact sheet, Atlanta, 2003, Centers for Disease Control and Prevention.

Hess D, DeBoer S: Emergency: ecstasy, *Am J Nurs* 102(4):45, 2002.

Keltner NL, Schwecke LH, Bostrom CE: *Psychiatric nursing,* ed 5, St Louis, 2007, Mosby.

NANDA International: *NANDA nursing diagnoses: definitions and classification 2003-2004,* Philadelphia, 2003, North American Nursing Diagnosis Association.

Chapter 29 Sexual Disorders
Suggestion for Further Reading

An article by Barbara Girardin titled "Is This Forensic Specialty for You?" (*RN* 64[12], 2001) offers an excellent insight into the world of sexual assault nurse examiners (SANEs) and their impact on victims of sexual assault.

References
American Psychiatric Association: *Diagnostic and statistical manual of mental disorders,* ed 4, text revision, Washington, DC, 2000, The Association.

Bell AP, Weinberg MS: *Homosexuality: a study of diversity among men and women,* New York, 1978, Simon & Schuster.

Coleman-Kennedy C, Pendley A: Assessment and diagnosis of sexual addiction, *J Am Psychiatr Nurs Assoc* 8(5):143, 2002.

Dessens AB and others: Prenatal exposure to anticonvulsants and psychosexual development, *Arch Sex Behav* 28(1):31, 1999.

Edelman CL, Mandle CL: *Health promotion throughout the life-span,* ed 6, St Louis, 2006, Mosby.

Fortinash KM, Holoday-Worret PA: *Psychiatric-mental health nursing,* ed 4, St Louis, 2008, Mosby.

Hockenberry M and others: *Wong's nursing care of infants and children,* ed 8, St Louis, 2007, Mosby.

Kinsey AC, Pomeroy WB, Martin EC: *Sexual behavior in the human female,* Philadelphia, 1953, WB Saunders.

Stuart GW, Laraia MT: *Principles and practice of psychiatric nursing,* ed 8, St Louis, 2005, Mosby.

Warner PH, Rowe MS, Whipple B: Shedding light on the sexual history, *Am J Nurs* 99(6):34, 1999.

Chapter 30 Personality Disorders
Suggestions for Further Reading

Internet Mental Health *(www.mentalhealth.com)* offers interesting information about the diagnosis and treatment of personality disorders. Other resources include Psychiatry On-line *(www.priory.co.uk/psych)* and National Mental Health Information Center *(www.mentalhealth.org).*

References
American Psychiatric Association: *Diagnostic and statistical manual of mental disorders,* ed 4, text revision, Washington, DC, 2000, The Association.

Fortinash KM, Holoday-Worret PA: *Psychiatric mental health nursing,* ed 4, St Louis, 2008, Mosby.

Gale Encyclopedia of Medicine: Personality disorders, *www.findarticles.com,* 1999.

Hockenberry M and others: *Wong's nursing care of infants and children,* ed 8, St Louis, 2007, Mosby.

Marshall LA, Cooke DJ: The childhood experience of psychopaths: a retrospective study of familial and societal factors, *J Personal Disord* 13(3):211, 1999.

Paris J: Personality disorders in sociocultural perspective, *J Personal Disord* 12(4):289, 1998.

Personality disorders: the anxious cluster, part I, *Harvard Mental Health Letter* 12(8):1, 1996.

Stuart GW, Laraia MT: *Principles and practice of psychiatric nursing,* ed 8, St Louis, 2005, Mosby.

Ward RK: Assessment and management of personality disorders, *Am Family Physician,* Oct 15, 2004.

Chapter 31 Schizophrenia and Other Psychoses
Suggestions for Further Reading

If you are interested in how people live with schizophrenia, read E. Fuller Torrey's *Surviving Schizophrenia: A Family Manual* (New York, 1983, Harper & Row).

The Schizophrenia Home Page (*www.schizophrenia.com*) offers much information relating to psychotic conditions and treatments.

References

American Psychiatric Association: *Diagnostic and statistical manual of mental disorders*, ed 4, text revision, Washington, DC, 2000, The Association.

Fortinash KM, Holoday-Worret PA: *Psychiatric mental health nursing*, ed 4, St Louis, 2008, Mosby.

Giger JN, Davidhizar RE: *Transcultural nursing: assessment and intervention*, ed 5, St Louis, 2008, Mosby.

Herbert W: Fearsome madness: schizophrenia remains frustratingly hard to control, *U.S. News & World Report* 125(6):53, 1998.

Hockenberry M and others: *Wong's nursing care of infants and children*, ed 8, St Louis, 2007, Mosby.

Kane JM, McGlashan TH: Treatment of schizophrenia, *Lancet* 346(8978):820, 1995.

Keltner NL, Folks DG: *Psychotropic drugs*, ed 4, St Louis, 2005, Mosby.

NIMH: How schizophrenia develops: major clues discovered, *National Institute of Mental Health*, Bethesda, Md, Department of Health & Human Services, October 17, 2007.

Peck RL, editor: Schizophrenia: not just a young person's disorder, *Behavioral Health Management* 22(2):29, 2002.

Schultz SK, Andreasen NC: Schizophrenia, *Lancet* 353(9):1425, 1999.

Stuart GW, Laraia MT: *Principles and practice of psychiatric nursing*, ed 8, St Louis, 2005, Mosby.

Torry EF and others: Prefrontal origin of schizophrenia in a subgroup of discordant monozygotic twins, *Schizophrenia Bull*, 20(3):423, 1994.

Chapter 32 Chronic Mental Health Disorders

Suggestions for Further Reading

Susan Muhlbauer's "Experience of Stigma by Families with Mentally Ill Members" (*J Am Psychiatr Nurs Assoc* 8[3]:76, 2002) describes some of the burdens placed on the families of persons with chronic, severe mental illness.

Websites with information about chronic mental illness include the Alliance for the Mentally Ill (www.schizophrenia.com) and Dual Diagnosis (www.erols.com).

References

Blaska B: What it's like to be a CMI, *Schizophr Bull* 17(1):173, 1991.

Editors: Management of serious mental illness, *www.medscape.com/pages*, 2003.

Farnam CR and others: Health status and risk factors of people with severe and persistent mental illness, *J Psychosoc Nurs* 37(6):16, 1999.

Fortinash KM, Holoday-Worret PA: *Psychiatric–mental health nursing*, ed 4, St Louis, 2008, Mosby.

HIV/AIDS Policy Fact Sheet: The HIV/AIDS epidemic in the united states, *The Henery J Kaiser Foundation*, September 2005.

Howd A: Trapped between the law and madness, *Insight in the News* 14(34):18, 1998.

O'Connor FW, Lovell D, Brown L: Implementing residential treatment for prison inmates with mental illness, *Arch Psychiatr Nurs* 16(5):232, 2002.

Stuart GW: *Pocket guide to psychiatric nursing*, ed 6, St Louis, 2005, Mosby.

Torrey EF, Zdanowicz MT: How freedom punishes the severely mentally ill, *USA Today*, July 7, 1999.

U.S. Census Bureau: *Statistical abstract of the United States: 2007*, ed 126, Washington, DC, 2006, www.census.gov/statab/www/

Chapter 33 Challenges for the Future

Suggestions for Further Reading

In the article "Understanding the Seven Stages of Change" (*Am J Nurs* 95[4]: 41, 1995), Jo Manion states that understanding the stages of change will help you survive and even grow from the change experience.

The Dynamics of Change at www.ncrel.org/sdrs/areas/issues lists 8 basic lessons learned from the change process.

Internet addresses for general mental health information include the American Psychological Association PsychNet (www.apa.org), Help! A Consumer's Guide to Mental Health (www.iComm.ca/madmagic/help), and Psychlink (www.psychlink.com).

References

Equal Employment Opportunity Commission: *A technical assistance manual on the employee provisions (Title 1) of the Americans with Disabilities Act*, Washington, DC, 1992, U.S. Government Printing Office.

Harrington SP: New bedlam: jails—not psychiatric hospitals—now care for the indigent mentally ill, *Humanist* 59(3):9, 1999.

Morrison M: *Professional skills for leadership: foundations of a successful career*, St Louis, 1993, Mosby.

NLCHP: *Homelessness & poverty in america*, National Law Center on Homelessness and Poverty, Washington, DC, 2007.

NAMI: *Grading the states 2006: executive summary*, National Alliance on Mental Illness, www.nami.org/Content/NavigationMenu, Accessed October 2, 2007.

NIMH: *Global survey reveals significant gap in meeting the world's mental health care needs*, National Institute of Mental Health, Bethesda, Md, Department of Health & Human Services, 2007a.

NIMH: *The numbers count: mental illness in America*, National Institute of Mental Health, Bethesda, Md, Department of Health & Human Services, 2007b.

Schofield R: Empowerment education for individuals with serious mental illness, *J Psychosoc Nurs* 36(11):35, 1998.

Torrey EF: *Out of the shadows: confronting America's mental illness crisis*, ed 2, New York, 1998, John Wiley & Sons.

Torrey EF, Zdanowicz MT: How freedom punishes the severely mentally ill, *USA Today*, July 7, 1999.

Illustration Credits

Chapter 1

1-2 William Hogarth, "The Rake in Bedlam," c. 1735. From the series entitled *The Rake's Progress*. Copyright The British Museum, London. **1-3, 1-4** courtesy U.S. National Library of Medicine, Bethesda, Md. **1-5** redrawn from U.S. National Library of Medicine, Bethesda, Md.

Chapter 2

2-1 Redrawn from Stroul BA: Community support systems for persons with long-term mental illnesses: a conceptual framework, *Psychosocial Rehabilitation Journal* 12(3):9, 1989.

Chapter 3

3-2 Redrawn from Stuart GW, Laraia MT: *Principles and practice of psychiatric nursing*, ed 7, St. Louis, 2001, Mosby.

Chapter 5

5-1 Data from Maslow A: *Motivation and personality*, ed 2, New York, 1970, Harper & Row. **5-2, 5-3** redrawn from Potter PA, Perry AG: *Basic nursing: a critical thinking approach*, ed 4, St. Louis, 1999, Mosby.

Chapter 6

6-2 A from Potter PA, Perry AG: *Fundamentals of nursing: concepts, process, and practice*, ed 6, St. Louis, 2005, Mosby.

Chapter 9

9-1 Courtesy Division of Psychiatric Nursing, Medical University of South Carolina.

Chapter 10

10-1 Redrawn from Rawlins RP, Williams SR, Beck CK: *Mental health–psychiatric nursing: a holistic life-cycle approach*, ed 3, St. Louis, 1993, Mosby. **10-2** redrawn from Sundeen SJ and others: *Nurse-client interaction: implementing the nursing process*, ed 6, St. Louis, 1998, Mosby. **10-3** redrawn from Smith S: *Communications in nursing: communicating assertively and responsibly in nursing—a guidebook*, ed 2, St. Louis, 1992, Mosby.

Chapter 12

12-1 Redrawn from Stuart GW, Laraia MT: *Principles and practice of psychiatric nursing*, ed 7, St. Louis, 2001, Mosby.

Chapter 13

13-1 Copyright © Cathy Lander-Goldberg, Lander Photographics, Inc., St. Louis.

Chapter 14

14-1 From Ezrin D and others: *Systematic endocrinology*, ed 2, New York, 1979, Harper & Row.

Chapter 16

16-2 A, B from Sorrentino SA, Gorek B: *Long-term care assistants*, ed 4, St. Louis, 2003, Mosby.

Chapter 20

20-1 Redrawn from Ebersole P, Hess P: *Toward healthy aging: human needs and nursing response*, ed 7, St. Louis, 2004, Mosby. **20-2** redrawn from Ebersole P, Hess P: *Geriatric nursing and healthy aging*, St. Louis, 2001, Mosby.

Chapter 21

21-1 Redrawn from Stuart GW, Laraia MT: *Principles and practice of psychiatric nursing*, ed 7, St. Louis, 2001, Mosby.

Chapter 22

22-2 From James S and others: *Nursing care of children: principles and practice*, ed 2, Philadelphia, 2002, Saunders. **22-3** from Hurwitz S: *Clinical pediatric dermatology: a textbook of skin disorders of children and adolescence*, ed 2, Philadelphia, 1993, Saunders.

Chapter 23

23-1 Redrawn from Stuart GW, Laraia MT: *Principles and practice of psychiatric nursing*, ed 7, St. Louis, 2001, Mosby. **23-2** from Williams SR: *Basic nutrition and diet therapy*, ed 10, St. Louis, 1995, Mosby. **23-3** from Seidel HM and others: *Mosby's guide to physical examination*, ed 5, St. Louis, 2002, Mosby. **23-4** modified from Biddle C, Oaster TRF: The nature of sleep, *AANA J* 58(1):36, 1990.

Chapter 24

24-1 Redrawn from Stuart GW, Laraia MT: *Principles and practice of psychiatric nursing*, ed 7, St. Louis, 2001, Mosby.

Chapter 25

25-2 From Wong DL: *Whaley and Wong's nursing care of infants and children*, ed 5, St. Louis, 1995, Mosby. **25-3** redrawn from Keltner NL, Schewecke LH, Bostrom CE: *Psychiatric nursing*, ed 3, St. Louis, 1999, Mosby.

Chapter 26

26-2 From Marx J and others: *Rosen's emergency medicine: concepts and clinical practice*, ed 6, St. Louis, 2006, Mosby. **26-3** redrawn from McFarland J, Parker B: Preventing abuse during pregnancy: an assessment and intervention protocol, *MCN: Am J Matern Child Nurs* 19(6):321, 1994.

Chapter 27

27-1 Redrawn from Stuart GW, Laraia MT: *Principles and practice of psychiatric nursing*, ed 7, St. Louis, 2001, Mosby. **27-2** Copyright © 2007 The History Place™. All rights reserved.

Chapter 28

28-1 From Streissguth AP: *Ciba Foundation symposium no. 105: mechanisms of alcohol damage in utero*. By permission of AP Streissguth and The Ciba Foundation, Pitman, London. **28-2, 28-3** data from U.S. Drug Enforcement Agency. **28-4** photo by Christopher B, Copyright © 2000 Erowid. worg, http://www.erowid.org.

Chapter 29

29-1 Redrawn from Stuart GW, Laraia MT: *Principles and practice of psychiatric nursing*, ed 7, St. Louis, 2001, Mosby. **29-2** redrawn from Kinsey AC, Pomeroy WB, Martin EC: *Sexual behavior in the human female*, Philadelphia, 1953, Saunders. **29-3** from Denney NW, Quadagno D: *Human sexuality*, ed 2, St. Louis, 1992, Mosby.

Chapter 30

30-1 Redrawn from Stuart GW, Laraia MT: *Principles and practice of psychiatric nursing*, ed 7, St. Louis, 2001, Mosby.

Chapter 31

31-1 Redrawn from Stuart GW, Laraia MT: *Principles and practice of psychiatric nursing*, ed 7, St. Louis, 2001, Mosby.

Glossary

The markings ˉ and ˘ above the vowels (a, e, i, o, and u) indicate the proper sounds of the vowels.

When ˉ is above a vowel its sound is long, that is, exactly like its name; for example:

> ā as in āpe
> ē as in ēven
> ī as in īce
> ō as in ōpen
> ū as in ūnit

The ˘ marking indicates a short vowel sound, as in the following examples:

> ă as in ăpple
> ĕ as in ĕvery
> ĭ as in ĭnterest
> ŏ as in pŏt
> ŭ as in ŭnder

A

abstinence Nonuse of an addictive substance or behavior.

abuse Process of causing an individual harm.

abused substances Chemicals that alter the individual's perception by affecting the central nervous system; also referred to as mind-altering substances.

acceptance Act of receiving or taking what is being offered or given.

acquired immunodeficiency syndrome (AIDS) A viral infection that prevents the body from warding off infectious diseases.

acting out Use of inappropriate, detrimental, or destructive behaviors to express current or past emotions.

acupuncture Insertion of fine needles into the skin at certain specific sites or meridians along the body to treat illness.

addiction Physical dependence on a drug that is taken or behavior that is performed despite the physical and psychosocial problems associated with its use.

addictive behaviors Obsessive-compulsive activities that take the form of certain repetitive behaviors, such as gambling, shopping, working, and engaging in excessive sexual activity.

adolescence Period of life between 11 and 21 years of age.

adolescent suicide Act of intentionally taking one's own life by a person between 11 and 21 years of age.

adulthood The period of life lasting from about 18 to approximately 65 years of age.

advocacy Process of providing a client with information, support, and feedback so that the client can make an informed decision.

affect Outward manifestation of a person's feelings or emotions.

affective Pertaining to emotion, mood, or feeling.

affective disorders Emotional states, ranging from deep depression to excited elation.

affective loss In dementia, the loss of mood, emotion, and personality.

ageism Practice of stereotyping older persons as feeble, dependent, and nonproductive.

From Chabner DE: *The language of medicine,* ed 7, Philadelphia, 2004, Saunders.

aggression Forceful attitude or action that is expressed physically, symbolically, or verbally.

aging Process of growing older.

agitation Behavior that is verbally or physically offensive.

agnosia Inability to recognize familiar environmental objects or people (stimuli).

agoraphobia Anxiety about possible situations (especially open or public places) in which a panic attack may occur.

AIDS Acquired immunodeficiency syndrome, a viral infection that prevents the body from warding off infectious diseases.

akathisia Inability to sit still, commonly caused by antipsychotic drugs.

akinesia Absence of movement, physically and mentally.

alcohol Ethanol (ETOH); the result of the fermentation or distillation of yeast and grains, malts, or fruits.

alcoholism Chronic disease caused by prolonged or excessive alcohol use.

alexithymia Difficulty in identifying and describing emotions.

allopathic Using medical and surgical methods to treat disease and injury; following the Disease Model.

alternative medicine Practices and treatments that are used instead of conventional (allopathic) medicine.

Alzheimer's disease (AD) Progressive, degenerative disorder that impedes the functioning of brain cells and synapses and results in impaired memory, thinking, and behavior.

ambivalence State in which an individual experiences conflicting feelings, attitudes, or drives.

amnesia Loss of memory that cannot be explained by normal forgetfulness.

amphetamines Class of drugs that act as central nervous system stimulants.

anger Normal emotional response to a perceived threat, frustration, or distressing event; occurs in response to an individual's frustration level or feelings of being threatened or losing control.

anhedonia Loss of interest or pleasure from previously enjoyed activities.

anorexia nervosa Severe disturbance in eating behavior that results in a body that is much lower than its ideal weight.

anticipatory grief The process of grieving before an actual event occurs.

antipsychotics Drugs used to treat the symptoms of major mental disorders.

antisocial personality Pervasive pattern of disregard for and violation of the rights of others.

anxiety Vague, uneasy feeling experienced by individuals in response to real or imagined stress.

anxiety disorder Psychic tension that interferes with a person's ability to perform activities of daily living.

anxiety state State that occurs when one's coping abilities are overwhelmed and emotional control is lost.

anxiety trait Learned component of the personality in which an individual reacts to relatively nonstressful situations with anxiety.

apathy Lack of feelings, emotions, concern, or interests.

aphasia Disorder in which language function is defective or absent; inability to speak or understand verbal messages.

aromatherapy The use of certain essential oils to promote health and well-being.

assault Any behavior that presents an immediate threat to another person.

assertiveness Ability to directly express one's feelings or needs in a way that respects the rights of other people and retains the individual's dignity.

assessment First step of the nursing process, which includes the gathering, clustering, and analysis of data relating to a client.

attention-deficit/hyperactivity disorder Cluster of behaviors associated with inattention and impulsive actions.

attitudes Ideas that help make up our points of view; one's outlook.

autism Pervasive developmental disorder of the brain. Symptoms appear during the first 3 years of life and include disturbances in physical, social, and language skills; abnormal responses to sensations; and abnormal ways of relating to people, objects, and events.

autonomic nervous system (ANS) System responsible for regulating the internal vital functions of the body, such as the cardiac and smooth muscles.

autonomy Ability to direct and control one's own activities and one's destiny.

avoidance behaviors Refusal to cope with anxiety-producing situations by ignoring them.

avoidant personality Extreme anxiety related to a fear of rejection and humiliation; to prevent possible rejection, individuals narrow their interests to a small range of activities with a very small, if any, support system.

ayurveda A healing system that was developed in India that focuses on the innate harmony of the body, mind, and spirit.

B

battering Repeated abuse of someone, usually a woman, child, or older person.

battery Unlawful use of force on a person.

behavior Manner of conducting oneself; one's actions.

belief Conviction that is mentally accepted as true whether or not it is based in fact.

beneficence Actively doing good.

bereavement Emotional and behavioral state of thoughts, feelings, and activities that follow a loss.

bereavement-related depression State of bereavement in which the griever feels the loss so intensely that despair, worthlessness, and depression overwhelm everything else in life.

binge eating Uncontrolled ingestion (in a certain period of time) of an amount of food that is definitely larger than most individuals would eat in similar circumstances.

bioelectromagnetic field (EMF) therapies The use of electromagnetic field energy to treat illness.

biofeedback A process that provides visual or auditory information about autonomic body functions.

bipolar disorder Behavioral problems associated with sudden, dramatic shifts in emotional extremes.

bisexuals Persons who are attracted to and engage in sexual activities with members of both genders.

body dysmorphic disorder Preoccupation with a physical difference or defect in one's body.

body image Person's subjective concept of his or her physical appearance.

borderline personality Instability in mood, thinking, behavior, personal relationships, and self-image.

bradykinesia Slowing down of body movements and mental state.

bulimia Uncontrolled ingestion of large amounts of food (called binge eating), followed by inappropriate methods to prevent weight gain (called purging).

C

caffeine Active ingredient of coffee, tea, and other beverages that stimulates the central nervous system.

calculation Ability to perform mathematical problems.

cannabis Leaves and flowers of the plant *Cannabis sativa;* also called marijuana.

caring Concern for the well-being of a person, demonstrated through attentive listening, comforting, honesty, acceptance, and sensitivity.

case management Assignment of a health care provider to assist a client in assessing health and social service systems and to ensure that all required services are obtained.

cataplexy Sudden episode of bilateral muscle weakness and loss of muscle tone that lasts for seconds to minutes.

catastrophic reactions Minor anxieties or frustrations that cascade into severe behavioral reactions in which the person becomes increasingly confused, agitated, and fearful and may wander, become noisy, act compulsively, or behave violently.

catchment area Delineated geographical region used for the planning of health care services.

central nervous system (CNS) Brain and spinal cord, which together control all the motor and sensory functions of the body.

cephalocaudal A pattern of growth and development in which the head of an organism develops first, followed by the extremities, and then feet.

change process Series of steps that result in a difference.

chelation Treatment using the chemical EDTA to bind with heavy metals and remove them from the body.

chemical dependency Psychophysiological state of being addicted to drugs or alcohol; also called addiction.

chemical restraint Antipsychotic medication; a medication that reduces or eliminates psychotic symptoms and quiets behavior.

chiropractic Treatment that uses manipulations to improve the relationship between body function and structure (the spine).

chronic mental illness The presence of one or more recurring psychiatric disorders that result in significantly impaired functional abilities.

chronicity Long-term, persistent difficulties; in chronic mental disorders, periods of relative comfort and ease of functioning, alternating with relapses into acute psychiatric states.

civil law Private law that functions to deal with relationships between individuals.

closed system Set of interacting, related units with rigid, impermeable boundaries that close out information and energy and eventually shorten survival.

cocaine Processed extract of the coca plant, which causes central nervous stimulation and intense feelings of well-being.

codes of ethics Statements encompassing the set of rules by which practitioners of a profession are expected to conform.

cognition Activities of the mind characterized by knowing, learning, judging, reasoning, and memory.

cognitive Pertaining to the mental processes of comprehension, judgment, memory, and reasoning.

commitment Personal bond to some course of action.

communication Reciprocal exchange of information, ideas, beliefs, feelings, and attitudes between two persons or among a group of persons.

communication disorders Problems with expressing and receiving messages, pronouncing words, and stuttering that interfere with a child's development.

communication style Rituals connected with greeting and departure, the lines of conversation, and the directness of communication.

community mental health centers Outpatient settings in which a comprehensive range of mental health services is made readily available to all members of a community.

community support systems (CSS) model Organized network of caring and trained people committed to assisting chronically mentally ill people to meet their needs within the community.

comorbidity (cooccurring) Two medical or psychiatric disorders present at the same time.

competent State of being able to make a choice, understand important information, appreciate one's own situation, and apply reasoning.

complementary medicine Practices and treatments that agree or "work with" allopathic therapies.

complicated grief Persistent yearning for a deceased person and other related symptoms that often occur without the signs of depression but are associated with impaired psychological functioning and disturbances of mood, sleep, and self-esteem.

compulsion Distressing recurring behavior that must be performed to reduce anxiety.

compulsive overeating Pattern of eating to lessen emotional discomfort, anxiety, or distress.

conative loss Loss of the ability to make and carry out plans.

conduct disorders Persistent patterns of unacceptable behaviors, which include defiance of authority, engaging in aggressive actions toward others, refusal to follow society's rules and norms, and violation of the rights of others.

confidentiality Sharing of client information only with those persons who are directly involved in the care of the client.

confusion A disruption in higher brain functions resulting in inaccurate interpretation of stimuli.

consistency Behaviors that imply being steady and regular, dependable.

consultation Process in which the assistance of a specialist is sought to help identify ways in which to cope effectively with client management problems.

contract law Division of private law that focuses on agreements between individuals or institutions.

controlled substances Certain drug classes manufactured, distributed, and dispensed according to the federal regulations of the 1970 Controlled Substances Act.

conversion disorder Somatoform disorder in which the individual presents with problems related to the sensory or motor functions.

coping mechanisms Any thought or action that is aimed at reducing stress.

countertransference Barrier in the therapeutic relationship based in the nurse's emotional responses to the client.

crack Type of processed cocaine made by combining cocaine with ammonia or baking soda and heating the mixture to remove the hydrochloride molecule, resulting in chips or chunks of highly addicting cocaine, called rocks.

criminal law Division of public law designed to protect the members of a society.

crisis Period of severe emotional disorganization resulting from a lack of appropriate coping mechanisms or supports.

crisis intervention Short-term, active therapy that provides emotional first aid for victims of trauma with the goal of assisting individuals and families in managing the immediate crisis situation and returning to precrisis levels of functioning.

cultural competence The process of continually learning about the cultures with which we work and developing cross-cultural therapeutic health care skills.

culture Set of learned values, beliefs, customs, and behaviors that is shared by a group of interacting individuals.

cyclothymic disorder Pattern of behaviors involving repeated mood swings, alternating between hypomania and depressive symptoms.

D

data collection Activities that elicit, retrieve, or discover information about a certain subject.

deceit Lying; act of representing as true something that is known to be false.

defamation Any false communication that results in harm.

defense mechanisms Unconscious, intrapsychic reaction that offers protection to the self from a stressful situation.

deinstitutionalization The transfer to a community setting of a patient who has been hospitalized for an extended period of time; a shift in the focus from the large, long-term institution to the community via the discharge of long-term patients and avoidance of unnecessary admissions.

delirium Change of consciousness that occurs over a short period of time.

delusions False beliefs that are resistant to reasoning or change.

dementia Loss of multiple abilities, including short- and long-term memory, language, and the ability to understand (conceptualize).

demonical exorcisms Religious ceremonies in which patients were physically punished to drive away the possessing spirit.

denial Psychological defense mechanism in which one refuses to acknowledge painful facts.

dependent personality Anxiety associated with separation and abandonment with a deep fear of rejection that expresses itself as the need to be cared for.

depersonalization Feeling of unreality and alienation from self with ego and self-concept disorganization.

depression Emotional state characterized by feelings of sadness, disappointment, and despair.

derealization Loss of ego boundaries; inability to tell where one's body ends and the environment begins.

designer drugs Substances created by underground chemists who alter the molecular structures of existing drugs.

detoxification The process of withdrawing a substance under medical supervision.

development Increasing ability in skills or functions.

dietary supplement A "dietary ingredient" supplement to the diet.

direct self-destructive behaviors Any form of active suicidal behavior, such as threats, gestures, or attempts to intentionally end one's life.

discharge planning Process whereby nurses help clients cope with the hurdles of illness or surgery through early identification of and intervention for potential problems following discharge from a health care facility.

disease Condition in which a physical dysfunction exists.

dissociation Disconnection from full awareness of self, time, or external circumstances.

dissociative disorder A disturbance in the normally interacting functions of consciousness: identity, memory, and perception.

dissociative identity disorder (DID) The presence of two or more identities or personalities that repeatedly take control of the individual's behavior.

disturbed communications Interference in communication related to the sending or receiving of messages, inadequate mastery of the language, insufficient information, or no opportunity for feedback.

disulfiram (Antabuse) A chemical that produces uncomfortable and possibly serious physical reactions when taken with alcohol.

domestic violence Aggressive behaviors directed toward significant others.

drug-induced parkinsonism Group of symptoms that mimic Parkinson's disease, including tremors, muscle rigidity, and difficulty with voluntary movements.

dual diagnosis In mental health, the presence of two or more psychiatric disorders, one commonly being substance abuse.

duty to warn Duty to protect potential victims from possible harm by a psychiatric client.

dying process Experience of progressing through several psychological stages before the actual death occurs, which allows people to cope with the overwhelming emotional reactions associated with losing loved ones.

dynamics Interactions among the various forces operating in any system.

dyskinesia Inability to execute voluntary movements.

dyslexia Impaired ability to read, sometimes accompanied by a mixing of letters or syllables in a word when speaking.

dyspareunia Pain associated with sexual intercourse.

dyssomnias Sleep disorders characterized by abnormalities in the amount, quality, or timing of sleep.

dysthymia Daily moderate depression that lasts for longer than 2 years.

dystonia Impaired muscle tone.

E

eating disorder Ongoing disturbance in behaviors associated with the ingestion of food.

ego In psychoanalysis, the part of the psyche that experiences and maintains conscious contact with reality; rational part of the personality; seat of mental processes such as perception and memory; develops defense mechanisms to cope with anxiety.

elder abuse Any action on the part of a caregiver to take advantage of an older adult, his or her emotional well-being, or his or her property.

electroconvulsive therapy (ECT) Artificial induction of a grand mal seizure by passing a controlled electrical current through electrodes applied to one or both temples.

elopement Unannounced leaving or running away from an inpatient health care institution.

emotion Nonintellectual reaction to various stimuli, based on individual's perceptions.

emotional abuse The rejection, criticism, terrorizing, and isolation of a significant other.

empathy Ability to recognize and share the emotions and states of mind of another and to understand the meaning and significance of that person's behavior.

encopresis Fecal incontinence in a child older than 4 years of age with no physical abnormalities; includes the repeated, usually voluntary, passage of feces in inappropriate places.

entrepreneur A self-employed person. In nursing, those who have established their own nurse-operated clinics, act as health care consultants, and provide a variety of health care services to business and industry.

enuresis Involuntary urinary incontinence of a child 5 years or older.

environmental control Ability of an individual to perceive and control his or her environment.

equilibrium Attempt of a system or organism to maintain a steady state or balance within itself and among other systems.

erotic Inducing sexual feelings.

ethical dilemmas Uncertainties or disagreements about the moral principles that endorse different courses of action.

ethics Set of rules or values that govern right behavior.

ethnicity Broad term that refers to socialization patterns, customs, and cultural habits of a particular group.

exacerbations Periods marked by an increase in the signs and symptoms and seriousness of a problem or disorder.

exhibitionism Exposure of one's genitals to an unsuspecting person followed by sexual arousal.

exploitation Use of another individual for selfish purposes, profit, or gain.

expressive therapy The use of creative activities to decrease stress.

extended family Household group consisting of parents, children, grandparents, and other family members.

external losses Those losses outside the individual that relate to objects, possessions, the environment, loved ones, and support.

extrapyramidal side effects (EPSEs) Abnormal involuntary movement disorders caused by a drug-induced imbalance between two major neurotransmitters, dopamine and acetylcholine, in portions of the brain.

Eye Movement Desensitization and Reprocessing (EMDR) Uses controlled eye movements to help reprocess traumatic memories.

F

factitious disorder Signs and symptoms that are intentionally produced so that one may assume the sick role.

failure Lack of success; neglect or omission.

false imprisonment Detention of a competent person against his or her will.

feedback Responses and intrapersonal communications of each person when messages are being sent and received.

felonies Crimes that are punishable by imprisonment or death.

flashbacks Vivid recollections of an event in which the individual relives a frightening, traumatic experience.

forensic evidence Objective information that is obtained from a victim and used in a court of law to determine guilt or innocence of an alleged perpetrator of violence.

fraud Act of giving false information with the knowledge that it will be acted on.

fugue Escape from reality; dissociative fugue: sudden, unexpected travel, with an inability to recall the past.

functional assessment Analysis of each client's abilities to perform the activities of daily living.

G

gangs Groups of people, generally adolescents, who act, look, and dress alike; share the same values; and follow similar codes of conduct.

gay Male or female homosexual.

gender identity The personal identity of being male or female that one carries.

gender perception A view of one's maleness or femaleness.

gender role Expected cultural and social patterns of behavior based on one's sex.

genuineness Quality of being open, honest, sincere; actively involved.

gerontophobia Fear of aging and refusal to accept elderly individuals into the mainstream of society.

gregarious Sociable, in need of the company of others.

grief Set of emotional reactions that accompany a loss.

grieving process The experience of coping with a significant loss.

growth The increase in physical size that follows organized and orderly patterns.

H

habituation Occurs when an individual depends on a substance to provide pleasure or relief from discomfort.

hallucinations False sensory inputs with no external stimuli in the form of smells, sounds, tastes, sight, or touch.

hallucinogen Chemical substance that alters one's reality.

health A state of physical, emotional, sociocultural, and spiritual well-being in which the psychological realms are in balance with the physical self in a state of homeostasis.

health-illness continuum Broad spectrum or scale by means of which a person's level of health can be described, ranging from high-level wellness to severe illness.

health maintenance organizations (HMOs) Groups of physicians, hospitals, and clinics who deliver health care to enrolled clients who pay a fixed, negotiated fee.

heroin A semisynthetic narcotic of opium.

heterosexual Person who expresses sexuality with members of the opposite gender.

histrionic personality Pattern of excessive emotional expression accompanied by attention-seeking behaviors.

hoarding Act of collecting and saving assorted, seemingly useless items.

holistic health care Philosophical concept designed to consider all aspects of human functioning and help clients achieve harmony within themselves and with others, nature, and the world.

homelessness Lack of a regular and adequate nighttime residence.

homeopathy A therapeutic method that uses natural substances in microdoses to relieve symptoms.

homeostasis Tendency of the body to achieve and maintain a steady internal state.

homicides The taking of others' lives: murders.

homosexuality Expression of sexual desire or preference for members of one's own gender.

hope Multidimensional dynamic life force characterized by an anticipated and confident yet uncertain expectation of achieving a future good.

hospice Philosophy of care for people with terminal illnesses or conditions and their loved ones.

hospitalization Placing of an ill or injured person into an inpatient health care facility that provides continuous nursing care and an organized medical staff.

humoral theory of disease Hippocrates' view that illness was the result of an imbalance of the body's humors of blood, phlegm, black bile, and yellow bile.

hypertensive crisis Condition in which the blood pressure rises to extreme levels; commonly caused by an interaction between monoamine oxidase inhibitors and other substances.

hypnosis The induction of a relaxed, trancelike state in which the individual is receptive to appropriate suggestions.

hypochondriasis Somatoform disorder in which one has an intense fear of or preoccupation with having a serious disease or medical condition based on a misinterpretation of body signs and symptoms.

hypomania Exaggerated sense of cheerfulness and well-being.

I

id In psychoanalysis the part of the psyche functioning in the unconscious that is the source of instinctive energy, impulses, and drives; based on the pleasure principle; has strong tendencies toward self-preservation.

ideas of reference Incorrect perceptions of causal events as having great or significant meaning; finding special, personal messages in everyday events.

identity diffusion Failure to bring various childhood identifications into an effective adult personality.

illness State of social, emotional, intellectual, and physical dysfunction.

illusions False perceptions of actual stimuli.

impulse control Ability to express one's emotions in appropriate or effective ways.

impulsivity Pattern of behavior in which actions are taken without forethought or regard to the consequences.

incest Inappropriate sexual activities with one or more members of one's family.

incongruent communications Interactions in which the verbal messages being sent do not match one's nonverbal communications.

indirect self-destructive behaviors Any behaviors that may result in harm to the individual's well-being or death in which people have no actual intention of ending their lives.

inferiority Feeling of being inadequate or less than others.

information overload Inability to process data because of their sheer volume.

informed consent Process of presenting clients with information about the benefits, risks, and side effects of specific treatments, thus enabling clients to make voluntary and competent decisions about their care.

inhalants Chemical substances that are introduced into the body by breathing in through the nose and mouth.

inpatient psychiatric care Health care facility that provides 24-hour/day care within a structured and protective setting.

insight The power or act of seeing into a situation; understanding the inner nature of things.

insomnia A disorder of falling asleep or maintaining a sound sleep.

Integrative medicine Uses the most effective practices and treatments from both conventional and alternative treatment systems with emphasis on interrelationship among body, mind, and spirit.

integrity State of wholeness, of being complete.

intermittent explosive disorder A failure to resist aggressive impulses that result in the destruction of property or assault of another living being.

internal losses Physical or emotional losses that involve some part of oneself.

interpersonal communications Interactions that occur between two or more persons consisting of the verbal and nonverbal messages that are sent and received during every interaction.

interview Purposeful, organized conversation with a client.

intoxication State of being under the influence of a chemical substance or drug.

intrapersonal communications Messages that are sent and received within oneself.

Introspection The process of looking into one's own mind.

invasion of privacy Violation of a person's space, body, belongings, or personal information.

involuntary admission Request for mental health services that is initiated by someone other than the client.

involvement The process of actively interacting with the environment and those persons within it.

J

judgment Ability to evaluate choices and make appropriate decisions.

L

la belle indifference Lack of concern or indifference about the nature or the implications of the signs and symptoms of a somatoform disorder.

laryngeal-pharyngeal dystonia Life-threatening side effect of antipsychotic medications that occurs when the muscles of the throat become rigid and the client begins to gag, choke, and become cyanotic. Respiratory distress and asphyxia result if immediate intervention does not occur.

laws Controls by which a society governs itself.

learning disorder Problems with learning to read, write, or calculate.

lesbian Woman who prefers homosexuality as a mode of sexual expression.

libel Written communication that results in harm.

libidinal energy Also called libido; psychic energy or instinctual drive associated with sexual desire, pleasure, or creativity.

life space Psychological field or space in which one moves, including oneself, other people, and objects.

limit setting Process of consistently reinforcing the established structure (rules, routine) of the therapeutic setting.

lithium Naturally occurring salt used to treat mania.

lobotomy Surgical procedure that disconnects the frontal lobes from the thalamus in the brain and results in a decrease in violent behaviors and mood swings.

loss Actual or potential state in which a valued object, person, or body part that was formerly present is lost or changed and can no longer be seen, felt, heard, known, or experienced.

lunacy Medieval term meaning a mental disorder caused by or relating to the moon.

M

machismo Compulsive masculinity evidenced by preoccupation with physical strength and athletic prowess, attempts to demonstrate daring, or violent and aggressive behaviors.

malingering Somatoform disorder in which one produces symptoms to meet a recognizable, external goal.

malpractice Failure to exercise an accepted degree of professional skill or learning, resulting in injury, loss, or damage.

mania Extreme emotional state characterized by excitement, great elation, overtalkativeness, increased motor activity, fleeting grandiose ideas, and agitated behaviors.

manic depression Behavioral problems caused by sudden, dramatic shifts in emotional extremes; older term for a bipolar disorder.

manipulation Controlling others for one's own purposes by influencing them in unfair or false ways.

marriage A legal state that bonds two people as a single-family unit.

masochism Sexual arousal achieved by being the recipient of pain, humiliation, or suffering.

massage The manipulation of muscles and connective tissue to relax the body and enhance well-being.

maturation Process of attaining complete physical and psychosocial development.

maturity The ability to accept responsibility for one's actions, delay gratification, and make priorities; the period in life from the end of adolescence until death.

meditation Techniques that share four common elements: concentration, retraining the attention to one item while excluding all other thoughts, mindfulness, and an altered state of consciousness.

memory Ability to recall past events, experience, and perceptions.

memory loss Natural part of the aging process relating to the inability to recall a certain detail or event.

mental health Relative state of mind in which a person who is healthy is able to cope with and adjust to the recurrent stresses of everyday living in an acceptable way.

mental health care team Group of professionally trained specialists who develop and implement comprehensive treatment plans for clients with mental or emotional problems.

mental illness (disorder) Any disturbance of psychic equilibrium that results in maladaptive behaviors and impaired functioning.

mental retardation Developmental disorder characterized by significantly below average intellectual level and limited abilities to function.

mentally healthy adult A person who can cope with and adjust to the recurrent stresses of daily living in an acceptable way.

methadone Narcotic used to treat long-term heroin addiction.

misdemeanors Crimes that are punishable by fines or imprisonment of less than 1 year.

model Example or pattern that provides a matrix or framework for a theory.

monoamine oxidase inhibitors (MAOIs) Antidepressant drugs that can produce serious drug and food interactions, such as cardiovascular and blood pressure reactions and central nervous system depression.

mood Subjective state of an individual's overall feelings.

mood disorder Prolonged emotional state that influences ones whole personality and life functioning.

morals Attitudes, beliefs, and values that define one's basis for right or wrong behavior.

mortality Condition of being subject to death.

mourning Process of working through or resolving one's grief.

multidisciplinary mental health care teams Teams composed of psychiatrists, social workers, psychologists, nurses, and other health care professionals who share their expertise and develop comprehensive therapeutic client care plans.

mutuality Process through which the client assumes an appropriate level of autonomy without blocking the provision of necessary health care services.

N

narcissistic personality Pattern of behavior characterized by ideas of grandiosity and the need to be admired; belief that one is special, unique, or extra important.

narcolepsy Uncommon sleep disorder in which an individual has repeated attacks of sleep.

narcotics Natural, semisynthetic, or synthetic chemical substances that act as central nervous system depressants.

naturopathy A whole medical system that views disease as an alteration in the process by which the body heals itself.

negative symptoms In schizophrenia, behaviors that indicate a lack of adaptive mechanisms, including flat affect, poor grooming, withdrawal, and poverty of speech.

neglect Lack of meeting a dependent person's (usually a child's) basic needs for food, clothing, shelter, love, and belonging.

negligence Omission or commission of an act that a reasonable and prudent person would or would not do.

neuroleptic malignant syndrome (NMS) Serious and potentially fatal extrapyramidal side effect of antipsychotic or neuroleptic medications.

neuron The basic unit of the nervous system whose function is to transmit electrical information to other nerve cells.

neuropeptides Neurotransmitters composed of amino acid strings that interact with the endocrine, immune, and nervous systems.

neurotransmitters Chemicals found in the nervous system that facilitate the transmission of energy and act as the body's chemical messenger system.

nicotine Addictive, active ingredient of tobacco.

noncompliance Informed decision made by a client not to follow a prescribed treatment program.

nonmaleficence The ethical principle that states "do no harm."

nontherapeutic communications Messages that hinder effective communications.

nonverbal communication Messages that are sent and received without the use of words, which include one's intrapersonal communications; the messages created through the body's motions and use of touch, space, and sight; unspoken interpersonal communications; and behaviors such as eye movement, gestures, movement of the body, expressions, posture, and eye contact.

norms Established rules of conduct that arise from a culture's behavioral standards.

nuclear family Household unit consisting of two parents and their offspring.

nurse case manager Professional nurse who works with psychiatrists to develop treatment plans tailored to each client's special needs.

nursing (therapeutic) process Organizational framework for the practice of nursing that uses the steps of assessment, nursing diagnosis, planning, implementation, and evaluation for the delivery of client care.

nurture Act or process to promote the development of persons or things.

O

obesity Abnormal increase in body fat; body weight that is more than 20% above one's ideal weight.

object constancy Awareness that a person or item still exists even though it cannot be perceived (seen, touched) at the time.

obsession Persistent, recurring, inappropriate, and distressing thoughts.

obsessive-compulsive personality Extreme anxiety about the uncertainty of the future; extremely orderly and overly preoccupied with details; devoted to work, has few leisure activities, and is consumed by the need for perfection.

oculogyric crisis Dystonic reaction, usually a side effect of psychotropic medication, in which the eyes involuntarily roll to the back of the head.

open system Set of interacting, related units with permeable boundaries through which matter, energy, and information pass.

outpatient mental health care Health care setting that provides comprehensive services for mentally ill clients within their home environments.

P

pain management Series of nursing interventions designed to assist clients in identifying, defining, and controlling pain.

panic attack Brief period of intense fear or discomfort accompanied by various physical and emotional reactions.

paranoia Suspicious system of thinking with delusions of persecution and grandeur; pattern of behaviors marked by suspiciousness and mistrust.

paraphilias Group of sexual variations that depart from society's traditional and acceptable modes of seeking sexual gratification.

parasomnias Sleep disorders characterized by abnormal behavioral or physical events during sleep.

parasuicidal behaviors Unsuccessful attempts and gestures of suicide that are associated with a low likelihood of success.

parasympathetic nervous system A branch of the autonomic nervous system designed to conserve energy and the sympathetic system's excitability. The main functions are to monitor and control the regulatory processes of the body, which it accomplishes by governing smooth muscle tone and glandular secretions.

parity Equality, uniformity, equal terms.

passive aggression Indirect expressions of anger through subtle, evasive, or manipulative behaviors.

passive suicide Act of taking one's own life by refusing to eat, drink, or cooperate with care.

Patient's Bill of Rights List of client's rights set forth by the American Hospital Association; offers some guidance and protection to clients by stating the responsibilities that a hospital and its staff have toward clients and their families during hospitalization; not a legally binding document.

peer groups Group of people of similar age, interests, and developmental levels.

perceptions Use of the senses to gain information.

peripheral nervous system (PNS) Thirty-one spinal nerves that originate in the spinal cord in addition to the 12 pairs of cranial nerves; further divided into a motor and an autonomic system.

perseveration Repeating of the same idea in response to different questions or interactions.

personal identity Composite of behavioral traits and characteristics by which one is recognized as an individual.

personality Unique pattern of attitudes and behaviors each individual develops to adapt to a particular environment and its standards.

personality disorder Enduring pattern of inner experience and behavior that deviates markedly from the expectations of the individual's culture, is pervasive and inflexible, has an onset in adolescence or early adulthood, is stable over time, and leads to distress or impairment.

personifications According to Harry Stack Sullivan, distorted images of certain relationships that spill over or transfer into other relationships.

pervasive developmental disorders Problems severe enough to affect several areas of a child's functioning (including difficulty with social interaction skills, communication skills, and learning) and behavior that is different from other children of the same age and developmental level.

phencyclidine (PCP) Drug developed for use as an animal tranquilizer; in humans, produces mild depression with low doses and a schizophrenic-like reaction with higher amounts.

phobia Unnatural fear of people, animals, objects, situations, or occurrences.

phototherapy Exposure of clients to full-spectrum light for certain periods during the day for the relief of depressive symptoms that occur during the winter months.

physical abuse Inflicted injury to a child, ranging from minor bruises and lacerations to severe trauma and death.

physiological stress response Mechanism that protects mammals during times of threat or illness; fight-or-flight response; a biochemical survival system designed to provide the body with the energy for fighting or fleeing.

pica Eating disorder characterized by ingestion of nonfood items, such as hair, string, or dirt for more than 1 month.

polysomnogram Device that monitors the client's electro-physical responses during sleep and includes such measurements as brain wave activity (electroencephalogram [EEG]), muscle movement (electromyogram [EMG]), and extraocular eye movements (electrooculogram [EOG]).

pornography Writings, pictures, or other messages that are intended to sexually arouse.

positive symptoms In schizophrenia, the signs related to maladaptive thoughts and behaviors, including hallucinations, speech problems, and bizarre behaviors.

postpartum depression A condition characterized by symptoms of tearfulness, irritability, hypochondria, sleeplessness, impairment of concentration, and headache in the days and weeks following childbirth.

posttraumatic stress disorder (PTSD) Problems that develop after a person experiences a psychologically distressing event; characterized by an oversensitivity or overinvolvement with stimuli that recall the traumatic event.

poverty Inability to secure the basic necessities of life, such as food, shelter, and clothing.

poverty of thought Lack of ability to produce new thoughts or follow a train of thought.

prayer An active process of appealing to a higher spiritual power.

preferred provider organizations (PPOs) Networks of physicians, hospitals, and clinics that agree to provide medical care for the organization's members at a discount.

prejudice Displacement of unacceptable impulses and behaviors onto a culturally different group.

primary gain Physical signs and symptoms of an illness used to relieve an individual's anxieties by masking inner emotional turmoil.

principle Standard or code that guides actions.

professional (nurse) practice acts A series of regulations that identify the limits and scope of practice and act as the legal framework for practice in that state.

prostitution The selling of sexual favors.

proximal-distal The pattern of growth and development in which growth occurs from near to far, midline to distal.

psyche Vital or spiritual aspect of the individual as opposed to the body or soma; total components of the id, ego, and superego, including all conscious and unconscious aspects.

psychiatric rehabilitation Multidisciplinary services that assist people with mental health problems to readjust and adapt to life in the community as actively and independently as possible; includes personal adjustment and social, residential, educational, and vocational services. Also called psychosocial rehabilitation.

psychoanalysis Branch of psychiatry founded by Sigmund Freud devoted to the study of the psychology of human behavior; also a therapy for certain emotional disorders that investigates the workings of the mind.

psychobiology Study of the biochemical foundations of thought, mood, emotion, affect, and behavior.

psychoneuroimmunology (PNI) The study of interactions among the body's central nervous system, its immune system, and aspects of the personality.

psychopath Person with an antisocial personality disorder and a pervasive pattern of disregard for and violation of the rights of others, often using deceit and manipulation.

psychophysical disorders Disorders in which stress-related problems result in physical signs and symptoms.

psychosis Inability to recognize reality, relate to others, or cope with life's demands.

psychosocial rehabilitation Multidisciplinary services that assist people with mental health problems to readjust and adapt to life in the community as actively and independently as possible; includes personal adjustment and social, residential, educational, and vocational services. Also called psychiatric rehabilitation.

psychosomatic illnesses Popular term that describes emotionally (psycho) related physical (somatic) disorders.

psychotherapeutic drugs Chemicals that affect the mind and treat the symptoms of mental-emotional illness.

psychotherapy Any of a large number of related methods of treating mental-emotional disorders by psychological techniques rather than by physical means.

puberty Period in life at which the ability to reproduce is developed, beginning with a 24- to 36-month growth spurt and ending when the reproductive system is mature.

purging Recurring inappropriate behaviors to prevent weight gain; usually associated with bulimia.

Q

qi gong A system of movement, regulation of breathing, and meditation designed to enhance the flow of qi (energy) throughout the body.

R

race Group of genetically related people who share certain physical characteristics.

rape Forced sexual assault.

rapport Dynamic process; an energy exchange between nurse and client that provides the background for all other nursing actions.

rational suicide Act of purposefully ending one's own life after conscious and rational deliberation.

reasonable and prudent care provider Principle by which the law judges a caregiver's actions by comparing what other caregivers would do in similar situations.

recidivism Relapse of a symptom, disease, or behavior pattern.

refugee A person who, because of war or persecution, flees from his or her home or country and seeks refuge elsewhere.

Reiki A life force energy that flows through one's body.

relapse The recurrence of substance-abusing behaviors after a significant period of abstinence.

religion Defined, organized, and practiced system of beliefs and practices usually involving a moral code.

religiosity Delusions of great spirituality; believing one has powers to communicate with God or be a spirit.

remissions In chronic mental illness, times of partial or complete disappearance of symptoms.

resistance Client's attempts to avoid recognizing or exploring anxiety-provoking material.

resource linkage Process of matching client's needs with the most appropriate community services.

responding strategies Therapeutic techniques that relate to the nurse's actions or interventions while communicating.

responsibility State of being answerable for acts or decisions and able to fulfill obligations.

right Power, privilege, or existence to which one has a just claim.

risk factor assessment Interview tool to identify risk factors that potentially present an immediate threat to the client.

role Expected pattern of behaviors associated with a certain position.

rumination disorder Uncommon problem of childhood involving regurgitating and rechewing food.

S

schizoid personality Personality that lacks the desire or willingness to become involved in a close relationship, prefers solitary activities, is emotionally restricted, and communicates emotional detachment, coldness, and a lack of concern for others.

schizophrenia Condition associated with disturbing thought patterns, behaviors, and loss of contact with reality to the point at which it impairs functioning.

schizotypal personality Interaction pattern of avoiding people with behaviors characterized by distortions and eccentricities (odd, strange, or peculiar actions).

seasonal affective disorder Levels of mild to moderate depression experienced during long winter days; symptoms begin to lift with the coming of spring.

secondary gain Situation in which the payoff for remaining ill outweighs the advantages of recovery and clients profit or avoid unpleasant situations by remaining ill.

self-awareness Consciousness of one's own individuality and personality.

self-concept All the attitudes, notions, beliefs, and convictions that make up an individual's self-knowledge, including perceptions of personal characteristics and abilities, interactions with other people and the environment, values associated with experiences and objects, and goals and ideals.

self-esteem Individual's judgment of his or her own worth.

self-ideal Personal standards of how one should behave.

self-injuries Attempts to harm or hurt oneself.

sensorium Part of the consciousness that perceives, sorts, and integrates information.

sexual abuse Intentional engaging of children or others in inappropriate or illegal sexual activities.

sexual addiction A progressive and chronic addiction characterized by patterns of compulsive sexual behavior despite negative consequences.

sexual disorder Disturbances in sexual desire or functioning that cause marked distress and interpersonal difficulties.

sexual dysfunction A disturbance anywhere in the four stages (appetite, excitement, orgasm, resolution) of the sexual response cycle.

sexual masochism Sexual arousal achieved by being receiver of pain (either physical or emotional), humiliation, or being made to suffer.

sexual orientation Individual's sexual attraction to others. Also called sexual preference.

sexual sadism Sexual arousal achieved by infliction of pain (either physical or emotional) or humiliation onto another person.

sexuality Combination of physical, chemical, psychological, and functional characteristics that are expressed by one's gender identity and sexual behaviors.

shaken baby syndrome Vigorous manual shaking of an infant who is being held by the extremities or shoulders, leading to whiplash-induced intracranial and intraocular bleeding and no external signs of head trauma.

sick role Actions and behaviors of a person who is ill and excused from everyday responsibilities.

signal anxiety Learned anxiety response to an anticipated event.

situational crisis Event or situation for which one is unprepared, resulting from environmental factors outside the individual.

situational depression Depressive responses tied to a specific event or situation that can be traced to a recognizable cause.

slander Verbal communications that result in harm.

sleep disorder Condition or problem that repeatedly disrupts an individual's pattern of sleep.

social isolation Removal of or withdrawal from the company and companionship of other people.

sociopath Person with an antisocial personality disorder and a pervasive pattern of disregard for and violation of the rights of others, often using deceit and manipulation. (See *psychopath*.)

soma The body, as distinguished from the mind or psyche.

somatic therapies Physical interventions that affect behavioral changes (e.g., electroconvulsive therapy).

somatization Act of focusing anxieties and emotional conflicts into physical symptoms.

somatoform disorder Disorder in which a child or adult has the signs and symptoms of illness or disease without a traceable physical cause.

speech cluttering Disorder of speech and language processing that results in unorganized, unrythmic, and frequently unintelligible speech.

spirituality A belief in a power greater than any human being.

spiritual dimension Broad term that includes an individual's belief in a higher power and a sense of meaning and purpose in life.

splitting Emotionally dividing staff members or other people by complimenting one group and degrading another; performed by clients.

standards of practice A set of guidelines that provide measurable criteria for care providers, clients, and others to evaluate the quality and effectiveness of health care; also called standards of care.

stereotype Oversimplified mental picture of a cultural group.

stigma A sign or mark of shame, disapproval, or disgrace, of being shunned or rejected.

stressor A nonspecific response of the body to any demand placed on it.

substance A drug of abuse, a medication, or a toxin.

substance (drug) abuse Inappropriate use of a drug, medication, or toxin whose use results in dependence, addiction, or withdrawal.

substance (chemical) dependency Occurs when a user must take his or her usual or an increasing dose of the drug to prevent the onset of withdrawal signs and symptoms.

substance use Act of taking a chemical substance.

suicidal attempts Serious self-directed actions that are intended to do harm to or end one's own life.

suicidal gestures Suicidal actions that result in little or no injury to oneself but communicate a message.

suicidal ideation Thoughts or fantasies of suicide that are expressed but have no definite intent.

suicidal threats Expressions of the intent to take one's life but without any action.

suicide Act of intentionally taking one's own life.

suicide precautions Standard interventions to prevent a suicide attempt from occurring.

suicidology Study of the nature of suicide.

sundown syndrome A group of behaviors characterized by confusion, agitation, and disruptive actions that occur in the late afternoon or evening. The cause is unknown, but sundowning is associated with dementia, loss of cognitive functions, and physical or social stressors.

superego In psychoanalysis, that part of the psyche, functioning mostly in the unconscious, that develops when the standards of the parents and society are incorporated into the ego.

surveillance Process of watching over adolescents to determine if they are safe, are behaving within acceptable limits, are making good decisions, or are in need of adult intervention.

sympathetic nervous system Division of the autonomic nervous system that prepares the body for immediate adaptation through the fight-or-flight mechanism.

T

tardive dyskinesia Drug-induced condition that produces involuntary, repeated movements of the muscles of the face, trunk, arms, and legs; usually occurs following a long period of antipsychotic drug use.

temperament Genetically linked biological bases that underlie moods, energy levels, and attitudes.

terminal illness Illness or condition likely to result in death.

territoriality The need to gain control over an area of space and claim it for oneself.

theory Statement that predicts, explains, or describes a relationship among events, concepts, or ideas.

therapeutic communications Interactions that focus on the client, foster the therapeutic relationship, and are specifically designed to achieve client outcomes.

therapeutic environment (milieu) Inpatient psychiatric setting that provides safe, stable surroundings that are structured to enhance the client's response to treatment.

therapeutic relationship Series of interactions initiated by the nurse with the purpose of providing corrective interpersonal experiences.

therapeutic touch A healing technique based upon the practice of laying on of hands, where the healing energies of the therapist encourage the client's body energies to return to a balanced state.

third-party payments Payments for medical costs made by someone other than the client, usually through an insurance company or government program, such as Medicare or Medicaid.

thought content What an individual is thinking.

thought processes How a person thinks, analyzes the world, and connects and organizes information.

tolerance Relating to drug use, a state in which increased amounts of the chemical are needed to produce the same effects that one dose once produced.

tort law Division of private law that relates to compensation for a legal wrong committed against the person or property of another.

torticollis Contraction of the cervical muscles that forces the neck into a twisted position.

traditional Chinese medicine (TCM) A whole medical system based on the view that the body is a delicate balance of opposing forces: yin and yang.

trance State resembling sleep in which consciousness remains but voluntary movement is lost, as in hypnosis.

transference Client's emotional response to the nurse based on earlier relationships with significant others.

transsexualism Discomfort with his or her biological gender and a desire to surgically change sexual anatomy and live as a member of the other gender.

transvestism Practice of dressing in opposite-gender clothing for sexual gratification.

traumatic stress reaction A series of behavioral and emotional responses following an overwhelmingly stressful event.

trust Risk-taking process whereby an individual's situation depends on the future behavior of another person.

V

vaginismus Persistent involuntary contractions of the perineal muscles around the outer third of the vagina whenever vaginal penetration is attempted.

value Dearly held belief about the worth of an idea, behavior, or item.

values clarification Method for discovering one's own values by assessing, exploring, and determining what those personal values are and how they affect personal decision making.

verbal communication Level of communication related to the spoken word, which includes the spoken and written word, use of language and symbols, and arrangement of words or phrases.

victimization Process of causing harm; children suffer more victimizations than do adults, including more conventional crime, more family violence, and some forms unique to children, such as family abduction, neglect, and abuse.

violence Any behavior that threatens or harms another person or his or her property.

voyeurism Sexual arousal achieved by observing unsuspecting persons who are disrobing, naked, or engaging in sexual activity.

W

whole medical systems Systems that are built on complete systems of theory and practice and include Western medicine, osteopathy, homeopathy, naturopathy, ayurveda, and Oriental medicine.

Index

The letter t indicates tables, f indicates figures, and b indicates boxes.

■

Review Worksheets

CHAPTER 1

The History of Mental Health Care

Student's Name _____

Date _____

1. Write your definition of mental health and mental illness.

   _____

   _____

   _____

Match the following people and their contributions:
   a. Hippocrates
   b. Plato
   c. Philippe Pinel
   d. Dorothea Dix
   e. Benjamin Rush
   f. Clifford Beers

2. _____ Surveyed conditions of mental hospitals in United States, Canada, and Scotland

3. _____ Wrote a book that started the mental hygiene movement

4. _____ Said life was a dynamic equilibrium maintained by the soul

5. _____ Wrote the first American textbook on psychiatry

6. _____ Viewed mental illness as the result of an imbalance of humors

7. _____ Freed the mentally ill in France from their chains

8. What made witch hunting so popular for 500 years?

   _____

   _____

   _____

Circle the correct answer:

9. Which legislative act called for a neighborhood-based mental health care delivery system?
   a. Mental Health Systems Act of 1977
   b. National Mental Health Act of 1946
   c. Omnibus Budget Reform Act of 1987
   d. Community Mental Health Centers Act of 1963

10. Which legislative act dramatically reduced federal funding for mental health and illness care?
    a. Mental Health Study Act of 1955
    b. Omnibus Budget Reconciliation Act of 1981
    c. Mental Health Systems Act of 1977
    d. Omnibus Budget Reform Act of 1987

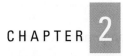

Current Mental Health Care Systems

Student's Name _____

Date _____

Define the following:

1. third-party payment

_____

2. preferred provider organization

_____

3. health maintenance organization

_____

4. diagnosis-related group

_____

Identify two factors that are considered when admitting a client to an inpatient psychiatric setting:

5. _____

6. _____

List two outpatient psychiatric care settings:

7. _____

8. _____

The client is a homeless, jobless, 25-year-old schizophrenic woman who thinks she may be pregnant. Using the community support systems model, determine which services would most benefit this client.

9. _____

10. _____

11. _____

12. _____

The client is being discharged from the hospital to the community where case management will be implemented. List four components of case management:

13. _____

14. _____

15. _____

16. _____

List two mental health problems associated with human immunodeficiency virus (HIV)/acquired immunodeficiency syndrome (AIDS):

17. _____

18. _____

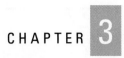

Ethical and Legal Issues

Student's Name _____

Date _____

Match the following terms and their definitions:
   a. laws
   b. rights
   c. morals
   d. nonmaleficence
   e. ethics
   f. values

1. _____ Serves as one's personal basis for right or wrong behaviors

2. _____ Power to which one has a just claim

3. _____ To do no harm

4. _____ Shared set of rules that govern right behavior

5. _____ Controls by which a society governs itself

Identify the ethical or legal principle being illustrated or violated:

6. _____ A man from the local newspaper calls and wants to know the condition of a client on the unit. The caregiver refuses to share any information with the reporter and notifies her supervisor.

7. _____ The nurse encourages the client to participate in informed decision making by answering his questions and providing him with educational materials.

8. _____ The care providers are careful to ensure that clients will not be harmed during care.

9. _____ Every caregiver on the unit is careful to treat each client equally, fairly, and respectfully.

10. _____ The technician charted that the client had a problem with drinking and, as a result, the client was fired from her job.

11. _____ The nurse locks the client in his room because of his constant wanderings.

Order the steps for resolving ethical dilemmas:

12. _____ Gather relevant information.

13. _____ Take action.

14. _____ Assume good will.

15. _____ List and order values.

16. _____ Identify all elements of the situation.

List three areas of potential liability for nurses and other care providers:

17. _____

18. _____

19. _____

Match the following examples with the appropriate tort:
   a. "She's a nasty old lady who bites."
   b. "If you don't cooperate, I'll call the techs and we will lock you up."
   c. Leaving a suicidal client unattended and he harms himself
   d. Searching a client's belongings without permission
   e. Charting a medication that was not actually given

20. _____ assault

21. _____ malpractice

22. _____ fraud

23. _____ slander

24. _____ invasion of privacy

CHAPTER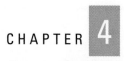

Sociocultural Issues

Student's Name _____

Date _____

Identify the term described:

1. _____ A group of people who share distinct physical characteristics
2. _____ Learned behavior patterns with shared values system
3. _____ Customs and cultural habits of a group
4. _____ An oversimplified mental picture of a cultural group
5. _____ An expected pattern of behavior associated with a certain position or rank

List four characteristics of culture:

6. _____

7. _____

8. _____

9. _____

You are about to perform a cultural communication assessment. Describe five areas that you will assess:

10. _____

11. _____

12. _____

13. _____

14. _____

List which area of the cultural assessment relates to each of the following statements:

15. "I practice Buddhism."

_____

16. "Pleasing the ancestors is more important than today's problems."

_____

17. He speaks Italian and Spanish.

_____

18. She visits an herbalist monthly.

_____

19. Women are not allowed to own property or drive cars.

_____

20. Describe how stereotyping can influence the care of mental health clients.

_____

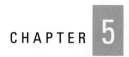
Theories and Therapies

Student's Name _____

Date _____

Match the therapy or theory with the statement that best describes it:

a. actualizing therapy   i. covert modeling
b. assertiveness training   j. social learning theory
c. coping skills therapies   k. behavior modification
d. client-centered therapy   l. sociocultural theory
e. Gestalt therapy   m. individual therapy
f. interpersonal therapy   n. stress adaptation theory
g. logotherapy   o. nursing theories
h. psychoanalysis   p. addiction theory

1. _____ Based on a person's need to search for meaning and values in life.

2. _____ People learn by observing the outcomes of various events and then comparing themselves with others.

3. _____ Uses dream analysis and free association to uncover unconscious conflicts.

4. _____ Used by therapists to define positive behaviors and develop programs with specific reinforcements to change the specified behaviors.

5. _____ Teaches clients how to develop more successful daily living skills.

6. _____ Describes physical responses of the body to stress and the processes by which they adapt.

7. _____ A process described as the act of mentally rehearsing an activity before actually engaging in the activity.

8. _____ The concept of self is developed through interactions with other people.

9. _____ Helps clients to uncover how their personifications (distorted images) affect their lives.

10. _____ The client directs the therapeutic relationship using the therapist as a guide to self-understanding.

11. _____ Teaches clients to express themselves in constructive, nonaggressive ways.

12. _____ Goal of therapy is self-actualization, not cure or relief of symptoms.

13. _____ Approaches human behavior from a helping point of view.

14. Describe how Maslow's theory is used in planning care for mentally ill clients.

_____

_____

_____

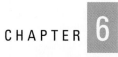

Complementary and Alternative Therapies

Student's Name _____

Date _____

Briefly describe the following:

1. Reiki

_____

2. integrative medicine

_____

3. massage therapy

_____

4. meditation

_____

5. acupuncture

_____

6. The student feels that therapeutic touch will benefit the client who is hallucinating. The nurse in charge will most likely say what? What is the nurse's reasoning for the decision?

_____

_____

_____

Identify three therapies that may be helpful in treating depression:

7. _____

8. _____

9. _____

Psychotherapeutic Drug Therapy

Student's Name _____

Date _____

1. Which of the following is a parasympathetic nervous system action?
   a. The pupils of the eye dilate.
   b. Saliva, tears, and respiratory and gastrointestinal secretions decrease.
   c. The smooth muscles of the lungs constrict and restrict airways.
   d. The blood vessels in the heart and skeletal muscles dilate.

2. The _____ prepares the body for immediate adaptation through the fight-or-flight response.
   a. central nervous system
   b. peripheral nervous system
   c. sympathetic nervous system
   d. parasympathetic nervous system

List the four responsibilities (client care guidelines) for clients receiving psychotherapeutic drug therapy:

3. _____

4. _____

5. _____

6. _____

Match the following terms and their definitions:
   a. benzodiazepines
   b. anticholinergic reaction
   c. extrapyramidal side effects (EPSEs)
   d. hypertensive crisis
   e. tricyclic drugs

7. _____ Treats depression

8. _____ Treats anxiety

9. _____ Dry mouth, blurred vision, sweating

10. _____ Akathisia, dyskinesia, akinesia

11. _____ Stiff neck, throbbing headache, tightness in the chest

12. What do you suspect is happening to the client who complains of feeling jittery, is unable to sit still, and has problems with eye movements?

_____

_____

_____

13. An informed decision made by a client not to follow the prescribed treatment program is called

_____

14. Why must salt intake be monitored in clients who are receiving lithium?
    a. Salt and water compete for lithium in the tissues.
    b. Salt and lithium compete for excretion in the kidney.
    c. Salt competes with lithium for detoxification in the liver.
    d. People who take lithium crave large amounts of salt.

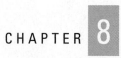

Skills and Principles of Mental Health Care

Student's Name _____

Date _____

State which principle of mental health care is being used in the following situations:

1. All clients will be at breakfast by 0800.

   _____

2. Mr. J. is practicing anger control by counting to 10 before he speaks out.

   _____

3. Caregiver Jane sits with a mute client for 15 minutes every morning.

   _____

4. Nurse Dan is not intimidated by Mr. Jones' rough appearance and salty mannerisms.

   _____

5. Miss Sally is expected to arrive for her appointment at 1300 every other day.

   _____

6. Sam states that he is being followed by the FBI. The caregiver responds with, "Tell me about it."

   _____

Rachel flunked a big test today because she stayed out late last night and had little time to study. She feels like a failure and is talking about leaving school. List three ways that she could grow from this experience:

7. _____

8. _____

9. _____

Helping boundaries help define the limits of caregivers' therapeutic actions. Identify whether the action is *within* or *outside* professional boundaries:

10. The caregiver braids the client's hair. _____

11. The caregiver shares family problems with the client. _____

12. The caregiver attends a party for clients, families, and staff. _____

13. The caregiver attends a party as the client's guest. _____

14. The caregiver teaches the client about problem solving. _____

15. The caregiver accepts a gift from the client. _____

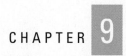

Mental Health Assessment Skills

Student's Name _____

Date _____

1. The purpose of the assessment step of the nursing (therapeutic) process is:

   _____

   _____

Identify the dimension (aspect) of the holistic assessment:

2. _____ The nurse performs a physical examination.

3. _____ The client describes his home and work life.

4. _____ The client describes her affect.

5. The purpose of the mental status examination is:

   _____

   _____

6. The purpose of a physical assessment (examination) for mental health clients is to discover any physical problems that can be treated medically because:

   _____

   _____

List 10 areas that are assessed with the mental status examination:

7. _____

8. _____

9. _____

10. _____

11. _____

12. _____

13. _____

14. _____

15. _____

16. _____

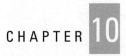

Therapeutic Communication

Student's Name _____

Date _____

List the communication as therapeutic (T) or nontherapeutic (NT):

1. _____ "Would you like to talk about it?"

2. _____ "Everything will be all right."

3. _____ "I'm glad you decided to do that."

4. _____ "You appear tense."

5. _____ "Dr. Dee is a very good psychiatrist. You should learn to trust him."

6. _____ "How did this make you feel?"

7. _____ "I'm not sure I understand."

8. A speech pattern that is associated with mentally ill clients in which the client shifts rapidly between unrelated ideas is called:

   _____

9. A nontherapeutic communication technique in which the caregiver responds with clichés or trite expressions is called:

   _____

10. _____ can identify hidden messages and agendas, minimize misunderstandings, and clarify messages.

11. Messages created through motions, eye contact and movement, gestures, use of touch, space, and sight are _____ communications.

12. Before clients feel safe enough to honestly share themselves, caregivers must:

    _____

    _____

Match the following terms with their definitions:
   a. responses of each person when messages are being sent and received
   b. rapid, confused delivery of unrhythmic speech patterns
   c. inability to read sometimes accompanied by a mixing of letters or syllables
   d. inability to speak
   e. use of the senses to gain information
   f. verbal messages not matching nonverbal communications

13. _____ Aphasia

14. _____ Dyslexia

15. _____ Speech cluttering

16. _____ Perception

17. _____ Feedback

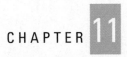

The Therapeutic Relationship

Student's Name _____

Date _____

Match the following terms and their definitions:

    a. trust

    b. empathy

    c. autonomy

    d. caring

    e. hope

1. _____ The ability to direct and control one's own activities

2. _____ Confident but uncertain view of the future

3. _____ Process in which one's situation depends on the future behavior of another person

4. _____ Energy that allows caregivers to accept and care for each client as a person

5. _____ Ability to share in the client's world

List four ways to develop caring abilities:

6. _____

7. _____

8. _____

9. _____

Identify the characteristic of the therapeutic relationship that is illustrated by the caregiver's behavior:

10. _____ The caregiver acknowledges the client as an individual who is worthy of respect.

11. _____ The caregiver actively works to improve his or her abilities to establish meaningful connections with clients.

12. _____ The caregiver knows that feelings and attitudes affect therapeutic relationships, so he or she works to develop an awareness of how his or her actions, gestures, and expressions affect other people.

Identify the phase of the therapeutic relationship, and fill in the blanks:

13. _____ Reviews progress toward meeting goal and prepares client for independence.

14. _____ Gathers data and explores own feelings about client.

15. _____ Caregiver and client establish a working agreement.

16. _____ Client and care provider work on meeting the mutually agreed-on goals.

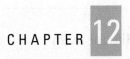

The Therapeutic Environment

Student's Name _____

Date _____

1. John S. is a 30-year-old man who has overdosed on methamphetamine. He states that he has wild thoughts and feels unable to control his behavior. Do you think he should be admitted to an inpatient environment? Explain your answer.

   _____

   _____

   _____

List three purposes of the inpatient therapeutic environment:

2. _____

3. _____

4. _____

Describe one intervention for each of the following client needs:

5. nourishment

   _____

6. personal hygiene

   _____

7. security

   _____

8. territory

   _____

9. communication

   _____

10. social relationships

    _____

11. acceptance

    _____

12. time

    _____

13. Repeated admissions to psychiatric inpatient facilities have become a way of life for many people with chronic mental illness. This situation is called:

_____

14. Clients who do not follow their prescribed courses of treatment are called:

_____

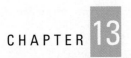

Problems of Childhood

Student's Name _____

Date _____

1. Temper tantrums are a common behavior in:
   a. infants
   b. 1- to 4-year-olds
   c. 5- to 9-year-olds
   d. children over 10 years old

2. The effects of poverty on children:
   a. are small and unimportant
   b. have little impact on their mental health
   c. have a strong impact on children's growth and development
   d. are not considered when making a diagnosis

3. Mental health assistance should be sought for parent-child conflicts when the:
   a. conflict worsens over a period of time
   b. parents are tired of dealing with the child
   c. child repeatedly threatens to run away
   d. child's behavior is out of control

4. One of the most frequent anxieties of young children is a fear of:
   a. strangers
   b. new people and places
   c. separation from their parents
   d. separation from a favorite object

5. Children with depression:
   a. become aggressive
   b. giggle continually
   c. lose interest in school and friends
   d. often stop talking and stare into space

6. Somatoform disorders are thought to be caused by:

   _____

7. Extremely traumatic events involving injury or threat to a child often result in the development of posttraumatic stress disorder (PTSD) because:

   _____

8. Children with enuresis can often be helped with:

   _____

9. Autism is diagnosed when the child has serious problems with:

_____

Three general therapeutic interventions for children with mental health problems are:

10. _____

11. _____

12. _____

CHAPTER 14

Problems of Adolescence

Student's Name _____

Date _____

1. Brian thinks through a problem by considering several options. He is learning to use and apply:

   _____

2. A teen's peer group has several important functions. The most important is:

   _____

3. When an adolescent's behaviors or problems impair performance (school, social, work) or threaten physical well-being, what is needed?

   _____

   _____

4. Describe the therapeutic intervention known as surveillance.

   _____

   _____

Match the following terms and their definitions:
- a. behavioral disorder
- b. emotional disorder
- c. eating disorder
- d. chemical dependency
- e. personality disorder
- f. sexual disorder
- g. psychotic disorder
- h. suicidal problems
- i. limit setting
- j. skill development

5. _____ Becomes preoccupied with ridding self of own characteristics and assuming those of the desired gender

6. _____ Anorexia nervosa or bulimia

7. _____ Symptoms: fighting, temper tantrums, running away from home, destroying property, and problems with authorities and school

8. _____ Thoughts or actions to take one's own life

9. _____ Problem solving, social interactions, working cooperatively in a group

10. _____ Moods ranging from depression to hyperactivity, anxiety

11. _____ Understanding the rules and consequences of breaking the rules

12. _____ Moves from experimenting to burnout

13. _____ Characterized by a loss of contact with reality

14. _____ A major characteristic: impulsivity, the drive to engage in acts harmful to self or others

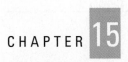

CHAPTER 15

Problems of Adulthood

Student's Name _____

Date _____

True (T) or False (F): The developmental tasks of adulthood include:

1. _____ learning to behave according to the rules

2. _____ valuing the contribution he or she has made throughout life

3. _____ committing to personal relationships

4. _____ developing a conscience

5. _____ becoming capable of living independently

6. Describe how a young adult's sense of personal identity affects his or her functioning.

_____

_____

7. How would you respond to a 20-year-old who wanted a baby so she would have someone to love her?

_____

_____

Describe three characteristics of a mentally healthy adult:

8. _____

9. _____

10. _____

11. Young adults are more likely to contract human immunodeficiency virus (HIV)/acquired immunodeficiency syndrome (AIDS) because:

_____

_____

12. The most important therapeutic tool in the prevention of HIV/AIDS is:

_____

_____

13. Beyond the diagnostic labels of mental illness lies:

_____

_____

14. Middle-age adults are faced with accepting:

_____

_____

Joe is a 23-year-old man with AIDS who has had sexual relationships with 12 women and 4 other men.

15. How many women has Joe put at risk for contracting HIV? _____

16. How many men has Joe put at risk for contracting HIV? _____

CHAPTER 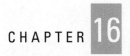 16

Problems of Late Adulthood

Student's Name _____

Date _____

1. After age _____ adults appear to age very little.

2. Adults who are rigid and do not continue learning, experience _____ more rapidly than those with active mental lives.

3. The practice of stereotyping older persons as feeble, dependent, and nonproductive is called

   _____.

4. Collecting and saving assorted, seemingly useless items is called _____.

5. According to Erikson, older adults with a sense of _____ are able to find order and meaning in their lives.

6. Although _____ begins to decline in the 40s, mental capabilities, such as judgment and wisdom, continue to improve as one grows older.

7. In older adults, physical problems can lead to changes in _____.

Match the following terms and their definitions:
a. gerontophobia	e. losses
b. financially vulnerable	f. dementia
c. substance abuse	g. depression
d. elder abuse	h. movement disorders

8. _____ Changes in occupation, living arrangements, physical function, death of a spouse

9. _____ Occurs most commonly with multiple prescriptions

10. _____ Fear of aging and refusal to accept elderly people

11. _____ Older adults who take other people "at their word" or are charmed out of their money

12. _____ Probably the most common mental health disorder of late adulthood

13. _____ Complication of long-term antipsychotic medication use

14. _____ Any action that takes advantage of an older person

15. Explain the concept of respect and its importance to geriatric health care.

   _____

   _____

   _____

CHAPTER 17

Cognitive Impairment, Alzheimer's Disease, and Dementia

Student's Name _____

Date _____

Match the following terms and their definitions:
- a. agnosia
- b. apraxia
- c. aphasia
- d. conative loss
- e. delirium
- f. dementia
- g. depression
- h. Alzheimer's disease

1. _____ A change of consciousness that occurs quickly

2. _____ The loss of the ability to make and carry out plans

3. _____ The loss of one's ability to use and understand a language

4. _____ The loss of the ability to perform everyday actions and activities

5. _____ The loss of multiple abilities, including memory, language, and the ability to think, understand, or conceptualize

6. _____ Loss of recognition of previously known or familiar people and objects

7. _____ Loss of multiple abilities, including memory, language, and the ability to think and understand (judgment and abstract thought)

List three general health care goals for the care of clients with Alzheimer's disease:

8. _____

9. _____

10. _____

Identify the stage of Alzheimer's disease in the descriptions below:
- a. Early stage
- b. Middle stage
- c. Late stage

11. _____ An inability to swallow increases the risk for developing pneumonia and malnutrition.

12. _____ Client develops aphasia, apraxia, and visual agnosia.

13. _____ Client begins to have difficulty performing activities of daily living.

14. _____ Behavior becomes further disorganized; and wandering, agitation, and physical aggression often occur.

15. _____ Individuals are social, but family members begin to report strange behaviors and mood swings.

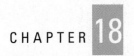

CHAPTER 18

Managing Anxiety

Student's Name _____

Date _____

Identify the level of anxiety (mild, moderate, severe, panic) for the following behaviors:

1. _____ After the news of her father's accident, Maria feels "overloaded." She begins to wring her hands, pace, and wander around the room moaning.

2. _____ Sam is awaiting the results of his examination. He appears to be calm and relaxed.

3. _____ Rose has just learned that she is being evicted from her home. She reacts by sitting immobilized. When questioned, she is unable to think or speak logically.

4. _____ Marian is preparing to free-climb a challenging mountain. She feels energized and concentrates on reaching her destination.

Describe maladaptive anxiety, and list two examples:

5. _____

6. _____

7. _____

List three behavioral addictions (compulsions):

8. _____

9. _____

10. _____

Identify two useful purposes of anxiety:

11. _____

12. _____

Indicate if the following interventions are therapeutic (T) or nontherapeutic (NT):

13. _____ Telling the client that everything will be all right as soon as the medication takes effect

14. _____ Teaching the client to problem solve

15. _____ Assessing every child for the presence of anxiety and stress

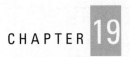

Illness and Hospitalization

Student's Name _____

Date _____

1. The experience of being hospitalized is a:
   a. developmental crisis
   b. personal crisis
   c. situational crisis
   d. maturational crisis

2. An individual's state of health:
   a. remains stable throughout life
   b. is constantly changing
   c. is in a state of disequilibrium
   d. changes through childhood and stabilizes as an adult

3. The stage of illness in which a person experiences symptoms is called the:
   a. first stage
   b. second stage
   c. third stage
   d. fourth stage

4. Nurses and other caregivers must always remember that _____ is just as important as good physical care.
   a. entertainment
   b. nutritional care
   c. financial arrangements
   d. psychosocial care

5. The way a person responds to the stresses of illness or hospitalization is based on:
   a. his or her insurance coverage
   b. how the person behaves when well
   c. how the person interprets the situation
   d. how the person treats his or her physicians and nurses

6. A refusal to acknowledge painful facts is called _____.

7. A feeling of having been mistreated, opposed, or injured is known as _____.

8. An overwhelming emotional state in which one is unable to process information is known as

   _____.

List the three stages of the hospitalization experience:

9. _____

10. _____

11. _____

List three ways in which care providers can support family members and significant others:

12. _____

13. _____

14. _____

CHAPTER 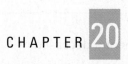 20

Loss and Grief

Student's Name _____

Date _____

Define the following terms:

1. external losses

_____

2. internal losses

_____

3. grief

_____

4. the grieving process

_____

5. mourning

_____

_____

List two types of dysfunctional (unresolved) grief:

6. _____

7. _____

List the five stages of dying, as defined by Elisabeth Kübler-Ross:

8. _____

9. _____

10. _____

11. _____

12. _____

13. Mary became a widow about 10 months ago. Although she seems to be adjusting well to the loss of her husband, lately she has been refusing invitations to social events. When visited by friends, she continually reminisces about her past. During her last visit, she told a friend that she was not really interested in any activities and would prefer to be left alone. Mary is suffering from:
    a. denial
    b. normal grief
    c. complicated grief
    d. complex grief

14. Health care providers should share in the grief experience with the loved ones of a deceased person, but they should remember that their primary goal is to:
    a. work through their own grief
    b. provide support for the grievers
    c. provide care for the body
    d. complete the documentation of the death

15. Mr. Clark is a 26-year-old man who was recently diagnosed with a fatal illness. During one of his visits to the clinic, he tells the medical assistant that he has decided to refuse further treatment for his condition. How will this decision change the goals of care for this client?
    a. The goal to cure the illness will remain the same.
    b. The goal will change to providing support for his choice.
    c. The goal will change to persuading him to reconsider his choice.
    d. The goal to keep him alive as long as possible will remain the same.

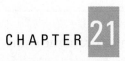

CHAPTER 21

Depression and Other Mood Disorders

Student's Name _____

Date _____

Identify the level of depression, and circle the correct answer:

1. Linda is a 22-year-old woman who has recently developed feelings of sadness and loss following a breakup with her boyfriend. She has noted no appetite or sleep changes.
   a. mild depression
   b. moderate depression
   c. severe depression
   d. she is feeling sorry for herself

2. Harold has become unable to concentrate or follow through with tasks. Lately even his appearance has begun to suffer. Today he spent the day staring at a blank television screen.
   a. mild depression
   b. moderate depression
   c. severe depression
   d. really bad depression

3. Rosie has to drag herself from chore to chore throughout the day. She feels helpless and ineffective when she has to care for her children. She believes there is no escape from her unhappy situation.
   a. mild depression
   b. moderate depression
   c. severe depression
   d. entrapment depression

4. Your client says that she has been taking antidepressants for 3 weeks and has not noted a difference. What do you tell her?

   _____

   _____

   _____

5. Toxicity should be suspected when lithium levels are above _____.

6. Describe the behaviors associated with hypomania.

   _____

   _____

   _____

7. The main characteristic of _____ is sudden or dramatic shifts in moods.

8. The drug classes most frequently used to treat mood disorders are _____ and _____.

List one therapeutic intervention for the following complaints:

9. Client experiences feelings of wanting to commit suicide.

_____

10. Client experiences excessive sweating after taking a tricyclic antidepressant.

_____

11. Client began antidepressant drug therapy 5 days ago. Today she has suddenly developed confusion and delirium.

_____

12. Conchita tells you that she cannot talk to other people because they will find out how stupid she really is.

_____

Rex has been taking lithium for about 3 months. Yesterday he urinated more than 4 quarts in less than 24 hours. List two interventions:

13 _____

14. _____

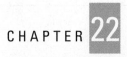

CHAPTER 22

Physical Problems, Psychological Sources

Student's Name _____

Date _____

Match the following terms and their definitions:
- a. primary gain
- b. secondary gain
- c. hypochondriasis
- d. conversion disorder
- e. malingering
- f. physiological stress response
- g. body dysmorphic disorder

1. _____ Intense fear of having a disease

2. _____ Often presents as seizure disorder in children under 10 years of age

3. _____ Relieves anxiety by masking inner emotional turmoil

4. _____ Produces symptoms to meet a recognizable goal

5. _____ Being relieved of responsibilities, having dependency needs met

6. _____ A preoccupation with a physical difference or defect in one's body

7. _____ The fight-or-flight response

8. The purpose of the physiological stress response is to:
   - a. decrease stress
   - b. keep hormone levels functional
   - c. protect the individual from anxiety
   - d. protect the individual from threat or illness

9. When the body is under continual or repeated stress, it responds by activating the fight-or-flight mechanism, which can result in:
   - a. an energized feeling
   - b. an emotional discharge
   - c. anger that is directed outward
   - d. physical signs and symptoms of an illness, disease, or disability

10. The _____ theory states that individuals are biochemically patterned to react to stress in childhood.

11. In somatoform disorders, the development of physical symptoms is the result of attempts to:

    _____

    _____

12. Because of the chronic nature of the disorder and the fact that they are "doctor shoppers," clients with _____ are difficult to treat.

List three therapeutic interventions for clients with somatoform disorders:

13. _____

14. _____

15. _____

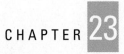

Eating and Sleeping Disorders

Student's Name _____

Date _____

Match the following terms and their definitions:

a. anorexia nervosa   f. narcolepsy
b. bulimia   g. parasomnia
c. obesity   h. dyssomnia
d. insomnia   i. polysomnogram
e. hypersomnia   j. sleep apnea

1. _____ An abnormality in the amount, quality, or timing of sleep

2. _____ A disorder of binge eating and use of inappropriate methods to prevent weight gain

3. _____ A disorder of falling or staying asleep

4. _____ Monitors the body's electrophysical responses during sleep

5. _____ A condition in which one refuses to maintain a normal body weight because of an intense fear of becoming fat

6. _____ Repeated attacks of sleep

7. _____ Excessive sleepiness

8. _____ Excessive body weight

9. _____ Abnormal behavior or physical events that happen during sleep

10. _____ Sleep problems that are caused by abnormal ventilation during sleep

11. The main goal for nurses and other health care providers in treating clients with eating disorders is:

_____

List three nursing diagnoses for clients with eating disorders:

12. _____

13. _____

14. _____

15. The mental health disorder with a high mortality rate is _____.

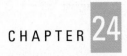

CHAPTER 24

Dissociative Disorders

Student's Name _____

Date _____

Complete the crossword puzzle:

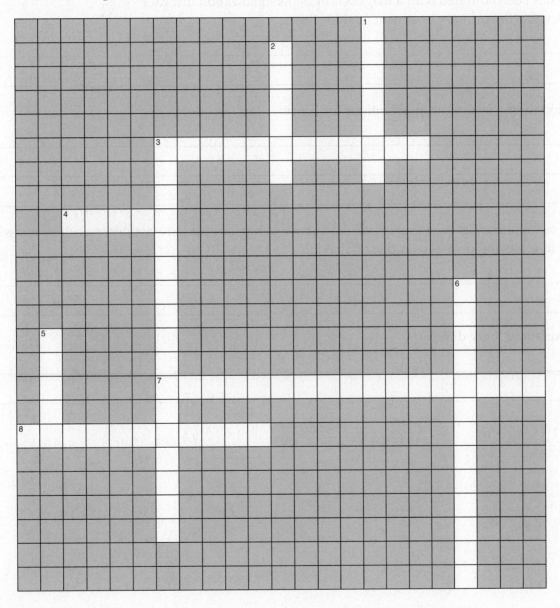

ACROSS

3. Disconnection from full awareness of self, time, and/or external circumstances
4. To escape or run away from reality
7. Failure to bring various childhood identifications into adult personality (two words)
8. Persons are able to struggle with life's problems while feeling good about living if this is healthy

DOWN

1. Loss of memory
2. A state resembling sleep, in which consciousness remains but voluntary movement is lost
3. During an episode, one feels detached or unconnected to the self
5. One of the main causes of dissociative disorders
6. Often expressed through various levels of anxiety and involves feelings of being weak, inadequate, and helpless (two or more words)

Bruce has been admitted with a diagnosis of depersonalization disorder:

9. Develop the primary treatment goal for Bruce.

_____

_____

Develop three therapeutic interventions for Bruce:

10. _____

11. _____

12. _____

Bruce has a history of engaging in self-destructive behaviors. Identify two interventions to assist Bruce in achieving control over these behaviors:

13. _____

14. _____

15. Explain identity diffusion.

_____

_____

Anger and Aggression

Student's Name _____

Date _____

1. Forceful behaviors that result in injury, abuse, or harm to another are called _____.
2. Children and adolescents often _____ in an attempt to establish and test the limits of appropriate behavior.
3. _____ is the abuse of members of one gender by members of another.
4. Models of anger and aggression that focus on the interactions of individuals within their social environment and locate the source of violence in interpersonal frustrations are based in the _____ group of theories.

Identify four factors that contribute to the use of aggressive behaviors:

5. _____

6. _____

7. _____

8. _____

Identify the stage in the assault cycle that most closely matches the listed behaviors:

9. _____ Cries, apologizes, tries to atone (make up) for behaviors

10. _____ Becomes restless and irritable, argues, paces

11. _____ Loses control, fights, kicks, bites, screams

12. _____ Loses ability to reason; becomes flushed or pale

Indicate if the following statements are true (T) or false (F):

13. _____ The most important intervention is to rapidly assess a potentially violent client.

14. _____ The use of restraints or seclusion is the last level of intervention for an aggressive client.

15. _____ The most therapeutic and experienced care providers never experience feelings of anger or aggression.

16. The client confides in a friend that she would like to punch her therapist in the face, then smiles sweetly when interacting with the therapist. The client is demonstrating:
    a. assertive behaviors
    b. active-aggressive behaviors
    c. passive-aggressive behaviors
    d. impulse-control behaviors

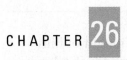

Outward-Focused Emotions: Violence

Student's Name _____

Date _____

1. Harm caused as a result of a failure to provide for basic needs or by placing an individual's health or welfare at unreasonable risk is called _____.

2. A term used to describe repeated physical abuse of someone, usually a woman, child, or elder, is _____.

3. _____ is the intentional misuse of someone or something that results in harm, injury, or trauma.

4. Information that is gathered for legal purposes and helps the law find and convict the perpetrator of a violent act or crime is called _____.

5. _____ is any behavior that threatens, harms, or injures a person or property.

6. _____ theories state that boys are socialized throughout their childhood to behave more aggressively and violently than girls.

7. A major care goal for victims of violence is _____.

8. The essential feature of _____ is the development of characteristic symptoms following exposure to extreme traumatic stressors.

9. Every caregiver needs to be alert for the possibility of _____ whenever there is a history of unexplained lethargy, fussiness, or irritability in an infant.

10. The most frequent abusers of the elderly are _____.

Case Scenario: Bonnie R., a 19-year-old mother of two, arrives in the emergency department with her 18-month-old son, Billy. She gives you a vague history of Billy being pushed off the bed by his older brother about 3 or 4 days ago. Since then Billy has been irritable and fussy. He refuses to eat and cries "all the time." Whenever Billy tries to walk, his left leg crumples and he falls. Because of his constant fussing, Bonnie admits to having "smacked him" yesterday so he would "stop screaming."

11. What information in Billy's history provides you with a clue to the possibility of child abuse?

_____

12. What information should your physical assessment include?

_____

13. What is the first priority of care for Billy at this time?

_____

As you assist the physician in placing Billy in traction, you become angry at the thought of Billy having to endure so much unnecessary pain. By the time Billy is finally settled, you are absolutely furious with Billy's mother.

14. How do you cope with these emotions and still remain therapeutic with Billy and his mother?

_____

_____

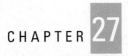

Inward-Focused Emotions: Suicide

Student's Name _____

Date _____

Identify the terms that best describe the behaviors characterized in the following statements:

1. _____ Jerry smokes cigarettes, drives his motorcycle too fast, and likes to feel the thrill of being chased by the police.

2. _____ Heather repeatedly scratches herself until she bleeds because the pain "lets me know I'm still here."

3. _____ Sam states that he will attempt suicide again, but he has not acted so far.

4. _____ Mary overdosed with sleeping medications because she "is tired of fighting."

5. _____ Yesterday, John gave his cherished car to his best friend. Last night he died from a gunshot wound to the head.

Indicate if the following statements are true (T) or false (F):

6. _____ Suicidal thoughts or intentions can exist in clients with any medical or mental health disorder.

7. _____ Suicide rates are lower in people who use drugs or alcohol.

8. _____ All suicidal persons are depressed.

9. _____ People who talk about suicide will not attempt to do it.

10. _____ It is harmful to discuss suicide with clients.

Case Scenario: David has recently lost his job, custody of his children, and his car because he was unable to make the monthly payments. He is being admitted following a week-long drinking binge. He has repeatedly stated that he would be better off dead.

11. The first priority for this client is:

_____

12. It has been assessed that David is a high suicide risk. The type of observation that he requires is called:

_____

13. Staff members attempt to make a "no–self-harm contract" with David. Explain a no–self-harm contract.

_____

14. David's nurse helps him to explore coping mechanisms that were successful in the past. The purpose of this is to:

_____

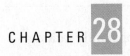
Substance-Related Disorders

Student's Name _____

Date _____

1. Physical dependence on a drug that is taken despite the problems associated with its use is called _____.

2. _____ occurs when an individual who was previously drug free returns to substance-abusing behaviors.

3. When a person is not using an addictive substance, he or she is practicing _____.

4. _____ occurs when increasingly larger amounts of a substance are required to produce the desired effect.

5. The incidence of _____ rises when women consume alcohol during pregnancy.

6. Older adults frequently abuse _____.

Identify the type of substance abused, and circle the correct answer:

7. Jerry has "chugged" large amounts of the substance and now is beginning to show signs of respiratory failure.
    a. antibiotics
    b. amphetamines
    c. alcohol
    d. inhalants

8. The physical assessment of Maria reveals constricted pupils, euphoria, and drowsiness.
    a. PCP (phencyclidine)
    b. heroin
    c. cocaine
    d. marijuana

9. After injecting or inhaling it, Jamie experiences intense feelings of well-being that last for less than 1 hour.
    a. alcohol
    b. acid
    c. caffeine
    d. cocaine

10. Stan had a flashback 2 weeks after taking:
    a. alcohol
    b. acid
    c. caffeine
    d. cocaine

11. Amber is unable to sit still, her pulse rate is over 120 beats/min, and she is constantly talking and fidgeting.
    a. alcohol
    b. acid
    c. amphetamines
    d. alfalfa

List four ways in which nurses and other care providers can act as therapeutic agents when caring for individuals with substance abuse problems:

12. _____

13. _____

14. _____

15. _____

CHAPTER 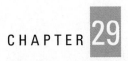 29

Sexual Disorders

Student's Name _____

Date _____

Identify the terms that most closely describe the behaviors characterized in the following statements:

1. _____ Prefers sexual relationships with persons of the opposite gender

2. _____ The practice of seeking sexual excitement from wearing the clothing of the opposite gender

3. _____ An inconsistency between the child's biological gender and his or her identity as a boy or girl

4. _____ A sexual behavior that departs from society's acceptable modes of seeking sexual gratification

5. _____ The process of establishing an integrated or complete identity as a homosexual

List four types of homosexual relationships:

6. _____

7. _____

8. _____

9. _____

Identify three theories that attempt to explain why an individual prefers a certain mode of sexual expression:

10. _____

11. _____

12. _____

13. Sexual addictions are characterized by:

_____

14. To effectively care for clients with sexual problems, care providers must first examine their own _____ and _____.

Personality Disorders

Student's Name _____

Date _____

Match the following terms and their definitions:

a. personality   e. paranoia
b. temperament   f. psychopath
c. dual diagnosis   g. impulsivity
d. manipulation   h. deceit

1. _____ A suspicious system of thinking with delusions of persecution and grandeur

2. _____ Controlling others for one's own purposes by influencing them in unfair or false ways

3. _____ Traits and attitudes that identify one as an individual

4. _____ The act of representing as true something that is actually known to be false

5. _____ The biological basis that underlies moods, energy levels, and attitudes

6. _____ Acting without forethought or regard to the consequences

7. _____ Suffering from two or more mental health problems or conditions

8. _____ A pattern of disregard for and violation of the rights of others

List three main characteristics of a personality disorder:

9. _____

10. _____

11. _____

12. Paul is unable to control his anger, acts impulsively, and abuses drugs. He has no friends but refuses to seek help. Why do clients like Paul with maladaptive social responses often not benefit from psychotherapy?

_____

_____

Identify three classes of medications used to treat clients who have been diagnosed with personality disorders:

13. _____

14. _____

15. _____

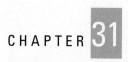

Schizophrenia and Other Psychoses

Student's Name _____

Date _____

Identify the terms that most closely describe the behaviors characterized in the following statements:

1. _____ Disorders marked by a loss of contact with reality

2. _____ Lack of energy or motivation

3. _____ Abnormal involuntary movement disorders caused by a drug-induced imbalance between two major neurotransmitters in the brain

4. _____ False sensory inputs with no external stimulus

5. _____ The idea that people or the media are talking about oneself

6. _____ Inability to recognize familiar environmental objects or people

7. _____ False perceptions of real objects or persons

8. _____ Inability to tell where one's body ends and the environment begins

9. _____ Lack of ability to produce new thoughts or follow a train of thought

10. Sam is delusional. Describe his behavior.

    _____

    _____

11. Lisa is sitting in the corner with her hand covering her mouth. She is whispering and giggling, and she appears to be deeply involved in a conversation, but no one is around. She is experiencing:

    _____

12. A potentially fatal extrapyramidal side effect of antipsychotic medications is:

    _____

The three major responsibilities when caring for clients who are receiving antipsychotic drug therapy are:

13. _____

14. _____

15. _____

CHAPTER 32

Chronic Mental Health Disorders

Student's Name _____

Date _____

1. Most chronic mental health problems are characterized by periods of _____ and _____.

2. Today, because of the process of _____, chronically mentally ill persons are cared for in the community.

Explain two goals of care for chronically mentally ill individuals:

3. _____

4. _____

5. Individuals with _____ are suffering from two psychiatric disorders, one of which is usually substance related.

List four psychological characteristics of chronic mental illness:

6. _____

7. _____

8. _____

9. _____

Indicate if the following statements are true (T) or false (F):

10. _____ People with chronic mental illness are unable to care for themselves.

11. _____ The sexual practices of chronically mentally troubled persons place them at an increased risk for contracting and transmitting human immunodeficiency virus (HIV)/acquired immunodeficiency syndrome (AIDS).

12. _____ Psychiatric rehabilitation programs teach severely mentally ill clients about the skills needed for proper nutrition, activity, and rest habits.

13. _____ It is inappropriate to ask a client to describe the meaning of his or her hallucinations.

14. _____ Mental health nursing is a critical component of every situation no matter what the diagnosis.

15. _____ Individuals with chronic mental health problems have higher rates of suicide.

16. _____ Many chronically mentally ill persons are homeless.

17. _____ Antianxiety agents help control hallucinations and other symptoms of psychosis.

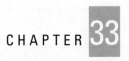

CHAPTER 33

Challenges for the Future

Student's Name _____

Date _____

List three treatment settings for clients with mental health problems:

1. _____

2. _____

3. _____

4. Children who are _____ experience serious threats to their current and future well-being.

5. The "old homeless" tended to be adult, unmarried _____ with an average age of _____ years old.

6. People with _____ make up about one third of the homeless population.

7. The _____ is a federal law that removes the employment barriers for people with mental or physical disabilities.

8. Mental problems that are limited to a specific cultural group of people are called _____.

9. Explain the meaning of "one paycheck away from poverty."

   _____

   _____

10. Children who are homeless for any length of time experience:

    _____

    _____

11. The Americans With Disabilities Act (ADA) of 1990 is a federal statute designed to:

    _____

    _____

12. Nurses who care for hospitalized clients begin _____ on admission.

13. Involving clients in treatment means every party must:

    _____

    _____

List the four measures of competency:

14. _____

15. _____

16. _____

17. _____

Indicate if the following statements are true (T) or false (F):

18. _____ Nurses can choose to be self-employed and establish their own practices.

19. _____ Supportive health care aides (HCAs) plan nursing care for the clients in their caseload.

20. _____ A basic concept of psychosocial rehabilitation is self-help.

21. _____ Under certain circumstances, change can be bad for people or organizations.

22. _____ Many people with human immunodeficiency virus (HIV) will demonstrate mental signs and symptoms before physical signs and symptoms.

23. _____ Change involves loss and discomfort.

24. _____ The first step in coping with unplanned change is to reset priorities.